a LANGE medical book

Basic & Clinical Biostatistics

Fifth edition

Susan E. White, PhD
Associate Professor Clinical
School of Health and Rehabilitation Sciences
The Ohio State University
Administrator of Analytics
The James Cancer Hospital at
The Ohio State University Wexner Medical Center

McGraw Hill

New York   Chicago   San Francisco   Athens   London   Madrid
Mexico City   Milan   New Delhi
Singapore   Sydney   Toronto

Notice

Medicine is an ever-changing science. As new research and clinical experience broaden our knowledge, changes in treatment and drug therapy are required. The authors and the publisher of this work have checked with sources believed to be reliable in their efforts to provide information that is complete and generally in accord with the standards accepted at the time of publication. However, in view of the possibility of human error or changes in medical sciences, neither the authors nor the publisher nor any other party who has been involved in the preparation or publication of this work warrants that the information contained herein is in every respect accurate or complete, and they disclaim all responsibility for any errors or omissions or for the results obtained from use of the information contained in this work. Readers are encouraged to confirm the information contained herein with other sources. For example and in particular, readers are advised to check the product information sheet included in the package of each drug they plan to administer to be certain that the information contained in this work is accurate and that changes have not been made in the recommended dose or in the contraindications for administration. This recommendation is of particular importance in connection with new or infrequently used drugs.

This book was set in Adobe Garamond Pro, Regular, 10/10.5 pt, by MPS Limited.
The editors were Jason Malley and Leah Carton.
The production supervisor was Richard Ruzycka.
Project management was provided by Poonam Bisht, MPS Limited.
The cover designer was W2 Design.
This book is printed on acid-free paper.

Library of Congress Cataloging-in-Publication Data
Names: White, Susan E., editor. | Preceded by (work): Dawson, Beth. Basic & clinical biostatistics.
Title: Basic & clinical biostatistics / editor, Susan E. White.
Other titles: Basic and clinical biostatistic
Description: Fifth edition. | New York : McGraw-Hill Companies, [2020] | Preceded by Basic & clinical biostatistics / Beth Dawson, Robert G. Trapp. 4th ed. 2004. | Includes bibliographical references and index.
Identifiers: LCCN 2019012807| ISBN 9781260455366 (adhesive - soft : alk. paper) | ISBN 9781260455373 (eISBN)
Subjects: | MESH: Biostatistics—methods | Biomedical Research
Classification: LCC QH323.5 | NLM WA 950 | DDC 610.1/5195—dc23 LC record available at https://nam05.safelinks. protection.outlook.com/?url=https%3A%2F%2Flccn.loc.gov%2F2019012807&data=01%7C01%7Cleah.carton%40m-heducation.com%7C1e1cc26f931143209d0b08d6b13099dd%7Cf919b1efc0c347358fca0928ec39d8d5%7C0&sdata=Xv2%2F36iSJXpK8qi7YAdT0MUktkXIqJGwI1TIyYGQE9Y%3D&reserved=0

McGraw-Hill Education books are available at special quantity discounts to use as premiums and sales promotions, or for use in corporate training programs. To contact a representative please visit the Contact Us pages at www.mhprofessional.com.

Contents

Preface

Basic & Clinical Biostatistics introduces the medical student, researcher, or practitioner to the study of statistics applied to medicine and other disciplines in the health field. The book covers the *basics* of biostatistics and quantitative methods in epidemiology and the *clinical* applications in evidence-based medicine and the decision-making methods. Particular emphasis is on study design and interpretation of results of research.

OBJECTIVE

The primary objective of this text is to provide the resources to help the reader become an informed user and consumer of statistics. This book should allow you to:

- Develop sound judgment about data applicable to clinical care.
- Read the clinical literature critically, understanding potential errors and fallacies contained therein, and apply confidently the results of medical studies to patient care.
- Interpret commonly used vital statistics and understand the ramifications of epidemiologic information for patient care and prevention of disease.
- Reach correct conclusions about diagnostic procedures and laboratory test results.
- Interpret manufacturers' information about drugs, instruments, and equipment.
- Evaluate study protocols and articles submitted for publication and actively participate in clinical research.
- Develop familiarity with well-known statistical software and interpret the computer output.

APPROACH & DISTINGUISHING FEATURES

The practitioner's interests, needs, and perspectives in mind during the preparation of this text. Thus, our approach embraces the following features:

- A genuine medical context is offered for the subject matter. After the introduction to different kinds of studies is presented in Chapter 2, subsequent chapters begin with several *Presenting Problems*—discussions of studies that have been published in the medical literature. These illustrate the methods discussed in the chapter and in some instances are continued through several chapters and in the exercises to develop a particular line of reasoning more fully.
- All example articles and datasets are available via open source access.
- Actual data from the *Presenting Problems* are used to illustrate the statistical methods.
- A focus on concepts is accomplished by using computer programs to analyze data and by presenting statistical calculations only to illustrate the logic behind certain statistical methods.
- The importance of sample size (power analysis) is emphasized, and computer programs to estimate sample size are illustrated.
- Information is organized from the perspective of the research question being asked.
- Terms are defined within the relevant text, whenever practical, because biostatistics may be a new language to you. In addition, a glossary of statistical and epidemiologic terms is provided at the end of the book.
- A table of all symbols used in the book is provided on the inside back cover.
- A simple classification scheme of study designs used in clinical research is discussed (Chapter 2). We employ this scheme throughout the book as we discuss the *Presenting Problems*.
- Flowcharts are used to relate research questions to appropriate statistical methods (inside front cover and Appendix C).
- A step-by-step explanation of how to read the medical literature critically (Chapter 13)—a necessity for the modern health professional—is provided.

- Evidence-based medicine and decision-making are addressed in a clinical context (Chapters 3 and 12). Clinicians will be called on increasingly to make decisions based on statistical information.
- Numerous end-of-chapter *Exercises* (Chapters 2 through 12) and their complete solutions (Appendix B) are provided.
- A posttest of multiple-choice questions (Chapter 13) similar to those used in course final examinations or licensure examinations is included.

SPECIAL FEATURES IN THIS EDITION

There are several important enhancements included in the fifth edition.

To facilitate and increase learning, each chapter (except Chapter 1) contains a set of *Key Concepts* to orient the reader to the important ideas discussed in the chapter.

- Many of the *Presenting Problems* have been updated with journal references that require the authors to provide access to the journal article and data through a creative commons license. The links to articles and datasets used for examples are detailed in the *Presenting Problem* summary at the beginning of each chapter.
- Material addressing best practices in data visualization is included in Chapter 3.
- All sample size calculations are now presented using G*Power, an open source program used widely for sample size calculation by researchers.
- Inclusion of output and exercise answers using R and R Commander—open source statistical applications that may be used across many computer operating systems (Windows, Mac, and Unix).

Susan E. White, PhD

Using R

R is a statistical computing package that is available via an open source license. R (R Core Team, 2019) may be downloaded from http://www.R-project.org.

The add-on R Commander provides new users with a graphical interface that makes using R far more intuitive.

R Commander (Fox and Bouchet-Valat 2019) may be downloaded from this site:
https://www.rcommander.com/
or
https://socialsciences.mcmaster.ca/jfox/Misc/Rcmdr/

There are also R Commander plug-ins that are used in the examples:
RcmdrPlugin.survival
RcmdrPlugin.aRnova

There are a number of excellent resources online to help you learn to use R and R Commander. Here is a short list:

R Commander an introduction: https://cran.r-project.org/doc/contrib/Karp-Rcommander-intro.pdf

Getting Started with R Commander: https://cran.r-project.org/web/packages/Rcmdr/vignettes/Getting-Started-with-the-Rcmdr.pdf

Introduction to Medical Research

The goal of this text is to provide you with the tools and skills you need to be a smart user and consumer of medical statistics. This goal has guided the selection of material and in the presentation of information. This chapter outlines the reasons physicians, medical students, and others in the health care field should know biostatistics. It also describes how the book is organized, what you can expect to find in each chapter, and how you can use it most profitably.

THE SCOPE OF BIOSTATISTICS & EPIDEMIOLOGY

The word "statistics" has several meanings: data or numbers, the process of analyzing the data, and the description of a field of study. It derives from the Latin word *status,* meaning "manner of standing" or "position." Statistics were first used by tax assessors to collect information for determining assets and assessing taxes—an unfortunate beginning and one the profession has not entirely lived down.

Everyone is familiar with the statistics used in baseball and other sports, such as a baseball player's batting average, a bowler's game point average, and a basketball player's free-throw percentage. In medicine, some of the statistics most often encountered are called means, standard deviations, proportions, and rates. Working with statistics involves using statistical methods that summarize data (to obtain, for example, means and standard deviations) and using statistical procedures to reach certain conclusions that can be applied to patient care or public health planning. The subject area of statistics is the set of all the statistical methods and procedures used by those who work with statistics. The application of statistics is broad indeed and includes business, marketing, economics, agriculture, education, psychology, sociology, anthropology, and biology, in addition to our special interest, medicine and other health care disciplines. The terms **biostatistics** and **biometrics** refer to the application of statistics in the health-related fields.

Although the focus of this text is biostatistics, some topics related to epidemiology are included as well.

The term "epidemiology" refers to the study of health and illness in human populations, or, more precisely, to the patterns of health or disease and the factors that influence these patterns; it is based on the Greek words for "upon" (*epi*) and "people" (*demos*). Once knowledge of the epidemiology of a disease is available, it is used to understand the cause of the disease, determine public health policy, and plan treatment. The application of population-based information to decision-making about individual patients is often referred to as **clinical epidemiology** and, more recently, **evidence-based medicine.** The tools and methods of biostatistics are an integral part of these disciplines.

BIOSTATISTICS IN MEDICINE

Clinicians must evaluate and use new information throughout their lives. The skills you learn in this text will assist in this process because they concern modern knowledge acquisition methods. The most important reasons for learning biostatistics are listed in the following subsections. (The most widely applicable reasons are mentioned first.)

Evaluating the Literature

Reading the literature begins early in the training of health professionals and continues throughout their careers. They must understand biostatistics to decide whether they can rely on the results presented in the literature. Journal editors try to screen out articles that are improperly designed or analyzed, but few have formal statistical training and they naturally focus on the content of the research rather than the method. Investigators for large, complex studies almost always consult statisticians for assistance in project design and data analysis, especially research funded by the National Institutes of Health and other national agencies and foundations. Even then it is important to be aware of possible shortcomings in the way a study is designed and carried out. In smaller research projects, investigators consult with statisticians less frequently, either because they are unaware of the need for statistical assistance or because the biostatistical resources are not readily available or affordable. The availability of easy-to-use computer programs to perform statistical analysis has been important in promoting the use of more complex methods. This same accessibility, however, enables people without the training or expertise in statistical methodology to report complicated analyses when they are not always appropriate.

The problems with studies in the medical literature have been amply documented. Sander Greenland's (2011) article on the misinterpretation in statistical testing in health risk assessment outlines errors in the reporting and interpretation of statistics in medical literature. The article includes a number of examples of erroneous conclusions surrounding the reporting of odds ratios and conclusions based on inadequate sample sizes. Much of the misinterpretation around the results of medical studies are in the reporting of statistical conclusions based on interferential methods such as hypothesis tests and p-values. Greenland's later work (2016) lists 25 misinterpretations of p-values, confidence intervals, and power commonly found in scientific literature.

The issue with misuse of p-values is so rampant that the American Statistical Association published a statement to guide the proper interpretation of p-values (Wasserstein and Lazar, 2016). The article outlines six principles that address the most common misconceptions around p-values:

1. P-values can indicate how incompatible the data are with a specified statistical model.
2. P-values do not measure the probability that the studied hypothesis is true, or the probability that the data were produced by random chance alone.
3. Scientific conclusions and business or policy decisions should not be based only on whether a p-value passes a specific threshold.
4. Proper inference requires full reporting and transparency.
5. A p-value, or statistical significance, does not measure the size of an effect or the importance of a result.
6. By itself, a p-value does not provide a good measure of evidence regarding a model or hypothesis.

Journals have also published a number of articles that suggest how practitioners could better report their research findings. Although these recommendations may result in improvements in the reporting of statistical results, the reader must assume the responsibility for determining whether the results of a published study are valid. The development of this book has been guided by the study designs and statistical methods found primarily in the medical literature, and topics were selected to provide the skills needed to determine whether a study is valid and should be believed. Chapter 13 focuses specifically on how to read the medical literature and provides checklists for flaws in studies and problems in analysis.

Applying Study Results to Patient Care

Applying the results of research to patient care is the major reason practicing clinicians read the medical literature. They want to know which diagnostic procedures are best, which methods of treatment are optimal, and how the treatment regimen should be designed and implemented. Of course, they also read journals to stay aware and up to date in medicine in general as well as in their specific area of interest. Chapters 3 and 12 discuss the application of techniques of evidence-based medicine to decisions about the care of individual patients.

Interpreting Vital Statistics: Physicians must be able to interpret vital statistics in order to diagnose and treat patients effectively. Vital statistics are based on data collected from the ongoing recording of vital events, such as births and deaths. A basic understanding of how vital statistics are determined, what they mean, and how they are used facilitates their use. Chapter 3 provides information on these statistics.

Understanding Epidemiologic Problems: Practitioners must understand epidemiologic problems because this information helps them make diagnoses and develop management plans for patients. Epidemiologic data reveal the prevalence of a disease, its variation by season of the year and by geographic location, and its relation to certain risk factors. In addition, epidemiology helps us understand how newly identified viruses and other infectious agents spread. This information helps society make informed decisions about the deployment of health resources, for example, whether a community should begin a surveillance program, whether a screening program is warranted and can be designed to be efficient and effective, and whether community resources should be used for specific health problems. Describing and using data in decision-making are highlighted in Chapters 3 and 12.

Interpreting Information about Drugs and Equipment: Physicians continually evaluate information about drugs and medical instruments and equipment. This material may be provided by company representatives, sent through the mail, or published in journals. Because of the high cost of developing drugs and medical instruments, companies do all they can to recoup their investments. To sell their products, a company must convince physicians that its products are better than those of its competitors. To make its point, a company uses graphs, charts, and the results of studies comparing its products with others on the market. Every chapter in this text is related to the skills needed to evaluate these materials, but Chapters 2, 3, and 13 are especially relevant.

Using Diagnostic Procedures: Identifying the correct diagnostic procedure to use is a necessity in making decisions about patient care. In addition to knowing the prevalence of a given disease, physicians must be aware of the sensitivity of a diagnostic test in detecting the disease when it is present and the frequency with which the test correctly indicates no disease in a well person. These characteristics are called the sensitivity and specificity of a diagnostic test. Information in Chapters 4 and 12 relates particularly to skills for interpreting diagnostic tests.

Being Informed: Keeping abreast of current trends and being critical about data are more general skills and ones that are difficult to measure. These skills are also not easy for anyone to acquire because many responsibilities compete for a professional's time. One of the by-products of working through this text is a heightened awareness of the many threats to the validity of information, that is, the importance of being alert for statements that do not seem quite right.

Appraising Guidelines: The number of guidelines for diagnosis and treatment has increased greatly in recent years. Practitioners caution that guidelines should not be accepted uncritically; although some are based on medical evidence, many represent the collective opinion of experts. A review of clinical practices guidelines between 1980 and 2007 by Alonso-Coello and colleagues (2010) found that the quality scores of the guidelines as measured by the AGREE Instrument improved somewhat over time, but remained in the moderate to low range.

Evaluating Study Protocols and Articles: Physicians and others in the health field who are associated with universities, medical schools, or major clinics are often called on to evaluate material submitted for publication in medical journals and to decide whether it should be published. Health practitioners, of course, have the expertise to evaluate the content of a protocol or article, but they often feel uncomfortable about critiquing the design and statistical methods of a study. No study, however important, will provide valid information about the practice of medicine and future research unless it is properly designed and analyzed. Careful attention to the concepts covered in this text will provide physicians with many of the skills necessary for evaluating the design of studies.

Participating in or Directing Research Projects: Clinicians participating in research will find knowledge about biostatistics and research methods indispensable. Residents in all specialties as well as other health care trainees are expected to show evidence of scholarly activity, and this often takes the form of a research project. The comprehensive coverage of topics in this text should provide most of them with the information they need to be active participants in all aspects of research.

THE DESIGN OF THIS BOOK

This text is both *basic* and *clinical* because both the basic concepts of biostatistics and the use of these concepts in clinical decision-making are emphasized. This comprehensive text covers the traditional topics in biostatistics plus the quantitative methods of epidemiology used in research. For example, commonly used ways to analyze survival data are included in Chapter 9; illustrations of computer analyses in chapters in which they are appropriate, because researchers today use computers to calculate statistics; and applications of the results of studies to the diagnosis of specific diseases and the care of individual patients, sometimes referred to as medical decision-making or evidence-based medicine.

The presentations of techniques and examples are illustrated using the statistical program R (R Core Team, 2018). R is a cross platform software program that is freely distributed on the terms of a GNU General Public License. Since the software is cross platform, the examples presented in the text may be replicated using computers that run Windows, macOS, or UNIX.

This text deemphasizes calculations and uses computer programs to illustrate the results of statistical tests. In most chapters, the calculations of some statistical procedures are included, primarily to illustrate the logic behind the tests, not because you will need to be able to perform the calculations yourself. Some exercises involve calculations because some students wish to work through a few problems in detail so as to understand the procedures better. The major focus of the text, however, is on the interpretation and use of research methods.

A word regarding the accuracy of the calculations is in order. Many examples and exercises require several steps. The accuracy of the final answer depends on the number of significant decimal places to which figures are extended at each step of the calculation. Calculators and computers, however, use a greater number of significant decimal places at each step and often yield an answer different from that obtained using only two or three significant digits. The difference will usually be small, but do not be concerned if your calculations vary slightly from the examples.

The examples used are taken from studies published in the medical literature. Occasionally, a subset of the data is used to illustrate a more complex procedure. In addition, the focus of an example may be on only one aspect of the data analyzed in a published study in order to illustrate a concept or statistical test. To explain certain concepts, tables and graphs are reproduced as they appear in a published study. These reproductions may contain symbols that are not discussed until a later chapter in this book. Simply ignore such symbols for the time being. The focus on published studies is based on two reasons: First, they convince readers of the relevance of statistical methods in medical research; and second, they provide an opportunity to learn about some interesting studies along with the statistics.

The presentation of techniques in this text often refer to both previous and upcoming chapters to help tie concepts together and point out connections. This technique requires to use definitions somewhat differently from many other statistical texts; that is, terms are often used within the context of a discussion without a precise definition. The definition is given later. Several examples appear in the foregoing discussions (e.g., vital statistics, means, standard deviations, proportions, rates, validity). Using terms properly within several contexts helps the reader learn complex ideas, and many ideas in statistics become clearer when viewed from different perspectives. Some terms are defined along the way, but providing definitions for every term would inhibit our ability to point out the connections between the ideas. To assist the reader, boldface type is used for terms (the first few times they are used) that appear in the Glossary of statistical and epidemiologic terms provided at the end of the book.

THE ORGANIZATION OF THIS BOOK

Each chapter begins with two components: **key concepts** and an introduction to the examples (presenting problems) covered in the chapter. The key concepts are intended to help readers organize and visualize the ideas to be discussed and then to identify the point at which each is discussed. At the conclusion of each chapter is a summary that integrates the statistical concepts with the presenting problems used to illustrate them. When flowcharts or diagrams are useful, they are included to help explain how different procedures are related and when they are relevant. The flowcharts are grouped in Appendix C for easy reference.

Patients come to their health care providers with various health problems. In describing their patients, these providers commonly say, "The patient presents with …" or "The patient's presenting problem is …" This terminology is used in this text to emphasize the similarity between medical practice and the research problems discussed in the medical literature. Almost all chapters begin with presenting problems that discuss studies taken directly from the medical literature; these research problems are used to illustrate the concepts and methods presented in the chapter. In chapters in which statistics are calculated (e.g., the mean in Chapter 3) or statistical procedures are explained (e.g., the t test in Chapters 5 and 6), data from the presenting problems are used in the calculations. The selection of presenting problems is intended to represent a broad array of interests, while being sure that the studies use the methods discussed.

Exercises are provided with all chapters (2–13); answers are given in Appendix B, most with complete solutions. A variety of exercises are included to meet the different needs of students. Some exercises call for calculating a statistic or a statistical test. Some focus on the presenting problems or other published studies and ask about the design (as in Chapter 2) or about the use of elements such as charts, graphs, tables, and statistical methods. Occasionally, exercises extend a concept discussed in the chapter. This additional development is not critical for all readers to understand, but it provides further insights for those who are interested. Some exercises refer to topics discussed in previous chapters to provide reminders and reinforcements.

The **symbols** used in statistics are sometimes a source of confusion. These symbols are listed on the inside back cover for ready access. When more than one symbol for the same item is encountered in the medical literature, the most common one is used and points out the others. Also, a Glossary of biostatistics and epidemiologic terms is provided at the end of the book (after Chapter 13).

ADDITIONAL RESOURCES

References are provided to other texts and journal articles for readers who want to learn more about a topic. With the growth of the Internet, many resources have become easily available for little or no cost. A number of statistical programs and resources are available on the Internet. Some of the programs are freeware, meaning that anyone may use them free of charge; others, called shareware, charge a relatively small fee for their use. Many of the software vendors have free products or software you can download and use for a restricted period of time.

The American Statistical Association (ASA) has a number of sections with a special emphasis, such as Teaching Statistics in the Health Sciences, Biometrics

Section, Statistical Education, and others. Many of these Section homepages contain links to statistical resources. The ASA homepage is http://www.amstat. org.

Dartmouth University has links to the impressive Chance Database http://www.dartmouth. edu/%7Echance/index.html, which contains many teaching resources and, in turn, many useful links to other resources.

The Medical University of South Carolina has links to a large number of evidence-based-medicine sites, including its own resources https://musc.libguides.com/ebp.

Study Designs in Medical Research

KEY CONCEPTS

 Study designs in medicine fall into two categories: studies in which subjects are observed, and studies in which the effect of an intervention is observed.

 Observational studies may be forward-looking (cohort), backward-looking (case–control), or looking at simultaneous events (cross-sectional). Cohort studies generally provide stronger evidence than the other two designs.

 Studies that examine patient outcomes are increasingly published in the literature; they focus on specific topics, such as resource utilization, functional status, quality of life, patient satisfaction, and cost-effectiveness.

 Studies with interventions are called experiments or clinical trials. They provide stronger evidence than observational studies.

 The single best way to minimize bias is to randomly select subjects in observational studies or randomly assign subjects to different treatment arms in clinical trials.

 Bias occurs when the way a study is designed or carried out causes an error in the results and conclusions. Bias can be due to the manner in which subjects are selected or data are collected and analyzed.

 Clinical trials without controls (subjects who do not receive the intervention) are difficult to interpret and do not provide strong evidence.

 Each study design has specific advantages and disadvantages.

This chapter introduces the different kinds of studies commonly used in medical research. Knowing how a study is designed is important for understanding the conclusions that can be drawn from it. Therefore, considerable attention will be devoted to the topic of study designs.

If you are familiar with the medical literature, you will recognize many of the terms used to describe different study designs. If you are just beginning to read the literature, you should not be dismayed by all the new terminology; there will be ample opportunity to review and become familiar with it. Also, the glossary at the end of the book defines the terms used here. In the final chapter of this book, study designs are reviewed within the context of reading journal articles, and pointers are given on how to look for possible biases that can occur in medical studies. Bias can be due to the manner in which patients are selected, data are collected and analyzed, or conclusions are drawn.

CLASSIFICATION OF STUDY DESIGNS

There are several different schemes for classifying study designs. The one most relevant in clinical applications divides studies into those in which the subjects were merely observed, sometimes called **observational studies,** and those in which some intervention was performed, generally called **experiments.** This approach is simple and reflects the sequence an investigation

Table 2–1. Classification of study designs.

I. Observational studies
  A. Descriptive or case–series
  B. Case–control studies (retrospective)
    1. Causes and incidence of disease
    2. Identification of risk factors
  C. Cross-sectional studies, surveys (prevalence)
    1. Disease description
    2. Diagnosis and staging
    3. Disease processes, mechanisms
  D. Cohort studies (prospective)
    1. Causes and incidence of disease
    2. Natural history, prognosis
    3. Identification of risk factors
  E. Historical cohort studies

II. Experimental studies
  A. Controlled trials
    1. Parallel or concurrent controls
      a. Randomized
      b. Not randomized
    2. Sequential controls
      a. Self-controlled
      b. Crossover
    3. External controls (including historical)
  B. Studies with no controls

III. Meta-analyses

sometimes takes. With a little practice, you should be able to read medical articles and classify studies according to the outline in Table 2–1 with little difficulty.

Each study design in Table 2–1 is illustrated in this chapter, using some of the studies that are presenting problems in upcoming chapters. In observational studies, one or more groups of patients are observed, and characteristics about the patients are recorded for analysis. Experimental studies involve an **intervention**—an investigator-controlled maneuver, such as a drug, a procedure, or a treatment—and interest lies in the effect the intervention has on study subjects. Of course, both observational and experimental studies may involve animals or objects, but most studies in medicine involve people.

OBSERVATIONAL STUDIES

Observational studies are of four main types: case–series, case–control, cross-sectional (including surveys), and cohort studies. When certain characteristics of a group (or series) of patients (or cases) are described in a published report, the result is called a **case–series study;** it is the simplest

design in which the author describes some interesting or intriguing observations that occurred for a small number of patients.

Case–series studies frequently lead to the generation of hypotheses that are subsequently investigated in a case–control, cross-sectional, or cohort study. These three types of studies are defined by the period of time the study covers and by the direction or focus of the research question. Cohort and case–control studies generally involve an extended period of time defined by the point when the study begins and the point when it ends; some process occurs, and a certain amount of time is required to assess it. For this reason, both cohort and case–control studies are sometimes also called **longitudinal studies.** The major difference between them is the direction of the inquiry or the focus of the research question: Cohort studies are forward-looking, from a risk factor to an outcome, whereas case–control studies are backward-looking, from an outcome to risk factors. The cross-sectional study analyzes data collected on a group of subjects at one time. If you would like a more detailed discussion of study designs used in medicine, a book by Hulley et al (2013) is devoted entirely to the design of clinical research. Garb (1996) and Burns and Grove (2014) discuss study design in medicine and nursing, respectively.

Case–Series Studies

A case–series report is a simple descriptive account of interesting characteristics observed in a group of patients. For example, Glazer et al (2016) presented information on a series of 21 patients with acinar cell carcinoma of the pancreas. The authors wanted to compare two treatments, a combination of surgery and adjuvant chemotherapy versus surgery only, to see which resulted in longer survival in both metastatic and nonmetastatic cancers. They concluded that a multidisciplinary approach to treat the disease may result in longer survival.

Case–series reports generally involve patients seen over a relatively short time. Generally, case–series studies do not include **control subjects,** persons who do not have the disease or condition being described. Some investigators would not include case–series in a list of types of studies because they are generally not planned studies and do not involve any research hypotheses. On occasion, however, investigators do include control subjects. We mention case–series studies because of their important descriptive role as a precursor to other studies.

Case–Control Studies

Case–control studies begin with the absence or presence of an outcome and then look backward in time to try to detect possible causes or risk factors that may have

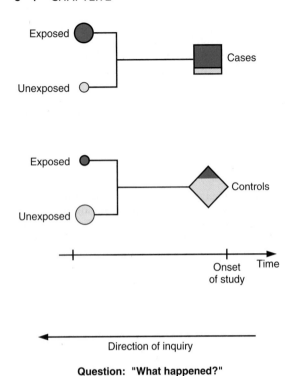

Figure 2–1. Schematic diagram of case–control study design. Shaded areas represent subjects exposed to the antecedent factor; unshaded areas correspond to unexposed subjects. Squares represent subjects with the outcome of interest; diamonds represent subjects without the outcome of interest. (Adapted with permission from Ilango K, Vijayakumar TM, Dubey GP, et al: An Enlarged Vision on Various Types of Study Design in Human Subjects, Global J Pharm 2012 Jan;6(3):216-221.)

been suggested in a case–series report. The *cases* in case–control studies are individuals selected on the basis of some disease or outcome; the *controls* are individuals without the disease or outcome. The history or previous events of both cases and controls are analyzed in an attempt to identify a characteristic or risk factor present in the cases' histories but not in the controls' histories.

Figure 2–1 illustrates that subjects in the study are chosen at the onset of the study after they are known to be either cases with the disease or outcome (squares) or controls without the disease or outcome (diamonds). The histories of cases and controls are examined over a previous period to detect the presence (shaded areas) or absence (unshaded areas) of predisposing characteristics or risk factors, or, if the disease is infectious, whether the subject has been exposed to the presumed infectious agent. In case–control designs, the nature of the inquiry is backward in time, as indicated by the

arrows pointing backward in Figure 2–1 to illustrate the backward, or retrospective, nature of the research process. We can characterize case–control studies as studies that ask "What happened?" In fact, they are sometimes called **retrospective studies** because of the direction of inquiry. Case–control studies are longitudinal as well, because the inquiry covers a period of time.

Cai and colleagues (2014) compared patients who had a surgical site infection (SSI) following total joint arthroplasty (cases) with patients who developed no infection (controls). The investigators found that Aquacel dressing use was associated with a lower rate of infection. The study found a number of variables that increased the odds of an SSI, including: age, body mass index, smoking history, thyroid and/or liver disease, and a history of steroid treatment.

Investigators sometimes use **matching** to associate controls with cases on characteristics such as age and sex. If an investigator feels that such characteristics are so important that an imbalance between the two groups of patients would affect any conclusions, they should employ matching. This process ensures that both groups will be similar with respect to important characteristics that may otherwise cloud or confound the conclusions.

Deciding whether a published study is a case–control study or a case–series report is not always easy. Confusion arises because both types of studies are generally conceived and written after the fact rather than having been planned. The easiest way to differentiate between them is to ask whether the author's purpose was to describe a phenomenon or to attempt to explain it by evaluating previous events. If the purpose is simple description, chances are the study is a case–series report.

Cross-Sectional Studies

The third type of observational study goes by all of the following names: cross-sectional studies, surveys, epidemiologic studies, and prevalence studies. We use the term "cross-sectional" because it is descriptive of the timeline and does not have the connotation that the terms "surveys" and "prevalence" do. **Cross-sectional studies** analyze data collected on a group of subjects at one time rather than over a period of time. Cross-sectional studies are designed to determine "What is happening?" right now. Subjects are selected and information is obtained in a short period of time (Figure 2–2; note the short timeline). Because they focus on a point in time, they are sometimes also called **prevalence** studies. Surveys and polls are generally cross-sectional studies, although surveys can be part of a cohort or case–control study if the survey data is collected from a subset of the subjects. Cross-sectional studies may be designed to address research questions raised by a case–series, or they may be done without a previous descriptive study.

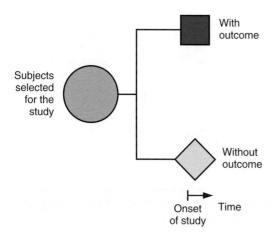

No direction of inquiry

Question: "What is happening?"

Figure 2–2. Schematic diagram of cross-sectional study design. Squares represent subjects with the outcome of interest; diamonds represent subjects without the outcome of interest. (Adapted with permission from Ilango K, Vijayakumar TM, Dubey GP, et al: An Enlarged Vision on Various Types of Study Design in Human Subjects, Global J Pharm 2012 Jan;6(3):216-221.)

Diagnosing or Staging a Disease: Anderson et al (2018) studied predictors of influenza in over 4,500 patients presenting to a hospital with flu-like symptoms from 2009 to 2014. They found that the most important symptoms for predicting influenza were cough, runny nose, chills, and body aches. They formulated a predictive model that was able to predict the presence/absence of the flu virus. Further, they tested the predictive value of a rapid influenza test versus virologically confirmed influenza cases.

Studying the Relationship Between Diseases: Poblador-Plou and her coinvestigators (2014) were interested in learning more about the relationship between dementia and other chronic diseases. Using electronic health records for patients identified with dementia, they were able to identify relationships with other chronic diseases such as Parkinson's disease, congestive heart failure, and others using a variety of statistical methods.

Establishing Norms: Knowledge of the range within which most patients fit is very useful to clinicians. Laboratories, of course, establish and then provide the normal limits of most diagnostic tests when they report the results for a given patient. Often these limits are established by testing people who are known to have normal values. We would not, for example, want to use people with diabetes mellitus to establish the norms for serum glucose levels. The results from the people known to have normal values are used to define the range that separates the lowest 2.5% of the values and the highest 2.5% of the values from the middle 95%. These values are called normal values, or norms.

Outside of the laboratory, there are many qualities for which normal ranges have not been established. This was true cognitive norms for Alzheimer's patients. Cognitive scores are an important tool used to detect patients with dementia, but may only be used if the distribution of normative scores is available. Kornak and colleagues (2018) analyzed data from the National Alzheimer's Coordinating Center (NACC). The investigators determined norms by exploring the relationships between age, sex, and other covariates to the cognitive scores for both normal subjects and those with dementia.

Surveys: Surveys are especially useful when the goal is to gain insight into a perplexing topic or to learn how people think and feel about an issue. Surveys are generally cross-sectional in design, but they can be used in case–control and cohort studies as well.

Monitoring the Future (MTF) is a longitudinal study that examines substance abuse in adolescents, college students, and adult high school graduates through age 55. Johnston et al (2018) compiled a summary of the data collected through 2017. They examined the trends in drug use including marijuana, bath salts, narcotics, tobacco, and alcohol based on 43,700 students in 360 secondary schools.

Interviews are sometimes used in surveys, especially when it is important to probe reasons or explanations more deeply than is possible with a written questionnaire. Interview surveys are also useful when the questions include topics that may require explanation due to complex topics or recalling particular events. The National Health Interview Survey (NHIS) has been conducted since 1962. The content and methodology of the survey has evolved over time to remain relevant and useful for research and investigation. The NHIS is an extensive survey that contains data regarding access to health care, cancer screening, health status, Internet, and email use as well as extensive sociodemographic data.

Many countries and states collect data on a variety of conditions to develop tumor registries, trauma, and databases of cases of infectious disease. Chaudhry and colleagues (2018) studied the number of cancer survivors based on the Ontario Cancer Registry (OCR) and health care administrative data. As cancer treatments advance, the number of survivors is increasing.

Understanding the number of survivors and their health status is an important public health question. The researchers included subjects with malignant cancer recorded in the OCR from 1964 to 2017. They found that 3% of the Ontario population were cancer survivors.

Cohort Studies

A **cohort** is a group of people who have something in common and who remain part of a group over an extended time. In medicine, the subjects in **cohort studies** are selected by some defining characteristic (or characteristics) suspected of being a precursor to or risk factor for a disease or health effect. Cohort studies ask the question "What will happen?" and thus, the direction in cohort studies is forward in time. Figure 2–3 illustrates the study design. Researchers select subjects at the onset of the study and then determine whether they have the risk factor or have been exposed. All subjects are followed over a certain period to observe the effect of the risk factor or exposure. Because the events

of interest transpire after the study has begun, these studies are sometimes called **prospective studies.**

Typical Cohort Studies: A classical cohort study with which most of you are probably familiar is the Framingham study of cardiovascular disease. This study was begun in 1948 to investigate factors associated with the development of atherosclerotic and hypertensive cardiovascular disease, for which Gordon and Kannel (1970) reported a comprehensive 20-year follow-up. More than 6,000 citizens in Framingham, Massachusetts, agreed to participate in this long-term study that involved follow-up interviews and physical examinations every 2 years. Many journal articles have been written about this cohort, and some of the children of the original subjects are now being followed as well.

Cohort studies often examine what happens to the disease over time—the natural history of the disease. Many studies have been based on the Framingham cohort; hundreds of journal articles are indexed by **MEDLINE.** Many studies deal with

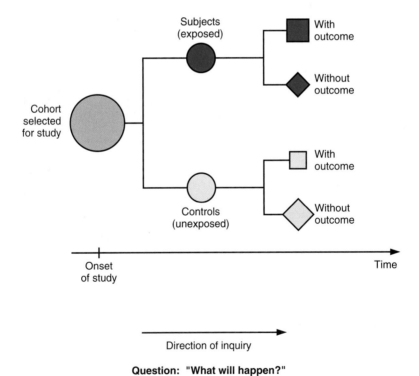

Figure 2–3. Schematic diagram of cohort study design. Shaded areas represent subjects exposed to the antecedent factor; unshaded areas correspond to unexposed subjects. Squares represent subjects with the outcome of interest; diamonds represent subjects without the outcome of interest. (Adapted with permission from Ilango K, Vijayakumar TM, Dubey GP, et al: An Enlarged Vision on Various Types of Study Design in Human Subjects, Global J Pharm 2012 Jan;6(3):216-221.)

cardiovascular-related conditions for which the study was designed, such as investigating cardiovascular biomarkers with heart failure (de Boer et al, 2018), but this very rich source of data is being used to study many other conditions as well. For instance, two recent articles examined treatable vascular disease and cognitive performance (van Eersel et al, 2019) and the relation of bone mass to hip fractures in women (McLean et al, 2018).

Although the Framingham Heart Study is very long term, many cohort studies follow subjects for a much shorter period. A presenting problem in Chapters 5 describes a cohort study to determine the effect of cholecystectomy on bowel habits and bile acid absorption (Dittrich et al, 2018). Thirteen subjects undergoing hypnosis were evaluated in three sessions at least 72 hours apart to detect changes such as EMG signals, peak muscle contraction, and M-wave amplitude.

Outcome Assessment: Increasingly, studies that assess medical outcomes are reported in the medical literature. Patient outcomes have always been of interest to health care providers; physicians and others in the health field are interested in how patients respond to different therapies and management regimens. There continues to be a growing focus on the ways in which patients view and value their health, the care they receive, and the results or outcomes of this care. The reasons for the increase in patient-focused health outcomes are complex, and some of the major ones are discussed later in this chapter.

Interest in outcome assessment was spurred by the Medical Outcomes Study (MOS), designed to determine whether variations in patient outcomes were related to the system of care, clinician specialty, and the technical and interpersonal skill of the clinician (Tarlov et al, 1989). Many subsequent studies looked at variations in outcomes in different geographic locations or among different ethnic groups that might result from access issues. In a cross-sectional study, Priede and colleagues (2018) studied models of social support in recently diagnosed cancer patients using the social support survey component of the MOS (MOS-SSS). They examined the results of the MOS-SSS and the Hospital Anxiety and Depression Scale (HADS) using factor analysis. The method allowed them to measure the structure of the survey and segment the questions into a five-factor model including: emotional, informational, tangible support, positive social interaction, and affection.

Functional status refers to a person's ability to perform their daily activities. Some researchers subdivide functional status into physical, emotional, mental, and social components (Gold et al, 1996). The 6-minute walk test (how far a person can walk in 6 minutes) was studied by Enright and colleagues (2003), and they recommended that the standards be adjusted for age, gender, height, and weight. Many instruments used to measure physical functional status have been developed to evaluate the extent of a patient's rehabilitation following injury or illness. These instruments are commonly called measures of activities of daily living (ADL). Cornelis and colleagues (2017) used the ADLS to aid in the early diagnosis of Alzheimer's disease.

Quality of life (QOL) is a broadly defined concept that includes subjective or objective judgments about all aspects of an individual's existence: health, economic status, environmental, and spiritual. Interest in measuring QOL was heightened when researchers realized that living a long time does not necessarily imply living a good life. QOL measures can help determine a patient's preferences for different health states and are often used to help decide among alternative approaches to medical management (Prigerson et al, 2015).

Patient satisfaction has been discussed for many years and has been shown to be highly associated with whether patients remain with the same physician provider and the degree to which they adhere to their treatment plan (Weingarten et al, 1995).

Patient satisfaction with medical care is influenced by a number of factors, not all of which are directly related to quality of care. The factors that influence patient satisfaction are often dependent on the reason for the contact. For example, Jacobs et al (2014) found that the most important factors driving patient satisfaction after total knee arthroplasty were extent of procedure and pain level post procedure as well as some demographic factors including race of the patient.

Cost-effectiveness and **cost–benefit analysis** are methods used to evaluate economic outcomes of interventions or different modes of treatment. Bagwell et al (2018) studied the effectiveness of intracapsular tonsillectomy and total tonsillectomy to treat pediatric obstructive sleep apnea (OSA). They used a decision tree model to simulate a model of choosing each of the two treatments. They found that when the recurrence rate of OSA was low (3.12%), partial tonsillectomy was more cost-effective. Cost-effectiveness analysis gives policy makers and health providers critical data needed to make informed judgments about interventions (Gold et al, 1996). A large number of questionnaires or instruments have been developed to measure outcomes. For quality of life, the most commonly used general-purpose instrument is the Medical Outcomes Study MOS 36-Item Short-Form Health Survey (SF-36). Originally developed at the RAND Corporation (Stewart et al, 1988), a refinement of the instrument has been validated and is now used worldwide to provide baseline measures and to monitor the results of medical care. The SF-36 provides a way to collect valid data and does not require very much time to complete. The 36 items are combined to produce a patient profile on eight concepts in addition to summary physical and mental health measures.

Many instruments are problem-specific. Cramer and Spilker (1998) provide a broad overview of approaches to QOL assessment, evaluations of outcomes, and pharmacoeconomic methods—both general purpose and disease-specific.

Some outcome studies address a whole host of topics, and we have used several as presenting problems in upcoming chapters. As efforts continue to contain costs of medical care while maintaining a high level of patient care, we expect to see many additional studies focusing on patient outcomes. The journal *Medical Care* is devoted exclusively to outcome studies.

Historical Cohort Studies: Many cohort studies are prospective; that is, they begin at a specific time, the presence or absence of the risk factor is determined, and then information about the outcome of interest is collected at some future time, as in the two studies described earlier. One can also undertake a cohort study

by using information collected in the past and kept in records or files.

For example, St. Sauver and colleagues (2015) studied the risk of developing multimorbidity using data from 123,716 residents of Olmsted County Minnesota. They defined multimorbidity as the development of at least 2 of the 20 chronic conditions selected by HHS. They found that the incidence of multimorbidity increased with age, but the number of people with more than one chronic condition was greater for those under 65 than 65 and older.

Some investigators call this type of study a **historical cohort study** or **retrospective cohort study** because historical information is used; that is, the events being evaluated actually occurred before the onset of the study (Figure 2–4). Note that the direction of the inquiry is still forward in time, from a possible cause or risk factor to an outcome. Studies that merely describe an investigator's experience with a group of patients and attempt to identify features associated with a good or bad outcome fall into this category, and many such studies are published in the medical literature.

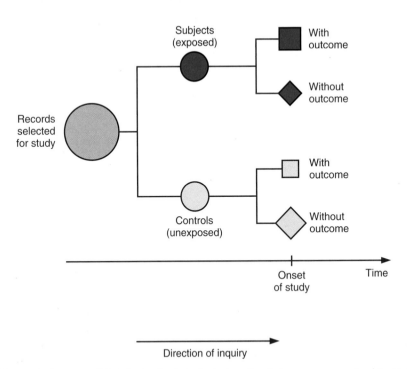

Figure 2–4. Schematic diagram of historical cohort study design. Shaded areas represent subjects exposed to the antecedent factor; unshaded areas correspond to unexposed subjects. Squares represent subjects with the outcome of interest; diamonds represent subjects without the outcome of interest. (Adapted with permission from Ilango K, Vijayakumar TM, Dubey GP, et al: An Enlarged Vision on Various Types of Study Design in Human Subjects, Global J Pharm 2012 Jan;6(3):216-221.)

The time relationship among the different observation study designs is illustrated in Figure 2–5. The figure shows the timing of surveys, which have no direction of inquiry, case–control designs, which look backward in time, and cohort studies, which look forward in time.

Comparison of Case–Control and Cohort Studies

Both case–control and cohort studies evaluate risks and causes of disease, and the design an investigator selects depends in part on the research question.

Moore and colleagues (2016) undertook a matched case–control study to look at the effectiveness of pneumonia vaccines in children. They examined 722 children with pneumonia and 2,991 controls. They found that 13-valent pneumococcal conjugate vaccine (PCV13) was highly effective against the disease.

As this illustration shows, a case–control study takes the outcome as the starting point of the inquiry and looks for precursors or risk factors; while a cohort study starts with a risk factor or exposure and looks at consequences.

Generally speaking, results from a well-designed cohort study carry more weight in understanding a disease than do results from a case–control study. A large number of possible biasing factors can play a role in case–control studies, and several of them are discussed at greater length in Chapter 13.

In spite of their shortcomings with respect to establishing causality, case–control studies are frequently used in medicine and can provide useful insights if well designed. They can be completed in a much shorter time than cohort studies and are correspondingly less expensive to undertake. Case–control studies are especially useful for studying rare conditions or diseases that may not manifest themselves for many years. In addition, they are valuable for testing an original premise; if the results of the case–control study are promising, the investigator can design and undertake a more involved cohort study.

EXPERIMENTAL STUDIES OR CLINICAL TRIALS

Experimental studies are generally easier to identify than observational studies in the medical literature. Authors of medical journal articles reporting experimental studies tend to state explicitly the type of study design used more often than do authors reporting observational studies. Experimental studies in medicine that involve humans are called **clinical trials** because their purpose is to draw conclusions about a particular procedure or treatment. Table 2–1 indicates that clinical trials fall into two categories: those with and those without controls.

Controlled trials are studies in which the experimental drug or procedure is compared with another drug or procedure, sometimes a placebo and sometimes the previously accepted treatment. Uncontrolled trials are studies in which the investigators' experience with the experimental drug or procedure is described, but the treatment is not compared with another treatment, at least not formally. Because the purpose of an experiment is to determine whether the intervention (treatment) makes a difference, studies with controls are much more likely than those without controls to detect whether the difference is due to the experimental treatment or to some other factor. Thus, controlled studies are viewed as having far greater validity in medicine than uncontrolled studies. The consolidated standard of reporting trials (CONSORT) guidelines reflect an effort to improve the reporting of clinical trials. The CONSORT statement was last updated in 2010 and may be found on the CONSORT Web site (www.consort-statement.org).

Trials with Independent Concurrent Controls

One way a trial can be controlled is to have two groups of subjects: one that receives the experimental procedure (the experimental group) and the other that receives the placebo or standard procedure (the control group; Figure 2–6). The experimental and control groups should be treated alike in all ways except for the procedure itself so that any differences between the groups will be due to the procedure and not to other

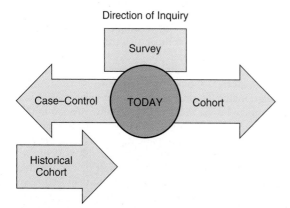

Figure 2–5. Schematic diagram of the time relationship among different observational study designs. The arrows represent the direction of the inquiry.

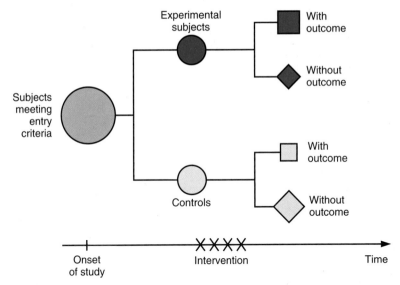

Experimental subjects

With outcome

Without outcome

Subjects meeting entry criteria

With outcome

Without outcome

Controls

Onset of study

Intervention

Time

Figure 2–6. Schematic diagram of randomized controlled trial design. Shaded areas represent subjects assigned to the treatment condition; unshaded areas correspond to subjects assigned to the control condition. Squares represent subjects with the outcome of interest; diamonds represent subjects without the outcome of interest.

factors. The best way to ensure that the groups are treated similarly is to plan interventions for both groups for the same time period in the same study. In this way, the study achieves **concurrent control.** To reduce the chances that subjects or investigators see what they expect to see, researchers can design **double-blind trials** in which neither subjects nor investigators know whether the subject is in the treatment or the control group. When only the subject is unaware, the study is called a **blind trial.** In some unusual situations, the study design may call for the investigator to be blinded even when the subject cannot be blinded. Blindedness is discussed in detail in Chapter 13. Another issue is how to assign some patients to the experimental condition and others to the control condition; the best method of assignment is random assignment. Methods for randomization are discussed in Chapter 4.

Randomized Controlled Trials: The **randomized controlled trial** is the epitome of all research designs because it provides the strongest evidence for concluding causation; it provides the best insurance that the result was due to the intervention.

One of the more noteworthy randomized trials is the Physicians' Health Study (Steering Committee of the Physicians' Health Study Research Group, 1989), which investigated the role of aspirin in reducing the risk of cardiovascular disease. One purpose was to learn whether aspirin in low doses reduces the mortality rate

from cardiovascular disease. Participants in this clinical trial were over 22,000 healthy male physicians who were randomly assigned to receive aspirin or placebo and were followed over an average period of 60 months. The investigators found that fewer physicians in the aspirin group experienced a myocardial infarction during the course of the study than did physicians in the group receiving placebo.

Nonrandomized Trials: Subjects are not always randomized to treatment options. Studies that do not use randomized assignment are generally referred to as **nonrandomized trials** or simply as clinical trials or comparative studies, with no mention of randomization. Many investigators believe that studies with nonrandomized controls are open to so many sources of bias that their conclusions are highly questionable. Studies using nonrandomized controls are considered to be much weaker because they do nothing to prevent bias in patient assignment. For instance, perhaps it is the stronger patients who receive the more aggressive treatment and the higher risk patients who are treated conservatively. An example of a nonrandomized study is a study comparing traditional lecture versus case-based learning and simulation in nurse education (Raurell-Torredà et al, 2014). The investigators studied 66 undergraduates enrolled in a traditional lecture and discussion course and 35 enrolled in a course that also included a case-based learning component. These two groups were then compared to

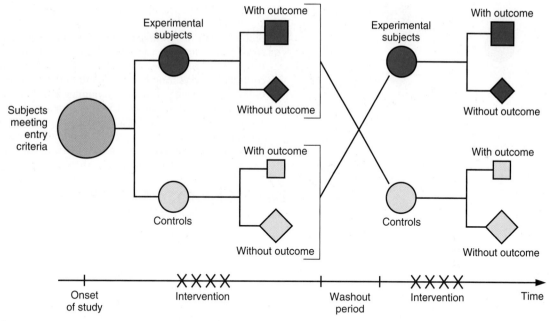

Figure 2–7. Schematic diagram of trial with crossover. Shaded areas represent subjects assigned to the treatment condition; unshaded areas correspond to subjects assigned to the control condition. Squares represent subjects with the outcome of interest; diamonds represent subjects without the outcome of interest.

59 continuing professional education (CPE) nurses with clinical experience. After administering a simulated clinical exam test, they found the intervention group (case-based learning) performed better than the traditional learning group.

Trials with Self-Controls

Moderate level of control can be obtained by using the same group of subjects for both experimental and control options. The study by Goto and colleagues (2018) examined the risk of acute exacerbation of COPD after bariatric surgery. They followed obese adults with COPD that underwent bariatric surgery. They compared the risk of an acute exacerbation in the 12-month period after surgery to months 13 to 24 before surgery. This type of study uses patients as their own controls and is called a **self-controlled study.** Studies with self-controls and no other control group are still vulnerable to the well-known Hawthorne effect, described by Roethlisberger and colleagues (1946), in which people change their behavior and sometimes improve simply because they receive special attention by being in a study and not because of the study intervention. These studies are similar to cohort studies except for the intervention or treatment that is involved.

The self-controlled study design can be modified to provide a combination of concurrent and self-controls. This design uses two groups of patients: one group is assigned to the experimental treatment, and the second group is assigned to the placebo or control treatment (Figure 2–7). After a time, the experimental treatment and placebo are withdrawn from both groups for a "washout" period. During the washout period, the patients generally receive no treatment. The groups are then given the alternative treatment; that is, the first group now receives the placebo, and the second group receives the experimental treatment. This design, called a **crossover study,** is powerful when used appropriately.

Trials with External Controls

The third method for controlling experiments is to use controls external to the study. Sometimes, the result of another investigator's research is used as a comparison. On other occasions, the controls are patients the investigator has previously treated in another manner, called **historical controls.** The study design is illustrated in Figure 2–8.

Historical controls are frequently used to study diseases for which cures do not yet exist and are used in oncology studies, although oncologic studies use concurrent controls when possible. In studies involving

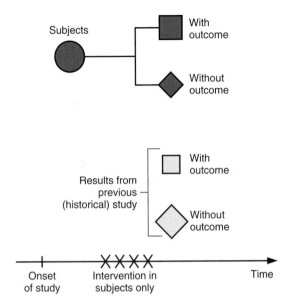

Figure 2–8. Schematic diagram of trial with external controls. Shaded areas represent subjects assigned to the treatment condition; unshaded areas correspond to patients cared for under the control condition. Squares represent subjects with the outcome of interest; diamonds represent subjects without the outcome of interest.

historical controls, researchers should evaluate whether other factors may have changed since the time the historical controls were treated; if so, any differences may be due to these other factors and not to the treatment.

Uncontrolled Studies

Not all studies involving interventions have controls, and by strict definition they are not really experiments or trials. For example, Bottegoni and associates (2016) reported the results of a trial of administering homologous platelet-rich plasma in elderly patients with knee osteoarthritis. Subjects were followed for a 2-month and 6-month visit after administration. The researchers found that there was some short-term clinical improvement after the treatment and that 90% of the patients were satisfied with the results 6 months after treatment. This study was an **uncontrolled study** because there were no comparisons with patients treated in another manner.

Uncontrolled studies are more likely to be used when the comparison involves a procedure than when it involves a drug. The major shortcoming of such studies is that investigators assume that the procedure used and described is the best one. The history of medicine is filled with examples in which one particular

treatment is recommended and then discontinued after a controlled clinical trial is undertaken. One significant problem with uncontrolled trials is that unproved procedures and therapies can become established, making it very difficult for researchers to undertake subsequent controlled studies. Another problem is finding a significant difference when it may be unfounded. Guyatt and colleagues (2000) identified 13 randomized trials and 17 observational studies in adolescent pregnancy prevention. Six of eight outcomes they examined showed a significant intervention effect in the observational studies, whereas the randomized studies showed no benefit.

META-ANALYSIS & REVIEW PAPERS

A type of study that does not fit specifically in either category of observation studies or experiments is called **meta-analysis**. Meta-analysis uses published information from other studies and combines the results so as to permit an overall conclusion. Meta-analysis is similar to review articles, but additionally includes a quantitative assessment and summary of the findings. It is possible to do a meta-analysis of observational studies or experiments; however, a meta-analysis should report the findings for these two types of study designs separately. This method is especially appropriate when the studies that have been reported have small numbers of subjects or come to different conclusions.

Finnerup and colleagues (2015) performed a meta-analysis of neuropathic pain in adults. The investigators wanted to know if topical or oral medications were more effective in treating pain. They found 229 studies that had addressed this question and combined the results in a statistical manner to reach an overall conclusion about their effectiveness—mainly that the evidence supporting the use of oral medications was stronger.

ADVANTAGES & DISADVANTAGES OF DIFFERENT STUDY DESIGNS

The previous sections introduced the major types of study designs used in medical research, broadly divided into experimental studies, or clinical trials, and observational studies (cohort, case–control, cross-sectional, and case–series designs). Each study design has certain advantages over the others as well as some specific disadvantages, which we discuss in the following sections.

Advantages & Disadvantages of Clinical Trials

The randomized clinical trial is the gold standard, or reference, in medicine; it is the design against which others are judged—because it provides the greatest justification for concluding causality and is subject to the least number of problems or biases. Clinical trials are the best type of study to use when the objective is to establish the efficacy of a treatment or a procedure. Clinical trials in which patients are randomly assigned to different treatments, or "arms," are the strongest design of all. One of the treatments is the experimental condition; another is the control condition. The control may be a placebo or a sham procedure; often, it is the treatment or procedure commonly used, called the standard of care or reference standard. A number of published articles have shown the tendency for non-randomized studies, especially those using historical controls, to be more likely to show a positive outcome, compared with randomized studies. In some situations, however, historical controls can and should be used. For instance, historical controls may be useful when preliminary studies are needed or when researchers are dealing with late treatment for an intractable disease, such as advanced cancer. Although clinical trials provide the greatest justification for determining causation, obstacles to using them include their great expense and long duration. For instance, a randomized trial comparing various treatments for carcinoma requires the investigators to follow the subjects for a long time. Another potential obstacle to using clinical trials occurs when certain practices become established and accepted by the medical community, even though they have not been properly justified. As a result, procedures become established that may be harmful to many patients, as evidenced by the controversy over silicone breast implants and the many different approaches to managing hypertension, many of which have never been subjected to a clinical trial that includes the most conservative treatment, diuretics.

Advantages & Disadvantages of Cohort Studies

Cohort studies are the design of choice for studying the causes of a condition, the course of a disease, or the risk factors because they are longitudinal and follow a group of subjects over a period of time. Causation generally cannot be proved with cohort studies because they are observational and do not involve interventions. However, because they follow a cohort of patients forward through time, they possess the correct time sequence to provide strong evidence for possible causes and effects, as in the smoking and lung cancer controversy. In well-designed cohort studies, investigators can control many sources of bias related to patient selection and recorded measurements.

The length of time required in a cohort study depends on the problem studied. With diseases that develop over a long period of time or with conditions that occur as a result of long-term exposure to some causative agent, many years are needed for study. Extended time periods make such studies costly. They also make it difficult for investigators to argue causation because other events occurring in the intervening period may have affected the outcome. For example, the long time between exposure and effect is one of the reasons it is difficult to study the possible relationship between environmental agents and various carcinomas. Cohort studies that require a long time to complete are especially vulnerable to problems associated with patient follow-up, particularly patient attrition (patients stop participating in the study) and patient migration (patients move to other communities). This is one reason that the Framingham study, with its rigorous methods of follow-up, is such a rich source of important information.

Advantages & Disadvantages of Case–Control Studies

Case–control studies are especially appropriate for studying rare diseases or events, for examining conditions that develop over a long time, and for investigating a preliminary hypothesis. They are generally the quickest and least expensive studies to undertake and are ideal for investigators who need to obtain some preliminary data prior to writing a proposal for a more complete, expensive, and time-consuming study. They are also a good choice for someone who needs to complete a clinical research project in a specific amount of time.

The advantages of case–control studies lead to their disadvantages. Of all study methods, they have the largest number of possible biases or errors, and they depend completely on high-quality existing records. Data availability for case–control studies sometimes requires compromises between what researchers wish to study and what they are able to study. One of the previous edition authors was involved in a study of elderly burn patients in which the goal was to determine risk factors for survival. The primary investigator wanted to collect data on fluid intake and output. He found, however, that not all of the existing patient records contained this information, and thus it was impossible to study the effect of this factor.

One of the greatest problems in a case–control study is selection of an appropriate control group. The cases in a case–control study are relatively easy to identify, but deciding on a group of persons who provide a relevant comparison is more difficult. Because of the problems inherent in choosing a control group in a case–control study, some statisticians have recommended the use of two control groups: one control group similar in some ways to the cases (e.g., having been hospitalized during the same period of time) and another control group of healthy subjects.

Advantages & Disadvantages of Cross-Sectional Studies

Cross-sectional studies are best for determining the status quo of a disease or condition, such as the prevalence of HIV in given populations, and for evaluating diagnostic procedures. Cross-sectional studies are similar to case–control studies in being relatively quick to complete, and they may be relatively inexpensive as well. Their primary disadvantage is that they provide only a "snapshot in time" of the disease or process, which may result in misleading information if the research question is really one of disease process. For example, clinicians used to believe that diastolic blood pressure, unlike systolic pressure, does not increase as patients grow older. This belief was based on cross-sectional studies that had shown mean diastolic blood pressure to be approximately 80 mm Hg in all age groups. In the Framingham cohort study, however, the patients who were followed over a period of several years were observed to have increased diastolic blood pressure as they grew older (Gordon et al, 1959).

This apparent contradiction is easier to understand if we consider what happens in an aging cohort. For example, suppose that the mean diastolic pressure in men aged 40 years is 80 mm Hg, although there is individual variation, with some men having a blood pressure as low as 60 mm Hg and others having a pressure as high as 100 mm Hg. Ten years later, there is an increase in diastolic pressure, although it is not an even increase; some men experience a greater increase than others. The men who were at the upper end of the blood pressure **distribution** 10 years earlier and who had experienced a larger increase have died in the intervening period, so they are no longer represented in a cross-sectional study. As a result, the mean diastolic pressure of the men still in the cohort at age 50 is about 80 mm Hg, even though individually their pressures are higher than they were 10 years earlier. Thus, a cohort study, not a cross-sectional study, provides the information leading to a correct understanding of the relationship between normal aging and physiologic processes such as diastolic blood pressure.

Surveys are generally cross-sectional studies. Most of the voter polls done prior to an election are one-time samplings of a group of citizens, and different results from week to week are based on different groups of people; that is, the same group of citizens is not followed to determine voting preferences through time. Similarly, consumer-oriented studies on customer satisfaction with automobiles, appliances, health care, and so on are cross-sectional.

A common problem with survey research is obtaining sufficiently large response rates; many people asked to participate in a survey decline because they are busy, not interested, and so forth. The conclusions are, therefore, based on a subset of people who agree to participate, and these people may not be **representative** of or similar to the entire population. The problem of representative participants is not confined to cross-sectional studies; it can be an issue in other studies whenever subjects are selected or asked to participate and decline or drop out. Another issue is the way questions are posed to participants; if questions are asked in a leading or emotionally inflammatory way, the responses may not truly represent the participants' feelings or opinions. We discuss issues with surveys more completely in Chapter 11.

Advantages & Disadvantages of Case–Series Studies

Case–series reports have two advantages: They are easy to write, and the observations may be extremely useful to investigators designing a study to evaluate causes or explanations of the observations. But as we noted previously, case–series studies are susceptible to many possible biases related to subject selection and characteristics observed. In general, you should view them as hypothesis-generating and not as conclusive.

SUMMARY

This chapter illustrates the study designs most frequently encountered in the medical literature. In medical research, subjects are observed or experiments are undertaken. Experiments involving humans are called trials. Experimental studies may also use animals and tissue, although we did not discuss them as a separate category; the comments pertaining to clinical trials are relevant to animal and tissue studies as well.

Each type of study discussed has advantages and disadvantages. Randomized, controlled clinical trials are the most powerful designs possible in medical research, but they are often expensive and time-consuming. Well-designed observational studies can provide useful insights on disease causation, even though they do not constitute proof of causes. Cohort studies are best for studying the natural progression of disease or risk factors for disease; case–control studies are much quicker and less expensive. Cross-sectional studies provide a snapshot of a disease or condition at one time, and we must be cautious in inferring disease progression from them. Surveys, if properly done, are useful in obtaining current opinions and practices. Case–series studies should be used only to raise questions for further research.

We have used several presenting problems from later chapters to illustrate different study designs. We will point out salient features in the design of the presenting problems as we go along, and we will return to the topic of study design again after all the prerequisites for evaluating the quality of journal articles have been presented.

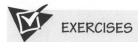 EXERCISES

Read the descriptions of the following studies and determine the study design used.

1. *Researchers wanted to determine if adding vancomycin to the protocol for shunt insertion would reduce the infection rate (van Lindert et al, 2018). The researchers compared patients with shunt insertions prior to the protocol change (263 procedures from January 2010 to December 2011) with those after the addition of vancomycin to the protocol (499 procedures from April 2012 to December 2015).*

2. *Priede and coworkers (2018) studied the level of psychological stress in newly diagnosed cancer patients using the MOS-SSS survey. Patients were recruited from December 2011 to October 2013.*

3. *The Prostate Cancer Outcomes Study was designed to investigate the patterns of cancer care and effects of treatment on quality of life. Hoffman and coworkers (2017) identified eligible cases from one SEER tumor registry. They surveyed 934 known survivors to assess treatment decision regret. Multivariate logistic regression was used to investigate the factors related to regret.*

4. *The relationship between exposure to benzodiazepine and Alzheimer's disease was investigated by Billioti de Gage and colleagues (2014). Subjects with Alzheimer's disease were matched with controls based on sex age group and duration of follow-up.*

5. *A study to determine whether radiation treatment with or without anti-androgen therapy in recurrent prostate cancer (Shipley et al, 2017). The primary outcome was overall survival.*

6. *Eckel et al (2018) reported on the relationship between transition from metabolic healthy to unhealthy status and association with cardiovascular disease. Subjects in the study were selected from the Nurses' Health Study originally completed in 1976; the study included 120,000 married female registered nurses, aged 30–55. The original survey provided information on the subjects' age, parental history of myocardial infarction, smoking status, height, weight, use of oral contraceptives or postmenopausal hormones, and history of myocardial infarction or angina pectoris, diabetes, hypertension, or high serum cholesterol levels. Follow-up surveys were every 2 years thereafter.*

7. **Group Exercise.** *The abuse of phenacetin, a common ingredient of analgesic drugs, can lead to kidney disease. There is also evidence that use of salicylate provides protection against cardiovascular disease. How would you design a study to examine the effects of these two drugs on mortality due to different causes and on cardiovascular morbidity?*

8. **Group Exercise.** *Select a study with an interesting topic, either one of the studies referred to in this chapter or from a current journal. Carefully examine the research question and decide which study design would be optimal to answer the question. Is that the study design used by the investigators? If so, were the investigators attentive to potential problems identified in this chapter? If not, what are the reasons for the study design used? Do they make sense?*

Summarizing Data & Presenting Data in Tables & Graphs

3

KEY CONCEPTS

 All observations of subjects in a study are evaluated on a scale of measurement that determines how the observations should be summarized, displayed, and analyzed.

 Nominal scales are used to categorize discrete characteristics.

 Ordinal scales categorize characteristics that have an inherent order.

 Numerical scales measure the amount or quantity of something.

 Means measure the middle of the distribution of a numerical characteristic.

 Medians measure the middle of the distribution of an ordinal characteristic or a numerical characteristic that is skewed.

 The standard deviation is a measure of the spread of observations around the mean and is used in many statistical procedures.

 The coefficient of variation is a measure of relative spread that permits the comparison of observations measured on different scales.

 Percentiles are useful to compare an individual observation with a norm.

 Stem-and-leaf plots are a combination of frequency tables and histograms that are useful in exploring the distribution of a set of observations.

 Frequency tables show the number of observations having a specific characteristic.

 Histograms, box plots, and frequency polygons display distributions of numerical observations.

 Proportions and percentages are used to summarize nominal and ordinal data.

 Rates describe the number of events that occur in a given period.

 Prevalence and incidence are two important measures of morbidity.

 Rates must be adjusted when populations being compared differ in an important confounding factor.

 The relationship between two numerical characteristics is described by the correlation.

 The relationship between two nominal characteristics is described by the risk ratio, odds ratio, and event rates.

 Number needed to treat is a useful indication of the effectiveness of a given therapy or procedure.

 Scatterplots illustrate the relationship between two numerical characteristics.

 Poorly designed graphs and tables mislead in the information they provide.

PRESENTING PROBLEMS

Presenting Problem 1

Life expectancy varies across regions of the United States. Davids et al (2014) examined the Community Health Status Indicators (CHSI) to Combat Obesity, Heart Disease, and Cancer to determine opportunities to improve health status and life expectancy based on known social determinants of health. They found a link between life expectancy and poverty, educational level, and the racial composition of the county.

The data may be accessed using the following link:

https://healthdata.gov/dataset/community-health-status-indicators-chsi-combat-obesity-heart-disease-and-cancer/resource

Details regarding the content of the data may be accessed here:

https://healthdata.gov/dataset/community-health-status-indicators-chsi-combat-obesity-heart-disease-and-cancer

Presenting Problem 2

Many patients with chronic diseases do not engage in self-management activities. Bos-Touwen and associates (2015) investigated the characteristics of patients that participate in self-management programs for a number of chronic diseases including: type-2 Diabetes Mellitus (DM-II), Chronic Obstructive Pulmonary Disease (COPD), Chronic Heart Failure (CHF), and Chronic Renal Disease (CRD). They used a survey tool called the 13-item Patient Activation Measure (PAM-13) as well as demographic, clinical, and psychosocial variables.

The data for this study is made public via the DRYAD data repository and may be accessed at this site:

https://datadryad.org/resource/doi:10.5061/dryad.jg413

Presenting Problem 3

Anderson et al (2018) studied predictors of influenza in over 4,500 patients presenting to a hospital with flu-like symptoms from 2009 to 2014. They found that the most important symptoms for predicting influenza were cough, runny nose, chills, and body aches. They formulated a predictive model that was able to predict the presence/absence of the flu virus. Further, they tested the predictive value of a rapid influenza test versus virologically confirmed influenza cases.

Anderson KB, Simasathien S, Watanaveeradej V, et al: Clinical and laboratory predictors of influenza infection among individuals with influenza-like illness presenting to an urban Thai hospital over a five-year period. PLOS ONE 2018;13(3): e0193050. https://doi.org/10.1371/journal.pone.0193050

The data may be accessed using the following link:

Anderson KB, Simasthien S, Watanaveeradej V, et al: Clinical and laboratory predictors of influenza infection among individuals with influenza-like illness presenting to an urban Thai hospital over a five-year period. Dryad Digital Repository 2018. https://doi.org/10.5061/dryad.t7n48

PURPOSE OF THE CHAPTER

This chapter introduces different kinds of data collected in medical research and demonstrates how to organize and present summaries of the data. Regardless of the particular research being done, investigators collect observations and generally want to transform them into tables or graphs or to present summary numbers, such as percentages or means. From a statistical perspective, it does not matter whether the observations are on people, animals, inanimate objects, or events. What matters is the kind of observations and the scale on which they are measured. These features determine the statistics used to summarize the data, called **descriptive statistics,** and the types of tables or graphs that best display and communicate the observations.

Data from open source health care datasets are used to illustrate the steps involved in calculating the statistics because seeing the steps helps most people understand procedures. However, most people will use a computer to analyze data. In fact, this and following chapters contain numerous illustrations from some commonly used statistical computer programs, including an open source statistical program called R. Readers are encouraged to download and install R so that the exercises presented here can be replicated.

SCALES OF MEASUREMENT

The scale for measuring a characteristic has implications for the way information is displayed and summarized. As we will see in later chapters, the **scale of measurement**—the precision with which a characteristic is measured—also determines the statistical methods for analyzing the data. The three scales of measurement that occur most often in medicine are nominal, ordinal, and numerical.

Nominal Scales

Nominal scales are used for the simplest level of measurement when data values fit into categories. A special case of the nominal scale indicates the presence or absence of an attribute. For example, in a mortality study, patients who die may be labeled with a 1 while those that live may be labeled with a 0. In this example, the observations are **dichotomous** or **binary** in that the outcome can take on only one of two values: yes or no (dead or alive). Although we talk about nominal data as being on the measurement scale, we do not actually measure nominal data; instead, we count the number of observations with or without the attribute of interest.

Many classifications in medical research are evaluated on a nominal scale. Outcomes of a medical treatment or surgical procedure, as well as the presence of possible risk factors, are often described as either occurring or not occurring. Outcomes may also be described with more than two categories, such as the classification of anemias as microcytic (including iron deficiency), macrocytic or megaloblastic (including vitamin B_{12} deficiency), and normocytic (often associated with chronic disease).

Data evaluated on a nominal scale are sometimes called **qualitative observations,** because they describe a quality of the person or thing studied, or **categorical observations,** because the values fit into categories. Nominal or qualitative data are generally described in terms of **percentages** or **proportions. Contingency tables** and **bar charts** are most often used to display this type of information and are presented in the section titled "Tables and Graphs for Nominal and Ordinal Data." The important attribute of nominal scale data is that the categories are not ordered; they are simply labeled categories that allow the research to tabulate a result or outcome.

Ordinal Scales

When an inherent order occurs among the categories, the observations are said to be measured on an **ordinal scale.** Observations are still classified, as with nominal scales, but some observations have *more* or are *greater than* other observations. Clinicians often use ordinal scales to determine a patient's amount of risk or the appropriate type of therapy. Tumors, for example, are staged according to their degree of development. The international classification for staging of carcinoma of the cervix is an ordinal scale from 0 to 4, in which stage 0 represents carcinoma in situ and stage 4 represents carcinoma extending beyond the pelvis or involving the mucosa of the bladder and rectum. The inherent order in this ordinal scale is, of course, that the prognosis for stage 4 is worse than that for stage 0.

Classifications based on the extent of disease are sometimes related to a patient's activity level. For example, rheumatoid arthritis is classified, according to the severity of disease, into four classes ranging from normal activity (class 1) to wheelchair-bound (class 4). Although order exists among categories in ordinal scales, the difference between two adjacent categories is not the same throughout the scale. To illustrate, Apgar scores, which describe the maturity of newborn infants, range from 0 to 10, with lower scores indicating depression of cardiorespiratory and neurologic functioning and higher scores indicating good functioning. The difference between scores of 8 and 9 probably does not have the same clinical implications as the difference between scores of 0 and 1.

Some scales consist of scores for multiple factors that are then added to get an overall index. An index frequently used to estimate the cardiac risk in noncardiac surgical procedures was developed by Goldman and his colleagues (1977, 1995). This index assigns points to a variety of risk factors, such as age over 70 years, history of an MI in the past 6 months, specific electrocardiogram abnormalities, and general physical status. The points are added to get an overall score from 0 to 53, which is used to indicate the risk of complications or death for different score levels.

A special type of ordered scale is a **rank-order scale,** in which observations are ranked from highest to lowest (or vice versa). For example, health providers could direct their education efforts aimed at the obstetric patient based on ranking the causes of low birthweight in infants, such as malnutrition, drug abuse, and inadequate prenatal care, from most common to least common. The duration of surgical procedures might be converted to a rank scale to obtain one measure of the difficulty of the procedure.

As with nominal scales, percentages and proportions are often used with ordinal scales. The entire set of data measured on an ordinal scale may be summarized by the **median** value, and we will describe how to find the median and what it means. Ordinal scales having a large number of values are sometimes treated as if they are numerical (see following section). The same types of tables and graphs used to display nominal data may also be used with ordinal data.

Numerical Scales

Observations for which the differences between numbers have meaning on a numerical scale are sometimes called **quantitative observations** because they measure the quantity of something. There are two types of numerical scales: continuous* (interval or ratio) and discrete scales. A **continuous scale** has values on a continuum (e.g., age); a **discrete scale** has values equal to integers (e.g., number of fractures).

If data need not be very precise, continuous data may be reported to the closest integer. Theoretically, however, more precise measurement is possible. Age is a continuous measure, and age recorded to the nearest year will generally suffice in studies of adults; however, for young children, age to the nearest month may be preferable. Other examples of continuous data include height, weight, length of time of survival, range of joint motion, and many laboratory values.

When a numerical observation can take on only integer values, the scale of measurement is discrete. For example, counts of things—number of pregnancies, number of previous operations, number of risk factors—are discrete measures.

Characteristics measured on a numerical scale are frequently displayed in a variety of tables and graphs. Means and standard deviations are generally used to summarize the values of numerical measures. We next examine ways to summarize and display numerical data and then return to the subject of ordinal and nominal data.

SUMMARIZING NUMERICAL DATA WITH NUMBERS

When an investigator collects many observations, such as activation score, body mass index (BMI), health status scores, and patient activation scores in the study by Bos-Touwen and colleagues (2015), numbers that summarize the data can communicate a lot of information.

Measures of the Middle

One of the most useful summary numbers is an indicator of the center of a distribution of observations—the

middle or average value. The three measures of central tendency used in medicine and epidemiology are the mean, the median, and, to a lesser extent, the mode. All three are used for numerical data, and the median is used for ordinal data as well.

Calculating Measures of Central Tendency

The Mean: Although several means may be mathematically calculated, the arithmetic, or simple, mean is used most frequently in statistics and is the one generally referred to by the term "mean." The **mean** is the arithmetic average of the observations. It is symbolized by $\overline{X}$ (called X-bar) and is calculated as follows: add the observations to obtain the sum and then divide by the number of observations.

The formula for the mean is written $\sum X/n$, where $\sum$ (Greek letter sigma) means to add, X represents the individual observations, and n is the number of observations.

Table 3–1 gives the value of the activation score, BMI, Activation Score, and SF-12 Total Score for 18 randomly selected patients in the self-management study (Bos-Touwen et al, 2015). (We will learn about random sampling in Chapter 4.) The mean activation score for these 18 patients is 53.0. The mean is used when the numbers can be added (i.e., when the characteristics are measured on a numerical scale); it should not ordinarily be used with ordinal data because of the arbitrary nature of an ordinal scale. The mean is sensitive to extreme values in a set of observations, especially when the sample size is fairly small. For example, the value of 75.3 for subject 1 and is relatively large compared with the others. If this value was not present, the mean would be 51.7 instead of 53.0.

$$\overline{X} = \frac{\sum X}{n} = \frac{75.3 + 56.4 + \ldots + 52.9}{18}$$

$$= \frac{954.7}{18} = 53.0$$

If the original observations are not available, the mean can be estimated from a frequency table. A **weighted average** is formed by multiplying each data value by the number of observations that have that value, adding the products, and dividing the sum by the number of observations. A frequency table of activation score observations is presented in Table 3–2, and we can use it to estimate the mean activation score for all 1,154 patients in the study. The weighted-average estimate

---

*Some statisticians differentiate interval scales (with an arbitrary zero point) from ratio scales (with an absolute zero point); examples are temperature on a Celsius scale (interval) and temperature on a Kelvin scale (ratio). Little difference exists, however, in how measures on these two scales are treated statistically, so we call them both simply numerical.

Table 3–1. Activation score for a random sample of 18 patients.

Subject ID	BMI	Activation Score	SF12 Total Score	Age
1	25.5	75.3	90.8	57
2	22.9	56.4	54.6	76
3	29.4	68.5	86.3	64
4	30.4	60.0	57.5	65
5	23.1	56.4	70.8	62
6	31.3	37.3	13.8	64
7	27.5	52.9	21.3	84
8	24.5	70.8	91.7	68
9	28.5	52.9	38.8	80
10	25.1	56.4	26.3	82
11	25.0	52.9	36.3	61
12	24.2	47.4	88.8	57
13	25.1	60.0	30.4	92
14	28.8	34.7	21.3	66
15	28.4	38.7	24.2	52
16	22.8	45.2	44.2	69
17	31.6	36.0	31.3	79
18	29.1	52.9	75.0	56

Data from Bos-Touwen I, Schuurmans M, Monninkhof EM, et al: Patient and disease characteristics associated with activation for self-management in patients with diabetes, chronic obstructive pulmonary disease, chronic heart failure and chronic renal disease: a cross-sectional survey study, PLoS One. 2015 May 7;10(5):e0126400.

Table 3–2. Frequency distribution of activation score in five-point intervals.

Activation Score	Count	Cumulative Count	Percent	Cumulative Percent
35 or less	11	11	0.95%	0.95%
35 up to 40	50	61	4.33%	5.29%
40 up to 45	148	209	12.82%	18.11%
45 up to 50	292	501	25.30%	43.41%
50 up to 55	130	631	11.27%	54.68%
55 up to 60	191	822	16.55%	71.23%
60 up to 65	151	973	13.08%	84.32%
65 up to 70	65	1038	5.63%	89.95%
70 up to 75	50	1088	4.33%	94.28%
75 up to 80	43	1131	3.73%	98.01%
80 or higher	23	1154	1.99%	100.00%

Data from Bos-Touwen I, Schuurmans M, Monninkhof EM, et al: Patient and disease characteristics associated with activation for self-management in patients with diabetes, chronic obstructive pulmonary disease, chronic heart failure and chronic renal disease: a cross-sectional survey study, PLoS One. 2015 May 7;10(5):e0126400.

of the mean, using the number of subjects and the midpoints in each interval, is

$$\frac{(32.5 \times 5) + (37.5 \times 28) \ldots + (82.5 \times 23)}{1154}$$

$$= \frac{62431.00}{1154} = 54.10$$

The value of the mean calculated from a frequency table is not always the same as the value obtained with raw numbers. In this example, the activation score means calculated from the raw numbers and the frequency table are very close. Investigators who calculate the mean for presentation in a paper or talk have the original observations, of course, and should use the exact formula. The formula for use with a frequency table is helpful when we, as readers of an article, do not have access to the raw data but want an estimate of the mean.

The Median: The **median** is the middle observation, that is, the point at which half the observations are smaller and half are larger. The median is sometimes symbolized by M or Md, but it has no conventional symbol. The procedure for calculating the median is as follows:

1. Arrange the observations from smallest to largest (or vice versa).
2. Count in to find the middle value. The median is the middle value for an odd number of observations; it is defined as the mean of the two middle values for an even number of observations.

For example, in rank order (from lowest to highest), the activation score values in Table 3–1 are as follows: 34.7, 36.0, 37.3, 38.7, 45.2, 47.4, 52.9, 52.9, 52.9, 52.9, 56.4, 56.4, 56.4, 60.0, 60.0, 68.5, 70.8, 75.3. For 18 observations, the median is the mean of the ninth and tenth values (52.9 and 52.9), or 52.9. The median tells us that half the activation score values in this group are less than 52.9 and half are greater than 52.9. We will learn later in this chapter that the median is easy to determine from a **stem-and-leaf plot** of the observations.

The median is less sensitive to extreme values than is the mean. For example, if the largest observation, 75.3, is excluded from the sample, the median would be the middle value, 52.9. The median is also used with ordinal observations.

The Mode: The **mode** is the value that occurs most frequently. It is commonly used for a large number of observations when the researcher wants to designate the value that occurs most often. The value 52.9 occurs most frequently among the data in Table 3–1. Therefore, the mode activation score is 52.9. When a set of data has two modes, it is called *bimodal.* For frequency tables or a small number of observations, the mode is sometimes estimated by the **modal class,** which is the interval having the largest number of observations. For the activation score data in Table 3–2, the modal class is 45 through 50 with 292 patients.

The Geometric Mean: Another measure of central tendency not used as often as the arithmetic mean or the median is the **geometric mean,** sometimes symbolized as GM or G. It is the nth root of the product of the n observations. In symbolic form, for n observations X_1, $X_2, X_3, \ldots X_n$, the geometric mean is

$$GM = \sqrt[n]{(X_1)(X_2)(X_3)\ldots(X_n)}$$

Taking the logarithm of both sides of the preceding equation, we see that the logarithm of the geometric mean is equal to the mean of the logarithms of the observations.

$$\log GM = \sum \frac{\log X}{n}$$

Find the mean, median, and mode for the activation score for all of the patients in the study by Bos-Touwen and colleagues (2015). Repeat for patients who did and did not have Chronic Renal Disease (disease = 4). Do you think the mean activation score is different for these two groups? In Chapter 6, we will learn how to answer this type of question.

Using Measures of Central Tendency: Which measure of central tendency is best with a particular set of observations? Two factors are important: the scale of measurement (ordinal or numerical) and the shape of the distribution of observations. Although distributions are discussed in more detail in Chapter 4, we consider here the notion of whether a distribution is symmetric about the mean or is skewed to the left or the right.

If outlying observations occur in only one direction—either a few small values or a few large ones—the distribution is said to be a **skewed distribution.** If the outlying values are small, the distribution is skewed to the left, or negatively skewed; if the outlying values are large, the distribution is skewed to the right, or positively skewed. A **symmetric distribution** has the same shape on both sides of the mean. Figure 3–1 gives examples of negatively skewed, positively skewed, and symmetric distributions.

The following facts help us as readers of articles know the shape of a distribution without actually seeing it.

1. If the mean and the median are equal, the distribution of observations is symmetric, generally as in Figures 3–1C and 3–1D.
2. If the mean is larger than the median, the distribution is skewed to the right, as in Figure 3–1B.
3. If the mean is smaller than the median, the distribution is skewed to the left, as in Figure 3–1A.

The following guidelines help us decide which measure of central tendency is best.

1. The mean is used for numerical data and for symmetric (not skewed) distributions.
2. The median is used for ordinal data or for numerical data if the distribution is heavily skewed.
3. The mode is used primarily for ordinal data and bimodal numeric distributions.
4. The geometric mean is generally used for observations measured on a logarithmic scale or data with moderate skewness.

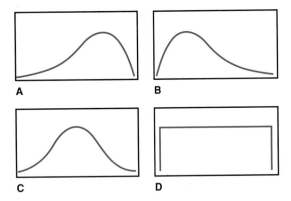

Figure 3–1. Shapes of common distributions of observations. **A:** Negatively skewed. **B:** Positively skewed. **C and D:** Symmetric.

Measures of Spread

Suppose all you know about the 18 randomly selected patients in Presenting Problem 1 is that the mean activation score is 53.0. Although the mean provides useful information, you have a better idea of the distribution of activation scores in these patients if you know something about the spread, or the variation, of the observations. Several statistics are used to describe the dispersion of data: range, standard deviation, coefficient of variation, percentile rank, and interquartile range. All are described in the following sections.

Calculating Measures of Spread

The Range: The **range** is the difference between the largest and the smallest observation. It is easy to determine once the data have been arranged in rank order. For example, the lowest activation score among the 18 patients is 34.7, and the highest is 75.3; thus, the range is 75.3 minus 34.7, or 40.6. Many authors give minimum and maximum values instead of the range, and in some ways these values are more useful.

The Standard Deviation: The standard deviation is the most commonly used measure of dispersion with medical and health data. Although its meaning and computation are somewhat complex, it is very important because it is used both to describe how observations cluster around the mean and in many statistical tests. Most of you will use a computer to determine the standard deviation, but the steps involved in its calculation are presented to give a greater understanding of the meaning of this statistic.

The **standard deviation** is a measure of the spread of data about their mean. Briefly looking at the logic behind this statistic, we need a measure of the "average" spread of the observations about the mean. Why not find the deviation of each observation from the mean, add these deviations, and divide the sum by n to form an analogy to the mean itself? The problem is that the sum of deviations about the mean is always zero (see Exercise 1). Why not use the absolute values of the deviations? The **absolute value** of a number ignores the sign of the number and is denoted by vertical bars on each side of the number. For example, the absolute value of 5, |5|, is 5, and the absolute value of −5, |−5|, is also 5. Although this approach avoids the zero-sum problem, it lacks some important statistical properties, and so is not used. Instead, the deviations are *squared* before adding them, and then the square root is found to express the standard deviation on the original scale of measurement. The standard deviation is symbolized as *SD*, *sd*, or simply *s* (in this text we use *SD*), and its formula is

$$SD = \sqrt{\frac{\sum(X - \bar{X})^2}{n - 1}}$$

The name of the statistic before the square root is taken is the **variance,** but the standard deviation is the statistic of primary interest because it is measured in the same units as the underlying data (the variance is measured in square units).

Using $n - 1$ instead of n in the denominator produces a more accurate (unbiased) estimate of the true population standard deviation and has desirable mathematical properties for statistical inferences.

The preceding formula for standard deviation, called the *definitional formula,* is not the easiest one for calculations. Another formula, the *computational formula,* is generally used instead. Because the standard deviation is generally computed using a computer, the illustrations in this text use the more meaningful but computationally less efficient formula. If you are curious, the computational formula is given in Exercise 7.

Now let's try a calculation. The activation score values for the 18 patients are repeated in Table 3–3 along with the computations needed. The steps follow:

1. Let X be the activation score for each patient, and find the mean: the mean is 53.04, as we calculated earlier.
2. Subtract the mean from each observation to form the deviations $X -$ mean.
3. Square each deviation to form $(X - \text{mean})^2$.
4. Add the squared deviations.
5. Divide the result in step 4 by $n - 1$; we have 138.48. This value is the variance.
6. Take the square root of the value in step 5 to find the standard deviation; we have 11.77.

Table 3–3. Calculations for standard deviation of activation score in a random sample of 18 patients.

Patient	X	$X - \bar{X}$	$(X - \bar{X})^2$
1	75.30	22.26	495.56
2	56.40	3.36	11.30
3	68.50	15.46	239.05
4	60.00	6.96	48.46
5	56.40	3.36	11.30
6	37.30	(15.74)	247.71
7	52.90	(0.14)	0.02
8	70.80	17.76	315.46
9	52.90	(0.14)	0.02
10	56.40	3.36	11.30
11	52.90	(0.14)	0.02
12	47.40	(5.64)	31.80
13	60.00	6.96	48.46
14	34.70	(18.34)	336.31
15	38.70	(14.34)	205.60
16	45.20	(7.84)	61.45
17	36.00	(17.04)	290.32
18	52.90	(0.14)	0.02
Sums	954.70		2354.14
Mean	53.04		

Data from Bos-Touwen I, Schuurmans M, Monninkhof EM, et al: Patient and disease characteristics associated with activation for self-management in patients with diabetes, chronic obstructive pulmonary disease, chronic heart failure and chronic renal disease: a cross-sectional survey study, PLoS One. 2015 May 7; 10(5):e0126400.

But note the relatively large squared deviation of 495.56 for patient 1 in Table 3–3. It contributes substantially to the variation in the data. The standard deviation of the remaining 17 patients (after eliminating patient 15) is smaller, 10.69, demonstrating the effect that outlying observations can have on the value of the standard deviation.

The standard deviation, like the mean, requires numerical data. Also, like the mean, the standard deviation is a very important statistic. First, it is an essential part of many **statistical tests** as we will see in later chapters. Second, the standard deviation is very useful in describing the spread of the observations about the mean value. Two rules of thumb when using the standard deviation are:

1. Regardless of how the observations are distributed, at least 75% of the values *always* lie between these two numbers: the *mean minus 2 standard deviations* and the *mean plus 2 standard deviations*. In the activation score example, the mean is 53.0 and the standard deviation is 11.77; therefore, at least 75% lie between 53.0 ± 2(11.77), or between 29.50 and 76.57. In this example, all of the 18 observations fall between these limits.

2. If the distribution of observations is **bell-shaped,** then even more can be said about the percentage of observations that lay between the mean and ±2 standard deviations. For a bell-shaped distribution, approximately:

67% of the observations lie between the mean ±1 standard deviation.

95% of the observations lie between the mean ±2 standard deviations.

99.7% of the observations lie between the mean ±3 standard deviations.

The standard deviation, along with the mean, can be helpful in determining skewness when only summary statistics are given: if the mean minus 2 SD contains zero (i.e., the mean is smaller than 2 SD), the observations are probably skewed.

Find the range and standard deviation of activation score for all of the patients in the Bos-Touwen and colleagues' study (2015). Repeat for patients with and without CRD. Are the distributions of activation score similar in these two groups of patients?

The Coefficient of Variation: The coefficient of variation (*CV*) is a useful measure of *relative* spread in data and is used frequently in the biologic sciences. For example, suppose Bos-Touwen and her colleagues (2015) wanted to compare the variability in activation score with the variability in BMI in the patients in their study. The mean and the standard deviation of activation score in the total sample are 51.10 and 10.80, respectively; for BMI, they are 27.55 and 4.58, respectively. A comparison of the standard deviations makes no sense because activation score and BMI are measured on much different scales. The coefficient of variation adjusts the scales so that a sensible comparison can be made.

The coefficient of variation is defined as the standard deviation divided by the mean times 100%. It produces a measure of relative variation—variation that is relative to the size of the mean. The formula for the **coefficient of variation** is

$$CV = \frac{SD}{\bar{X}}(100\%)$$

From this formula, the *CV* for activation score is (10.80/54.10)(100%) = 20.0%, and the *CV* for BMI is (4.58/27.55)(100%) = 16.6%. We can, therefore, conclude that the *relative* variation in activation score is greater than the variation in BMI. A frequent application of the coefficient of variation in the health field is in laboratory testing and quality control procedures.

Find the coefficient of variation for activation score for patients who did and did not have CRD in the Bos-Touwen and colleagues' study.

Percentiles: A **percentile** is the percentage of a distribution that is equal to or below a particular number. For example, consider the standard physical growth chart for girls from birth to 36 months old given in Figure 3–2. For girls 21 months of age, the 95th percentile of weight is 12 kg, as noted by the arrow in the chart. This percentile means that among 21-month-old girls, 95% weigh 12 kg or less and only 5% weigh more than 12 kg. The 50th percentile is, of course, the same value as the median; for 21-month-old girls, the median or 50th percentile weight is approximately 10.6 kg.

Percentiles are often used to compare an individual value with a norm. They are extensively used to develop and interpret physical growth charts and measurements of ability and intelligence. They also determine normal ranges of laboratory values; the "normal limits" of many laboratory values are set by the 2.5th and 97.5th percentiles, so that the normal limits contain the central 95% of the distribution.

Interquartile Range: A measure of variation that makes use of percentiles is the **interquartile range,** defined as the difference between the 25th and 75th percentiles, also called the **first** and **third quartiles,** respectively. The interquartile range contains the central 50% of observations. For example, the interquartile range of weights of girls who are 9 months of age (see Figure 3–2) is the difference between 7.5 kg (the 75th percentile) and 6.5 kg (the 25th percentile); that is, 50% of infant girls weigh between 6.5 kg and 7.5 kg at 9 months of age.

Using Different Measures of Dispersion: The following guidelines are useful in deciding which measure of dispersion is most appropriate for a given set of data.

1. The standard deviation is used when the mean is used (i.e., with symmetric numerical data).
2. Percentiles and the interquartile range are used in two situations:
   a. When the median is used (i.e., with ordinal data or with skewed numerical data).
   b. When the mean is used but the objective is to compare individual observations with a set of norms.
3. The interquartile range is used to describe the central 50% of a distribution, regardless of its shape.

4. The range is used with numerical data when the purpose is to emphasize extreme values.
5. The coefficient of variation is used when the intent is to compare distributions measured on different scales.

DISPLAYING NUMERICAL DATA IN TABLES & GRAPHS

We all know the saying, "A picture is worth 1,000 words," and researchers in the health field certainly make frequent use of graphic and pictorial displays of data. Numerical data may be presented in a variety of ways, and the dataset associated with Presenting Problem 1 regarding patient self-management will be used to demonstrate them.

Stem-and-Leaf Plots

Stem-and-leaf plots are graphs developed in 1977 by Tukey, a statistician interested in meaningful ways to communicate by visual display. They provide a convenient means of tallying the observations and can be used as a direct display of data or as a preliminary step in constructing a frequency table. The data reporting the age of the patients in the patient self-management study will be used to demonstrate a stem-and-leaf plot.

The first step in organizing data for a stem-and-leaf plot is to decide on the number of subdivisions, called classes or intervals (it should generally be between 6 and 14; more details on this decision are given in the following section). Initially, we categorize observations by 5s, from 50 to 55, 56 to 60, 61 to 65, and so on. The scores from the sample of 18 patients displayed in Table 3–1 will be used to demonstrate the details in constructing the plot.

To form a **stem-and-leaf plot,** draw a vertical line, and place the first digits of each class—called the stem—on the left side of the line, as in Table 3–4. The numbers on the right side of the vertical line represent the second digit of each observation; they are the leaves. The steps in building a stem-and-leaf plot are as follows:

1. Take the score of the first person, 57, and write the second digit, 7, or leaf, on the *right* side of the vertical line, opposite the first digit, or stem, corresponding to 56 to 60.
2. For the second person, write the 6 (leaf) on the right side of the vertical line opposite 76 to 80 (stem).
3. For the third person, write the 4 (leaf) opposite 61 to 65 (stem).

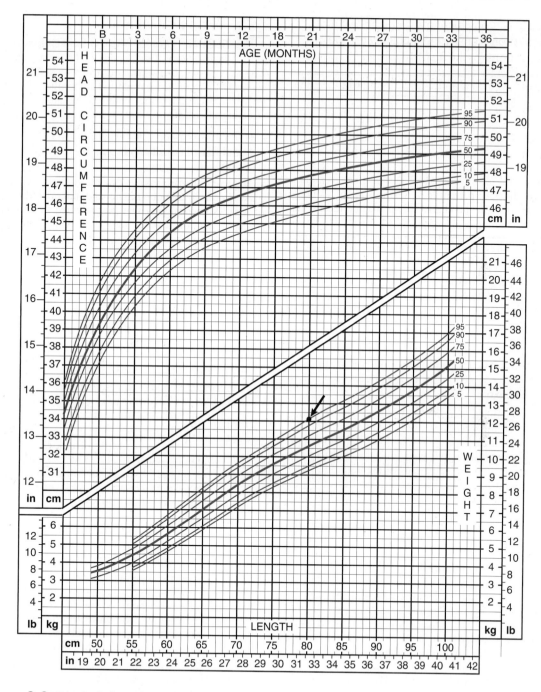

Figure 3–2. Standard physical growth chart. (Reproduced with permission from National Center for Health Statistics in collaboration with National Center for Chronic Disease Prevention and Health Promotion (2000). http:/www.cdc.gov/growthcharts)

Table 3–4. Constructing a stem-and-leaf plot of activation scores using 5-point categories: Observations for the first 10 subjects.

Stem	Leaves
51 to 55	2
56 to 60	6 7 7
61 to 65	1 2 4 4
66 to 70	5 6 8 9
71 to 75	
76 to 80	6 9
81 to 85	0 2 4
86 to 90	
91 to 95	2

Data from Bos-Touwen I, Schuurmans M, Monninkhof EM, et al: Patient and disease characteristics associated with activation for self-management in patients with diabetes, chronic obstructive pulmonary disease, chronic heart failure and chronic renal disease: a cross-sectional survey study, PLoS One. 2015 May 7;10(5):e0126400.

4. For the fourth person, write the 5 (leaf) opposite 61 to 65 (stem) next to the previous score of 3; and so on.

The complete stem-and-leaf plot for the activation score of all the subjects is given in Table 3–5. The plot both provides a tally of observations and shows how the ages are distributed. First, only the first digit of the stem is displayed. One can tell the minimum value of the stem from the first leaf displayed in each row. Note that the leaves for stems 5 through 8 end with a "+ ###," which indicates that there was not sufficient space to show all of the leaves. Stem-and-leaf plots work best with a smaller sample that is available in this study. Although all of the leaves are not displayed, the distribution appears to be bimodal.

The choice of class widths of 5 points is reasonable, although we usually prefer to avoid having many empty classes at the high end of the scale. It is generally preferred to have equal class widths and to avoid open-ended intervals, such as 30 or higher, although some might choose to combine the higher classes in the final plot.

Usually, the leaves are reordered from lowest to highest within each class. After the reordering, it is easy to locate the median of the distribution by simply counting in from either end.

Use the data file and R to generate stem-and-leaf plots with the data on activation score separately for patients who did and did not have CRD in the Bos-Touwen and colleagues' study (2015).

Frequency Tables

Scientific journals often present information in frequency distributions or frequency tables. The scale of the observations must first be divided into classes, as in stem-and-leaf plots. The number of observations in each class is then counted. The steps for constructing a frequency table are as follows:

1. Identify the largest and smallest observations.
2. Subtract the smallest observation from the largest to obtain the **range.**
3. Determine the number of classes. Common sense is usually adequate for making this decision, but the following guidelines may be helpful.
   a. Between 6 and 14 classes is generally adequate to provide enough information without being overly detailed.
   b. The number of classes should be large enough to demonstrate the shape of the distribution but not so many that minor fluctuations are noticeable.
4. One approach is to divide the range of observations by the number of classes to obtain the width of the classes. For some applications, deciding on the class width first may make more sense; then use the class width to determine the number of classes. The following are some guidelines for determining class width.
   a. **Class limits** (beginning and ending numbers) must not overlap. For example, they must be stated as "40 to 49" or "40 up to 50," not as "40 to 50" or "50 to 60." Otherwise, we cannot tell the class to which an observation of 50 belongs.
   b. If possible, class widths should be equal. Unequal class widths present graphing problems and should be used only when large gaps occur in the data.
   c. If possible, open-ended classes at the upper or lower end of the range should be avoided because they do not accurately communicate the range of the observations. We used open-ended classes in Table 3–2 when we had the categories of 35 or less and 80 or higher.
   d. If possible, class limits should be chosen so that most of the observations in the class are closer to the midpoint of the class than to either end of the class. Doing so results in a better estimate of the raw data mean when the weighted mean is calculated from a frequency table (see the section titled, "The Mean" and Exercise 3).

Table 3–5. Stem-and-leaf plot of activation scores using 5-point categories.

```
> stem(activation_score)

  The decimal point is 1 digit(s) to the right of the |

   2 | 4
   2 |
   3 | 0124
   3 | 55555566666666667777777777777999999999999999999999999999
   4 | 000000000000000000000000000000222222222222222222222222222222222222222+68
   4 | 5555555555555555555555555555555555555555555555555555555555555555555555+212
   5 | 333333333333333333333333333333333333333333333333333333333333333333+50
   5 | 66666666666666666666666666666666666666666666666666666666666666666+111
   6 | 0000000000000000000000000000000000000000000000000000000000000000000+71
   6 | 6666666666666666666666666666666666666666669999999999999999999999999
   7 | 11111111111111111111111111111111113333333333333333333
   7 | 555555555555555555555555558888888888888888888888
   8 | 000033333333
   8 | 6666
   9 | 2222222

> |
```

Data from Bos-Touwen I, Schuurmans M, Monninkhof EM, et al: Patient and disease characteristics associated with activation for self-management in patients with diabetes, chronic obstructive pulmonary disease, chronic heart failure and chronic renal disease: a cross-sectional survey study, PLoS One. 2015 May 7;10(5):e0126400.

5. Tally the number of observations in each class. If you are constructing a stem-and-leaf plot, the actual value of the observation is noted. If you are constructing a frequency table, you need use only the number of observations that fall within the class.

Computer programs generally list each value, along with its frequency. Users of the programs must designate the class limits if they want to form frequency tables for values in specific intervals, such as in Table 3–2, by recoding the original observations.

Some tables present only frequencies (number of patients or subjects); others present percentages as well. **Percentages** are found by dividing the number of observations in a given class, n_i, by the total number of observations, n, and then multiplying by 100. For example, for the activation score class from 40 to 45 in Table 3–2, the percentage is

$$\frac{n_i}{n} \times 100 = \frac{148}{1154} \text{ or } 12.82\%$$

For some applications, cumulative frequencies, or percentages, are desirable. The **cumulative frequency** is the percentage of observations for a given value plus that for all lower values. The cumulative value in the last column of Table 3–2, for instance, shows that almost 90% of patients had an activation score less than 70. Table 3–6 is a frequency table that displays the scores for male and female patients. The methodology for producing Table 3–6 is the same as Table 3–2, but the data points are segmented by gender prior to creating the table.

Histograms, Box Plots, & Frequency Polygons

Graphs are used extensively in medicine—in journals, in presentations at professional meetings, and in advertising literature. Graphic devices especially useful in medicine are histograms, box plots, error plots, line graphs, and scatterplots.

Histograms: A histogram of the age in the study of self-management is shown in Figure 3–3. **Histograms** usually present the measure of interest along the X-axis and the number or percentage of observations along the Y-axis. Whether numbers or percentages are used depends on the purpose of the histogram. For example, percentages are needed when two histograms based on different numbers of subjects are compared.

Note that the area of each bar is in proportion to the percentage of observations in that interval; for example, the 199 observations in the range between 65 and 69 account for 199/1154, or 17.2%, of the area covered by this histogram. A histogram therefore communicates information about *area*, one reason the width of classes

Table 3–6. Frequency table for activation scores.

Category	Count	Cumulative Count	Percent	Cumulative Percent
		A. Activation Score for Male Patients		
35 or less	7	7	1.01%	1.01%
35 up to 40	24	31	3.46%	4.47%
40 up to 45	88	119	12.68%	17.15%
45 up to 50	176	295	25.36%	42.51%
50 up to 55	76	371	10.95%	53.46%
55 up to 60	115	486	16.57%	70.03%
60 up to 65	92	578	13.26%	83.29%
65 up to 70	46	624	6.63%	89.91%
70 up to 75	25	649	3.60%	93.52%
75 up to 80	29	678	4.18%	97.69%
80 or higher	16	694	2.31%	100.00%
		B. Activation Score for Female Patients		
35 or less	4	4	0.87%	0.87%
35 up to 40	26	30	5.68%	6.55%
40 up to 45	59	89	12.88%	19.43%
45 up to 50	115	204	25.11%	44.54%
50 up to 55	54	258	11.79%	56.33%
55 up to 60	76	334	16.59%	72.93%
60 up to 65	59	393	12.88%	85.81%
65 up to 70	19	412	4.15%	89.96%
70 up to 75	25	437	5.46%	95.41%
75 up to 80	14	451	3.06%	98.47%
80 or higher	7	458	1.53%	100.00%

Data from Bos-Touwen I, Schuurmans M, Monninkhof EM, et al: Patient and disease characteristics associated with activation for self-management in patients with diabetes, chronic obstructive pulmonary disease, chronic heart failure and chronic renal disease: a cross-sectional survey study, PLoS One. 2015 May 7;10(5):e0126400.

should be equal; otherwise the heights of columns in the histogram must be appropriately modified to maintain the correct area. For example, in Figure 3–3, if the lowest class were 10 score points wide (from 25 to 35) and all other classes remained 5 score points wide, 4 observations would fall in the interval. The height of the column for that interval should then be only 2 units (instead of 4 units) to compensate for its doubled width.

Box Plots: A **box plot,** sometimes called a **box-and-whisker plot** by Tukey (1977), is another way to display information when the objective is to illustrate certain locations in the distribution. The median age is 70, the 75th percentile is 78, and the 25th percentile is 63.

A box plot of the age of the subjects is given in Figure 3–4. A box is drawn with the top at the third quartile and the bottom at the first quartile; quartiles are sometimes referred to as *hinges* in box plots. The length of the box is a visual representation of the interquartile range, representing the middle 50% of the data. The width of the box is chosen to be pleasing esthetically. The location of the midpoint or median of the distribution is indicated with a horizontal line in the box. Finally, straight lines, or *whiskers,* extend 1.5 times the interquartile range above and below the 75th and 25th percentiles. Any values above or below the whiskers are called outliers.

Box plots communicate a great deal of information; for example, we can easily see from Figure 3–4 that the subject ages range from about 30 to about 90 (actually, from 28 to 92). Half of the score changes were between about 65 and 80, and the median is a little larger than 70. There are eight outlying values.

Use the data file to generate box plots for age separately for patients with and without CRD in

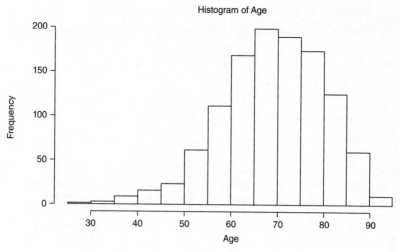

Figure 3–3. **Histogram of patient age.** (Data from Bos-Touwen I, Schuurmans M, Monninkhof EM, et al: Patient and disease characteristics associated with activation for self-management in patients with diabetes, chronic obstructive pulmonary disease, chronic heart failure and chronic renal disease: a cross-sectional survey study, PLoS One. 2015 May 7;10(5):e0126400.)

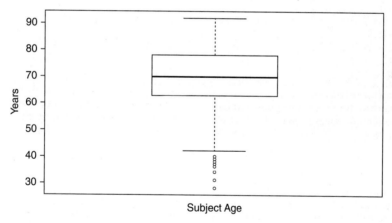

Figure 3–4. **Box plot of subject age.** (Data from Bos-Touwen I, Schuurmans M, Monninkhof EM, et al: Patient and disease characteristics associated with activation for self-management in patients with diabetes, chronic obstructive pulmonary disease, chronic heart failure and chronic renal disease: a cross-sectional survey study, PLoS One. 2015 May 7;10(5):e0126400.)

the Bos-Touwen and colleagues' study (2015). Do these graphs enhance your understanding of the distributions?

Frequency Polygons: Frequency polygons are line graphs similar to histograms and are especially useful when comparing two distributions on the same graph. As a first step in constructing a frequency polygon, a stem-and-leaf plot or frequency table is generated. Table 3–6 contains the frequencies activation score for male and female subjects.

Figure 3–5 is a histogram based on the frequencies for patients who had a pulmonary embolism (PE) with a frequency polygon superimposed on it. It demonstrates that frequency polygons are constructed by connecting the midpoints of the columns of a histogram. Therefore, the same guidelines hold for constructing frequency polygons as for constructing frequency tables

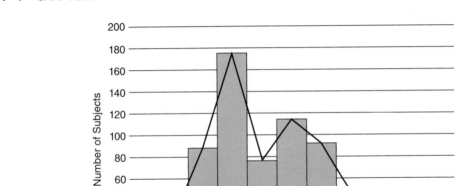

Figure 3–5. Frequency polygon of activation score for patients with a pulmonary embolism. (Data from Bos-Touwen I, Schuurmans M, Monninkhof EM, et al: Patient and disease characteristics associated with activation for self-management in patients with diabetes, chronic obstructive pulmonary disease, chronic heart failure and chronic renal disease: a cross-sectional survey study, PLoS One. 2015 May 7;10(5):e0126400.)

and histograms. Note that the line extends from the midpoint of the first and last columns to the X-axis in order to close up both ends of the distribution and indicate zero frequency of any values beyond the extremes. Because frequency polygons are based on a histogram, they also portray area.

Graphs Comparing Two or More Groups: Merely looking at the numbers in Table 3–6 is insufficient for deciding if the distributions of activation score are similar for male and female subjects. Several methods are useful for comparing distributions.

Box plots are very effective when there is more than one group and are shown for activation score among male and female patients in Figure 3–6. The distributions of the activation score are similar, although more variability exists in female subjects, and the median score is the same for both genders. Does a difference exist between the two groups? We will have to wait until Chapter 6 to learn the answer.

Percentage polygons are also useful for comparing two frequency distributions. Percentage polygons for activation score in both male and female subjects are illustrated in Figure 3–7. Frequencies must be converted to percentages when the groups being compared have unequal numbers of observations, and this

conversion has been made for Figure 3–7. The distribution of activation score does not appear to be very different for the two patient groups; most of the area in one polygon is overlapped by that in the other. Thus, the visual message of box plots and frequency polygons is consistent.

Another type of graph often used in the medical literature is an error bar plot. Figure 3–8 contains error bars for male and female subjects. The circle designates the mean, and the bars illustrate the standard deviation, although some authors use the mean and standard error (a value smaller than the standard deviation, discussed in Chapter 4). We recommend using standard deviations and discuss this issue further in Chapter 4. The error bars indicate the similarity of the distributions, just as the percentage polygons and the box plots do.

Look at Figures 3–6, 3–7, and 3–8 and decide which one you think provides the most useful information.

SUMMARIZING NOMINAL & ORDINAL DATA WITH NUMBERS

When observations are measured on a **nominal,** or **categorical,** scale, the methods just discussed are not appropriate. Characteristics measured on a nominal scale do not have numerical values but are counts

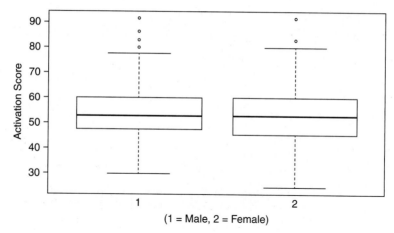

Figure 3–6. Box plot of activation score for male and female subjects. (Data from Bos-Touwen I, Schuurmans M, Monninkhof EM, et al: Patient and disease characteristics associated with activation for self-management in patients with diabetes, chronic obstructive pulmonary disease, chronic heart failure and chronic renal disease: a cross-sectional survey study, PLoS One. 2015 May 7;10(5):e0126400.)

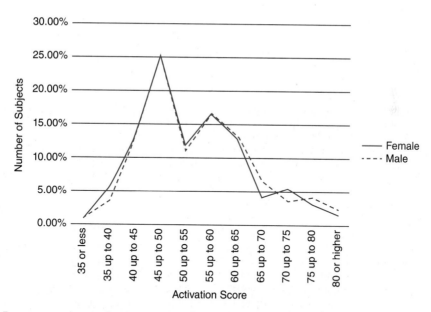

Figure 3–7. Frequency polygon of activation score for male and female patients. (Data from Bos-Touwen I, Schuurmans M, Monninkhof EM, et al: Patient and disease characteristics associated with activation for self-management in patients with diabetes, chronic obstructive pulmonary disease, chronic heart failure and chronic renal disease: a cross-sectional survey study, PLoS One. 2015 May 7;10(5):e0126400.)

or frequencies of occurrence. The study on influenza symptoms included a number of symptoms experienced by subjects that may be related to influenza. A number of the variables in the study, including symptoms such as fever, coughing, and so on, are **dichotomous,** or **binary,** meaning that only two categories are possible. In this section, we examine measures that can be used with such observations.

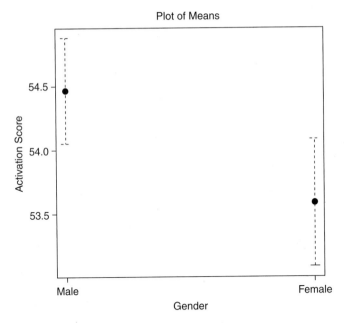

Figure 3–8. Error bar charts of activation score for male and female patients. (Data from Bos-Touwen I, Schuurmans M, Monninkhof EM, et al: Patient and disease characteristics associated with activation for self-management in patients with diabetes, chronic obstructive pulmonary disease, chronic heart failure and chronic renal disease: a cross-sectional survey study, PLoS One. 2015 May 7;10(5):e0126400.)

Ways to Describe Nominal Data

Nominal data can be summarized using several methods: proportions, percentages, ratios, and rates. To illustrate these measures, we will use the numbers of patients who were diagnosed with influenza based on whether or not they received a flu vaccine in the last 12 months; the data are given in Table 3–7.

Proportions and Percentages: A proportion is the number, *a*, of observations with a given characteristic (such as those diagnosed with influenza) divided by the total number of observations, *a* + *b*, in a given group (such as those who received a flu vaccine). That is,

$$\text{Proportion} = \frac{a}{a+b}$$

A proportion is always defined as a *part* divided by the *whole* and is useful for ordinal and numerical data as well as nominal data, especially when the observations have been placed in a frequency table. In the influenza study, the proportion of patients receiving the flu vaccine that were ultimately diagnosed with the flu is 210/959 = 0.219, and the proportion without a vaccine that were diagnosed with the flu is 1283/3610 = 0.355.

A **percentage** is simply the proportion multiplied by 100%.

Ratios and Rates: A **ratio** is the number of observations in a group with a given characteristic divided by the number of observations without the given characteristic:

$$\text{Ratio} = \frac{a}{b}$$

A ratio is always defined as a *part* divided by another *part*. For example, among patients who were vaccinated, the ratio of those who were diagnosed with the flu and those that were not is 210/749 = 0.280. Other familiar ratios in medicine include ratios of the three components of cholesterol (HDL, LDL, triglycerides), such as the LDL/HDL ratio.

Rates are similar to proportions except that a multiplier (e.g., 1,000, 10,000, or 100,000) is used, and they are computed over a specified period of time. The multiplier is called the *base,* and the formula is

$$\text{Rate} = \frac{a}{a+b} \times \text{Base}$$

Table 3–7. Influenza diagnosis by whether or not the patient received a flu vaccine in the last 12 months.

	Influenza Diagnosis		
	Yes	No	Total
Influenza Vaccine			
Yes	210	749	959
No	1283	2327	3610

Data from Anderson KB, Simasathien S, Watanaveeradej V, et al: Clinical and laboratory predictors of influenza infection among individuals with influenza-like illness presenting to an urban Thai hospital over a five-year period, PLoS One. 2018 Mar 7;13(3): e0193050.

For example, if a study lasted exactly 1 year and the proportion of patients with a given condition was 0.002, the rate *per 10,000 patients* would be (0.002) × (10,000), or 20 per 10,000 patients per year.

Vital Statistics Rates

Rates are very important in epidemiology and evidence-based medicine; they are the basis of the calculation of vital statistics, which describe the health status of populations. Some of the most commonly used rates are briefly defined in the following sections.

Mortality Rates: Mortality rates provide a standard way to compare numbers of deaths occurring in different populations, deaths due to different diseases in the same population, or deaths at different periods of time. The numerator in a mortality rate is the number of people who died during a given period of time, and the denominator is the number of people who were at risk of dying during the same period. Because the denominator is often difficult to obtain, the number of people alive in the population halfway through the time period is frequently used as an estimate. Table 3–8 gives death data from *Vital Statistics of the United States.*

A crude rate is a rate computed over all individuals in a given population. For example, the crude annual mortality rate in the entire population from Table 3–8 is 849.3 per 100,000 in 2016. The **sex-specific mortality rate** for males is 880.2 during that same year, and for females it is 819.3 per 100,000. Comparing the sex-specific mortality rates across the years given in Table 3–8, the mortality rate appears to have increased for women. Does this make sense, or could there be another explanation? Consider that a larger number of older women may have been living in 2016 than in previous years. This hypothesis can be examined by adjusting the mortality rates for the age of people at risk. When age-adjusted rates are examined in Table 3–8, we see that the rates have been declining as we would expect. We talk more about adjusting rates in the section of that title.

Cause-specific mortality rates measure deaths in a population from a specific disease or adverse event. Comparing cause-specific mortality rates over a period of time helps epidemiologists to determine possible predisposing factors in the development of disease as well as to make projections about future trends.

Other commonly used mortality rates are infant mortality rate and case fatality rate. The infant mortality rate, sometimes used as an indicator of the level of general health care in a population, is the number of infants who die before 1 year of age per 1,000 live births. The case fatality rate is the number of deaths from a specific disease occurring in a given period divided by the number of individuals with the specified disease during the same period.

Morbidity Rates: Morbidity rates are similar to mortality rates, but many epidemiologists think they provide a more direct measure of health status in a population. The **morbidity rate** is the number of individuals who develop a disease in a given period of time divided by the number of people in the population at risk.

Prevalence and incidence are two important measures frequently used in medicine and epidemiology. **Prevalence** is defined as the number of individuals with a given disease at a given point in time divided by the population at risk for that disease at that time. **Incidence** is defined as the number of new cases that have occurred during a given interval of time divided by the population at risk at the beginning of the time interval. (Because prevalence does not involve a period of time, it is actually a proportion, but is often mistakenly termed a rate.) The term "incidence" is sometimes used erroneously when the term "prevalence" is meant. One way to distinguish between them is to look for units: An incidence rate should always be expressed in terms of a unit of time.

We can draw an analogy between prevalence and incidence and two of the study designs discussed in Chapter 2. Prevalence is like a snapshot in time, as is a cross-sectional study. In fact, some cross-sectional studies are called prevalence studies by epidemiologists. Incidence, on the other hand, requires a period of time to transpire, similar to cohort studies. Recall that cohort studies begin at a given time and continue to examine outcomes over the specified length of the study.

Epidemiologists use prevalence and incidence rates to evaluate disease patterns and make future projections. For example, diabetes mellitus has an increasing

Table 3–8. Number of deaths, death rates, and age-adjusted death rates, by race and sex: United States 2010–2016.[a]

	All			Non-Hispanic White			Non-Hispanic Black		
Year	All	Male	Female	All	Male	Female	All	Male	Female
Number of Deaths in the United States: 2010–2016									
2016	2,744,248	1,400,232	1,344,016	2,133,463	1,077,362	1,056,101	326,810	168,750	158,060
2015	2,712,630	1,373,404	1,339,226	2,123,631	1,063,705	1,059,926	315,254	161,850	153,404
2014	2,626,418	1,328,241	1,298,177	2,066,949	1,035,345	1,031,604	303,844	154,836	149,008
2013	2,596,993	1,306,034	1,290,959	2,052,660	1,021,135	1,031,525	299,227	152,661	146,566
2012	2,543,279	1,273,722	1,269,557	2,016,896	998,832	1,018,064	291,179	148,344	142,835
2011	2,515,458	1,254,978	1,260,480	2,006,319	989,835	1,016,484	286,797	145,052	141,745
2010	2,468,435	1,232,432	1,236,003	1,969,916	971,604	998,312	283,438	143,824	139,614
Death Rates in the United States per 100,000: 2010–2016									
2016	849.3	880.2	819.3	1059.7	1085.6	1034.6	775.5	836.2	719.7
2015	844.0	868.0	820.7	1055.3	1072.5	1038.5	754.6	809.4	704.3
2014	823.7	846.4	801.7	1028.1	1045.4	1011.3	735.4	783.3	691.4
2013	821.5	839.1	804.4	1021.6	1032.1	1011.5	733.4	782.5	688.4
2012	810.2	824.5	796.4	1004.9	1011.2	998.8	720.9	768.5	677.3
2011	807.3	818.7	796.3	1001.0	1004.1	998.1	718.0	760.4	679.2
2010	799.5	812.0	787.4	984.3	987.5	981.2	718.7	764.5	676.9
Age-Adjusted Death Rates in the United States per 100,000: 2010–2016									
2016	728.8	861.0	617.5	749.0	879.5	637.2	882.8	1081.2	734.1
2015	733.1	863.2	624.2	753.2	881.3	644.1	876.1	1070.1	731.0
2014	724.6	855.1	616.7	742.8	872.3	633.8	870.7	1060.3	731.2
2013	731.9	863.6	623.5	747.1	876.8	638.4	885.2	1083.3	740.6
2012	732.8	865.1	624.7	745.8	876.2	637.6	887.1	1086.4	742.1
2011	741.3	875.3	632.4	754.3	887.2	644.6	901.6	1098.3	759.8
2010	747.0	887.1	634.9	755.0	892.5	643.3	920.4	1131.7	770.8

[a]Crude rates on an annual basis per 100,000 population in specified group; age-adjusted rates per 100,000 U.S. standard million population. Rates are based on populations enumerated as of April 1 for census years and estimated as of July 1 for all other years. Excludes deaths of nonresidents of the United States.

Data from Xu JQ, Murphy SL, Kochanek KD, et al: Deaths: Final data for 2016. National Vital Statistics Reports; vol 67 no 5. Hyattsville, MD: National Center for Health Statistics. 2018.

Table 3–9. Infant mortality rate adjustment: Direct method.

	Developed Country				Developing Country			
	Infants Born		Deaths		Infants Born		Deaths	
Birthweight	N (in 1,000s)	%	No.	Rate	N (in 1,000s)	%	No.	Rate
<1,500 g	20	10	870	43.5	30	21	1,860	62.0
1,500–2,499 g	30	15	480	16.0	45	32	900	20.0
≥2,500 g	150	75	1,050	7.0	65	47	585	9.0
Total	200		2,400	12.0	140		3,345	23.9

prevalence even though the annual incidence rate of approximately 230 cases per 100,000 has remained relatively stable over the past several years. The reason for the difference is that once this disease occurs, an individual continues to have diabetes for the remainder of their life; but advances in care of diabetic patients have led to greater longevity for these patients. In contrast, for diseases with a short duration (e.g., influenza) or with an early mortality (e.g., pancreatic cancer), the incidence rate is generally larger than the prevalence.

⑯ Adjusting Rates

We can use crude rates to make comparisons between two different populations only if the populations are similar in all characteristics that might affect the rate. For example, if the populations are different or **confounded** by factors such as age, gender, or race, then age-, gender-, or race-specific rates must be used, or the crude rates must be adjusted; otherwise, comparisons will not be valid.

Rates in medicine are commonly adjusted for age. Often, two populations of interest have different age distributions; yet many characteristics studied in medicine are affected by age, becoming either more or less frequent as individuals grow older. If the two populations are to be compared, the rates must be adjusted to reflect what they would be had their age distributions been similar.

Direct Method of Adjusting Rates: As an illustration, suppose a researcher compares the infant mortality rates from a developed country with those from a developing country and concludes that the mortality rate in the developing country is almost twice as high as the rate in the developed country. Is this conclusion misleading; are confounding factors affecting infant mortality that might contribute to different distributions in the two countries? A relationship between birthweight and mortality certainly exists, and in this example, a valid comparison of mortality rates requires that the distribution of birthweight be similar in the two countries. Hypothetical data are given in Table 3–9.

The crude infant mortality rate for the developed country is 12.0 per 1,000 infants; for the developing country, it is 23.9 per 1,000. The specific rates for the developing country are higher in all birthweight categories. However, the two distributions of birthweight are not the same: The percentage of low-birthweight infants (<2,500 g) is more than twice as high in the developing country as in the developed country. Because birthweight of infants and infant mortality are related, we cannot determine how much of the difference in crude mortality rates between the countries is due to differences in weight-specific mortality and how much is due to the developing country's higher proportion of low-birthweight babies. In this case, the mortality rates must be standardized or adjusted so that they are independent of the distribution of birthweight.[†]

Determining an **adjusted rate** is a relatively simple process when information such as that in Table 3–9 is available. For each population, we must know the specific rates. Note that the crude rate in each country is actually a *weighted average* of the specific rates, with the *number of infants* born in each birthweight category used as the *weights*. For example, the crude mortality rate in the developed country is 2,400/200,000 = 0.012, or 12 per 1,000, and is equal to

$$\frac{\sum(\text{Rate} \times N)}{\text{Total } N} = \frac{(43.5 \times 20) + (16.0 \times 30) + (7.0 \times 150)}{20 + 30 + 150}$$

$$= \frac{2400}{200}, \text{ or } 12 \text{ per } 1000$$

Because the goal of adjusting rates is to have them reflect similar distributions, the numbers in each category from one population, called the *reference*

[†]Of course, factors other than birthweight may affect mortality, and it is important to remember that correcting for one factor may not correct for others.

Table 3–10. Infant mortality rate adjustment: Indirect method.

| Birthweight | Number of Infants Born (in 1,000s) | | Specific Death Rates per 1,000 in Standard Population |
	Developed Country	Developing Country	
<1,500	20	30	50.0
1,500–2,499 g	30	45	20.0
≥2,500 g	150	65	10.0
Number of Deaths	2,400	3,345	

population, are used as the weights to form weighted averages for both populations. Which population is chosen as the standard does not matter; in fact, a set of frequencies corresponding to a totally separate reference population may be used. The point is that the same set of numbers must be applied to both populations.

For example, if the numbers of infants born in each birthweight category in the developed country are used as the standard and applied to the specific rates in the developing country, we obtain

$$\text{Adjusted rate} = \frac{\sum \text{Rate} \times N \text{ in standard}}{\text{Total } N \text{ in standard}}$$

$$= \frac{(62.0 \times 20) + (20.0 \times 30) + (9.0 \times 150)}{20 + 30 + 150}$$

$$= \frac{3190}{200}, \text{ or } 15.95 \text{ per } 1000$$

The adjusted mortality rate in the developing country would therefore be 15.95 per 1,000 (rather than 23.9 per 1,000) if the proportions of infant birthweight were distributed as they are in the developed country.

To use this method of adjusting rates, you must know the specific rates for each category in the populations to be adjusted and the frequencies in the reference population for the factor being adjusted. This method is known as the **direct method of rate standardization.**

Indirect Method of Adjusting Rates: Sometimes specific rates are not available in the populations being compared. If the frequencies of the adjusting factor, such as age or birthweight, are known for each population, and any set of specific rates is available (either for one of the populations being compared or for still another population), an indirect method may be used to adjust rates. The indirect method results in the **standardized mortality ratio,** defined as the number of observed deaths divided by the number of expected deaths.

To illustrate, suppose the distribution of birthweight is available for both the developed and the developing countries, but we have specific death rates only for another population, denoted the

Standard Population in Table 3–10. The expected number of deaths is calculated in *each* population by using the specific rates from the standard population. For the developed country, the expected number of deaths is

$$(50.0 \times 20) + (20.0 \times 30) + (10.0 \times 150) = 3100$$

In the developing country, the expected number of deaths is

$$(50.0 \times 30) + (20.0 \times 45) + (10.0 \times 65) = 3050$$

The standard mortality ratio (the observed number of deaths divided by the expected number) for the developed country is $2,400/3,100 = 0.77$. For the developing country, the standard mortality ratio is $3,345/3,050 = 1.10$. If the standard mortality ratio is greater than 1, as in the developing country, the population of interest has a mortality rate greater than that of the standard population. If the standard mortality rate is less than 1, as in the developed country, the mortality rate is less than that of the standard population. Thus, the indirect method allows us to make a relative comparison; in contrast, the direct method allows us to make a direct comparison. If rates for one of the populations of interest are known, these rates may be used.

TABLES & GRAPHS FOR NOMINAL & ORDINAL DATA

We describe some of the more common methods for summarizing nominal and ordinal data in this section. To illustrate how to construct tables for nominal data, consider the observations given in Table 3–11 for the 28 of the patients included in the influenza study in Presenting Problem 3. The simplest way to present nominal data (or ordinal data, if there are not too many points on the scale) is to list the categories in one column of the table and the **frequency** (counts) or percentage of observations in another column. Table 3–12 shows a simple way of presenting data for the number of patients who did or did not have a sore throat at the time of diagnosis of Flu A/H3.

Table 3–11. Data on 28 patients with Flu A/H3 diagnosis after receiving a flu vaccine in the last 12 months.

ID	Age	Fever	Cough	Sore Throat	Difficulty Breathing
1	70	Yes	Yes	No	No
2	70	Yes	Yes	Yes	Yes
3	75	Yes	Yes	Yes	Yes
4	93	Yes	Yes	Yes	No
5	69	No	Yes	Yes	Yes
6	85	Yes	Yes	No	Yes
7	80	Yes	Yes	Yes	Yes
8	26	Yes	Yes	Yes	No
9	33	Yes	Yes	Yes	No
10	81	Yes	Yes	Yes	No
11	42	Yes	Yes	Yes	Yes
12	74	Yes	Yes	Yes	Yes
13	55	Yes	Yes	No	Yes
14	86	Yes	Yes	No	No
15	71	Yes	Yes	Yes	No
16	89	No	Yes	Yes	Yes
17	81	No	Yes	Yes	Yes
18	82	No	Yes	Yes	Yes
19	82	Yes	Yes	No	Yes
20	71	Yes	Yes	Yes	No
21	32	No	Yes	Yes	No
22	30	Yes	Yes	Yes	Yes
23	29	Yes	Yes	No	No
24	78	Yes	Yes	No	No
25	58	Yes	Yes	No	Yes
26	26	Yes	Yes	No	Yes
27	51	Yes	Yes	Yes	Yes
28	69	Yes	Yes	Yes	No

Data from Anderson KB, Simasathien S, Watanaveeradej V, et al: Clinical and laboratory predictors of influenza infection among individuals with influenza-like illness presenting to an urban Thai hospital over a five-year period, PLoS One. 2018 Mar 7; 13(3):e0193050.

Table 3–12. Table for frequency of sore throat in patients with Flu A/H3 diagnosis after receiving a flu vaccine in the last 12 months.

Sore Throat	Number of Patients
Yes	19
No	9

Data from Anderson KB, Simasathien S, Watanaveeradej V, et al: Clinical and laboratory predictors of influenza infection among individuals with influenza-like illness presenting to an urban Thai hospital over a five-year period, PLoS One. 2018 Mar 7;13(3): e0193050.

When two characteristics on a nominal scale are examined, a common way to display the data is in a **contingency table,** in which observations are classified according to several factors. Suppose we want to know the number of patients that had both a sore throat and difficulty breathing at time of diagnosis. The first step is to list the categories to appear in the table: patients with/without a sore throat and patients with/without difficulty breathing (Table 3–13). Tallies are placed for each patient who meets the criterion. Patient 1 has a tally in the cell "No sore throat with no difficulty breathing"; patient 2 has a tally in the cell "Sore throat and difficulty breathing"; and so on. Tallies for the 28 patients are listed in Table 3–13.

The sum of the tallies in each cell is then used to construct a contingency table such as Table 3–14, which contains cell counts for all 28 patients in the study.

For a graphic display of nominal or ordinal data, bar charts are commonly used. In a **bar chart,** counts or percentages of the characteristic in different categories are shown as bars. The investigators in this example could have used a bar chart to present the number of patients with and without hematuria sore throat, as illustrated in Figure 3–9. The categories of sore throat (yes or no) are placed along the horizontal, or *X*-axis, and the number of patients with and without difficulty breathing along the vertical, or *Y*-axis. Bar charts may also have the categories along the vertical axis and the numbers along the horizontal axis.

Other graphic devices such as pie charts and pictographs are often used in newspapers, magazines, and advertising brochures. They are occasionally used in the health field to display such resource information as the portion of the gross national product devoted to health expenditures or the geographic distribution of primary-care physicians.

Table 3–13. Step 1 in constructing contingency table for patients with and without a sore throat and difficulty breathing.

Category	Tally
Sore throat with difficulty breathing	///////////
Sore throat without difficulty breathing	/////////
No sore throat with difficulty breathing	/////
No sore throat without difficulty breathing	////

Data from Anderson KB, Simasathien S, Watanaveeradej V, et al: Clinical and laboratory predictors of influenza infection among individuals with influenza-like illness presenting to an urban Thai hospital over a five-year period, PLoS One. 2018 Mar 7;13(3): e0193050.

Table 3–14. Contingency table for patients with and without a sore throat and difficulty breathing.

Sore Throat	No Difficulty Breathing	Difficulty Breathing
No	4	5
Yes	8	11

Data from Anderson KB, Simasathien S, Watanaveeradej V, et al: Clinical and laboratory predictors of influenza infection among individuals with influenza-like illness presenting to an urban Thai hospital over a five-year period, PLoS One. 2018 Mar 7;13(3): e0193050.

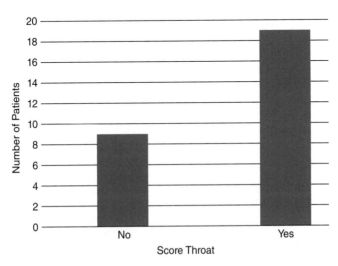

Figure 3–9. Illustration of a bar chart. (Data from Anderson KB, Simasathien S, Watanaveeradej V, et al: Clinical and laboratory predictors of influenza infection among individuals with influenza-like illness presenting to an urban Thai hospital over a five-year period, PLoS One. 2018 Mar 7;13(3):e0193050.)

DESCRIBING RELATIONSHIPS BETWEEN TWO CHARACTERISTICS

Much of the research in medicine concerns the relationship between two or more characteristics. The following discussion focuses on examining the relationship between two variables measured on the same scale when both are numerical, both are ordinal, or both are nominal.

The Relationship Between Two Numerical Characteristics

In Presenting Problem 2, Bos-Touwen and associates (2015) wanted to estimate the relationship between the activation scores and function status (SF-12). The **correlation coefficient** (sometimes called the Pearson product moment correlation coefficient, named for the statistician who defined it) is one measure of the relationship between two numerical characteristics, symbolized by X and Y. Table 3–15 gives the information needed to calculate the correlation between activation scores and SF-12. The formula for the correlation coefficient, symbolized by r, is

$$ r = \frac{\sum (X - \bar{X})(Y - \bar{Y})}{\sqrt{\sum (X - \bar{X})^2 \sum (Y - \bar{Y})^2}} $$

As with the standard deviation, we give the formula and computation for illustration purposes only and, for that reason, use the definitional rather than the computational formula. Using the data from Table 3–15, we obtain a correlation of

$$ r = \frac{3749.886}{\sqrt{(2354.1428)(12638.2427)}} $$

$$ = \frac{3749.8866}{5454.5603} = 0.6875 $$

Interpreting Correlation Coefficients

What does a correlation of 0.69 between activation scores and SF12 scores mean? (Correlations are generally reported to two decimal places.) Chapter 8 discusses methods used to tell whether a statistically

Table 3–15. Calculation for correlation coefficient between activation score (X) and SF-12 score (Y) for random sample of patients in Presenting Problem 2.[a]

Patient	X	Y	$(X - \bar{X})$	$(Y - \bar{Y})$	$(X - \bar{X})^2$	$(Y - \bar{Y})^2$	$(X - \bar{X})(Y - \bar{Y})$
1	75.3	90.8	22.2611	40.6713	495.5571	1,654.1543	905.3882
2	56.4	54.6	3.3611	4.4213	11.2971	19.5479	14.8605
3	68.5	86.3	15.4611	36.0880	239.0460	1,302.3411	557.9600
4	60.0	57.5	6.9611	7.3380	48.4571	53.8457	51.0804
5	56.4	70.8	3.3611	20.6713	11.2971	427.3025	69.4785
6	37.3	13.8	(15.7389)	(36.4120)	247.7126	1,325.8364	573.0850
7	52.9	21.3	(0.1389)	(28.9120)	0.0193	835.9059	4.0156
8	70.8	91.7	17.7611	41.5046	315.4571	1,722.6343	737.1683
9	52.9	38.8	(0.1389)	(11.4120)	0.0193	130.2346	1.5850
10	56.4	26.3	3.3611	(23.9120)	11.2971	571.7855	(80.3710)
11	52.9	36.3	(0.1389)	(13.9120)	0.0193	193.5448	1.9322
12	47.4	88.8	(5.6389)	38.5880	31.7971	1,489.0309	(217.5932)
13	60.0	30.4	6.9611	(19.7454)	48.4571	389.8797	(137.4497)
14	34.7	21.3	(18.3389)	(28.9120)	336.3148	835.9059	530.2146
15	38.7	24.2	(14.3389)	(25.9954)	205.6037	675.7593	372.7447
16	45.2	44.2	(7.8389)	(5.9954)	61.4482	35.9445	46.9970
17	36.0	31.3	(17.0389)	(18.9120)	290.3237	357.6651	322.2401
18	52.9	75.0	(0.1389)	24.8380	0.0193	616.9244	(3.4497)
Sum	954.7	902.9	(0.0000)	(0.0000)	2,354.1428	12,638.2427	3,749.8866
Average	53.0	50.2					

[a]Values are reported to four decimal places to minimize round-off error.
Data from Bos-Touwen I, Schuurmans M, Monninkhof EM, et al: Patient and disease characteristics associated with activation for self-management in patients with diabetes, chronic obstructive pulmonary disease, chronic heart failure and chronic renal disease: a cross-sectional survey study, PLoS One. 2015 May 7;10(5):e0126400.

significant relationship exists; for now, we will discuss some characteristics of the correlation coefficient that will help us interpret its numerical value.

The correlation coefficient always ranges from -1 to $+1$, with -1 describing a perfect negative linear (straight-line) relationship and $+1$ describing a perfect positive linear relationship. A correlation of 0 means no linear relationship exists between the two variables.

Sometimes the correlation is squared (r^2) to form a useful statistic called the **coefficient of determination** or **r-squared,** and we recommend this practice. For the activation score data, the coefficient of determination is $(0.69)^2$, or 0.48. This means that 48% of the variability in one of the measures, such as SF12 scores, may be accounted for (or predicted) by knowing the value of the other measure, activation score.

Several other characteristics of the correlation coefficient deserve mention. The value of the correlation coefficient is independent of the particular units used to measure the variables. Suppose two medical students measure the heights and weights of a group of preschool children to determine the correlation between height and weight. They measure the children's height in centimeters and record their weight in kilograms, and they calculate a correlation coefficient equal to 0.70. What would the correlation be if they had used inches and pounds instead? It would, of course, still be 0.70, because the denominator in the formula for the correlation coefficient adjusts for the scale of the units.

The value of the correlation coefficient is markedly influenced by outlying values, just as is the standard deviation. Thus, the correlation does not describe the relationship between two variables well when the distribution of either variable is skewed or contains outlying values. In this situation, a **transformation** of the data that changes the scale of measurement and moderates the effect of outliers (see Chapter 5) or the Spearman correlation can be used.

People first learning about the correlation coefficient often ask, "How large should a correlation be?" The answer depends on the application. For example, when physical characteristics are measured and good measuring devices are available, as in many physical sciences, high correlations are possible. Measurement in the biologic sciences, however, often involves characteristics that are less well defined and measuring devices that are imprecise; in such cases, lower correlations may occur. Colton (1974) gives the following crude rule of thumb for interpreting the size of correlations:

> *Correlations from 0 to 0.25 (or −0.25) indicate little or no relationship; those from 0.25 to 0.50 (or −0.25 to −0.50) indicate a fair degree of relationship; those from 0.50 to 0.75 (or −0.50 to −0.75) a moderate to good relationship; and those greater than 0.75 (or −0.75) a very good to excellent relationship.*

Colton cautions against correlations higher than 0.95 in the biologic sciences because of the inherent variability in most biologic characteristics. When you encounter a high correlation, you should ask whether it is an error or an artifact or, perhaps, the result of combining two populations (illustrated in Chapter 8). An example of an artifact is when the number of pounds patients lose in the first week of a diet program is correlated with the number of pounds they lose during the entire 2-month program.

The correlation coefficient measures only a straight-line relationship; two characteristics may, in fact, have a strong curvilinear relationship, even though the correlation is quite small. Therefore, when you analyze relationships between two characteristics, always plot the data as we do in the section titled, "Graphs for Two Characteristics." A plot will help you detect outliers and skewed distributions.

Finally, "correlation does not imply causation." The statement that one characteristic causes another must be justified on the basis of experimental observations or logical argument, not because of the size of a correlation coefficient.

Use R and find the correlation between activation score and BMI using the Bos-Touwen and colleagues' study (2015). Interpret the correlation using the guidelines just described.

The Relationship Between Two Ordinal Characteristics

The **Spearman rank correlation,** sometimes called Spearman's rho (also named for the statistician who defined it), is frequently used to describe the relationship between two ordinal (or one ordinal and one numerical) characteristics. It is also appropriate to use with numerical observations that are skewed with extreme observations. The calculation of the Spearman rank correlation, symbolized as r_s, involves rank-ordering the values on each of the characteristics from lowest to highest; the ranks are then treated as though they were the actual values themselves. Although the formula is simple when no ties occur in the values, the computation is quite tedious. Because the calculation is available on many computer programs, we postpone its illustration until Chapter 8, where it is discussed in greater detail.

 ## The Relationship Between Two Nominal Characteristics

In studies involving two characteristics, the primary interest may be in whether they are significantly related (discussed in Chapter 6) or the magnitude of the relationship, such as the relationship between a risk factor and occurrence of a given outcome. Two ratios used to estimate such a relationship are the **relative risk** and the **odds ratio,** both often referred to as **risk ratios.** For example, in Presenting Problem 3, the investigators may wish to learn whether receiving a flu vaccine reduces the "risk" that symptomatic patients are later diagnosed with the flu. In the context of this discussion, we introduce some of the important concepts and terms that are increasingly used in the medical and health literature, including the useful notion of the number of patients who need to be treated in order to observe one positive outcome.

Experimental and Control Event Rates: Important concepts in the computation of measures of risk are called the event rates. Using the notation in Table 3–16, we are interested in the event of a disease occurring. The experimental event rate (EER) is the proportion of people with the risk factor who have or develop the disease, or $A/(A + B)$. The control event rate (CER) is the proportion of people without the risk factor who have or develop the disease, or $C/(C + D)$.

The Relative Risk: The relative risk, or risk ratio, of a disease, symbolized by RR, is the ratio of the incidence

Table 3–16. Table arrangement and formulas for several important measures of risk.

	Disease	No Disease	
Risk factor present	A	B	$A + B$
Risk factor absent	C	D	$C + D$
	$A + C$	$B + D$	

Experimental event rate $(EER) = \dfrac{A}{(A + B)}$

Control event rate $(CER) = \dfrac{C}{(C + D)}$

Absolute risk reduction $(ARR) = |\,EER - CER\,|$

Number needed to treat $(NNT) = \dfrac{1}{ARR}$

Relative risk reduction $(RRR) = \dfrac{|EER - CER|}{CER} = ARR/CER$

Relative risk $(RR)\dfrac{EER}{CER} = \dfrac{A/(A + B)}{C/(C + D)}$

Odds ratio $(OR) = \dfrac{[A/(A + C)]/[C/(A + C)]}{[B/(B + D)]/[D/(B + D)]} = \dfrac{A/C}{B/D} = \dfrac{AD}{BC}$

in people with the risk factor (exposed persons) to the incidence in people without the risk factor (nonexposed persons). It can, therefore, be found by dividing the EER by the CER.

Table 3–14 gives data on the number of patients receiving a flu vaccine and whether or not the subject was diagnosed with the flu. In this study, the flu vaccine assumes the role of the risk factor. The EER is the incidence of flu in patients who were vaccinated, or $210/959 = 0.2190$; the CER is the incidence of flu in those who were not vaccinated, or $1{,}283/3{,}610 = 0.3554$. The relative risk of flu diagnosis with a vaccine, compared with flu diagnosis without a vaccine, is therefore

$$RR = \frac{EER}{CER} = \frac{A/(A + B)}{C/(C + D)} = \frac{210/959}{1283/3610}$$

$$= \frac{0.2190}{0.3554} = 0.616$$

Because fewer rate of flu diagnosis for patients with a vaccine is lower than that without, the relative risk is less than 1. If we take the reciprocal and look at the relative risk of having the flu in the group not vaccinated, the relative risk is $1/0.62 = 1.61$. Thus, patients without a flu vaccine were 1.6 times more likely to be diagnosed with the flu than the vaccinated group.

The relative risk is calculated only from a cohort study or a clinical trial in which a group of subjects with the risk factor and a group without it are first identified and then followed through time to determine which persons develop the outcome of interest. In this situation, the investigator determines the number of subjects in each group.

Absolute Risk Reduction: The **absolute risk reduction (ARR)** provides a way to assess the reduction in risk compared with the baseline risk. In the flu study (see Table 3–17), the experimental event rate for flu in the vaccinated group was 0.2190, and the control event rate was 0.3554 in the nonvaccinated group. The ARR is the absolute value of the difference between these two event rates:

$$ARR = |\,0.2190 - 0.3554\,| = |\,-0.1364\,| = 0.1364$$

A good way to interpret these numbers is to think about them in terms of events per 10,000 people. Then the risk of flu is 219 ($0.219 \times 10{,}000$) in a group with the vaccine and 355 ($0.355 \times 10{,}000$) in a group without, and the absolute risk reduction is 1,364 per 10,000 people.

 Number Needed to Treat: An added advantage of interpreting risk data in terms of absolute risk reduction is that its reciprocal, 1/

Table 3–17. Summary of flu diagnosis by vaccine status.

Flu Vaccine	Flu Diagnosis		Grand Total
	Yes	No	
	(A)	(B)	
Yes	210	749	959
	(C)	(D)	
No	1,283	2,327	3,610
Grand Total	1,493	3,076	4,569

Data from Anderson KB, Simasathien S, Watanaveeradej V, et al: Clinical and laboratory predictors of influenza infection among individuals with influenza-like illness presenting to an urban Thai hospital over a five-year period, PLoS One. 2018 Mar 7;13(3): e0193050.

Table 3–18. Summary of Benzodiazepine use and Alzheimer's status.

	Cases [with Alzheimer's disease] ($n = 1,796$)	Controls ($n = 7,184$)	Odds Ratio (95% CI)
Benzodiazepine ever used	894	2,873	1.5 (1.4–1.7)
Benzodiazepine daily doses			
1–90	234	1051	1.1 (0.9–1.3)
91–180	70	257	1.3 (1.0–1.8)
>180	590	1565	1.8 (1.6–2.1)

Data from Billioti de Gage S, Moride Y, Ducruet T, et al: Benzodiazepine use and risk of Alzheimer's disease: case-control study, BMJ. 2014 Sep 9;349:g5205.

ARR, is the **number needed to treat (NNT)** in order to prevent one event. The number of people that need to be treated to avoid one flu case is then 1/0.1364, or 7.3 (about 7 people). This type of information helps clinicians evaluate the relative risks and benefits of a particular treatment. Based on the risks associated with the flu vaccine, do you think it is a good idea to vaccinate 7 people in order to prevent one of them from having the flu?

Absolute Risk Increase and Number Needed to Harm: Some treatments or procedures increase the risk for a serious undesirable side effect or outcome. In this situation, the (absolute value of the) difference between the EER and the CER is termed the **absolute risk increase (ARI).** The CDC (2017) reports the risk of Guillain-Barre' Syndrome (GBS) as 1 to 2 cases per million people increase in risk after a flu vaccine (0.000002 using the higher estimate). This is the ARI for GBS. The reciprocal of the absolute risk increase, 1/ARI, is called the **number needed to harm (NNH).** Based on the CDC estimates, the NNH = 1/ARI = 500,000. Based on the magnitude of this NNH and the NNT of 7 to prevent one flu case, the statistics favor the dissemination of the vaccine.

Relative Risk Reduction: A related concept, the **relative risk reduction (RRR),** is also presented in the literature. This measure gives the amount of risk reduction relative to the baseline risk; that is, the EER minus the CER all divided by the control (baseline) event rate, CER. The RRR in the flu vaccine study is

$$RRR = \frac{|\,EER - CER\,|}{CER}$$

$$= \frac{0.1364}{0.3554} = 0.3838$$

or approximately 38%. The relative risk reduction tells us that, relative to the baseline risk of 355 flu diagnoses in 10,000 people, giving the vaccine reduces the risk by 38%.

Many clinicians feel that the absolute risk reduction is a more valuable index than the relative risk reduction because its reciprocal is the number needed to treat. If a journal article gives only the relative risk reduction, it can (fairly easily) be converted to the absolute risk reduction by multiplying by the control event rate, a value that is almost always given in an article. For instance, 0.3838 × 0.3554 is 0.1364, the same value we calculated earlier for the ARR.

The Odds Ratio: The odds ratio provides a way to look at risk in case–control studies. The study by Billioti de Gage and coworkers (2014) in which the use of benzodiazepine was studied serves as an example for the use of the odds ratio. Summarized data from this study are given in Table 3–18. The **odds ratio (OR)** is the odds that a person with an adverse outcome was at risk divided by the odds that a person without an adverse outcome was at risk. The odds ratio is easy to calculate when the observations are given in a 2 × 2 table. The numbers of subjects with an Alzheimer's disease diagnosis in Table 3–18 are rearranged and given in Table 3–19.

In this study, the odds that a subject with Alzheimer's used benzodiazepine are

$$\frac{894\,/\,1796}{902\,/\,1796} = \frac{894}{902} = 0.9911$$

Table 3–19. Data for odds ratio benzodiazepine ever used.

Benzodiazepine Group	With Alzheimer's	Without Alzheimer's	Total
Used	894	2,873	3,767
Never used	902	4,311	5,213
Total	1,796	7,184	

Data from Billioti de Gage S, Moride Y, Ducruet T, et al: Benzodiazepine use and risk of Alzheimer's disease: case-control study, BMJ. 2014 Sep 9;349:g5205.

and the odds that a subject without Alzheimer's used benzodiazepine are

$$\frac{2873 / 7184}{4311 / 7184} = \frac{2873}{4311} = 0.6664$$

Putting these two odds together to obtain the odds ratio gives

$$\frac{0.9911}{0.6664} = 1.487 \approx 1.5$$

An odds ratio of 1.5 means that a subject in the benzodiazepine group is 1.5 times more likely to develop Alzheimer's disease than a subject with no exposure.

The odds ratio is also called the cross-product ratio because it can be defined as the ratio of the product of the diagonals in a 2 × 2 table:

$$\frac{(894)(4311)}{(2873)(902)} = 1.487$$

In case–control studies, the investigator decides how many subjects with and without the disease will be studied. This is the opposite from cohort studies and clinical trials, in which the investigator decides the number of subjects with and without the risk factor. The odds ratio should, therefore, be used with case–control studies.

GRAPHS FOR TWO CHARACTERISTICS

Most studies in medicine involve more than one characteristic, and graphs displaying the +relationship between two characteristics are common in the literature. No graphs are commonly used for displaying a relationship between two characteristics when both are measured on a nominal scale; the numbers are simply presented in contingency tables. When one of the characteristics is nominal and the other is numerical, the data can be displayed in box plots like the one in Figure 3–6 or error plots, as in Figure 3–8.

Also common in medicine is the use of **bivariate plots** (also called **scatterplots** or scatter diagrams) to illustrate the relationship between two characteristics when both are measured on a numerical scale. In the study by Bos-Touwen and associates (2015), information was collected on the patient activation measure (PAM-13) and as well as the Short Form Health Survey (SF-12). Box 3–1 contains a scatterplot of activation scores and SF12 total scores for the sample of 18 subjects presented in Table 3–15. A scatterplot is constructed by drawing X- and Y-axes; the characteristic hypothesized to explain or predict or the one that occurs first (sometimes called the risk factor) is placed on the X-axis. The characteristic or outcome to be explained or predicted or the one that occurs second is placed on the Y-axis. In applications in which a noncausal relationship is hypothesized, placement for the X- and Y-axes does not matter. Each observation is represented by a small circle; for example, the circle in the lower right in the graph in Box 3–1 represents subject 6, who had an activation score of 37.3 and a SF-12 total score of 13.8. More information on interpreting scatterplots is presented in Chapter 8, but we see here that the data in Box 3–1 suggest the possibility of a positive relationship between the two scores. At this point, we cannot say whether the relationship is significant or one that simply occurs by chance; this topic is covered in Chapter 8.

As a final note, there is a correspondence between the size of the correlation coefficient and a **scatterplot** of the observations. We also included in Box 3–1 the output from Excel giving the correlation coefficient. Recall that a correlation of 0.69 indicates a moderate to good relationship between the two scores. When the correlation is near 0, the shape of the pattern of observations is more or less circular or scattered. As the value of the correlation gets closer to +1 or −1, the shape becomes more elliptical, until, at +1 and −1, the observations fall directly on a straight line. With a correlation of 0.69, we expect a scatter plot of the data to be somewhat oval-shaped, as it is in Box 3–1.

Whether to use tables or graphs is generally based on the purpose of the presentation of the data. Tables give

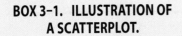

BOX 3–1. ILLUSTRATION OF A SCATTERPLOT.

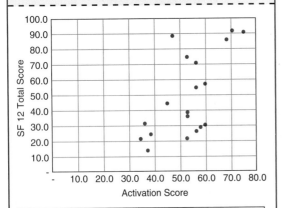

Pearson Correlation		
	Activation Score	**SF 12 Total Score**
Activation Score	1.00	0.69
SF 12 Total Score	0.69	1.00

Data from *Bos-Touwen* I, Schuurmans M, Monninkhof EM, et al: Patient and disease characteristics associated with activation for self-management in patients with diabetes, chronic obstructive pulmonary disease, chronic heart failure and chronic renal disease: a cross-sectional survey study, PLoS One. 2015 May 7;10(5):e0126400.

more detail and can display information about more characteristics, but they take longer to read and synthesize. Graphs present an easy-to-interpret picture of the data and are appropriate when the goal is to illustrate the distribution or frequencies without specific details.

Data Visualization Considerations

Charts and graphs can be generally thought of as data visualizations. The purpose of visualizations is to present the results of a study for publication or presentation in a way that allows the reader or audience to immediately grasp your message. We have reviewed a number of data visualization types in this chapter. In this section, we will consider the aspects of a chart or graph that may make it easier for the user to interpret. Most journals limit the number of figures included in a manuscript, so the selection of the ones with the most impact is critically important in ensuring that your efforts are accepted by the journal and cited by other authors—both important measures of success in the academic and clinical community.

Stephen Few (2018) gives guidance for selection of the proper graph to use for a variety of data types and comparisons. The graph types include scatter plots, line plots, bar charts and box plots. His graph selection matrix may be downloaded from here: http://www.perceptualedge.com/images/Effective_Chart_Design.pdf. In Few's book *Now You See It: Simple Visualization Techniques for Quantitative Analysis* (2009), he presents a number of methods for data presentation. His main message though is to keep the visualizations as simple and clean as possible. Few believes that graphs and charts have one of two primary purposes: communicating relationships between variables or communicating variation. If we keep those two purposes in mind along with his premise of keeping the display simple and clean, the quality of data visualizations can be improved immensely.

In designing data visualizations, authors should consider a number of **pre-attentive attributes** that the reader will experience when viewing the graph or chart. Pre-attentive attributes are processed much faster by the brain when presented. Ware (2013) discusses four pre-attentive visual properties that can enhance the reader's understanding of a graph or chart: color, form, movement, and special positioning. Few (2016) expanding on that concept by further defining form as properties such as length, width, shape, orientation, and angle. He also expands color into the properties of hue, lightness, saturation, and intensity.

These properties can be leveraged to enhance the messaging in data visualizations. Data visualization software tools are becoming more popular and include many functions that allow the user to optimize their charts and graphs. Software such as Tableau, Qlik, and Microsoft's Power Business Intelligence application are excellent examples. Excel also may be used to create effective charts and graphs.

Examples of using pre-attentive attributes to enhance data visualizations include:

1. Highlighting or changing the shape of important points in a scatter plot. Compare Figures 3–10A and B. This is an example of displaying the relationship between variables. Which plot highlights the outlier point better?

2. Ordering of categories in a bar chart. Consider Figures 3–11A and B. This is an example of showing variation. Which chart is easier to interpret if you would like to communicate the distribution of the patients by age group? What if you want to show the top three age groups?

3. Size (length and width) and positioning are both demonstrated in Figure 3–12. This visualization allows the reader to see the relationship between three variables: activation score, age, and SF-12 score. Notice that older patients tend to have lower SF-12 scores (smaller bubbles) and lower activation scores. What other trends can you see in this chart? (Note that the scale in this chart was modified to allow illustration of the technique.)

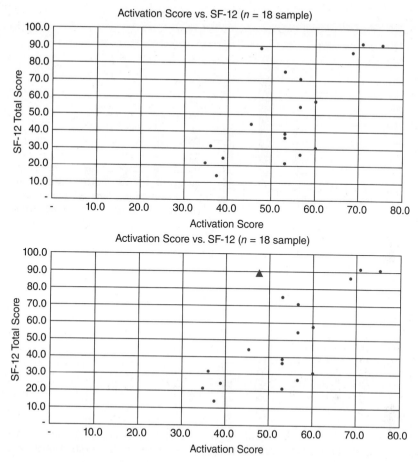

Figure 3–10. Illustration of effect of highlighting points. (Data from Bos-Touwen I, Schuurmans M, Monninkhof EM, et al: Patient and disease characteristics associated with activation for self-management in patients with diabetes, chronic obstructive pulmonary disease, chronic heart failure and chronic renal disease: a cross-sectional survey study, PLoS One. 2015 May 7;10(5):e0126400.)

The format of this text does not allow examples of the utilization of color, but it can be a very effective way to convey a message in chart. For example, gradient colors from dark red to lighter red to light green to dark green can convey a message to desirable to undesirable values. Color charts often require a surcharge in journals and, therefore, should always be used in an intention manner to convey a message.

EXAMPLES OF MISLEADING CHARTS & GRAPHS

The quality of charts and graphs published in the medical literature is higher than that in similar displays in the popular press. The most significant problem with graphs (and tables as well) in medical journal articles is their complexity. Many authors attempt to present too much information in a single display, and it may take the reader a long time to make sense of it.

The purpose of tables and graphs is to present information (often based on large numbers of observations) in a concise way so that observers can comprehend and remember it more easily. Charts, tables, and graphs should be simple and easily understood by the reader, and concise but complete labels and legends should accompany them.

Knowing about common errors helps you correctly interpret information in articles and presentations. We illustrate four errors we have seen with sufficient frequency to warrant their discussion. We use hypothetical examples and do not imply that they necessarily occurred in the Presenting Problems used in this text.

A researcher can make a change appear more or less dramatic by selecting a starting time for a graph, either

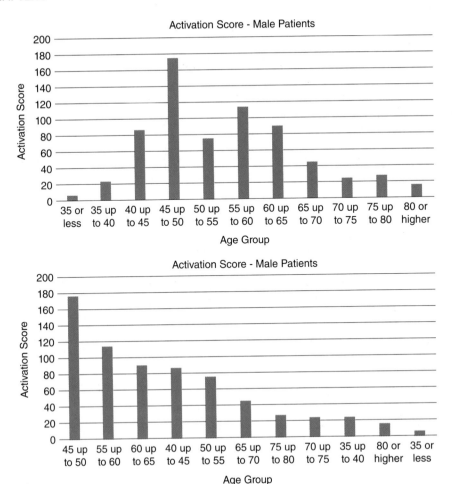

Figure 3–11. Illustration of effect of ordering of categories in a bar chart. (Data from Bos-Touwen I, Schuurmans M, Monninkhof EM, et al: Patient and disease characteristics associated with activation for self-management in patients with diabetes, chronic obstructive pulmonary disease, chronic heart failure and chronic renal disease: a cross-sectional survey study, PLoS One. 2015 May 7;10(5):e0126400.)

before or after the change begins. Figure 3–13A shows the decrease in annual mortality from a disease, beginning in 1960 and continuing with the projected mortality through 2010. The major decrease in mortality from this disease occurred in the 1970s. Although not incorrect, a graph that begins in 1980 (Figure 3–13B) deemphasizes the decrease and implies that the change has been small.

If the values on the *Y*-axis are large, the entire scale cannot be drawn. For example, suppose an investigator wants to illustrate the number of deaths from cancer, beginning in 1960 (when there were 200,000 deaths) to the year 2010 (when 600,000 deaths are projected). Even if the vertical scale is in thousands of deaths, it

must range from 200 to 600. If the *Y*-axis is not interrupted, the implied message is inaccurate; a misunderstanding of the scale makes the change appear larger than it really is. This error, called **suppression of zero,** is common in histograms and line graphs. Figure 3–14A illustrates the effect of suppression of zero on the number of deaths from cancer per year; Figure 3–14B illustrates the correct construction. The error of suppression of zero is more serious on the *Y*-axis than on the *X*-axis, because the scale on the *Y*-axis represents the magnitude of the characteristic of interest. Many researchers today use computer programs to generate their graphics. Some programs make it difficult to control the scale of the *Y*-axis (and the *X*-axis as well).

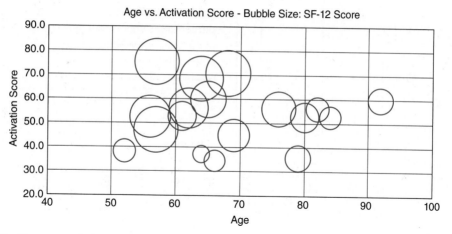

Figure 3–12. Illustration of effect of size (length and width) and positioning in a graph. (Data from Bos-Touwen I, Schuurmans M, Monninkhof EM, et al: Patient and disease characteristics associated with activation for self-management in patients with diabetes, chronic obstructive pulmonary disease, chronic heart failure and chronic renal disease: a cross-sectional survey study, PLoS One. 2015 May 7;10(5):e0126400.)

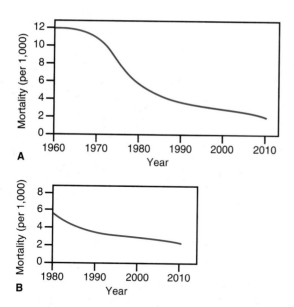

Figure 3–13. Illustration of effect of portraying change at two different times. **A:** Mortality from a disease since 1960. **B:** Mortality from a disease since 1980.

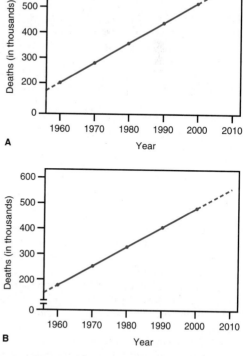

Figure 3–14. Illustration of effect of suppression of zero on Y-axis in graphs showing deaths from cancer. **A:** No break in the line on Y-axis. **B:** Break in the line correctly placed on Y-axis.

As readers, we therefore need to be vigilant and not be unintentionally misled by this practice.

The magnitude of change can also be enhanced or minimized by the choice of scale on the vertical axis.

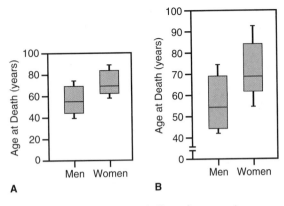

Figure 3–15. Illustration of effect of suppressing or stretching the scale in plots showing age at death. **A:** Suppressing the scale. **B:** Stretching the scale.

For example, suppose a researcher wishes to compare the ages at death in a group of men and a group of women. Figure 3–15A, by suppressing the scale, indicates that the ages of men and women at death are similar; Figure 3–15B, by stretching the scale, magnifies the differences in age at death between men and women.

Our final example is a table that gives irrelevant percentages, a somewhat common error. Suppose that the investigators are interested in the relationship between levels of patient compliance and their type of insurance coverage. When two or more measures are of interest, the purpose of the study generally determines which measure is viewed within the context of the other. Table 3–20A shows the percentage of patients with different types of insurance coverage within three levels of patient compliance, so the percentages in each column total 100%. The percentages in Table 3–20A make sense if the investigator wishes to compare the type of insurance coverage of patients who have specific levels of compliance; it is possible to conclude, for example, that 35% of patients with low levels of compliance have no insurance.

Contrast this interpretation with that obtained if percentages are calculated within insurance status, as in Table 3–20B, in which percentages in each row total 100%. From Table 3–20B, one can conclude that 55% of patients with no insurance coverage have a low level of compliance. In other words, the format of the table should reflect the questions asked in the study. If one measure is examined to see whether it explains another measure, such as insurance status explaining compliance, investigators should present percentages within the explanatory measure.

Table 3–20. Effect of calculating column percentages versus row percentages for study of compliance with medication versus insurance coverage.

A. Percentages Based on Level of Compliance (Column %)			
	Level of Compliance with Medication		
Insurance Coverage	**Low**	**Medium**	**High**
Medicaid	30	20	15
Medicare	20	25	30
Medicaid and Medicare	5	5	5
Other insurance	10	30	40
No insurance	35	20	10

B. Percentages Based on Insurance Coverage (Row %)			
Medicaid	45	30	25
Medicare	25	35	40
Medicaid and Medicare	33	33	33
Other insurance	15	35	50
No insurance	55	30	15

SUMMARY

This chapter presents two important biostatistical concepts: the different scales of measurement influence the methods for summarizing and displaying information. Some of the summary measures we introduce in this chapter form the basis of statistical tests illustrated in subsequent chapters.

The simplest level of measurement is a nominal scale, also called a categorical, or qualitative, scale. Nominal scales measure characteristics that can be classified into categories; the number of observations in each category is counted. Proportions, ratios, and percentages are commonly used to summarize categorical data. Nominal characteristics are displayed in contingency tables and in bar charts.

Ordinal scales are used for characteristics that have an underlying order. The differences between values on the scale are not equal throughout the scale. Examples are many disease staging schemes, which have four or five categories corresponding to the severity of the disease. Medians, percentiles, and ranges are the summary measures of choice because they are less affected by out-lying measurements. Ordinal characteristics, like nominal characteristics, are displayed in contingency tables and bar charts.

Numerical scales are the highest level of measurement; they are also called interval, ratio or quantitative scales. Characteristics measured on a numerical scale can be continuous (taking on any value on the number line) or discrete (taking on only integer values).

The mean should be used with observations that have a symmetric distribution. The median, also a measure of the middle, is used with ordinal observations or numerical observations that have a skewed distribution. When the mean is appropriate for describing the middle, the standard deviation is appropriate for describing the spread, or variation, of the observations. The value of the standard deviation is affected by outlying or skewed values, so percentiles or the interquartile range should be used with observations for which the median is appropriate. The range gives information on the extreme values, but alone it does not provide insight into how the observations are distributed.

An easy way to determine whether the distribution of observations is symmetric or skewed is to create a histogram or box plot. Other graphic methods include frequency polygons or line graphs, and error plots. Although each method provides information on the distribution of the observations, box plots are especially useful as concise displays because they show at a glance the distribution of the values. Stem-and-leaf plots combine features of frequency tables and histograms; they show the frequencies as well as the shape of the distribution. Frequency tables summarize numerical observations; the scale is divided into classes, and the number of observations in each class is counted. Both frequencies and percentages are commonly used in frequency tables.

When measurements consist of one nominal and one numerical characteristic, frequency polygons, box plots, and error plots illustrate the distribution of numerical observations for each value of the nominal characteristic.

The correlation coefficient indicates the degree of the linear relationship between the two characteristics on the same group of individuals. Spearman's rank correlation is used with skewed or ordinal observations. When the characteristics are measured on a nominal scale and proportions are calculated to describe them, the relative risk or the odds ratio may be used to measure the relationship between two characteristics.

The data from the study by Bos-Touwen and colleagues (2015), Presenting Problem 2, was used to illustrate the calculation of common statistics for summarizing data, such as the mean, median, and standard deviation, and to provide some useful ways of displaying data in graphs.

The results of the study by Anderson and colleagues (2018) on screening for domestic violence (Presenting Problem 3) were used to illustrate that proportions and percentages can be used interchangeably to describe the relationship of a part to the whole; ratios relate the two parts themselves. When a proportion is calculated over time, the result is called a rate. Some of the rates commonly used in medicine were defined and illustrated. For comparison of rates from two different populations, the populations must be similar with respect to characteristics that might affect the rate; adjusted rates are necessary when these characteristics differ between the populations. In medicine, rates are frequently adjusted for disparities in age. Contingency tables display two nominal characteristics measured on the same set of subjects. Bar charts are an effective way to illustrate nominal data.

EXERCISES

1. Show that the sum of the deviations from the mean is equal to 0. Demonstrate this fact by finding the sum of the deviations for activation score variation in Table 3–3.

2. Bos-Touwen et al analyzed SF-12 score data from 1,154 patients. Using the dataset found here: https://doi.org/10.5061/dryad.jg413, complete the following:

   a. Calculate the mean and standard deviation of SF-12 Total Score (SF12_total_score).

   b. Generate a frequency table of SF12_total_score for patients using the following categories: 0 to 20, 21 to 40, 41 to 60, 61 to 80, 81 to 100.

   c. Generate box plots of SF12_total_score according to gender.

3. Again, using the Bos-Touwen dataset, generate a frequency table of mean, median, minimum, and maximum SF12_total_score for patients in age categories. Use the age categories: and the Numerical Summary procedure in R Commander. There are 1,129 patients for whom both age and heart rate variation are available. Estimate the overall mean age of the patients. Estimate the overall SF12_total_score. Compare each to the mean calculated with R. Which is more accurate? Why?

4. Use the data from the Anderson study found: https://doi.org/10.5061/dryad.t7n to form a 2 × 2 contingency table for the frequencies of

flu diagnosis Flu_final_posneg) in columns and which setting the patient presented (Collection_site). After you have found the numbers in the cells, use the R Commander program to find the odds ratio.

5. What is the most likely shape of the distribution of observations in the following studies?

   a. The age of subjects in a study of patients with Crohn's disease.

   b. The number of babies delivered by all physicians who delivered babies in a large city during the past year.

   c. The number of patients transferred to a tertiary care hospital by other hospitals in the region.

6. Draw frequency polygons to compare men and women SF-12 Total scores on in the study by Bos-Touwen and coworkers (2015). What do you conclude?

7. The computational formula for the standard deviation is

$$SD = \sqrt{\frac{\sum x^2 - \frac{(\sum x)^2}{n}}{n-1}}$$

Illustrate that the value of the standard deviation calculated from this formula is equivalent to that found with the definitional formula using shock index data in Table 3–3. From the section titled, "The Standard Deviation," the value of the standard deviation of activation score using the definitional formula is 10.80. (Use the sums in Table 3–3 to save some calculations.)

8. What measures of central tendency and dispersion are the most appropriate to use with the following sets of data?

   a. Salaries of 125 physicians in a clinic

   b. The test scores of all medical students taking USLME Step I of the National Board Examination in a given year

   c. Serum sodium levels of healthy individuals

   d. Number of tender joints in 30 joints evaluated on a standard examination for disease activity in rheumatoid arthritis patients

   e. Presence of diarrhea in a group of infants

   f. The disease stages for a group of patients with Reye's syndrome (six stages, ranging from 0 = alert wakefulness to 5 = unarousable, flaccid paralysis, areflexia, pupils unresponsive)

   g. The age at onset of breast cancer in females

   h. The number of pills left in subjects' medicine bottles when investigators in a study counted the pills to evaluate compliance in taking medication

9. The correlation between activation score and SF-12 total score is 0.27 (Bos-Touwen et al, 2015) and between age and SF-12 total score is −0.19. How do you interpret these values?

10. Refer to Figure 3–2 to answer the following questions:

    a. What is the mean weight of girls 24 months old?

    b. What is the 90th percentile for head circumference for 12-month-old girls?

    c. What is the fifth percentile in weight for 12-month-old girls?

11. Find the coefficient of variation of mean change in activation score for men and women using the data from Bos-Touwen and colleagues (2015). Does one sex have greater relative variation in the activation score?

12. From their own experiences in an urban public hospital, Kaku and Lowenstein (1990) noted that stroke related to recreational drug use was occurring more frequently in young people. To investigate the problem, they identified all patients between 15 and 44 years of age admitted to a given hospital and selected sex- and age-matched controls from patients admitted to the hospital with acute medical or surgical conditions for which recreational drug abuse has not been shown to be a risk factor. Data are given in Table 3–21. What is the odds ratio?

Table 3–21. Data for odds ratio for stroke with history of drug abuse.

	Stroke	Control
Drug Abuse	73	18
No Drug Abuse	141	196
Total	214	214

Data from Kaku DA, Lowenstein DH: Emergence of recreational drug abuse as a major risk factor for stroke in young adults, Ann Intern Med. 1990 Dec 1;113(11):821-827.

13. **Group Exercise.** Obtain a copy of the study by Moore and colleagues (1991) from your medical library, and answer the following questions:

  a. What was the purpose of this study?

  b. What was the study design?

  c. Why were two groups of patients used in the study?

  d. Examine the box plots in the article's Figure 3–1. What conclusions are possible from the plots?

  e. Examine the box plots in the article's Figure 3–2. What do these plots tell you about pH levels in normal healthy men?

14. Group Exercise. It is important that scales recommended to physicians for use in assessing risk or making management decisions be shown to be reliable and valid. Select an area of interest, and consult some journal articles that describe scales or decision rules. Evaluate whether the authors presented adequate evidence for the reproducibility and validity of these scales. What kind of reproducibility was established? What type of validity? Are these sufficient to warrant the use of the scale? (For example, if you are interested in assessing surgical risk for noncardiac surgery, you can consult the articles on an index of cardiac risk by Goldman [1995] and Goldman and associates [1977], as well as a follow-up report of an index developed by Detsky and colleagues [1986].)

Probability & Related Topics for Making Inferences About Data

4

KEY CONCEPTS

 Probability is an important concept in statistics. Both objective and subjective probabilities are used in the medical field.

 Basic definitions include the concept of an event or outcome. A number of essential rules tell us how to combine the probabilities of events.

 Bayes' theorem relates to the concept of conditional probability—the probability of an outcome depending on an earlier outcome. Bayes' theorem is part of the reasoning process when interpreting diagnostic procedures.

 Populations are rarely studied; instead, researchers study samples.

 Several methods of sampling are used in medical research; a key issue is that any method should be random.

 When researchers select random samples and then make measurements, the result is a random variable. This process makes statistical tests and inferences possible.

 The binomial distribution is used to determine the probability of yes/no events—the number of times a given outcome occurs in a given number of attempts.

 The Poisson distribution is used to determine the probability of rare events.

 The normal distribution is used to find the probability that an outcome occurs when the observations have a bell-shaped distribution. It is used in many statistical procedures.

 If many random samples are drawn from a population, a statistic, such as the mean, follows a distribution called a sampling distribution.

 The central limit theorem tells us that means of observations, regardless of how they are distributed, begin to follow a normal distribution as the sample size increases. This is one of the reasons the normal distribution is so important in statistics.

 It is important to know the difference between the standard deviation, which describes the spread of individual observations, from the standard error of the mean, which describes the spread of the mean observations.

 One of the purposes of statistics is to use a sample to estimate something about the population. Estimates form the basis of statistical tests.

 Confidence intervals can be formed around an estimate to tell us how much the estimate would vary in repeated samples.

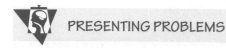

PRESENTING PROBLEMS

Presenting Problem 1

The World Health Organization (WHO) collects influenza rates worldwide. The CDC collects the statistics for the United States and territories. The data collection is completed weekly through the NREVSS collaborating laboratories. The data for the 2017–2018 flu season is used as a Presenting Problem to demonstrate the concepts of probability and displayed in Table 4–1.

The full data for this and other flu seasons may be found here:

https://www.cdc.gov/flu/weekly/

Presenting Problem 2

A local blood bank was asked to provide information on the distribution of blood types among males and females. This information is useful in illustrating some basic principles in probability theory. The results are given in "Basic Definitions and Rules of Probability."

Presenting Problem 3

In the United States, prostate cancer is the second leading cause of death among men who die of neoplasia, accounting for 12.3% of cancer deaths. Men who are treated surgically with a radical prostatectomy are often also treated with salvage radiation therapy. Shipley and colleagues (2017) investigated the utility of adding anti-androgen therapy along with radiation therapy might result in longer survival.

Shipley WU, Seiferheld W, Lukka HR, et al: Radiation with or without Antiandrogen Therapy in Recurrent Prostate Cancer. New England J Med 2017; 376(5):417–428,

https://www.nejm.org/doi/full/10.1056/ NEJMoa1607529.

Presenting Problem 4

The Coronary Artery Surgery Study was a classic study in 1983; it was a prospective, randomized, multicenter collaborative trial of medical and surgical therapy in subsets of patients with stable ischemic heart disease. This classic study established that the 10-year survival rate in this group of patients was equally good in the medically treated and surgically (coronary revascularization) treated groups (Alderman et al 1990). A second part of the study compared the effects of medical and surgical treatment on the quality of life.

Over a 5-year period, 780 patients with stable ischemic heart disease were subdivided into three clinical subsets (groups A, B, and C). Patients within each subset were randomly assigned to either medical or surgical treatment. All patients enrolled had 50% or greater stenosis of the left main coronary artery or 70% or greater stenosis of the other operable vessels. In addition, group A had mild angina and an ejection fraction of at least 50%; group B had mild angina and an ejection fraction less than 50%; group C had no angina after myocardial infarction. History, examination, and treadmill testing were done at 6, 18, and 60 months; a follow-up questionnaire was completed at 6-month intervals. Quality of life was evaluated by assessing chest pain status; heart

Table 4–1. Summary of flu virus type by age group for the 2017–2018 season.

| Age Group | Virus | | | | | Total |
| | Flu A | | Flu B | | | |
	Count	Column %	Count	Column %		
0–4 yr	2,989	9%	952	7%		3,941
5–24 yr	7,489	22%	4,296	31%		11,785
25–64 yr	11,403	33%	4,618	33%		16,021
65+ yr	12,448	36%	4,096	29%		16,544
Total	34,329	100%	13,962	100%		48,291

Reproduced with permission from Centers for Disease Control and Prevention. Availble at https://www. cdc.gov/flu/weekly/

failure; activity limitation; employment status; recreational status; drug therapy; number of hospitalizations; and risk factor alteration, such as smoking status, BP control, and cholesterol level. Data on number of hospitalizations after mean follow-up of 11 years will be used to illustrate the Poisson probability distribution (Rogers et al 1990).

PURPOSE OF THE CHAPTER

The previous chapter presented methods for summarizing information from studies: graphs, plots, and summary statistics. A major reason for performing clinical research, however, is to generalize the findings from the set of observations on one group of subjects to others who are similar to those subjects. Shipley and colleagues (2017) concluded that antiandrogen therapy with daily bicalutamide combined with salvage radiation therapy resulted in longer overall survival than radiation therapy and a placebo. This conclusion was based on their study and follow-up for a median of 13 years of 760 men. Studying all patients in the world with T2 and T3 tumors with no nodal involvement is neither possible nor desirable; therefore, the investigators made **inferences** to a larger **population** of patients on the basis of their study of a **sample** of patients. They cannot be sure that men with a specific tumor or course of radiation treatment will respond to treatment as the average man did in this study, but they can use the data to find the **probability** of a positive response.

The concepts in this chapter will enable you to understand what investigators mean when they make statements like the following:

- *The difference between treatment and control groups was tested by using a t test and found to be significantly greater than zero.*
- *An α value of 0.01 was used for all statistical tests.*
- *The sample sizes were determined to give 90% power of detecting a difference of 30% between treatment and control groups.*

Many of the concepts underlying statistical inference are not easily absorbed in a first reading. This chapter should be reviewed again after completing Chapters 5 through 9 to solidify understanding of the concepts. It should be easier to understand the basic ideas of inference using this approach.

THE MEANING OF THE TERM "PROBABILITY"

Assume that an experiment can be repeated many times, with each replication (repetition) called a **trial** and assume that one or more outcomes can result from each trial. Then, the **probability** of a given outcome is the number of times that outcome occurs divided by the total number of trials. If the outcome is sure to occur, it has a probability of 1; if an outcome cannot occur, its probability is 0.

An estimate of probability may be determined empirically, or it may be based on a theoretical model. We know that the probability of flipping a fair coin and getting tails is 0.50, or 50%. If a coin is flipped ten times, there is no guarantee, of course, that exactly five tails will be observed; the proportion of tails can range from 0 to 1, although in most cases we expect it to be closer to 0.50 than to 0 or 1. If the coin is flipped 100 times, the chances are even better that the proportion of tails will be close to 0.50, and with 1,000 flips, the chances are better still. As the number of flips becomes larger, the proportion of coin flips that result in tails approaches 0.50; therefore, the probability of tails on any one flip is 0.50.

This definition of probability is sometimes called objective probability, as opposed to **subjective probability,** which reflects a person's opinion, hunch, or best guess about whether an outcome will occur. Subjective probabilities are important in medicine because they form the basis of a physician's opinion about whether a patient has a specific disease. In Chapter 12, we discuss how this estimate, based on information gained in the history and physical examination, changes as the result of diagnostic procedures. Quinn et al (2017) discuss the way physicians use probability in speaking to patients.

Basic Definitions & Rules of Probability

Probability concepts are helpful for understanding and interpreting data presented in tables and graphs in published articles. In addition, the concept of probability lets us make statements about how much confidence we have in such estimates as means, proportions, or relative risks (introduced in the previous chapter). Understanding probability is essential for understanding the meaning of p values given in journal articles.

We use two examples to illustrate some definitions and rules for determining probabilities: Presenting Problem 1 on influenza disease (Table 4–1) and the information given in Table 4–2 on gender and blood type. All illustrations of probability assume the observation has been randomly selected from a population of observations. We discuss these concepts in more detail in the next section.

In probability, an **experiment** is defined as any planned process of data collection. For Presenting Problem 1, the experiment is the process of determining the type of virus in patients with influenza.

Table 4–2. Distribution of blood type by gender.

Blood Type	Probabilities		
	Males	Females	Total
O	0.21	0.21	0.42
A	0.215	0.215	0.43
B	0.055	0.055	0.11
AB	0.02	0.02	0.04
Total	0.50	0.50	1.00

An experiment consists of a number of independent **trials** (replications) under the same conditions; in this example, a trial consists of determining the type of virus for an individual person. Each trial can result in one of two outcomes: A or B.

The probability of a particular outcome, say outcome A, is written $P(A)$. For example, in Table 4–1, if outcome A is Virus A, the probability that a randomly selected person from the study has Influenza Type A is

$$P(\text{Influenza Type A}) = \frac{34,329}{48,291} = 0.71$$

In Presenting Problem 2, the probabilities of different outcomes are already computed. The outcomes of each trial to determine blood type are O, A, B, and AB. From Table 4–2, the probability that a randomly selected person has type A blood is

$$P(\text{type A}) = 0.43$$

The blood type data illustrate two important features of probability:

1. The probability of each outcome (blood type) is greater than or equal to 0.
2. The sum of the probabilities of the various outcomes is 1.

Events may be defined either as a single outcome or a set of outcomes. For example, the outcomes for the type of influenza virus is A or B, but we may wish to define an event as having Type A and having an age of less than 25. The event of Type A virus and under 25 years of age contains the two outcomes of virus type; the value for 0–4 years and 5–24 years.

Sometimes, we want to know the probability that an event will not happen; an event opposite to the event of interest is called a **complementary event.** For example, the complementary event to "having Flu virus A"

is "not having Flu virus A." The probability of the complement is

$$P(\text{complement of Flu Virus A}) = P(\text{Flu Virus B})$$

$$= \frac{13,962}{48,291} = 0.29$$

Note that the probability of a complementary event may also be found as 1 minus the probability of the event itself, and this calculation may be easier in some situations.

Mutually Exclusive Events & the Addition Rule

Two or more events are **mutually exclusive** if the occurrence of one precludes the occurrence of the others. For example, a person cannot have both blood type O and blood type A. By definition, all complementary events are also mutually exclusive; however, events can be mutually exclusive without being complementary if three or more events are possible.

As we indicated earlier, what constitutes an event is a matter of definition. Let us define the experiment in Presenting Problem 2 so that each outcome (blood type O, A, B, or AB) is a separate event. The probability of two mutually exclusive events occurring is the probability that either one event occurs *or* the other event occurs. This probability is found by adding the probabilities of the two events, which is called the **addition rule** for probabilities. For example, the probability that a randomly selected person has either blood type O or blood type A is

$$P(\text{O or A}) = P(\text{O}) + P(\text{A})$$

$$= 0.42 + 0.43 = 0.85$$

Does the addition rule work for more than two events? The answer is yes, as long as they are all mutually exclusive. We discuss the approach to use with nonmutually exclusive events in the section titled, "Nonmutually Exclusive Events and the Modified Addition Rule."

Independent Events & the Multiplication Rule

Two different events are **independent events** if the outcome of one event has no effect on the outcome of the second. Using the blood type example, let us also define a second event as the gender of the person; this event consists of the outcomes male and female.

In this example, gender and blood type are independent events; the sex of a person does not affect the person's blood type, and vice versa. The probability of two independent events is the probability that both events occur and is found by multiplying the probabilities of the two events, which is called the **multiplication rule** for probabilities. The probability of being male and of having blood type O is

$$P(\text{male and blood type O}) = P(\text{male}) \times P(\text{blood type O})$$

$$= 0.50 \times 0.42 = 0.21$$

The probability of being male, 0.50, and the probability of having blood type O, 0.42, are both called *marginal probabilities* because they appear on the margins of a probability table. The probability of being male and of having blood type O, 0.21, is called a **joint probability;** it is the probability of both male and type O occurring jointly.

Is having the Type B flu virus independent from the age group in the CDC data? Table 4–1 gives the data we need to answer to this question. If two events are independent, the product of the marginal probabilities will equal the joint probability in all instances. To show that two events are not independent, we need to demonstrate only one instance in which the product of the marginal probabilities is not equal to the joint probability. For example, to show that having Type B flu virus and age group 5–24 are not independent, find the joint probability of a randomly selected person having Type B flu and being in the Age group 5–24. Table 4–1 shows that

$$P(\text{Type B Virus and Age group 5–24}) = \frac{4,296}{48,291} = 0.089$$

However, the product of the marginal probabilities does not yield the same result; that is,

$$P(\text{Type B Virus}) \times P(\text{Age group 5–24}) = \frac{13,962}{48,291} \times \frac{11,785}{48,291}$$

$$= 0.289 \times 0.244 - 0.070 \neq 0.089$$

We could show that the product of the marginal probabilities is not equal to the joint probability for any of the combinations in this example, but we need to show only one instance to prove that two events are not independent.

Nonindependent Events & the Modified Multiplication Rule

Finding the joint probability of two events when they are not independent is a bit more complex than simply multiplying the two marginal probabilities. When two events are not independent, the occurrence of one event depends on whether the other event has occurred. Let *A* stand for the event "Virus A" and *B* for the event "Age Group 65+". We want to know the probability of event *A* given event *B*, written $P(A \mid B)$ where the vertical line, |, is read as "given." In other words, we want to know the probability of event *A*, assuming that event *B* has happened. From the data in Table 4–1, the probability of Virus A, given that the subject is in the 65+ age group is,

$$P(\text{Virus A}|\text{Age Group 65+}) = \frac{12,488}{16,544} = 0.752$$

This probability, called a **conditional probability,** is the probability of one event given that another event has occurred. Put another way, the probability of a patient having Virus A is conditional on the Age group of the subject; it is substituted for $P(\text{Virus A})$ in the multiplication rule. If we put these expressions together, we can find the joint probability of having Virus A *and* being in the age group 65+:

$$P(\text{Virus A and Age Group 65+}) = P(\text{Virus A}|\text{Age Group 65+})$$

$$\times P(\text{Age Group 65+})$$

$$= \frac{12,448}{16,544} \times \frac{16,544}{48,291}$$

$$= 0.752 \times 0.343 = 0.258$$

The probability of having Virus A in the Age Group 65+ can also be determined by finding the conditional probability of contracting the disease in age group 65+, given known Virus A, and substituting that expression in the multiplication rule for $P(\text{Age group 65+})$. To illustrate,

$$P(\text{Virus A and Age Group 65+})$$

$$= P(\text{Age Group 65+ and Virus A})$$

$$= P(\text{Age Group 65+}|\text{Virus A}) \times P(\text{Virus A})$$

$$= \frac{12,448}{34,329} \times \frac{34,329}{48,291} = 0.363 \times 0.711 = 0.258$$

Nonmutually Exclusive Events & the Modified Addition Rule

Remember that two or more mutually exclusive events cannot occur together, and the addition rule applies for the calculation of the probability that one or another of the events occurs. Now we find the probability that either of two events occurs when they are not mutually exclusive. For example, gender and blood type O are **nonmutually exclusive events** because the occurrence of one does not preclude the occurrence of the other. The addition rule must be modified in this situation; otherwise, the probability that both events occur will be added into the calculation twice.

In Table 4–2, the probability of being male is 0.50 and the probability of blood type O is 0.42. The probability of being male *or* of having blood type O is not $0.50 + 0.42$, however, because the males with type O blood are counted in both the male and blood type O probabilities. The joint probability of being male *and* having blood type O, 0.21, must therefore be subtracted. The calculation is

$$P(\text{male or type O}) = P(\text{male}) + P(\text{type O})$$
$$-P(\text{male and type O})$$
$$= 0.50 + 0.42 - 0.21$$
$$= 0.71$$

Of course, if we do not know that $P(\text{male } and \text{ type O}) = 0.21$, we must use the multiplication rule (for independent events, in this case) to determine this probability.

Summary of Rules & an Extension

Let us summarize the rules presented thus far so we can extend them to obtain a particularly useful rule for combining probabilities called **Bayes' theorem.** Remember that questions about mutual exclusiveness use the word "or" and the addition rule; questions about independence use the word "and" and the multiplication rule. We use letters to represent events; *A, B, C,* and *D* are four different events with probability $P(A)$, $P(B)$, $P(C)$, and $P(D)$.

The **addition rule** for the occurrence of either of two or more events is as follows: If *A, B,* and *C* are mutually exclusive, then

$$P(A \text{ or } B \text{ or } C) = P(A) + P(B) + P(C)$$

If two events such as *A* and *D* are not mutually exclusive, then

$$P(A \text{ or } D) = P(A) + P(D) - P(A \text{ and } D)$$

The[*] **multiplication rule** for the occurrence of both of two or more events is as follows: If *A, B,* and *C* are independent, then

$$P(A \text{ and } B \text{ and } C) = P(A) \times P(B) \times P(C)$$

If two events such as *B* and *D* are not independent, then

$$P(B \text{ and } D) = P(B \mid D) \times P(D)$$
$$\text{or}$$
$$P(D \text{ and } B) = P(D \mid B) \times P(B)$$

The multiplication rule for probabilities when events are not independent can be used to derive one form of an important formula called Bayes' theorem. Because $P(B \text{ and } D)$ equals both $P(B \mid D) \times P(D)$ and $P(B) \times P(D \mid B)$, these latter two expressions are equal. Assuming $P(B)$ and $P(D)$ are not equal to zero, we can solve for one in terms of the other, as follows:

$$P(B \mid D) \times P(D) = P(D \mid B) \times P(B)$$
$$\text{Then}$$
$$P(B \mid D) = \frac{P(D \mid B) \times P(B)}{P(D)}$$

which is found by dividing both sides of the equation by $P(D)$. Similarly,

$$P(D \mid B) = \frac{P(B \mid D) \times P(D)}{P(B)}$$

In the equation for $P(B \mid D)$, $P(B)$ in the right-hand side of the equation is sometimes called the **prior probability,** because its value is known prior to the calculation; $P(B \mid D)$ is called the **posterior probability,** because its value is known only after the calculation.

The two formulas of Bayes' theorem are important because investigators frequently know only one of the pertinent probabilities and must determine the other. Examples are diagnosis and management, discussed in detail in Chapter 12.

A Comment on Terminology

Although in everyday use the terms **probability, odds,** and **likelihood** are sometimes used synonymously, mathematicians do not use them that way. **Odds** is

---

[*]The probability of three or more events that are not mutually exclusive or not independent involves complex calculations beyond the scope of this book. Interested readers can consult any introductory book on probability.

defined as the probability that an event occurs divided by the probability the event does not occur. For example, the odds that a person has blood type O are $0.42/(1 - 0.42) = 0.72$ to 1, but "to 1" is not always stated explicitly. This interpretation is consistent with the meaning of the odds ratio, discussed in Chapter 3. It is also consistent with the use of odds in gaming events such as football games and horse races.

Likelihood may be related to Bayes' theorem for conditional probabilities. Suppose a physician is trying to determine which of three likely diseases a patient has: myocardial infarction, pneumonia, or reflux esophagitis. Chest pain can appear with any one of these three diseases; and the physician needs to know the probability that chest pain occurs with myocardial infarction, the probability that chest pain occurs with pneumonia, and the probability that chest pain occurs with reflux esophagitis. The probabilities of a given outcome (chest pain) when evaluated under different hypotheses (myocardial infarction, pneumonia, and reflux esophagitis) are called likelihoods of the hypotheses (or diseases).

POPULATIONS & SAMPLES

A major purpose of doing research is to infer, or generalize, from a sample to a larger population. This process of **inference** is accomplished by using statistical methods based on probability. **Population** is the term statisticians use to describe a large set or collection of items that have something in common. In the health field, population generally refers to patients or other living organisms, but the term can also be used to denote collections of inanimate objects, such as sets of autopsy reports, hospital charges, or birth certificates. A **sample** is a subset of the population, selected so as to be representative of the larger population.

There are many good reasons for studying a sample instead of an entire population, and the four commonly used methods for selecting a sample are discussed in this section. Before turning to those topics, however, we note that the term "population" is frequently misused to describe what is, in fact, a sample. For example, researchers sometimes refer to the "population of patients in this study." After you have read this book, you will be able to spot such errors when you see them in the medical literature. If you want more information, Levy and Lemeshow (1999) provide a comprehensive treatment of sampling.

Reasons for Sampling

There are at least six reasons to study samples instead of populations:

1. Samples can be studied *more quickly* than populations. Speed can be important if a physician needs to determine something quickly, such as a vaccine or treatment for a new disease.

2. A study of a sample is *less expensive* than studying an entire population, because a smaller number of items or subjects are examined. This consideration is especially important in the design of large studies that require a lengthy follow-up.

3. A study of an entire population (census) is *impossible* in most situations. Sometimes, the process of the study destroys or depletes the item being studied. For example, in a study of cartilage healing in limbs of rats after 6 weeks of limb immobilization, the animals may be sacrificed in order to perform histologic studies. On other occasions, the desire is to infer to future events, such as the study of men with prostate cancer. In these cases, a study of a population is impossible.

4. Sample results are often *more accurate* than results-based observations of a population. For samples, more time and resources can be spent on training the people who perform observations and collect data. In addition, more expensive procedures that improve accuracy can be used for a sample because fewer procedures are required.

5. If samples are properly selected, probability methods can be used to *estimate the error* in the resulting statistics. It is this aspect of sampling that permits investigators to make probability statements about observations in a study.

6. Samples can be selected to *reduce heterogeneity*. For example, systemic lupus erythematosus (SLE) has many clinical manifestations, resulting in a heterogeneous population. A sample of the population with specified characteristics is more appropriate than the entire population for the study of certain aspects of the disease.

To summarize, bigger does not always mean better in terms of sample sizes. Thus, investigators must plan the sample size appropriate for their study prior to beginning research. This process is called determining the **power** of a study and is discussed in detail in later chapters.

Methods of Sampling

The best way to ensure that a sample will lead to reliable and valid inferences is to use probability samples, in which the probability of being included in the sample is known for each subject in the population. Four commonly used probability sampling methods in medicine are simple random sampling, systematic sampling, stratified sampling, and cluster sampling, all of which use random processes.

The following example illustrates each method: Consider a physician applying for a grant for a study that involves measuring the tracheal diameter on radiographs. The physician wants to convince the granting agency that these measurements are reliable. To estimate **intrarater reliability,** the physician will select a sample of chest x-ray films from those performed during the previous year, remeasure the tracheal diameter, and compare the new measurement with the original one on file in the patient's chart. The physician has a population of 3,400 radiographs, and we assume that the physician has learned that a sample of 200 films is sufficient to provide an accurate estimate of intrarater reliability. Now, the physician must select the sample for the reliability study.

Simple Random Sampling: A **simple random sample** is one in which every subject (every film in the example) has an equal probability of being selected for the study. The recommended way to select a simple random sample is to use a table of random numbers or a computer-generated list of random numbers. For this approach, each x-ray film must have an identification (ID) number, and a list of ID numbers, called a sampling frame, must be available. For the sake of simplicity, assume that the radiographs are numbered from 1 to 3,400. Using a random number table or computer program to generate a set of random numbers, the physician can select the first 200 digits between 1 and 3,400. A computer program such as Excel or R may be used to generate a sequence of 3,400 random numbers. Each random number corresponds on a radiograph as demonstrated in Table 4–3. The series can then be sorted by the random number values. The first 200 radiograph sequence numbers will be a random sample of 200 from the total population of 3,400.

Systematic Sampling: A **systematic random sample** is one in which every *k*th item is selected; *k* is determined by dividing the number of items in the sampling frame by the desired sample size. For example, 3,400 radiographs divided by 200 is 17, so every 17th x-ray film is sampled. In this approach, we must select a number randomly between 1 and 17 first, and we then select every 17th film. Suppose we randomly select the number 12 from a random number table or computer program. Then, the systematic sample consists of radiographs with ID numbers 12, 29, 46, 63, 80, and so on; each subsequent number is determined by adding 17 to the last ID number.

Systematic sampling should not be used when a cyclic repetition is inherent in the sampling frame. For example, systemic sampling is not appropriate for selecting months of the year in a study of the frequency of different types of accidents, because some accidents

Table 4–3. Random numbers assigned to radiograph sequence numbers.

Radiograph #	Random #
1	0.9034895
2	0.3532915
3	0.7992323
4	0.4648716
5	0.6079091
6	0.3868423
7	0.5667295
8	0.9136576
9	0.8125268
10	0.2458116
11	0.4230705
12	0.5088833
13	0.0600749
...	...
3389	0.0556582
3390	0.4113534
3391	0.4749432
3392	0.7383921
3393	0.5820639
3394	0.6768157
3395	0.8973512
3396	0.8412195
3397	0.7896784
3398	0.8220758
3399	0.6395098
3400	0.4819353

occur more often at certain times of the year. For instance, skiing injuries and automobile accidents most often occur in cold-weather months, whereas swimming injuries and farming accidents most often occur in warm-weather months.

Stratified Sampling: A **stratified random sample** is one in which the population is first divided into relevant strata (subgroups), and a random sample is then selected from each stratum. In the radiograph example, the physician may wish to stratify on the age of patients, because the trachea varies in size with age and measuring the diameter accurately in young patients may be difficult. The population of radiographs may be divided into infants younger than 1 year old, children from 1 year old to less than 6 years old, children from 6 to younger than 16 years old, and subjects 16 years of age or older; a random sample is then selected from each age stratum. Other commonly used strata in medicine besides age include gender of patient, severity or stage of disease, and duration of disease. Characteristics used to stratify should be related to the measurement of interest, in which case stratified random sampling is the most efficient, meaning that it requires the smallest sample size.

Cluster Sampling: A **cluster random sample** results from a two-stage process in which the population is divided into clusters and a subset of the clusters is randomly selected. Clusters are commonly based on geographic areas or districts, so this approach is used more often in epidemiologic research than in clinical studies. For example, the sample for a household survey taken in a city may be selected by using city blocks as clusters; a random sample of city blocks is selected, and all households (or a random sample of households) within the selected city blocks are surveyed. In multicenter trials, the institutions selected to participate in the study constitute the clusters; patients from each institution can be selected using another random-sampling procedure. Cluster sampling is somewhat less efficient than the other sampling methods because it requires a larger sample size, but in some situations, such as in multicenter trials, it is the method of choice for obtaining adequate numbers of patients.

Nonprobability Sampling: The sampling methods just discussed are all based on probability, but nonprobability sampling methods also exist, such as convenience samples or quota samples. **Nonprobability samples** are those in which the probability that a subject is selected is unknown and may reflect selection biases of the person doing the study; they do not fulfill the requirements of randomness needed to estimate sampling errors. When we use the term "sample" in the context of observational studies, we will assume that the sample has been randomly selected in an appropriate way.

Random Assignment: Random sampling methods are used when a sample of subjects is selected from a population of possible subjects in observational studies, such as cohort, case–control, and cross-sectional studies. In experimental studies such as randomized clinical trials, subjects are first selected for inclusion in the study on the basis of appropriate criteria; they are then assigned to different treatment modalities. If the assignment of subjects to treatments is done by using random methods, the process is called **random assignment.** Random assignment may also occur by randomly assigning treatments to subjects. In either case, random assignment helps ensure that the groups receiving the different treatment modalities are as similar as possible. Thus, any differences in outcome at the conclusion of the study are more likely to be the result of differences in the treatments used in the study rather than differences in the compositions of the groups.

Random assignment is best carried out by using random numbers. As an example, consider the DIETFITS study (Gardner et al 2018), in which patients meeting the entry criteria were divided into clinical subsets and then randomly assigned to either a healthy low-fat (HLF) diet or treatment health low-carbohydrate (HLC) diet. Random assignment in this study could have been accomplished by using a list of random numbers (obtained from a computer or a random number table) and assigning the random numbers to patients as they entered the trial. If a study involves several investigators at different sites, such as in a multicenter trial, the investigator preparing to enter an eligible patient in the study may call a central office to learn which treatment assignment is next. As an alternative, separately randomized lists may be generated for each site. Of course, in **double-blind** studies, someone other than the investigator must keep the list of random assignments.

Suppose investigators in the DIETFITS study wanted an equal number of patients at each site participating in the study. For this design, the assignment of random numbers might have been balanced within blocks of patients of a predetermined size. For example, balancing patients within blocks of 12 would guarantee that every time 12 patients entered the study at a given site, 6 patients received the medical treatment and 6 received the surgical treatment. Within the block of 12 patients, however, assignment would be random until 6 patients were assigned to one or the other of the treatments.

A study design may match subjects on important characteristics, such as gender, age group, or severity of disease, and then make the random assignment. This stratified assignment controls for possible confounding effects of the characteristic(s); it is equivalent to stratified random sampling in observational studies.

Many types of biases may result in studies in which patients are not randomly assigned to treatment modalities. For instance, early studies comparing medical and surgical treatment for coronary artery disease did not randomly assign patients to treatments and were criticized as a result. Some critics claimed that sicker patients were not candidates for surgery, and thus the group receiving surgery was biased by having healthier subjects. Other critics stated that the healthier patients were given medical treatment because their disease was not as serious as that of the sicker patients. In nonrandomized studies, the problem is determining which biases are operating and which conclusions are appropriate. A description of different kinds of biases that threaten the validity of studies is given in Chapter 13.

Using and Interpreting Random Samples: In actual clinical studies, patients are not always randomly selected from the population from which the investigator wishes to infer. Instead, the clinical researcher often

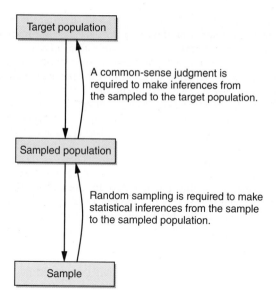

Figure 4–1. Target and sampled populations.

uses all patients at hand who meet the entry criteria for the study. This practical procedure is used especially when studies involve rather uncommon conditions. Colton (1974) makes a useful distinction between the target population and the sampled population. The **target population** is the population to which the investigator wishes to generalize; the **sampled population** is the population from which the sample was actually drawn. Figure 4–1 presents a scheme of these concepts.

For example, Shipley and colleagues (2017), in Presenting Problem 3, clearly wished to generalize their findings about survival to all men with recurrent prostate cancer, such as patients who live in other locations and perhaps even patients who do not yet have the disease. The sample was the set of patients with T2 and T3 tumors undergoing a prostatectomy with a lymphadenectomy between 1998 and 2003. Statistical inference permits generalization from the sample to the population sampled. In order to make inferences from the population sampled to the target population, we must ask whether the population sampled is representative of the target population. A **population** (or sample) is **representative** of the target population if the distribution of important characteristics in the sampled population is the same as that in the target population. This judgment is clinical, not statistical. It points to the importance of always reading the Method section of journal articles to learn what population was actually sampled so that you can determine the representativeness of that population.

Table 4–4. Commonly used symbols for parameters and statistics.

Characteristic	Parameter Symbol	Statistical Symbol
Mean	μ	$\bar{X}$
Standard deviation	σ	SD
Variance	σ^2	s^2
Correlation	ρ	r
Proportion	π	p

Population Parameters & Sample Statistics

Statisticians use precise language to describe characteristics of populations and samples. Measures of central tendency and variation, such as the mean and the standard deviation, are fixed and invariant characteristics in populations and are called **parameters.** In samples, however, the observed mean or standard deviation calculated on the basis of the sample information is actually an estimate of the population mean or standard deviation; these estimates are called **statistics.** Statisticians customarily use Greek letters for population parameters and Roman letters for sample statistics. Some of the frequently encountered symbols used in this text are summarized in Table 4–4.

RANDOM VARIABLES & PROBABILITY DISTRIBUTIONS

The characteristic of interest in a study is called a **variable.** The term "variable" makes sense because the value of the characteristic varies from one subject to another. This variation results from inherent biologic variation among individuals and from errors, called measurement errors, made in measuring and recording a subject's value on a characteristic. A **random variable** is a variable in a study in which subjects are randomly selected. If the subjects in Presenting Problem 1 are a random sample selected from a larger population of citizens, then age group, and type of virus are examples of random variables.

Just as values of characteristics, such as type of virus or PSA level, can be summarized in frequency distributions, values of a random variable can be summarized in a frequency distribution called a **probability distribution.** For example, if X is a random variable defined as the PSA level prior to treatment in Presenting Problem 3, X can take on any value between 0.1 and 2,500; and we can determine the probability that the random variable X has any given value or range of values. For instance, Shipley reports that 405 of the 760 subjects had a PSA level of <0.7 ng/mL at trial entry. This data may be used to estimate the probability of a PSA value of <0.7 in the study population: 405/760 = 0.533. In some applications, a formula or rule will adequately describe a distribution; the formula can then be used to calculate the probability of interest. In other situations, a theoretical probability distribution provides a good fit to the distribution of the variable of interest.

Several theoretical probability distributions are important in statistics, and we shall examine three that are useful in medicine. Both the binomial and the Poisson are *discrete* probability distributions; that is, the associated random variable takes only integer values, 0, 1, 2, ..., *n*. The normal (Gaussian) distribution is a *continuous* probability distribution; that is, the associated random variable has values measured on a continuous scale. We will examine the binomial and Poisson distributions briefly, using examples from the Presenting Problems to illustrate each; then we will discuss the normal distribution in greater detail.

The Binomial Distribution

Suppose an event can have only binary outcomes (e.g., yes and no, or positive and negative), denoted *A* and *B*. The probability of *A* is denoted by π, or $P(A) = \pi$, and this probability stays the same each time the event occurs. The probability of *B* must, therefore, be $1 - \pi$, because *B* occurs if *A* does not. If an experiment involving this event is repeated *n* times and the outcome is independent from one trial to another, what is the probability that outcome *A* occurs exactly *X* times? Or equivalently, what proportion of the *n* outcomes will be *A*? These questions frequently are of interest, especially in basic science research, and they can be answered with the binomial distribution.

Basic principles of the binomial distribution were developed by the seventeenth-century Swiss mathematician Jakob Bernoulli, who made many contributions to probability theory. He was the author of what is generally acknowledged as the first book devoted to probability, published in 1713. In fact, in his honor, each trial involving a binomial probability is sometimes called a Bernoulli trial, and a sequence of trials is called a Bernoulli process. The **binomial distribution** gives the probability that a specified outcome occurs in a given number of independent trials. The binomial distribution can be used to model the inheritability of a particular trait in genetics, to estimate the occurrence of a specific reaction (e.g., the single packet, or quantal release, of acetylcholine at the neuromuscular junction), or to estimate the death of a cancer cell in an in vitro test of a new chemotherapeutic agent.

We use the information collected by Shipley and colleagues (2017) in Presenting Problem 3 to illustrate the binomial distribution. Assume, for a moment,

that the entire population of men with recurrent prostate cancer and a pretreatment PSA <0.7 was studied, and the probability of 12-year survival is equal to 0.8 (we use 0.8 for computational convenience, rather than 0.81 as reported in the study) for patients in the placebo group. Let *S* represent the event of 12-year survival and *D* represent death before 12 years; then, $\pi = P(S) = 0.8$ and $1 - \pi = P(D) = 0.2$. Consider a group of $n = 2$ men with a localized prostate tumor and a pretreatment PSA <0.7. What is the probability that exactly two men live 12 years? That exactly one lives 12 years? That none lives 12 years? These probabilities are found by using the multiplication and addition rules outlined earlier in this chapter.

The probability that exactly two men live 12 years is found by using the multiplication rule for independent events. We know that $P(S) = 0.8$ for patient 1 and $P(S) = 0.8$ for patient 2. Because the survival of one patient is independent from (has no effect on) the survival of the other patient, the probability of *both* surviving is

P(S for patient 1 and S for patient 2) = P(S)P(s)

$$= (0.8)(0.8) = 0.64$$

The event of exactly one patient living 12 years can occur in two ways: event 1: patient 1 survives 12 years and patient 2 does not, or event 2: patient 2 survives 12 years and patient 1 does not. These two events are mutually exclusive; therefore, after using the multiplication rule to obtain the probability of each event, we can use the addition rule for mutually exclusive events to combine the probabilities as follows:

P(S for patient 1 and D for patient 2) = P(S)P(D)

$$= (0.8)(0.2)$$

$$= 0.16$$

and

P(D for patient 1 and S for patient 2) = P(D)P(S)

$$= (0.2)(0.8)$$

$$= 0.16$$

Therefore,

P(event 1 or event 2) = 0.16 + 0.16

$$= 0.32$$

Finally, the probability that neither lives 12 years is

P(D for patient 1 and D for patient 2) = P(D)P(D)

$$= (0.2)(0.2)$$

$$= 0.04$$

Table 4–5. Summary of probabilities for two patients.

Outcome			
First Patient	Second Patient	Number of Ways to Occur	Probability
S	S	1	$0.8 \times 0.8 = 0.64$
D	S	2	$2 \times 0.8 \times 0.2 = 0.32$
S	D		
D	D	1	$0.2 \times 0.2 = 0.04$

These computational steps are summarized in Table 4–5. Note that the total probability is

$$(0.8)^2 + 2(0.8)(0.2) + (0.2)^2 = 1.0$$

which you may recognize as the binomial formula, $(a + b)^2 = a^2 + 2ab + b^2$.

The same process can be applied for a group of patients of any size or for any number of trials, but it becomes quite tedious. An easier technique is to use the formula for the binomial distribution, which follows. The probability of X outcomes in a group of size n, if each outcome has probability π and is independent from all other outcomes, is given by

$$P(X) = \frac{n!}{X!(n - X)!} \pi^X (1 - \pi)^{n-X}$$

where ! is the symbol for factorial; $n!$ is called n factorial and is equal to the product $n(n - 1)(n - 2) \ldots (3)(2)(1)$. For example, $4! = (4)(3)(2)(1) = 24$. The number $0!$ is defined as 1. The symbol π^X indicates that the probability is raised to the power X, and $(1 - \pi)^{n-X}$ means that 1 minus the probability is raised to the power $n - X$. The expression $n!/[X!(n - X)!]$ is sometimes referred to as the formula for combinations because it gives the number of combinations (or assortments) of X items possible among the n items in the group.

To verify that the probability that exactly $X = 1$ of $n = 2$ patients survives 12 years is 0.32, we use the formula:

$$P(1) = \frac{2!}{1!(2 - 1)!} (0.8)^1 (1 - 0.8)^{2-1}$$

$$= \frac{(2)(1)}{1(1)} (0.8)(0.2)$$

$$= 2(0.8)(0.2)$$

$$= 0.32$$

To summarize, the binomial distribution is useful for answering questions about the probability of X number of occurrences in n independent trials when there is a constant probability π of success on each trial. For example, suppose a new series of men with prostate tumors is begun with ten patients. We can use the binomial distribution to calculate the probability that any particular number of them will survive 12 years. For instance, the probability that all ten will survive 12 years is

$$P(10) = \frac{10!}{10!(10 - 10)!} (0.8)^{10} (1 - 0.8)^{10-10}$$

$$= \frac{10!}{(10!)(0!)} (0.8)^{10} (0.2)^0$$

$$= (1)(0.8)^{10}(1)$$

$$= 0.107$$

Similarly, the probability that exactly eight patients will survive 12 years is

$$P(8) = \frac{10!}{8!(10 - 8)!} (0.8)^8 (1 - 0.8)^{10-8}$$

$$= \frac{10(9)(8!)}{(8!)(2!)} (0.8)^8 (0.2)^2$$

$$= \frac{10(9)}{(2)(1)} (0.168)(0.04)$$

$$= (45)(0.168)(0.04)$$

$$= 0.302$$

Table 4–6 lists the probabilities for $X = 0, 1, 2, 3, \ldots, 10$; a plot of the binomial distribution when $n = 10$ and $\pi = 0.8$ is given in Figure 4–2. The mean of the binomial distribution is $n\pi$; so $(10)(0.8) = 8$ is the mean number of patients surviving 12 years in this example. The standard deviation is

$$\sqrt{n\pi(1 - \pi)}$$

which for this example is

$$\sqrt{10(0.8)(0.2)} = 1.265$$

Thus, the only two pieces of information needed to define a binomial distribution are n and π, which are called the parameters of the binomial distribution. Studies involving dichotomous, or binary, variables often use a proportion rather than a number (e.g., the proportion of patients surviving a given length of time rather than the number of patients). When a proportion is used instead of a number of successes, the

Table 4–6. Probabilities for binomial distribution with $n = 10$ and $\pi = 0.8$.

Number of Patients Surviving	$\dfrac{n!}{X!(n-X)!}$	π^X	$(1-\pi)^{n-X}$	$P(X)^a$
0	1	1	0.0000001	0
1	10	0.8	0.0000005	0
2	45	0.64	0.0000026	0.0001
3	120	0.512	0.0000128	0.0008
4	210	0.410	0.000064	0.0055
5	252	0.328	0.00032	0.0264
6	210	0.262	0.0016	0.0881
7	120	0.210	0.008	0.2013
8	45	0.168	0.04	0.3020
9	10	0.134	0.2	0.2684
10	1	0.107	1	0.1074

^{a}Rounded to four decimal places.

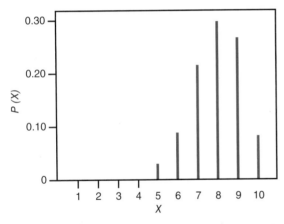

Figure 4–2. Binomial distribution for $n = 10$ and $\pi = 0.8$.

same two pieces of information (n and π) are needed. Because the proportion is found by dividing X by n or equivalently multiplying n by π; however, the mean of the distribution of the proportion becomes π, and the standard deviation becomes

$$\sqrt{\frac{\pi(1-\pi)}{n}}$$

Even using the formula for the binomial distribution becomes time-consuming, especially if the numbers are large. Also, the formula gives the probability

of observing exactly X successes, and interest frequently lies in knowing the probability of X or more successes or of X or less successes. For example, to find the probability that eight or more patients will survive 12 or more years, we must use the formula to find the separate probabilities that eight will survive, nine will survive, and ten will survive and then sum these results; from Table 4–6, we obtain $P(X \geq 8) = P(X = 8) + P(X = 9) + P(X = 10) = 0.3020 + 0.2684 + 0.1074 = 0.6778$. Tables giving probabilities for the binomial distribution are presented in many elementary texts. Much research in the health field is conducted with sample sizes large enough to use an approximation to the binomial distribution; this approximation is discussed in Chapter 5.

The Poisson Distribution

The Poisson distribution is named for the French mathematician who derived it, Siméon D. Poisson. Like the binomial, the Poisson distribution is a discrete distribution applicable when the outcome is the number of times an event occurs. The **Poisson distribution** can be used to determine the probability of rare events; it gives the probability that an outcome occurs a specified number of times when the number of trials is large and the probability of any one occurrence is small. For instance, the Poisson distribution is used to plan the number of beds a hospital needs in its intensive care unit, the number of ambulances needed on call, or the number of operators needed on a switchboard to ensure that an adequate number of resources is available. It can also be used to model the number of cells in a given volume of fluid, the number of bacterial colonies growing in a certain amount of medium, or the emission of radioactive particles from a specified amount of radioactive material.

Consider a random variable representing the number of times an event occurs in a given time or space interval. Then the probability of exactly X occurrences is given by the formula:

$$P(X) = \frac{\lambda^X e^{-\lambda}}{X!}$$

in which λ (the lowercase Greek letter lambda) is the value of both the mean and the variance of the Poisson distribution, and e is the base of the natural logarithms, equal to 2.718. The term λ is called the parameter of the Poisson distribution, just as n and π are the parameters of the binomial distribution. Only one piece of information, λ, is therefore needed to characterize any given Poisson distribution.

A random variable having a Poisson distribution was used in the Coronary Artery Surgery Study (Rogers et al 1990) summarized in Presenting Problem 4.

The number of hospitalizations for each group of patients (medical and surgical) followed Poisson distributions. This model is appropriate because the chance that a patient goes into the hospital during any one time interval is small and can be assumed to be independent from patient to patient. After mean follow-up of 11 years, the 390 patients randomized to the medical group were hospitalized a total of 1,256 times; the 390 patients randomized to the surgical group were hospitalized a total of 1,487 times. The mean number of hospitalizations for medical patients is 1,256/390 = 3.22, and the mean for the surgical patients is 1,487/390 = 3.81. We can use this information and the formula for the Poisson model to calculate probabilities of numbers of hospitalizations. For example, the probability that a patient in the medical group has zero hospitalizations is

$$P(X = 0) = \frac{3.22^0 e^{-3.22}}{0!}$$

$$= \frac{(1)(0.04)}{1}$$

$$= 0.04$$

The probability that a patient has exactly one hospitalization is

$$P(X = 1) = \frac{3.22^1 e^{-3.22}}{1!}$$

$$= \frac{(3.22)(0.04)}{1}$$

$$= 0.129$$

The calculations for the Poisson distribution when $\lambda = 3.22$ and $X = 0, 1, 2 \ldots, 7$ are given in Table 4–7.

Figure 4–3 is a graph of the Poisson distribution for $\lambda = 3.22$. The mean of the distribution is between 3 and 4 (actually, it is 3.22). Note the slight positive skew of the Poisson distribution; the skew becomes more pronounced as λ becomes smaller.

The Normal (Gaussian) Distribution

We now turn to the most famous probability distribution in statistics, called the normal, or Gaussian, distribution (or bell-shaped curve). The normal curve was first discovered by French mathematician Abraham de Moivre and published in 1733. Two mathematician-astronomers, however, Pierre-Simon Laplace from France and Karl Friedrich Gauss from Germany, were responsible for establishing the scientific principles of the normal distribution. Many consider Laplace to have made the greatest contributions to

Table 4–7. Probabilities for Poisson distribution with $\lambda = 3.22$.

Number of Hospitalizations (x)	3.22^x	$e^{-3.22}$	X!	$P(X)^a$
0	1	0.040	0	0.040
1	3.22	0.040	1	0.129
2	10.37	0.040	2	0.207
3	33.39	0.040	6	0.223
4	107.50	0.040	24	0.179
5	346.16	0.040	120	0.115
6	1114.64	0.040	720	0.062
7	3589.15	0.040	5040	0.028

^{a}Rounded to three decimal places.

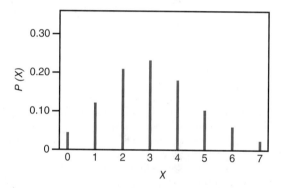

Figure 4–3. Poisson distribution for $\lambda = 3.22$.

probability theory, but Gauss' name was given to the distribution after he applied it to the theory of the motions of heavenly bodies. Some statisticians prefer to use the term *Gaussian* instead of "normal" because the latter term has the unfortunate (and incorrect) connotation that the normal curve describes the way characteristics are distributed in populations composed of "normal"—as opposed to sick—individuals. We use the term "normal" in this text, however, because it is more frequently used in the medical literature.

Describing the Normal Distribution: The normal distribution is continuous, so it can take on any value (not just integers, as do the binomial and Poisson distributions). It is a smooth, bell-shaped curve and is symmetric about the mean of the distribution, symbolized by μ (Greek letter mu). The curve is shown in Figure 4–4. The standard deviation of the distribution is symbolized by σ (Greek letter sigma); σ is the horizontal distance between the mean and the point of inflection on the curve. The point of inflection is the

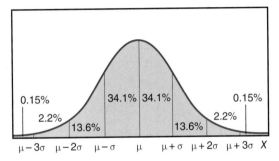

Figure 4–4. Normal distribution and percentage of area under the curve.

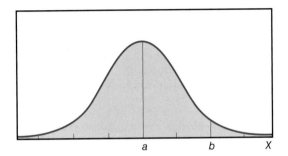

Figure 4–5. Area under a normal curve between *a* and *b*.

point where the curve changes from convex to concave. The mean and the standard deviation (or variance) are the two parameters of the normal distribution and completely determine the location on the number line and the shape of a normal curve. Thus, many different normal curves are possible, one each for every value of the mean and the standard deviation. Because the normal distribution is a probability distribution, the area under the curve is equal to 1. (Recall that one of the properties of probability is that the sum of the probabilities for any given set of events is equal to 1.) Because it is a **symmetric distribution,** half the area is on the left of the mean and half is on the right.

Given a random variable X that can take on any value between negative and positive infinity ($-\infty$ and $+\infty$), (∞ represents infinity), the formula for the normal distribution is as follows:

$$\frac{1}{\sqrt{2\pi\sigma^2}}\exp\left[-\frac{1}{2}\left(\frac{X-\mu}{\sigma}\right)^2\right]$$

where exp stands for the base e of the natural logarithm and $\pi \approx 3.1416$. The function depends only on the mean μ and standard deviation σ because they are the only components that vary.

Because the area under the curve is equal to 1, we can use the curve for calculating probabilities. For example, to find the probability that an observation falls between a and b on the curve in Figure 4–5, we integrate the preceding equation between a and b, where $-\infty$ is given the value a and $+\infty$ is given the value b. (Integration is a mathematical technique in calculus used to find area under a curve.)

The Standard Normal(z) Distribution: Fortunately, there is no need to integrate this function because tables for it are available. So that we do not need a different table for every value of μ and σ. However, we use the **standard normal curve (distribution),** which has a

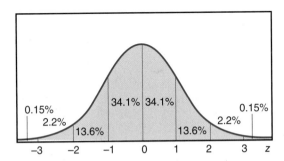

Figure 4–6. Standard normal (z) distribution.

mean of 0 and a standard deviation of 1, as shown in Figure 4–6. This curve is also called the **z distribution.** Table A–2 (see Appendix A) gives the area under the curve between $-z$ and $+z$, the sum of the areas to the left of $-z$ and the right of $+z$, and the area to either the left of $-z$ or the right of $+z$.

Before we use Table A–2, look at the standard normal distribution in Figure 4–6 and estimate the proportion (or percentage) of these areas:

1. Above 1
2. Below −1
3. Above 2
4. Below −2
5. Between −1 and 1
6. Between −2 and 2

Now turn to Table A–2 and find the designated areas. The answers follow.

1. 0.159 of the area is to the right of 1 (from the fourth column in Table A–2).
2. Table A–2 does not list values for z less than 0; however, because the distribution is symmetric about 0, the area below −1 is the same as the area to the right of 1, which is 0.159.

3. 0.023 of the area is to the right of 2 (from the fourth column in Table A–2).

4. The same reasoning as in answer 2 applies here; so 0.023 of the area is to the left of −2.

5. 0.683 of the area is between −1 and 1 (from the second column in Table A–2).

6. 0.954 of the area is between −2 and 2 (from the second column in Table A–2).

When the mean of a Gaussian distribution is not 0 and the standard deviation is not 1, a simple transformation, called the **z transformation,** must be made so that we can use the standard normal table. The z transformation expresses the deviation from the mean in standard deviation units. That is, any normal distribution can be transformed to the standard normal distribution by using the following steps:

1. Move the distribution up or down the number line so that the mean is 0. This step is accomplished by subtracting the mean μ from the value for X.

2. Make the distribution either narrower or wider so that the standard deviation is equal to 1. This step is accomplished by dividing by σ.

To summarize, the transformed value is

$$z = \frac{X - \mu}{\sigma}$$

and is variously called a **z score,** a normal deviate, a standard score, or a **critical ratio.**

Examples Using the Standard Normal Distribution: To illustrate the standard normal distribution, we consider Presenting Problem 2 from Chapter 3. Recall that the topic of that study was an assessment of patient activation. The variable BMI is approximately normally distributed and is used in the following examples. To facilitate computations, we assume BMI in normal healthy individuals is normally distributed with $\mu = 27.5$ and $\sigma = 4.6$. Make the appropriate transformations to answer the following questions. (*Hint:* Make sketches of the distribution to be sure you are finding the correct area.)

1. What area of the curve is above 32.1?

2. What area of the curve is above 36.7?

3. What area of the curve is between 18.3 and 36.7?

4. What area of the curve is above 41.3?

5. What area of the curve is either below 13.7 or above 41.3?

6. What is the value of BMI that divides the area under the curve into the lower 95% and the upper 5%?

7. What is the value of BMI that divides the area under the curve into the lower 97.5% and the upper 2.5%?

The answers, referring to the sketches in Figure 4–7, are shown in the following list.

1. $z = (32.1 - 27.5)/4.6 = 1.00$, and the area above 1.00 is 0.159. So 15.9% of normal healthy individuals have a BMI above 1 standard deviation (>32.1).

2. $z = (36.7 - 27.5)/4.6 = 2.00$, and the area above 2.00 is 0.023. So 2.3% have a BMI above 2 standard deviations (>36.7).

3. $z_1 = (18.3 - 27.5)/4.6 = -2.00$, and $z_2 = (36.7 - 27.5)/4.6 = 2.00$; the area between −2 and +2 is 0.954. So 95.4% have a systolic BP between −2 and +2 standard deviations (between 18.3 and 36.7).

4. $z = (41.3 - 27.5)/4.6 = 3.00$, and the area above 3.00 is 0.001. So only 0.1% have a BMI above 3 standard deviations (>41.3).

5. $z_1 = (13.7 - 27.5)/4.6 = -3.00$, and $z_2 = 3.00$; the area below −3 and above +3 is 0.003. So only 0.3% have a BMI either below or above 3 standard deviations (<13.7 or >41.3).

6. This problem is a bit more difficult and must be worked backward. The value of z, obtained from Table A–2, that divides the lower 0.95 of the area from the upper 0.05 is 1.645. Substituting this value for z in the formula and solving for X yields

$$z = \frac{X - \mu}{\sigma}$$

$$1.645 = \frac{X - 27.5}{4.6}$$

$$X = 1.645 \times 4.6 + 27.5 = 35.06$$

A BMI of 35.06 is therefore at the 95th percentile. So 95% of normal, healthy people have a BMI of 35.06 or lower.

7. Working backward again, we obtain the value 1.96 for z. Substituting and solving for X yields

$$1.96 = \frac{X - 120}{10}$$

$$19.6 = X - 120$$

$$139.6 = X$$

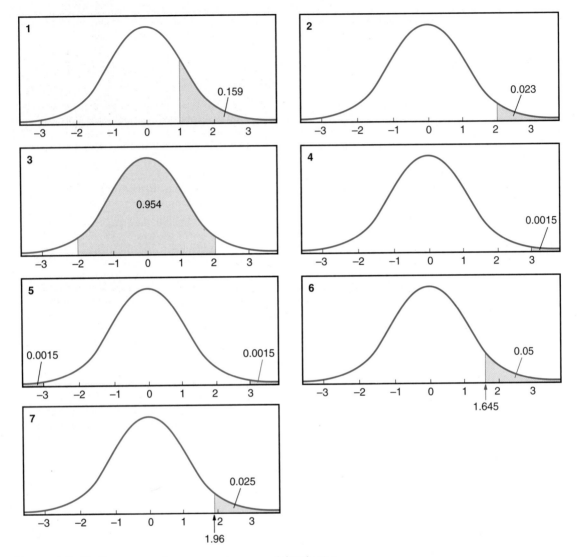

Figure 4–7. Finding areas under a curve using normal distribution.

$$1.96 = \frac{X - 27.5}{4.6}$$

$$X = 1.96 \times 4.6 + 27.5 = 36.52$$

Thus, a BMI of 36.52 divides the distribution of normal, healthy individuals into the lower 97.5% and the upper 2.5%.

From the results of the previous exercises, we can state some important guidelines for using the normal distribution. As mentioned in Chapter 3, the normal distribution has the following distinguishing features:

1. The mean ± 1 standard deviation contains approximately 66.7% of the area under the normal curve.

2. The mean ± 2 standard deviations contains approximately 95% of the area under the normal curve.

3. The mean ± 3 standard deviations contains approximately 99.7% of the area under the normal curve.

Although these features indicate that the normal distribution is a valuable tool in statistics, its value goes beyond merely describing distributions. In actuality, few characteristics are normally distributed. In some populations, data are positively skewed: More people are found with BMI above 27.5 than below. Elveback and coworkers (1970) showed that many common laboratory values are not normally distributed; consequently, using the mean ±2 SD may cause substantially more or less than 5% of the population to lie outside 2 standard deviations. Used judiciously, however, the three guidelines are good rules of thumb about characteristics that have approximately normal distributions.

The major importance of the normal distribution is in the role it plays in statistical inference. In the next section, we show that the normal distribution forms the basis for making statistical inferences even when the population is not normally distributed. The following point is very important and will be made several times: Statistical inference generally involves mean values of a population, not values related to individuals. The examples we just discussed deal with individuals and, if we are to make probability statements about individuals using the mean and standard deviation rules, the distribution of the characteristic of interest must be approximately normally distributed.

SAMPLING DISTRIBUTIONS

We just learned that the binomial, Poisson, and normal distributions can be used to determine how likely it is that any specific measurement is in the population. Now we turn to another type of distribution, called a **sampling distribution,** that is very important in statistics. Understanding sampling distributions is essential for grasping the logic underlying the prototypical statements from the literature. After we have a basic comprehension of sampling distributions, we will have the tools to learn about **estimation** and **hypothesis testing,** methods that permit investigators to generalize study results to the population that the sample represents. Throughout, we assume that the sample has been selected using one of the proper methods of random sampling discussed in the section titled, "Populations and Samples."

The distribution of individual observations is very different from the distribution of means, which is called a **sampling distribution.** Gelber and colleagues (1997) collected data on heart rate variation to deep breathing and the Valsalva ratio in order to establish population norms. A national sample of 490 subjects was the basis of establishing norm values for heart rate variation, but clearly the authors wished to generalize from this sample to all healthy adults. If another sample of 490 healthy individuals were evaluated, it is unlikely that exactly this distribution would be observed.

Although the focus in this study was on the normal range, defined by the central 95% of the observed distribution, the researchers were also interested in the mean heart rate variation. The mean in another sample is likely to be less (or more) than the 50.17 observed in their sample, and they might wish to know how much the mean can be expected to differ. To find out, they could randomly select many samples from the target population of patients, compute the mean in each sample, and then examine the distribution of means to estimate the amount of variation that can be expected from one sample to another. This distribution of means is called the **sampling distribution** of the mean. It would be very tedious, however, to have to take many samples in order to estimate the variability of the mean. The sampling distribution of the mean has several desirable characteristics, not the least of which is that it permits us to answer questions about a mean with only one sample.

In the following section, we use a simple hypothetical example to illustrate how a sampling distribution can be generated. Then we show that we need not generate a sampling distribution in practice; instead, we can use statistical theory to answer questions about a single observed mean.

The Sampling Distribution of the Mean

Four features define a sampling distribution. The first is the statistic of interest, for example, the mean, standard deviation, or proportion. Because the sampling distribution of the mean plays such a key role in statistics, we use it to illustrate the concept. The second defining feature is a random selection of the sample. The third—and very important—feature is the size of the random sample. The fourth feature is specification of the population being sampled.

To illustrate, suppose a physician is trying to decide whether to begin mailing reminders to patients who have waited more than a year to schedule their annual examination. The physician reviews the files of all patients who came in for an annual checkup during the past month and determines how many months had passed since their previous visit. To keep calculations simple, we use a very small population size of five patients. Table 4–8 lists the number of months since the last examination for the five patients in this population. The following discussion presents details about generating and using a sampling distribution for this example.

Generating a Sampling Distribution: To generate a sampling distribution from the population of five patients, we select all possible samples of two patients per sample and calculate the mean number of months

Table 4–8. Population of months since last examination.

Patient	Number of Months Since Last Examination
1	12
2	13
3	14
4	15
5	16

Table 4–9. Twenty-five samples of size 2 patients each.

Sample	Patients Selected	Number of Months for Each	Mean
1	1, 1	12, 12	12.0
2	1, 2	12, 13	12.5
3	1, 3	12, 14	13.0
4	1, 4	12, 15	13.5
5	1, 5	12, 16	14.0
6	2, 1	13, 12	12.5
7	2, 2	13, 13	13.0
8	2, 3	13, 14	13.5
9	2, 4	13, 15	14.0
10	2, 5	13, 16	14.5
11	3, 1	14, 12	13.0
12	3, 2	14, 13	13.5
13	3, 3	14, 14	14.0
14	3, 4	14, 15	14.5
15	3, 5	14, 16	15.0
16	4, 1	15, 12	13.5
17	4, 2	15, 13	14.0
18	4, 3	15, 14	14.5
19	4, 4	15, 15	15.0
20	4, 5	15, 16	15.5
21	5, 1	16, 12	14.0
22	5, 2	16, 13	14.5
23	5, 3	16, 14	15.0
24	5, 4	16, 15	15.5
25	5, 5	16, 16	16.0

since the last examination for each sample. For a population of five, 25 different possible samples of two can be selected. That is, patient 1 (12 months since last checkup) can be selected as the first observation and returned to the sample; then, patient 1 (12 months), or patient 2 (13 months), or patient 3 (14 months), and so on, can be selected as the second observation. The 25 different possible samples and the mean number of months since the patient's last visit for each sample are given in Table 4–9.

Comparing the Population Distribution with the Sampling Distribution: Figure 4–8 is a graph of the population of patients and the number of months since their last examination. The probability distribution in this population is *uniform,* because every length of time has the same (or uniform) probability of occurrence; because of its shape, this distribution is also referred to as *rectangular.* The mean in this population is 14 months, and the standard deviation is 1.41 months (see Exercise 8).

Figure 4–9 is a graph of the sampling distribution of the mean number of months since the last visit for a sample of size 2. The sampling distribution of means is certainly not uniform; it is shaped somewhat like a pyramid. The following are three important characteristics of this sampling distribution:

1. The mean of the 25 separate means is 14 months, the same as the mean in the population.
2. The variability in the sampling distribution of means is less than the variability in the original population. The standard deviation in the population is 1.41; the standard deviation of the means is 1.00.

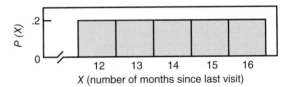

Figure 4–8. Distribution of population values of number of months since last office visit (data from Table 4–8).

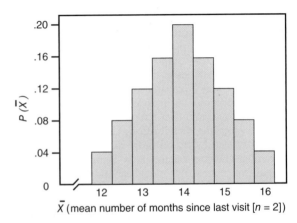

Figure 4–9. Distribution of mean number of months since last office visit for $n = 2$ (data from Table 4–9).

3. The shape of the sampling distribution of means, even for a sample of size 2, is beginning to "approach" the shape of the normal distribution, although the shape of the population distribution is rectangular, not normal.

Using the Sampling Distribution: The sampling distribution of the mean is extremely useful because it allows us to make statements about the probability that specific observations will occur. For example, using the sampling distribution in Figure 4–9, we can ask questions such as "If the mean number of months since the previous checkup is really 14, how likely is a random sample of $n = 2$ patients in which the mean is 15 or more months?" From the sampling distribution, we see that a mean of 15 or more can occur 6 times out of 25, or 24% of the time. A random sample with a mean of 15 or more is, therefore, not all that unusual.

In medical studies, the sampling distribution of the mean can answer questions such as "If there really is no difference between the therapies, how often would the observed outcome (or something more extreme) occur simply by chance?"

The Central Limit Theorem

Generating the sampling distribution for the mean each time an investigator wants to ask a statistical question would be too time-consuming, but this process is not necessary. Instead, statistical theory can be used to determine the sampling distribution of the mean in any particular situation. These properties of the sampling distribution are the basis for one of the most important theorems in statistics, called the central limit theorem. A mathematical proof of the central limit theorem is not possible in this text, but we will advance some empirical arguments that hopefully convince you that the theory is valid. The following list details the features of the **central limit theorem.**

Given a population with mean μ and standard deviation σ, the sampling distribution of the mean based on repeated random samples of size n has the following properties:

1. The mean of the sampling distribution, or the mean of the means, is equal to the population mean μ based on the individual observations.

2. The standard deviation in the sampling distribution of the mean is equal to $\sigma/\sqrt{n}$. This quantity, called the **standard error of the mean (SEM),** plays an important role in many of the statistical procedures discussed in several later chapters. The standard error of the mean is variously written as

$$\sigma_{\bar{x}}, SD_{\bar{x}}, SE_{\bar{x}}, SEM$$

or sometimes simply *SE,* if it is clear the mean is being referred to.

3. If the distribution in the population is normal, then the sampling distribution of the mean is also normal. More importantly, for sufficiently large sample sizes, the sampling distribution of the mean is approximately normally distributed, *regardless* of the shape of the original population distribution.

The central limit theorem is illustrated for four different population distributions in Figure 4–10. In row A, the shape of the population distribution is uniform, or rectangular, as in our example of the number of months since a previous physical examination. Row B is a bimodal distribution in which extreme values of the random variable are more likely to occur than middle values. Results from opinion polls in which people rate their agreement with political issues sometimes have this distribution, especially if the issue polarizes people. Bimodal distributions also occur in biology when two populations are mixed, as they are for ages of people who have Crohn's disease. Modal ages for these populations are mid-20s and late 40s to early 50s. In row C, the distribution is negatively skewed because of some small outlying values. This distribution can model a random variable, such as age of patients diagnosed with breast cancer. Finally, row D is similar to the normal distribution.

The second column of distributions in Figure 4–10 illustrates the sampling distributions of the mean when samples of size 2 are randomly selected from the parent populations. In row A, the pyramid shape is the same as in the example on months since a patient's last examination. Note that, even for the bimodal population distribution in row B, the sampling distribution of means begins to approach the shape of the normal distribution. This bell shape is more evident in the third column of Figure 4–10, in which the sampling distributions are based on sample sizes of 10. Finally, in the fourth row, for sample sizes of 30, all sampling distributions resemble the normal distribution.

A sample of 30 is commonly used as a cutoff value because sampling distributions of the mean based on sample sizes of 30 or more are considered to be normally distributed. A sample this large is not always needed, however. If the parent population is normally distributed, the *means of samples of any size* will be normally distributed. In non-normal parent populations, large sample sizes are required with extremely skewed population distributions; smaller sample sizes can be used with moderately skewed distributions. Fortunately, guidelines about sample sizes have been developed, and they will be pointed out as they arise in our discussion.

Distribution in the Population   Sampling Distribution of the Mean, $\bar{X}$

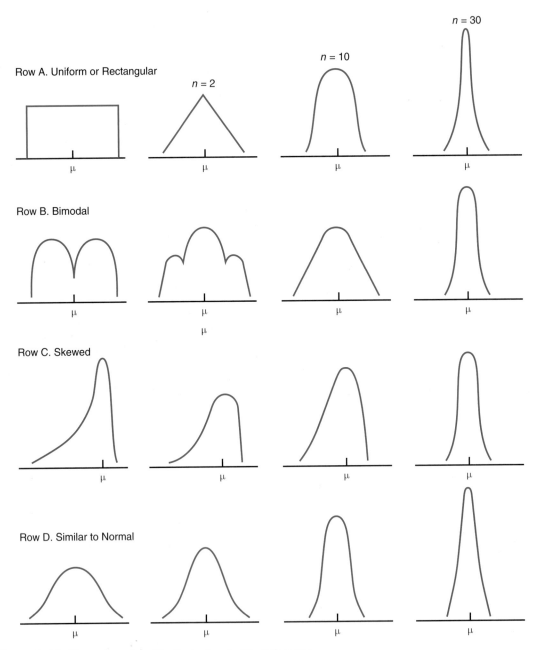

Figure 4–10. Illustration of ramifications of central limit theorem.

In Figure 4–10, also note that in every case the mean of the sampling distributions is the same as the mean of the parent population distribution. The variability of the means decreases as the sample size increases, however, so the standard error of the mean decreases as well. Another feature to note is that the relationship between sample size and standard error of the mean is not linear; it is based on the square root of the sample size, not the sample size itself. It is therefore necessary to quadruple, not double, the sample size in order to reduce the standard error by half.

Points to Remember

Several points deserve reemphasis. In practice, selecting repeated samples of size n and generating a sampling distribution for the mean is not necessary. Instead, only one sample is selected, the sample mean is calculated (as an estimate of the population mean), and, if the sample size is 30 or more, the central limit theorem is invoked to argue that the sampling distribution of the mean is known and does not need to be generated. Then, because the mean has a known distribution, statistical questions can be addressed.

Standard Deviation versus Standard Error: The value σ measures the standard deviation in the population and is based on measurements of individuals. That is, the standard deviation tells us how much variability can be expected among *individuals.* The standard error of the mean, however, is the standard deviation of the means in a sampling distribution; it tells us how much variability can be expected among *means* in future samples.

For example, earlier in this chapter, we used the fact that BMI is approximately normally distributed in normal healthy populations, with mean 27.5 and standard deviation 4.6, to illustrate how areas under the curve are related to probabilities. We also demonstrated that the interval defined by the mean ± 2 SD contains approximately 95% of the individual observations when the observations have a normal distribution. Because the central limit theorem tells us that a sample mean is normally distributed (when the sample size is 30 or more), we can use these same properties to relate areas under the normal curve to probabilities when the sample mean instead of an individual value is of interest. Also, we will soon see that the interval defined by the sample mean ± 2 SE generally contains about 95% of the *means* (not the individuals) that would be observed if samples of the same size were repeatedly selected.

The Use of the Standard Deviation in Research Reports: Authors of research reports sometimes present data in terms of the mean and standard deviation. At other times, authors report the mean and standard error of the mean. This practice is especially prominent in graphs. Although some journal editors now require authors to use the standard deviation (Bartko, 1985), many articles still use the standard error of the mean. There are two reasons for increasing use of the standard deviation instead of the standard error. First, the standard error is a function of the sample size, so it can be made smaller simply by increasing n. Second, the interval (mean ± 2 SE) will contain approximately 95% of the *means* of samples, but it will never contain 95% of the observations on *individuals;* in the latter situation, the mean ± 2 SD is needed. By definition, the standard error pertains to means, not to individuals. When physicians consider applying research results, they generally wish to apply them to individuals in their practice, not to groups of individuals. The standard deviation is, therefore, generally the more appropriate measure to report.

Other Sampling Distributions: Statistics other than the mean, such as standard deviations, medians, proportions, and correlations, also have sampling distributions. In each case, the statistical issue is the same: How can the statistic of interest be expected to vary across different samples of the same size?

Although the sampling distribution of the mean is approximately normally distributed, the sampling distributions of most other statistics are not. In fact, the sampling distribution of the mean assumes that the value of the population standard deviation σ is known. In actuality, it is rarely known; therefore, the population standard deviation is estimated by the sample standard deviation SD, and the SD is used in place of the population value in the calculation of the standard error; that is, the standard error in the population is estimated by

$$SE_{\bar{x}} = \frac{SD}{\sqrt{n}}$$

When the SD is used, the sampling distribution of the mean actually follows a **t distribution** instead of the normal distribution. This important distribution is similar to the normal distribution and is discussed in detail in Chapters 5 and 6.

As other examples, the sampling distribution of the ratio of two variances (squared standard deviations) follows an **F distribution,** a theoretical distribution presented in Chapters 6 and 7. The proportion, which is based on the binomial distribution, is normally distributed under certain circumstances, as we shall see in Chapter 5. For the correlation to follow the normal distribution, a transformation must be applied, as illustrated in Chapter 8. Nevertheless, one property that all sampling distributions have in common is having a standard error, and the variation of the statistic in its sampling distribution is called the standard error of the statistic. Thus, the standard error of the mean is just one of many standard errors, albeit the one most commonly used in medical research.

Applications Using the Sampling Distribution of the Mean

Let us turn to some applications of the concepts introduced so far in this chapter. Recall that the **critical ratio** (or z score) transforms a normally distributed random variable with mean μ and standard deviation σ to the standard normal (z) distribution with mean 0 and standard deviation 1 by subtracting the mean and dividing by the standard deviation:

$$z = \frac{X - \mu}{\sigma}$$

When we are interested in the mean rather than individual observations, the mean itself is the entity transformed. According to the central limit theorem, the mean of the sampling distribution is still μ, but the standard deviation of the mean is the standard error of the mean. The critical ratio that transforms a mean to have distribution with mean 0 and standard deviation 1 is, therefore,

$$z = \frac{\bar{X} - \mu}{\sigma/\sqrt{n}}$$

The use of the critical ratio is illustrated in the following examples.

Example 1: Suppose a health care provider studies a randomly selected group of 25 men and women between 20 and 39 years of age and finds that their mean systolic BP is 124 mm Hg. How often would a sample of 25 patients have a mean systolic BP this high or higher? If we assume that systolic BP is a normally distributed random variable with a known mean of 120 mm Hg and a standard deviation of 10 mm Hg in the population of normal healthy adults. The provider's question is equivalent to asking: If repeated samples of 25 individuals are randomly selected from the population, what proportion of samples will have *mean* values greater than 124 mm Hg?

Solution: The sampling distribution of the mean is normal because the population of BPs is normally distributed. The mean is 120 mm Hg, and the SE (based on the known standard deviation) is equal to $\bar{X} = 10/5 = 2$. Therefore, the critical ratio is

$$z = \frac{124 - 120}{10/\sqrt{25}} = \frac{4}{2} = 2.0$$

From column 4 of Table A–2 (Appendix A) for the normal curve, the proportion of the z distribution area above 2.0 is 0.023; therefore, 2.3% of random samples

with $n = 25$ can be expected to have a mean systolic BP of 124 mm Hg or higher. Figure 4–11A illustrates how the distribution of means is transformed to the critical ratio.

Example 2: Suppose a health care provider wants to detect adverse effects on systolic BP in a random sample of 25 patients using a drug that causes vasoconstriction. The provider decides that a mean systolic BP in the upper 5% of the distribution is cause for alarm; therefore, the provider must determine the value that divides the upper 5% of the sampling distribution from the lower 95%.

Solution: The solution to this example requires working backward from the area under the standard normal curve to find the value of the mean. The value of z that divides the area into the lower 95% and the upper 5% is 1.645 (we find 0.05 in column 4 of Table A–2 and read 1.645 in column 1). Substituting this value for z in the critical ratio and then solving for the mean yields

$$1.645 = \frac{(\bar{X} - 120)}{10/\sqrt{25}} = \frac{\bar{X} - 120}{2}$$

$$\text{and} \quad (1.645)(2) + 120 = \bar{X} \quad \text{or} \quad \bar{X} = 123.29$$

A mean systolic BP of 123.29 is the value that divides the sampling distribution into the lower 95% and the upper 5%. So, there is cause for alarm if the mean in the sample of 25 patients surpasses this value (see Figure 4–11B).

Example 3: Continuing with Examples 1 and 2, suppose the health care provider does not know how many patients should be included in a study of the drug's effect. After some consideration, the provider decides that, 90% of the time, the mean systolic BP in the sample of patients must not rise above 122 mm Hg. How large a random sample is required so that 90% of the means in samples of this size will be 122 mm Hg or less?

Solution: The answer to this question requires determining n so that only 10% of the sample means exceed $\mu = 120$ by 2 or more, that is, $X - \mu = 2$. The value of z in Table A–2 that divides the area into the lower 90% and the upper 10% is 1.28. Using $z = 1.28$ and solving for n yields

$$1.28 = \frac{122 - 120}{10/\sqrt{n}} = \frac{(2)(\sqrt{n})}{10}$$

Therefore,

$$\frac{(1.28)(10)}{2} = \sqrt{n} \quad \text{or} \quad \sqrt{n} = 6.40$$

$$\text{and} \quad n = 6.40^2 = 40.96$$

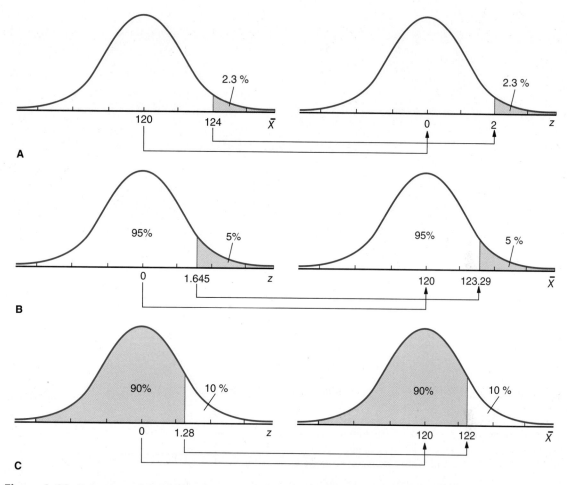

Figure 4–11. Using normal distribution to draw conclusions about systolic BP in healthy adults.

Thus, a random sample of 41 individuals is needed for a sampling distribution of means in which no more than 10% of the mean systolic BPs are above 122 mm Hg (see Figure 4–11C).

Example 4: A study based on a sample of 580 individuals found a mean heart rate variation of 49.7 beats/min with a standard deviation of 23.4. What proportion of *individuals* can be expected to have a heart rate variation between 27 and 73, assuming a normal distribution?

Solution: This question involves individuals, and the critical ratio for individual values of X must be used. To simplify calculations, we round off the mean to 50 and the standard deviation to 23. The transformed values of the z distribution for $X = 27$ and $X = 73$ are

$$z = \frac{X - \mu}{\sigma} = \frac{27 - 50}{23} = \frac{-23}{23} = 1.00$$

$$\text{and} \quad z = \frac{X - \mu}{\sigma} = \frac{73 - 50}{23} = \frac{23}{23} = 1.00$$

The proportion of area under the normal curve between -1 and $+1$, from Table A–2, column 2, is 0.683. Therefore, 68.3% of normal healthy individuals can be expected to have a heart rate variation between 27 and 73 (Figure 4–12A).

Example 5: If repeated samples of six healthy individuals are randomly selected in the Example 4, what proportion will have a *mean* Po_2 between 27 and 73 beats/min?

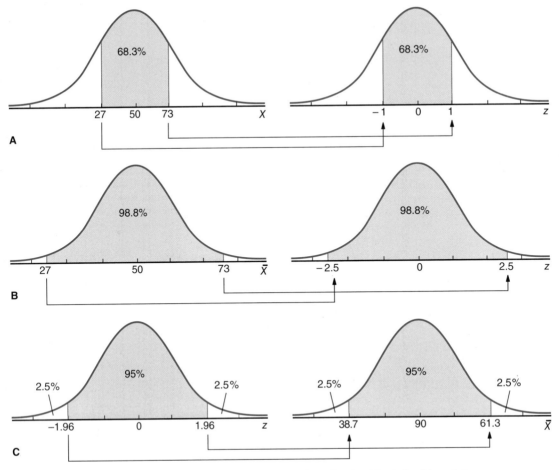

Figure 4–12. Using normal distribution to draw conclusions about levels of Po_2 in healthy adults.

Solution: This question concerns means, not individuals, so the critical ratio for means must be used to find appropriate areas under the curve. For $\bar{X} = 27$,

$$Z = \frac{\bar{X} - \mu}{\sigma/\sqrt{n}}$$

$$= \frac{27 - 50}{23/\sqrt{6}}$$

$$= \frac{-23}{23/2.5}$$

$$= -2.5$$

Similarly, for $\bar{X} = 73$, $z = +2.5$. We must, therefore, find the area between -2.5 and $+2.5$. From Table A–2, the area is 0.988. Therefore, 98.8% of the area lies

between ± 2.5, and 98.8% of the mean heart rate variation values in samples with six subjects will fall between 27 and 73 beats/min (see Figure 4–12B).

Examples 4 and 5 illustrate the contrast between drawing conclusions about individuals and drawing conclusions about means.

Example 6: For 100 healthy individuals in repeated samples, what proportion of the samples will have mean values between 27 and 73 beats/min?

Solution: We will not do computations for this example; from the previous calculations, we can see that the proportion of means is very large. (The z values are ± 10, which go beyond the scale of Table A–2.)

Example 7: What mean value of heart rate variation divides the sampling distribution for 16 individuals into the central 95% and the upper and lower 2.5%?

Solution: The value of z is ± 1.96 from Table A–2. First we substitute -1.96 in the critical ratio to get

$$-1.96 = \frac{\bar{X} - 50}{23/\sqrt{16}} \quad \text{and} \quad -1.96\left(\frac{23}{4}\right)$$

$$+50 = 38.73 = \bar{X}$$

Similarly, using $+1.96$ gives $X = 61.27$. Thus, 61.27 beats/min divides the upper 2.5% of the sampling distribution of heart rate variation from the remainder of the distribution, and 38.73 beats/min divides the lower 2.5% from the remainder (see Figure 4–12C).

Example 8: What size sample is needed to ensure that 95% of the sample means for heart rate variation will be within 3 beats/min of the population mean?

Solution: To obtain the central 95% of any normal distribution, we use $z = 1.96$, as in Example 7. Substituting 1.96 into the formula for z and solving for n yields

$$1.96 = \frac{3}{23/\sqrt{n}} \quad \text{or} \quad \sqrt{n} = \frac{(1.96)(23)}{3} = 15.03$$

$$\text{and} \quad n = (15.03)^2 = 225.8, \quad \text{or} \quad 226$$

Thus, a sample of 226 individuals is needed to ensure that 95% of the sample means are within 3 beats/min of the population mean. Note that sample sizes are always rounded up to the next whole number.

These examples illustrate how the normal distribution can be used to draw conclusions about distributions of individuals and of means. Although some questions were deliberately contrived to illustrate the concepts, the important point is to understand the logic involved in these solutions. The exercises provide additional practice in solving problems of these types.

ESTIMATION & HYPOTHESIS TESTING

We discussed the process of making inferences from data in this chapter, and now we can begin to illustrate the inference process itself. There are two approaches to statistical inference: estimating parameters and testing hypotheses.

The Need for Estimates

Suppose we wish to evaluate the relationship between toxic reactions to drugs and fractures resulting from falls among elderly patients. For logistic and economic reasons, we cannot study the entire population of elderly patients to determine the proportion who have toxic drug reactions and fractures. Instead, we conduct a cohort study with a random sample of elderly patients followed for a specified period. The proportion of patients in the sample who experience drug reactions and fractures can be determined and used as an estimate of the proportion of drug reactions and fractures in the population; that is, the sample proportion is an estimate of the population proportion π.

In another study, we may be interested in the mean rather than the proportion, so the mean in the sample is used as an estimate of the mean population μ. For example, in a study of a low-calorie diet for weight loss, suppose the mean weight loss in a random sample of patients is 20 lb; this value is an estimate of the mean weight loss in the population of subjects represented by the sample.

Both the sample proportion and the sample mean are called **point estimates** because they involve a specific number rather than an interval or a range. Other point estimates are the sample standard deviation SD as an estimate of σ and the sample correlation r as an estimate of the population correlation ρ.

Properties of Good Estimates

A good estimate should have certain properties; one is that it should be **unbiased,** meaning that systematic error does not occur. Recall that when we developed a sampling distribution for the mean, we found that the mean of the mean values in the sampling distribution is equal to the population mean. Thus, the mean of a sampling distribution of means is an unbiased estimate. Both the mean and the median are unbiased estimates of the population mean μ. However, the sample standard deviation SD is not an unbiased estimate of the population standard deviation σ if n is used in the denominator. Recall that the formula for SD uses $n - 1$ in the denominator (see Chapter 3). Using n in the denominator of SD produces an estimate of σ that is systematically too small; using $n - 1$ makes the SD an unbiased estimate of σ.

Another property of a good estimate is small variability from one sample to another; this property is called *minimum variance.* One reason the mean is used more often than the median as a measure of central tendency is that the standard error of the median is approximately 25% larger than the standard error of the mean when the distribution of observations is approximately normal. Thus, the median has greater variability from one sample to another, and the chances are greater, in any one sample, of obtaining a median value that is farther away from the population mean than the sample mean. For this reason, the mean is the recommended statistic when the distribution of observations follows a normal distribution. (If the distribution of observations is quite skewed, however, the median is the better statistic, as we discussed in Chapter 3, because the median has minimum variance in skewed distributions.)

Confidence Intervals and Confidence Limits: Sometimes, instead of giving a simple point estimate, investigators wish to indicate the variability the estimate would have in other samples. To indicate this variability, they use interval estimates. A shortcoming of point estimates, such as a mean weight loss of 20 lb, is that they do not have an associated probability indicating how likely the value is. In contrast, we can associate a probability with interval estimates, such as the interval from, say, 15 to 25 lb. Interval estimates are called **confidence intervals;** they define an upper limit (25 lb) and a lower limit (15 lb) with an associated probability. The ends of the confidence interval (15 and 25 lb) are called the **confidence limits.**

Confidence intervals can be established for any population parameter. You may commonly encounter confidence intervals for the mean, proportion, relative risk, odds ratio, and correlation, as well as for the difference between two means, two proportions, and so on. Confidence intervals for these parameters will be introduced in subsequent chapters.

Hypothesis Testing

As with estimation and confidence limits, the purpose of a **hypothesis test** is to permit generalizations from a sample to the population from which it came. Both statistical hypothesis testing and estimation make certain assumptions about the population and then use probabilities to estimate the likelihood of the results obtained in the sample, given the assumptions about the population. Again, both assume a random sample has been properly selected.

Statistical hypothesis testing involves stating a null hypothesis and an alternative hypothesis and then doing a statistical test to see which hypothesis should be concluded. Generally the goal is to disprove the null hypothesis and accept the alternative. Like the term "probability," the term "hypothesis" has a more precise meaning in statistics than in everyday use, as we will see in the following chapters.

The next several chapters will help clarify the ideas presented in this chapter, because we shall reiterate the concepts and illustrate the process of estimation and hypothesis testing using a variety of published studies. Although these concepts are difficult to understand, they become easier with practice.

SUMMARY

This chapter focused on several concepts that explain why the results of one study involving a certain set of subjects can be used to draw conclusions about other similar subjects. These concepts include probability, sampling, probability distributions, and sampling distributions. We began with examples to illustrate how the rules for calculating probabilities can help us determine the distribution of characteristics in samples of people (e.g., the distribution of blood types in men and women; the distribution of heart rate variation).

The addition rule, multiplication rule, and modifications of these rules for nonmutually exclusive and nonindependent events were also illustrated. The addition rule is used to add the probabilities of two or more mutually exclusive events. If the events are not mutually exclusive, the probability of their joint occurrence must be subtracted from the sum. The multiplication rule is used to multiply the probabilities of two or more independent events. If the events are not independent, they are said to be conditional; Bayes' theorem is used to obtain the probability of conditional events. Application of the multiplication rule allowed us to conclude that gender and blood type are independently distributed in humans. The site of infection, however, was not independent from the time during an epidemic at which an individual contracted serogroup B meningococcal disease.

The advantages and disadvantages of different methods of random sampling were illustrated for a study involving the measurement of tracheal diameters. A simple random sample was obtained by randomly selecting radiographs corresponding to random numbers taken from a random number table. Systematic sampling was illustrated by selecting each 17th x-ray film. We noted that systematic sampling is easy to use and is appropriate as long as there is no cyclical component to the data. Radiographs from different age groups were used to illustrate stratified random sampling. Stratified sampling is the most efficient method and is, therefore, used in many large studies. In clinical trials, investigators must randomly assign patients to experimental and control conditions (rather than randomly select patients) so that biases threatening the validity of the study conclusions are minimized.

Three important probability distributions were presented: binomial, Poisson, and normal (Gaussian). The binomial distribution is used to model events that have a binary outcome (i.e., either the outcome occurs or it does not) and to determine the probability of outcomes of interest. We used the binomial distribution to obtain the probabilities that a specified number of men with localized prostate tumor survive at least 5 years.

The Poisson distribution is used to determine probabilities for rare events. In the CASS study of coronary artery disease, hospitalization of patients during the 10-year follow-up period was relatively rare. We calculated the probability of hospitalization for patients randomly assigned to medical treatment. Exercise 5 asks for calculations for similar probabilities for the surgical group.

The normal distribution is used to determine the probability of characteristics measured on a continuous numerical scale. When the distribution of the characteristics is approximately bell-shaped, the normal distribution can be used to show how representative or extreme an observation is. the normal distribution was used to determine percentages of the population expected to have systolic BPs above and below certain levels. The level of systolic BP that divides the population of normal, healthy adults into the lower 95% and the upper 5% was identified using the normal distribution tables.

Estimation and hypothesis testing are two methods for making inferences about a value in a population of subjects by using observations from a random sample of subjects. In subsequent chapters, we illustrate both confidence intervals and hypothesis tests. We also demonstrate the consistency of conclusions drawn regardless of the approach used.

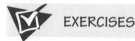

EXERCISES

1. a. Show that gender and blood type are independent; that is, that the joint probability is the product of the two marginal probabilities for each cell in Table 4–2.

   b. What happens if you use the multiplication rule with conditional probability when two events are independent? Use the gender and blood type data for males, type O, to illustrate this point.

2. The term "aplastic anemia" refers to a severe pancytopenia (anemia, neutropenia, thrombocytopenia) resulting from an acellular or markedly hypocellular bone marrow. Patients with severe disease have a high risk of dying from bleeding or infections. Allogeneic bone marrow transplantation is probably the treatment of choice for patients under 40 years of age with severe disease who have a human leukocyte antigen (HLA)-matched donor.
   Researchers reported results of bone marrow transplantation into 50 patients with severe aplastic anemia who did not receive a

transfusion of blood products until just before the marrow transplantation (Anasetti et al 1986). The probability of 10-year survival in this group of nontransfused patients was 82%; the survival rate was 43–50% for patients studied earlier who had received multiple transfusions. Table 4–10 gives the incidence of acute graft-versus-host disease, chronic graft-versus-host disease, and death in subgroups of patients defined according to serum titers of antibodies to cytomegalovirus from this study. Use the table to answer the following questions.

   a. What is the probability of chronic graft-versus-host disease?

   b. What is the probability of acute graft-versus-host disease?

   c. If a patient seroconverts, what is the probability that the patient has acute graft-versus-host disease?

   d. How likely is it that a patient who died was seropositive?

   e. What proportion of patients was seronegative? If this value were the actual proportion in the population, how likely would it be for 4 of 8 new patients to be seronegative?

3. Refer to Table 4–1 on the 48,291 patients for the distribution of flu virus A and B. Assume a patient is selected at random from the patients in this study.

   a. What is the probability a patient selected at random had flu virus A?

   b. What is the probability a patient selected at random the age group 25–64 years old had flu virus B?

4. A plastic surgeon wants to compare the number of successful skin grafts in her series of burn patients with the number in other burn patients. A literature survey indicates that approximately 30% of the grafts become infected but that 80% survive. She has had 7 of 8 skin grafts survive in her series of patients and has had one infection.

   a. How likely is only 1 out of 8 infections?

   b. How likely is survival in 7 of 8 grafts?

5. Use the Poisson distribution to estimate the probability that a surgical patient would have five hospitalizations in 10 years of follow-up if a sample of 390 surgical patients had a total of 1,487 hospitalizations.

6. The values of serum sodium in healthy adults approximately follow a normal distribution with

a mean of 141 mEq/L and a standard deviation of 3 mEq/L.

  a. What is the probability that a normal healthy adult will have a serum sodium value above 147 mEq/L?

  b. What is the probability that a normal healthy adult will have a serum sodium value below 130 mEq/L?

  c. What is the probability that a normal healthy adult will have a serum sodium value between 132 and 150 mEq/L?

  d. What serum sodium level is necessary to put someone in the top 1% of the distribution?

  e. What serum sodium level is necessary to put someone in the bottom 10% of the distribution?

7. Calculate the binomial distribution for each set of parameters: $n = 6$, $\pi = 0.1$; $n = 6$, $\pi = 0.3$; $n = 6$, $\pi = 0.5$. Draw a graph of each distribution, and state your conclusions about the shapes.

8. a. Calculate the mean and the standard deviation of the number of months since a patient's last office visit from Table 4–8.

  b. Calculate the mean and the standard deviation of the sampling distribution of the mean number of months from Table 4–9. Verify that the standard deviation in the sampling distribution of means (SE) is equal to the standard deviation in the population (found in part A) divided by the square root of the sample size, 2.

9. Assume that serum chloride has a mean of 100 mEq/L and a standard deviation of 3 in normal healthy populations.

  a. What proportion of the population has serum chloride levels greater than 103 and less than 97 mEq/L?

  b. If repeated samples of 36 were selected, what proportion of them would have means less than 99 and greater than 101 mEq/L?

10. The relationship between alcohol consumption and psoriasis is unclear. Some studies have suggested that psoriasis is more common among people who are heavy alcohol drinkers, but this opinion is not universally accepted. To clarify the nature of the association between alcohol intake and psoriasis, Poikolainen and colleagues (1990) undertook a case–control study of patients between the ages of 19 and 50 who were seen in outpatient clinics. Cases were men who had psoriasis, and controls were men who had other skin diseases. Subjects completed questionnaires assessing their life styles and alcohol consumption for the 12 months before

Table 4–10. Incidence of graft-versus-host disease.

Condition	Sero-negative[a]	Sero-converters[b]	Sero-positive[c]
Acute graft-versus-host disease	$\frac{6}{17}$	$\frac{2}{18}$	$\frac{2}{12}$
Chronic graft-versus-host disease	$\frac{7}{17}$	$\frac{3}{18}$	$\frac{2}{12}$
Death	$\frac{3}{17}$	$\frac{3}{18}$	$\frac{2}{12}$

[a]Patients who had titers of less than 1:8 before transplant and never showed consistent titer increases. One patient received marrow from a cytomegalovirus seropositive donor and 16 patients, from seronegative donors.
[b]Initially seronegative patients who became seropositive within 100 days after transplant. Six patients received marrow from cytomegalovirus seropositive donors and 10 from cytomegalovirus seronegative donors. Serum titers in 2 donors were not determined for antibodies to cytomegalovirus.
[c]Patients with titers of more than 1:8 before transplant. Within this group, seven patients had fourfold increases in serum titers of antibodies to cytomegalovirus and one other patient showed cultures of virus within 3 months of transplantation. Two of the eight patients developed acute graft-versus-host disease, one had chronic graft-versus-host disease, and one died.
Reproduced with permission from Anasetti C, Doney KC, Storb R, et al: Marrow transplantation for severe aplastic anemia. Long-term outcome in fifty "untransfused" patients, *Ann Intern Med.* 1986 Apr;104(4):461–466.

Table 4–11. Alcohol intake (g/day) and frequency of intoxication (times/year) before onset of skin disease among patients with psoriasis and controls.

	Mean	SEM	Number of Cases	p value[a]
Alcohol intake:				
Patients with psoriasis	42.9	7.2	142	0.004
Controls	21.0	2.1	265	
Frequency of intoxication				
Patients with psoriasis	61.6	6.2	131	0.007
Controls	42.6	3.3	247	

[a]Two-sided *t*-test; separate variance estimate.
Reproduced with permission from Poikolainen K, Reunala T, Karvonen J, et al: Alcohol intake: a risk factor for psoriasis in young and middle aged men? *BMJ.* 1990 Mar 24;300(6727):780–783.

the onset of disease and for the 12 months immediately before the study. Use the information in Table 4–11 on the frequency of intoxication among patients with psoriasis.

a. What is the probability a patient selected at random from the group of 131 will be intoxicated more than twice a week, assuming the standard deviation is the actual population value σ? Hint: Remember to convert the standard error to the standard deviation.

b. How many times a year would a patient need to be intoxicated in order to be in the top 5% of all patients?

11. The Association of American Medical Colleges reported that the debt in 2002 for graduates from U.S. medical schools was: mean $104,000 and median $100,000; 5% of the graduates had a debt of $200,000 or higher. Assuming debt is normally distributed, what is the approximate value of the standard deviation?

Research Questions About One Group

KEY CONCEPTS

 Three factors help determine whether an observed estimate, such as the mean, is different from a norm: the size of the difference, the degree of variability, and the sample size.

 The t distribution is similar to the z distribution, especially as sample sizes exceed 30, and t is generally used in medicine when asking questions about means.

 Confidence intervals are common in the literature; they are used to determine the confidence with which we can assume future estimates (such as the mean) will vary in future studies.

 The logic behind statistical hypothesis tests is somewhat backward, generally assuming there is no difference and hoping to show that a difference exists.

 Several assumptions are required to use the t distribution for confidence intervals or hypothesis tests.

 Tests of hypothesis are another way to approach statistical inference; a somewhat rigid approach with six steps is recommended.

 Confidence intervals and statistical tests lead to the same conclusions, but confidence intervals actually provide more information and are being increasingly recommended as the best way to present results.

 In hypothesis testing, we err if we conclude there is a difference when none exists (type I, or α, error), as well as when we conclude there is not a difference when one does exist (type II, or β, error).

 Power is the complement of a type II, or β, error: it is concluding there is a difference when one does exist. Power depends on several factors, including the sample size. It is truly a key concept in statistics because it is critical that researchers have a large enough sample to detect a difference if one exists.

 The p value first assumes that the null hypothesis is true and then indicates the probability of obtaining a result as or more extreme than the one observed. In more straightforward language, the p value is the probability that the observed result occurred by chance alone.

 The z distribution, sometimes called the z approximation to the binomial, is used to form confidence intervals and test hypotheses about a proportion.

 The width of confidence intervals (CI) depends on the confidence value: 99% CI are wider than 95% CI because 99% CI provide greater confidence.

 Paired, or before-and-after, studies are very useful for detecting changes that might otherwise be obscured by variation within subjects, because each subject is their own control.

 Paired studies are analyzed by evaluating the differences themselves. For numerical variables, the paired t test is appropriate.

 The kappa κ statistic is used to compare the agreement between two independent judges or methods when observations are being categorized.

The McNemar test is the counterpart to the paired t test when observations are nominal instead of numerical.

 The sign test can be used to test medians (instead of means) if the distribution of observations is skewed.

 The Wilcoxon signed rank test is an excellent alternative to the paired t test if the observations are not normally distributed.

 To estimate the needed sample size for a study, we need to specify the level of significance (often 0.05), the desired level of power (generally 80%), the size of the difference in order to be of clinical importance, and an estimate of the standard deviation.

 It is possible to estimate sample sizes needed, but it is much more efficient to use one of the statistical power packages, such as GPower.

 PRESENTING PROBLEMS

Presenting Problem 1

Rabago and colleagues (2015) wanted to determine the minimum detectable change in gait patterns under various types of perturbation. They collected data from 20 participants and measured their stride width, step length, and stride time under a number of visual and cognitive distractions.

The article and data may be accessed using the following links:

Rabago CA, Dingwell JB, Wilken JM: Reliability and minimum detectable change of temporal-spatial, kinematic, and dynamic stability measures during perturbed gait. PLOS ONE 2015;10(11):e0142083.

https://doi.org/10.1371/journal.pone.0142083

Rabago CA, Dingwell JB, Wilken JM: Reliability and minimum detectable change of temporal-spatial, kinematic, and dynamic stability measures during perturbed gait. Dryad Digital Repository 2015.

https://doi.org/10.5061/dryad.bn987

Presenting Problem 2

Cerebrospinal fluid (CSF) shunt infections occur in 5–15%. Van Lindert and colleagues (2018) added topical vancomycin to the existing shunt protocol. This study assesses the efficacy of this change in protocol in reducing the infection rate for a number of age cohorts.

The article and data may be accessed using the following links:

van Lindert EJ, Bilsen Mv, Flier Mvd, et al: Topical vancomycin reduces the cerebrospinal fluid shunt infection rate: A retrospective cohort study. PLOS ONE 2018;13(1):e0190249.

https://doi.org/10.1371/journal.pone.0190249

van Lindert EJ, van Bilsen M, van der Flier M, et al: Topical vancomycin reduces the cerebrospinal fluid shunt infection rate: a retrospective cohort study. Dryad Digital Repository 2018.

https://doi.org/10.5061/dryad.ch304

Presenting Problem 3

The study by Dittrich et al (2018) investigated the impact of hypnotic suggestion on knee extensor muscle activity for subjects at rest and after exercise. They recruited 13 volunteers that participated in both control and hypnosis sessions in a random order. They measured maximal voluntary contraction (MVC) force and M-ware amplitude (mV) as the primary outcome variables.

The article and data may be accessed using the following links:

Dittrich N, Agostino D, Antonini Philippe R, Guglielmo LGA, Place N: Effect of hypnotic suggestion on knee extensor neuromuscular properties in resting and fatigued states. PLoS ONE 2018;13(4) e0195437.

https://doi.org/10.1371/journal.pone.0195437

Data:
https://zenodo.org/record/1213604#.XB5n-1xKiUl

Presenting Problem 4

Leone and colleagues (2013) studied the inter-rater agreement for detecting indicators of multiple sclerosis using color-Doppler sonographic studies. This study included 38 patients with multiple sclerosis and 55 controls that were age matched within 5 years. The evaluations were performed by eight sonographers based on five criteria documents by Zamboni (2011).

The article and data may be accessed using the following links:

Leone MA, Raymkulova O, Lucenti A, et al: A reliability study of colour-Doppler sonography for the diagnosis of chronic cerebrospinal venous insufficiency shows low inter-rater agreement. BMJ Open 2013;3(11):e003508.

https://doi.org/10.1136/bmjopen-2013-003508

Leone MA, Raymkulova O, Lucenti A, et al: A reliability study of colour-Doppler sonography for the diagnosis of chronic cerebrospinal venous insufficiency shows low inter-rater agreement. Dryad Digital Repository 2013.

https://doi.org/10.5061/dryad.7k048

PURPOSE OF THE CHAPTER

The methods in Chapter 3 are often called **descriptive statistics** because they help investigators describe and summarize data. Chapter 4 provided the basic probability concepts needed to evaluate data using statistical methods. Without probability theory, researchers could not make statements about populations without studying everyone in the population—clearly an undesirable and often impossible task. The study of **inferential statistics** begins in this chapter; these are the statistical methods used to draw conclusions from a sample and make inferences to the entire population. In all the Presenting Problems in this and future chapters dealing with inferential methods, we assume the investigators selected a random sample of individuals to study from a larger population to which they wanted to generalize.

The focus of this chapter is research questions that involve *one group of subjects* who are measured on one or two occasions. The best statistical approach may depend on the way the research question is posed and the assumptions the researcher is willing to make.

The material reviewing confidence intervals and hypothesis testing in this chapter is intended to introduce the logic behind these two approaches. Some of the traditional topics associated with hypothesis testing are also discussed, such as the errors that can be made, and the interpretation of *p* values. In subsequent chapters, the presentation of the procedures is streamlined, but it is worthwhile to emphasize the details in this chapter to help reinforce the concepts.

Surveys of statistical methods used in journals indicate that the *t* test is one of the most commonly used statistical methods. The percentages of articles that use the *t* test range from 10% to more than 60%. Thiese and colleagues (2015) noted a number of problems in using statistical methods including the *t* test. Thus, being able to evaluate the use of tests comparing means—whether they are used properly and how to interpret the results—is an important skill for medical practitioners.

The presentation here departs from some of the traditional texts and presents formulas in terms of sample statistics rather than population parameters. The formulas that best reflect the concepts rather than the ones that are easiest to calculate are used here, for the very reason that calculations are not the important issue due to the ease of accessing computer programs to perform the calculations.

MEAN IN ONE GROUP WHEN THE OBSERVATIONS ARE NORMALLY DISTRIBUTED

Introduction to Questions About Means

Rabago and colleagues (2015) wanted to determine the minimum detectable change in gait patterns under various types of perturbation. They collected data from 20 participants and measured their stride width, step length, and stride time under a number of conditions. Research questions that may be addressed by this data include: (1) How sure are we that the average step length is 0.68 m? (2) Is the step length of the subjects different under no perturbation (NOP) versus visual perturbation (VIS)? These questions may be answered using the *t* distribution to form confidence limits and perform statistical tests to answer this kind of research questions.

Before discussing research questions involving means, let's think about what it takes to convince us that a mean in a study is significantly different from a norm or population mean. In comparing the mean step length is different with VIS, what evidence is needed to conclude that step length is really different in the VIS group and not just a random occurrence? If the mean step length is much larger or smaller in the NOP group than the mean reported for the VIS group, such as the situation in Figure 5–1A, we will probably conclude that the difference is real. What if the difference is relatively moderate, as is the situation in Figure 5–1B?

What other factors can help us? Figure 5–1B gives a clue: The sample values vary substantially, compared with Figure 5–1A, in which there is less variation. A smaller standard deviation may lead to a real difference, even though the difference is relatively small.

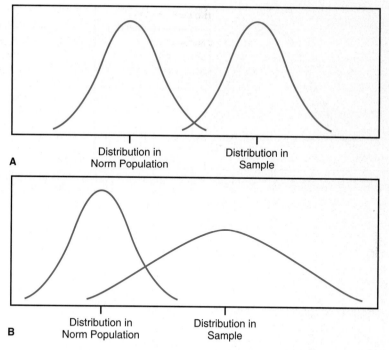

Figure 5–1. Comparison of distributions.

For the variability to be small, subjects must be relatively similar (homogeneous) and the method of measurement must be relatively precise. In contrast, if the characteristic measured varies widely from one person to another or if the measuring device is relatively crude, the standard deviations will be greater, and we will need to observe a greater difference to be convinced that the difference is real and not just a random occurrence.

Another factor is the number of patients included in the sample. Most people have greater intuitive confidence in findings that are based on a larger rather than a smaller sample, and there are sound statistical reasons for this confidence as demonstrated later in this chapter.

To summarize, three factors play a role in deciding whether an observed mean differs from a norm: (1) the difference between the observed mean and the norm, (2) the amount of variability among subjects, and (3) the number of subjects in the study. We will see later in this chapter that the first two factors are important when we want to estimate the needed sample size before beginning a study.

Introduction to the *t* Distribution

The *t* test is used a great deal in all areas of science. The *t* distribution is similar in shape to the *z* distribution introduced in the previous chapter, and one of its major uses is to answer research questions about

means. Because we use the *t* distribution and the *t* test in several chapters, we need a basic understanding of *t*.

The *t* test is sometimes called "Student's *t* test" after the person who first studied the distribution of means from small samples in 1890. Student was really a mathematician named William Gosset who worked for the Guinness Brewery; he was forced to use the pseudonym Student because of company policy prohibiting employees from publishing their work. Gosset discovered that when observations come from a normal distribution, the means are normally distributed *only if the true standard deviation in the population is known.* When the true standard deviation is not known and researchers use the sample standard deviation in its place, the means are no longer normally distributed. Gosset named the distribution of means when the sample standard deviation is used the *t* distribution.

If you think about it, you will recognize that we almost always use samples instead of populations in medical research. As a result, we seldom know the true standard deviation and almost always use the sample standard deviation. Our conclusions are, therefore, more likely to be accurate if we use the *t* distribution rather than the normal distribution, although the difference between *t* and *z* becomes very small when *n* is greater than 30.

The formula (or critical ratio) for the *t* test has the observed mean minus the hypothesized value of the

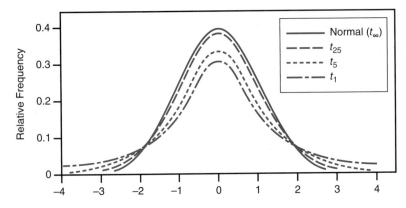

Figure 5–2. *t* distribution with 1, 5, and 25 df and standard normal (*z*) distribution.

population mean (μ) in the numerator, and the standard error of the mean in the denominator. The symbol μ stands for the true mean in the population; it is the Greek letter mu, pronounced "mew." The formula for the *t* test is

$$t = \frac{\bar{X} - \mu}{SD / \sqrt{n}}$$
$$= \frac{\bar{X} - \mu}{SE}$$

We know the standard normal, or *z*, distribution is symmetric with a mean of 0 and a standard deviation of 1. The *t* distribution is also symmetric and has a mean of 0, but its standard deviation is larger than 1. The precise size of the standard deviation depends on a complex concept related to the sample size, called **degrees of freedom (df)**, which is related to the number of times sample information is used. Because sample information is used once to estimate the standard deviation, the *t* distribution for one group, it has $n - 1$ df.

Because the *t* distribution has a larger standard deviation, it is wider and its tails are higher than those for the *z* distribution. As the sample size increases to 30 or more, the df also increases, and the *t* distribution becomes almost the same as the standard normal distribution, and either *t* or *z* can be used. Generally, the *t* distribution is used in medicine, even when the sample size is 30 or greater, and we will follow that practice in this book. Computer programs can be used to generate *t* distributions for different sample sizes in order to compare them, as we did in Figure 5–2.

When using the *t* distribution to answer research questions, we need to find the area under the curve, just as with the *z* distribution. The area can be found by using calculus to integrate a mathematical function, but fortunately we do not need to do

so. Formerly, statisticians used tables (as we do when illustrating some points in this book), but today most of us use computer programs. Table A–3 in Appendix A gives the critical values for the *t* distribution corresponding to areas in the tail of the distribution equal to 0.10, 0.05, 0.02, 0.01, and 0.001 for two-tailed, or two-sided, tests (half that size for one-tailed tests or one-sided tests).

We assume that the observations are normally distributed in order to use the *t* distribution. When the observations are not normally distributed, a nonparametric statistical test, called the sign test, is used instead; see the section titled, "What to Do When Observations Are Not Normally Distributed."

The *t* Distribution and Confidence Intervals About the Mean in One Group

Confidence intervals are used increasingly for research involving means, proportions, and other statistics in medicine, and we will encounter them in subsequent chapters. Thus, it is important to understand the basics. The general format for confidence intervals for one mean is

Observed mean ± (Confidence coefficient)
×(A measure of variability of the mean)

The confidence coefficient is a number related to the level of confidence required; typical values are 90%, 95%, and 99%, with 95% being the most common. Refer to Table A–3 to find the confidence coefficients. For 95% confidence, we want the value that separates the central 95% of the distribution from the 5% in the two tails; with 10 df, this value is 2.228. As the sample size becomes very large, the confidence coefficient for a 95% confidence interval is the same as the *z* distribution, 1.96, as shown in the bottom line of Table A–3. Recall from Chapter 4 that the standard error of the mean (SE) is the standard deviation divided by the square root of the sample size and is used to estimate how much the mean can be expected to vary from one sample to another. Using as the observed (sample) mean, the formula for a 95% confidence interval for the true mean is

$$\bar{X} \pm t\frac{SD}{\sqrt{n}} = \bar{X} \pm t \times SE$$

where t stands for the confidence coefficient (critical value from the t distribution), which, as we saw earlier, depends on the df (which in turn depends on the sample size) and the level of confidence.

Using the data from Rabago and colleagues (2015) in Table 5–1 for step length with no perturbation for male subjects, we discover that the mean is 0.68 m and the standard deviation is 0.04 m. The df for the mean in a single group is $n - 1$, or $20 - 1 = 19$ in

Table 5–1. Stride length.

Subjects	Sex	Age	Height (m)	Weight (kg)	No Perturbation	Physical Perturbation	Cognitive Perturbation	Visual Perturbation
					Stride Length			
1	F	18	1.65	70	0.59	0.57	0.59	0.56
2	M	19	1.803	70.5	0.71	0.67	0.69	0.67
3	M	19	1.78	88	0.70	0.66	0.68	0.68
4	M	19	1.74	77.3	0.71	0.65	0.68	0.61
5	F	31	1.5	75.7	0.62	0.59	0.63	0.60
6	M	26	1.865	82.3	0.71	0.69	0.70	0.69
7	M	23	1.829	95.3	0.67	0.65	0.68	0.66
8	M	19	1.71	72.7	0.64	0.63	0.64	0.61
9	M	28	1.76	96.6	0.70	0.68	0.70	0.67
10	M	30	1.75	77.8	0.71	0.68	0.73	0.70
11	M	23	1.74	81.5	0.67	0.67	0.69	0.65
12	M	28	1.82	91.5	0.74	0.69	0.73	0.69
13	M	32	1.86	82	0.66	0.62	0.67	0.64
14	F	23	1.69	64.5	0.66	0.62	0.67	0.54
15	F	25	1.85	67	0.70	0.63	0.70	0.67
16	F	28	1.68	77.5	0.67	0.63	0.67	0.63
17	M	43	1.63	67	0.61	0.60	0.58	0.56
18	M	23	1.84	72.5	0.71	0.66	0.72	0.69
19	M	25	1.835	87.5	0.65	0.62	0.65	0.63
20	M	39	1.82	82	0.69	0.66	0.68	0.64
Count		20	20	20	20	20	20	20
Mean		26.05	1.76	78.96	0.68	0.64	0.67	0.64
Median		25.00	1.77	77.65	0.68	0.65	0.68	0.64
Standard Dev		6.67	0.09	9.38	0.04	0.03	0.04	0.05

Summary Statistics for Males

Count		15	15	15	15	15	15	15
Mean		26.40	1.79	81.63	0.68	0.65	0.68	0.65
Median		25.00	1.80	82.00	0.70	0.66	0.68	0.66
Standard Dev		7.27	0.06	8.94	0.03	0.03	0.04	0.04

Summary Statistics for Females

Count		5	5	5	5	5	5	5
Mean		25.00	1.67	70.94	0.65	0.61	0.65	0.60
Median		24.00	1.69	68.50	0.66	0.62	0.67	0.59
Standard Dev		4.95	0.12	5.56	0.04	0.03	0.04	0.05

our example. In Table A–3, the value corresponding to 95% confidence limits and 19 degrees of freedom is 2.093. Using these numbers in the preceding formula, we get

$$\bar{X} \pm t \frac{SD}{\sqrt{n}}$$

$$0.68 \pm 2.093 \frac{0.04}{\sqrt{20}}$$

$$0.68 \pm 2.093 \times 0.009$$

$$0.68 \pm 0.02$$

or approximately 0.66 to 0.70 m. We interpret this confidence interval as follows: in other samples of walkers, Rabago and coworkers (or other researchers) would almost always observe mean step length different from the one in this study. They would not know the true mean, of course. If they calculated a 95% confidence interval for each mean, 95% of these confidence intervals would contain the true mean. They can therefore have 95% confidence that the interval from 0.66 to 0.70 m contains the actual mean step length in adults. Using 0.66 to 0.70 m to express the confidence interval is better than 0.66 to 0.70 m, which can become confusing if the interval appears to have subtraction or a negative sign included in the interval.

Medical researchers often use error graphs to illustrate means and confidence intervals. There is nothing sacred about 95% confidence intervals; they simply are the ones most often reported in the medical literature. If researchers want to be more confident that the interval contains the true mean, they can use a 99% confidence interval. Will this interval be wider or narrower than the interval corresponding to 95% confidence?

The *t* Distribution and Testing Hypotheses About the Mean in One Group

Some investigators test hypotheses instead of finding and reporting confidence intervals. The conclusions are the *same*, regardless of which method is used. More and more, statisticians recommend confidence intervals because they actually provide more information than hypothesis tests. Some researchers still prefer hypothesis tests, possibly because tests have been used traditionally. We will return to this point after we illustrate the procedure for testing a hypothesis concerning the mean in a single sample.

As with confidence limits, the purpose of a **hypothesis test** is to permit generalizations from a sample to

the population from which the sample was selected. Both statistical hypothesis testing and estimation make certain assumptions about the population and then use probabilities to estimate the likelihood of the results obtained in the sample, given these assumptions.

To illustrate hypothesis testing, we use the step length data from Rabago and coworkers (2015) in Table 5–1. We use these observations to test whether the mean step length for male subjects in this study is different from the mean step length reported by Sekiya and Nagasaki (1998) for males (0.66), assumed to be the norm for the purposes of this example. Another way to state the research question is: On average, subjects studied by Rabago and coworkers have the different step lengths than the norm.

Statistical hypothesis testing seems to be the reverse of our nonstatistical thinking. We first assume that the mean step length is the same as the norm (0.66), and then we find the probability of observing mean step length for male subjects equal to 0.68 m in a sample of 15 male subjects, given this assumption. If the probability is large, we conclude that the assumption is justified and the mean step length in the Rabago study is not statistically different from the norm. If the probability is small—such as 1 out of 20 (0.05) or 1 out of 100 (0.01)—we conclude that the assumption is not justified and that there really is a difference; that is, male subjects in the Rabago and coworkers study have a mean step length different from the norm. Following a brief discussion of the assumptions we make when using the *t* distribution, we will use the Rabago and coworkers' study to illustrate the steps in hypothesis testing.

Assumptions in Using the *t* Distribution

For the *t* distribution or the *t* test to be used, observations should be normally distributed. Many computer programs, such as R and SPSS, are able to overlay a plot of the normal distribution on a histogram of the data. Often it is possible to look at a histogram or a box-and-whisker plot and make a judgment call. Sometimes we know the distribution of the data from past research, and we can decide whether the assumption of normality is reasonable. This assumption can be tested empirically by plotting the observations on a normal probability graph, called a Lilliefors graph (Conover, 1999), or using several statistical tests of normality. SPSS has a routine to test normality that is part of the Explore Plots option. In R, the density plot of the data may be produced as well as tests of normality such as the Shapiro-Wilks test. It is always a good idea to plot data before beginning the analysis in case some strange values are present that need to be investigated.

You may wonder why normality matters. What happens if the t distribution is used for observations that are not normally distributed? With 30 or more observations, the central limit theorem (Chapter 4) tells us that means are normally distributed, regardless of the distribution of the original observations. So, for research questions concerning the mean, the central limit theorem basically says that we do not need to worry about the underlying distribution with reasonable sample sizes. However, using the t distribution with observations that are not normally distributed and when the sample size is fewer than 30 can lead to confidence intervals that are too narrow. In this situation, we erroneously conclude that the true mean falls in a narrower range than is really the case. If the observations deviate from the normal distribution in only minor ways, the t distribution can be used anyway, because it is **robust** for non-normal data. (Robustness means we can draw the proper conclusion even when all our assumptions are not met.)

HYPOTHESIS TESTING

We now illustrate the steps in testing a hypothesis and discuss some related concepts using data from the study by Rabago and coworkers.

Steps in Hypothesis Testing

 A statistical hypothesis is a statement of belief about population parameters. Like the term "probability," the term "hypothesis" has a more precise meaning in statistics than in everyday use. **Step 1: State the research question in terms of statistical hypotheses.** The **null hypothesis,** symbolized by H_0, is a statement claiming that there is no difference between the assumed or hypothesized value and the population mean; **null** means "no difference." The **alternative hypothesis,** which we symbolize by H_1 (some textbooks use H_A) is a statement that disagrees with the null hypothesis.

If the null hypothesis is rejected as a result of sample evidence, then the alternative hypothesis is concluded. If the evidence is insufficient to reject the null hypothesis, it is retained but *not* accepted per se. Scientists distinguish between not rejecting and accepting the null hypothesis; they argue that a better study may be designed in which the null hypothesis will be rejected. Traditionally, we therefore do not accept the null hypothesis from current evidence; we merely state that it cannot be rejected.

For the Rabago and coworkers' study, the null and alternative hypotheses are as follows:

H_0: The mean step length for males in the study, μ_1, is not different from the norm (mean in Sekiya), μ_0, written $\mu_1 = \mu_0$.

H_1: The mean step length for males in the Rabago study, μ_1, is different from the norm (mean in Sekiya), μ_0, and written $\mu_1 \neq \mu_0$. (Recall that μ stands for the true mean in the population.)

These hypotheses are for a **two-tailed** (or nondirectional) test: The null hypothesis will be rejected if mean step length is sufficiently greater than 0.66 m or if it is sufficiently less than 0.66 m. A two-tailed test is appropriate when investigators do not have an a priori expectation for the value in the sample; they want to know if the sample mean differs from the population mean in either direction.

A **one-tailed** (or directional) test can be used when investigators have an expectation about the sample value, and they want to test only whether it is larger or smaller than the mean in the population. Examples of an alternative hypothesis are:

H_1: The mean step length for males in the Rabago and coworkers' study, μ_1, is larger than the norm, μ_0, and sometimes written $\mu_1 > \mu_0$

or

H_1: The mean step length for males in the Rabago and coworkers' study, μ_1, is smaller than the norm, μ_0, sometimes written as $\mu_1 < \mu_0$.

A one-tailed test has the advantage over a two-tailed test of obtaining statistical significance with a smaller departure from the hypothesized value, because there is interest in only one direction. Whenever a one-tailed test is used, it should therefore make sense that the investigators really were interested in a departure in only one direction before the data were examined. The disadvantage of a one-tailed test is that once investigators commit themselves to this approach, they are obligated to test only in the hypothesized direction. If, for some unexpected reason, the sample mean departs from the population mean in the opposite direction, the investigators cannot rightly claim the departure as significant. Medical researchers often need to be able to test for possible unexpected adverse effects as well as the anticipated positive effects, so they most frequently choose a two-tailed hypothesis even though they have an expectation about the direction of the departure. A graphic representation of a one-tailed and a two-tailed test is given in Figures 5–3A, B, and C.

Step 2: Decide on the appropriate test statistic. Some texts use the term "critical ratio" to refer to **test statistics.** Choosing the right test statistic is a major topic in statistics, and subsequent chapters focus on which test statistics are appropriate for answering specific kinds of research questions.

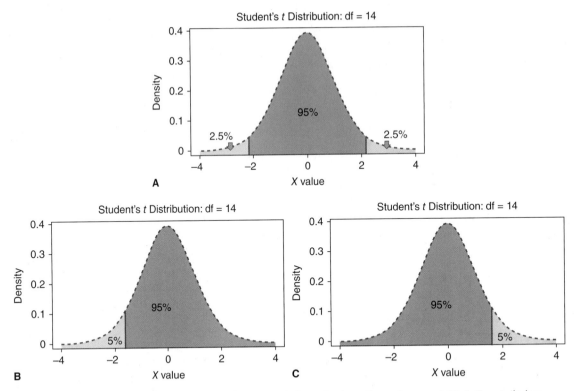

Figure 5–3. Defining areas of acceptance and rejection in hypothesis testing using $\alpha = 0.05$. **A:** Two-tailed or nondirectional. **B:** One-tailed or directional lower tail. **C:** One-tailed or directional upper tail.

Each test statistic has a probability distribution. In this example, the appropriate test statistic is based on the *t* distribution because we want to make inferences about a mean and do not know the population standard deviation. The *t* test is the test statistic for testing one mean; it is the difference between the sample mean and the hypothesized mean (μ_o) divided by the standard error.

$$t = \frac{\bar{X} - \mu_o}{s/\sqrt{n}} = \frac{\bar{X} - \mu_o}{SE}$$

Step 3: Select the level of significance for the statistical test. The **level of significance,** when chosen before the statistical test is performed, is called the **alpha value,** denoted by α (Greek letter alpha); it gives the probability of incorrectly rejecting the null hypothesis when it is actually true (and concluding there is a difference when there is not). This probability should be small, because we do not want to reject the null hypothesis when it is true. For example, $\alpha = 0.05$ means there is a 5% chance of incorrectly rejecting the null hypothesis. Traditional values used for α are 0.05, 0.01, and 0.001. An α of 0.05 will be used in this example.

Step 4: Determine the value the test statistic must attain to be declared significant. This significant value is also called the **critical value** of the test statistic. Determining the critical value is simple (we already found it when we calculated a 95% confidence interval), but detailing the reasoning behind the process is instructive. Each test statistic has a distribution; the distribution of the test statistic is divided into an area of (hypothesis) acceptance and an area of (hypothesis) rejection. The critical value is the dividing line between the areas.

An illustration should help clarify the idea. The test statistic in our example follows the *t* distribution; α is 0.05; and a two-tailed test was specified. Thus, the area of acceptance is the central 95% of the *t* distribution, and the areas of rejection are the 2.5% areas in each tail (see Figure 5–3A). From Table A–3, the value of *t* (with $n - 1$ or $15 - 1 = 14$ df) that defines the central 95% area is between -2.145 and 2.145, as we found for the 95% confidence interval. Thus, the portion of the curve below -2.145 contains the lower 2.5% of the area of the *t* distribution with 14 df, and the portion above $+2.145$ contains the upper 2.5% of the area.

The null hypothesis (that the mean step length for males of the group studied by Rabago and coworkers is equal to 0.66 m the norm) for this example will therefore be rejected if the critical value of the test statistic is less than -2.145 or if it is greater than $+2.145$.

In practice, however, almost everyone uses computers to do their statistical analyses. As a result, researchers do not usually look up the critical value before doing a statistical test. Although researchers need to decide beforehand the alpha level, they will use to conclude significance, in practice they wait and see the more exact **p value** calculated by the computer program. We discuss the p value in the following sections.

Step 5: Perform the calculation. To summarize, the mean step length among the 15 male subjects studied by Rabago and coworkers was 0.68 m with standard deviation 0.03 and standard error 0.01.[*] We compare this value with the assumed population value of 0.66 m. Substituting these values in the test statistic yields

$$t = \frac{\bar{X} - \mu_o}{SE} = \frac{0.68 - 0.66}{0.01} = 2.00$$

Step 6: Draw and state the conclusion. Stating the conclusion in words is important because, in our experience, people learning statistics sometimes focus on the mechanics of hypothesis testing but have difficulty applying the concepts. In our example, the observed value for t is 2.00. (Typically, the value of test statistics is reported to two decimal places.) Referring to Figure 5–3A, we can see that 2.00 falls within the acceptance area of the distribution. The decision is, therefore, not to reject the null hypothesis that the mean step length for males in the study by Rabago et al equals the norm reported in the Sekiya study. Another way to state the conclusion is that we do not reject the hypothesis that the sample of step length values could come from a population with mean step length of 0.66 m. This means that, on average, the step lengths observed in male subjects by Rabago et al are not statistically significantly different from the normative value from the Sekiya study. The probability of observing a mean step length of 0.68 m in a random sample of 15 males, if the true mean is actually 0.66 m, is greater than 0.05, the alpha value chosen for the test.

---

[*]Where does the value of 0.01 come from? Recall from Chapter 4 that the standard error of the mean, *SE,* is the standard deviation of the mean, not the standard deviation of the original observations. We calculate the standard error of the mean by dividing the standard deviation by the square root of the sample size:

Equivalence of Confidence Intervals and Hypothesis Tests: Now, let us examine the correspondence between hypothesis tests and confidence intervals. The results from the hypothesis test lead us to conclude that the mean step length in males studied by Rabago and coworkers is not different from the norm (0.66 m), using an α value of 0.05. A 95% confidence interval for mean step length based on the Rabago study is:

$$0.68 \pm 2.145 \times 0.01$$

$$0.68 \pm 0.02$$

$$(0.66, 0.70)$$

Note that 0.66, the value from the Sekiya study, is contained within the interval; therefore, we can conclude that the mean in the Rabago study could well be 0.66, even though the observed mean intake was 0.68 m. When we compare the two approaches, we see that the df, $15 - 1 = 14$, are the same, the critical value of t is the same, ± 2.145, and the conclusions are the same. The only difference is that the confidence interval gives us an idea of the range within which the mean could occur by chance. In other words, confidence intervals give more information than hypothesis tests yet are no more costly in terms of work; thus, we get more for our money, so to speak.

There is every indication that more and more results will be presented using confidence intervals. For example, the *British Medical Journal* has established the policy of having its authors use confidence intervals instead of hypothesis tests if confidence intervals are appropriate to their study (Gardner and Altman, 1986; 1989). To provide practice with both approaches to statistical inference, we will use both hypothesis tests and confidence intervals throughout the remaining chapters.

Replicate our findings using R. Also find the 99% confidence interval. Is it narrower or wider? Why?

Errors in Hypothesis Tests

Two errors can be made in testing a hypothesis. In step 3, we tacitly referred to one of these errors—rejecting the null hypothesis when it is true—as a consideration when selecting the significance level α for the test. This error results in our concluding a difference when none exists. Another error is also possible: *not* rejecting the null hypothesis when it is actually false. This error results in our concluding that *no* difference exists when one really does. Table 5–2 summarizes these errors. The situation marked by I, called a **type I error** (see the upper right box), is rejecting the null hypothesis when it is really true; α is the probability of making a type I error. In the study of children's mean energy intake, a type I

Table 5–2. Correct decisions and errors in hypothesis testing.

		True Situation	
		Difference Exists (H_1)	No Difference (H_0)
Conclusion from hypothesis test	Difference Exists (Reject H_0)	* (Power or $1 - \beta$)	I (Type I error, or α error)
	No Difference (Do not reject H_0)	II (Type II error, or β error)	*

Table 5–3. Shunt infection rates with and without vancomycin.

	Previous Protocol				New Protocol			
Age Group	n	Number of Infections	% with Infection	95% CI	n	Number of Infections	% with Infection	95% CI
≤1 yr	47	8	17.0%	(6.3%, 27.8%)	52	5	9.6%	(1.6%, 17.6%)
1–17 yrs	84	2	2.4%	(−0.9%, 5.6%)	146	5	3.4%	(0.5%, 6.4%)
≥17 yrs	132	8	6.1%	(2.0%, 10.1%)	301	5	1.7%	(0.2%, 3.1%)

Data from van Lindert EJ, van Bilsen M, van der Flier M, et al: Topical vancomycin reduces the cerebrospinal fluid shunt infection rate: a retrospective cohort study, *PLoS One.* 2018 Jan 9;13(1):e0190249.

error would be concluding that the mean step length in the sample studied by Rabago and coworkers is different from the norm (rejecting the null hypothesis) when, in fact, it is not.

A **type II error** occurs in the situation marked by II (see lower left box in Table 5–3); this error is failing to reject the null hypothesis when it is false (or not concluding a difference exists when it does). The probability of a type II error is denoted by β (Greek letter beta). In the step length example, a type II error would be concluding that the mean step length in the Rabago study is not different from that in norm (not rejecting the null hypothesis) when the mean step length was, in fact, actually different from the norm.

The situations marked by the asterisk (*) are correct decisions. The upper left box in Table 5–3 correctly rejects the null hypothesis when a difference exists; this situation is also called the power of the test, a concept we will discuss in the next section. Finally, the lower right box is the situation in which we correctly retain the null hypothesis when there is no difference.

Power

Power is important in hypothesis testing. **Power** is the probability of rejecting the null hypothesis when it is indeed false. Power is the ability of a study to detect a true difference. Obviously, high power is a valuable attribute for a study, because all investigators want to detect a significant result if it is present. Power is calculated as $(1 - \beta)$ or $(1 - a$ type II error) and is intimately related to the sample size used

in the study. The importance of addressing the issue of the power of a study cannot be overemphasized—it is essential in designing a valid study. Power is discussed in more detail in the following sections where programs for estimating sample sizes are illustrated and in subsequent chapters.

p Values

Another vital concept related to significance and to the α level is the **p value,** commonly reported in medical journals. The p value is related to a hypothesis test (although sometimes p values are stated along with confidence intervals); it is the probability of obtaining a result as extreme as (or more extreme than) the one observed, *if* the null hypothesis is true. Some people like to think of the p value as the probability that the observed result is due to chance alone. The p value is calculated *after* the statistical test has been performed; if the p value is less than α, the null hypothesis is rejected.

Referring to the test using the Rabago data, the p value cannot be precisely obtained from Table A–3 because not all probabilities are included in the table. We need to extrapolate in these situations. For 14 df $\alpha = 0.10$, the critical value is approximately 1.761 and for $\alpha = 0.05$ it is 2.145. We could report the p value as $p > 0.05$ to indicate that the significance level is more than 0.05. It is easier and more precise to use a computer program to do this calculation, however. Using Excel to find the two-tailed p value is 0.065, consistent with our conclusion that $P > 0.05$.

Some authors report that the p value is less than some traditional value such as 0.05 or 0.01; however, more authors now report the precise p value produced by computer programs. The practice of reporting values less than some traditional value was established prior to the availability of computers, when statistical tables such as those in Appendix A were the only source of probabilities. Reporting the actual p value communicates the significance of the findings more precisely. We prefer this practice; using the arbitrary traditional values may lead an investigator (or reader of a journal article) to conclude that a result is significant when $p = 0.05$ but is not significant when $p = 0.06$, a dubious distinction.

Analogies to Hypothesis Testing

Analogies often help us better understand new or complex topics. Certain features of diagnostic testing, such as sensitivity and specificity, provide a straightforward analogy to hypothesis testing. A type I error, incorrectly concluding significance when the result is not significant, is similar to a false-positive test that incorrectly indicates the presence of a disease when it is absent. Similarly, a type II error, incorrectly concluding no significance when the result is significant, is analogous to a false-negative test that incorrectly indicates the absence of disease when it is present. The power of a statistical test, the ability to detect significance when a result is significant, corresponds to the sensitivity of a diagnostic test: the test's ability to detect a disease that is present. We may say we want the statistical test to be sensitive to detecting significance when it should be detected. We illustrate diagnostic testing concepts in detail in Chapter 12.

Another analogy is to the U.S. legal system. Assuming that the null hypothesis is true until proven false is like assuming that a person is innocent until proven guilty. Just as it is the responsibility of the prosecution to present evidence that the accused person is guilty, the investigator must provide evidence that the null hypothesis is false. In the legal system, in order to avoid a type I error of convicting an innocent person, the prosecution must provide evidence to convince jurors "beyond a reasonable doubt" that the accused is guilty before the null hypothesis of innocence can be rejected. In research, the evidence for a false null hypothesis must be so strong that the probability of incorrectly rejecting the null hypothesis is very small, typically, but not always, less than 0.05.

The U.S. legal system opts to err in the direction of setting a guilty person free rather than unfairly convicting an innocent person. In scientific inquiry, the tradition is to prefer the error of missing a significant difference (arguing, perhaps, that others will come along and design a better study) to the error of incorrectly concluding significance when a result is not significant. These two errors are, of course, related to each other. If a society decides to reduce the number of guilty people that go free, it must increase the chances that innocent people will be convicted. Similarly, an investigator who wishes to decrease the probability of missing a significant difference by decreasing β necessarily increases the probability α of falsely concluding a difference. The way the legal system can simultaneously reduce both types of errors is by requiring more evidence for a decision. Likewise, the way simultaneously to reduce both type I and type II errors in scientific research is by increasing the sample size n. When that is not possible—because the study is exploratory, the problem studied is rare, or the costs are too high—the investigator must carefully evaluate the values for α and β and make a judicious decision.

RESEARCH QUESTIONS ABOUT A PROPORTION IN ONE GROUP

When a study uses nominal or binary (yes/no) data, the results are generally reported as proportions or percentages (see Chapter 3). In medicine we sometimes observe a single group and want to compare the proportion of subjects having a certain characteristic with some well-accepted standard or norm. For example, van Lindert and colleagues (2018) in Presenting Problem 2 wanted to examine the efficacy adding vancomycin to the protocol when placing cerebrospinal fluid (CSF) shunts. Findings from this study are given in Table 5–3.

The binomial distribution introduced in Chapter 4 can be used to determine confidence limits or to test hypotheses about the observed proportion. Recall that the **binomial distribution** is appropriate when a specific number of independent trials is conducted (symbolized by n), each with the same probability of success (symbolized by the Greek letter π), and this probability can be interpreted as the proportion of people with or without the characteristic we are interested in. Applied to the data in this study, each shunt placement is considered a trial, and the probability of having an infection in the ≤ 1 year age group is $8/47 = 0.170$.

The binomial distribution has some interesting features, and we can take advantage of these. Figure 5–4 shows the binomial distribution when the population proportion π is 0.2 and 0.4 for sample sizes of 5, 10, and 25. We see that the distribution becomes more bell-shaped as the sample size increases and as the proportion approaches 0.5. This result should not be surprising because a proportion is actually a special case of a mean in which successes equal 1 and failures equal 0, and the central limit theorem states that the sampling distribution of means for large samples resembles the

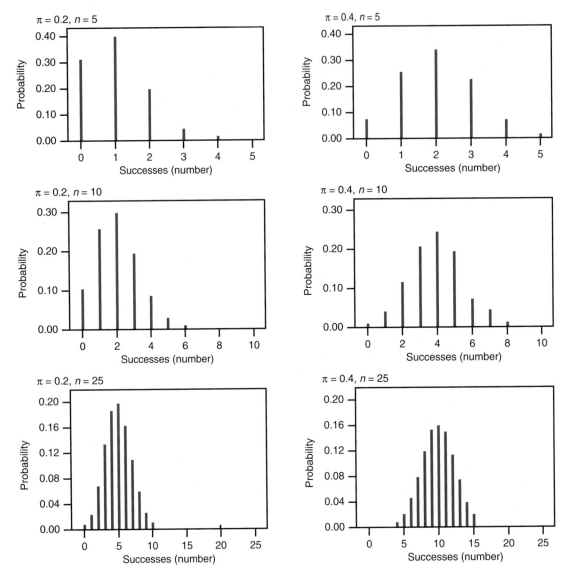

Figure 5–4. Probability distributions for the binomial when $\pi = 0.2$ and 0.4.

normal distribution. These observations lead naturally to the idea of using the standard normal, or z, distribution as an approximation to the binomial distribution.

Confidence Intervals for a Proportion of Subjects

In the study by van Lindert and colleagues (2018), the proportion of people with an infection after shunt placement in the ≤1 year age group was 0.170 under the previous protocol. Of course,

0.170 is only an estimate of the unknown true proportion in the entire population in this age group of who could have a CSF shunt placed. How much do you think the proportion of patients with a successful outcome would vary from one sample to another? We can use the sampling distribution for proportions from large samples to help answer this question. Recall from Chapter 4 that, in order to use a sampling distribution, we need to know the mean and standard error. For a proportion, the mean is simply the proportion itself (symbolized as π in the population and lowercase p in the sample), and the standard error is the square root of $\pi(1-\pi)$ divided by n in the population or $p(1-p)$ divided by n in the sample; that is, the standard error is

$$\sqrt{\frac{\pi(1-\pi)}{n}} \text{ or } \sqrt{\frac{p(1-p)}{n}}$$

Then the 95% confidence limits for the true population proportion π are given by

Observed proportion $\pm 1.96 \times$ Standard error

of the observed proportion

or

$$p \pm 1.96 \times \sqrt{\frac{p(1-p)}{n}}$$

Where did 1.96 come from? From Appendix A–2, we find that 1.96 is the value that separates the central 95% of the area under the standard normal, or z, distribution from the 2.5% in each tail. The only requirement is that the product of the proportion and the sample size (pn) be greater than 5 and that $(1-p)n$ be greater than 5 as well. Using the preceding formula, the 95% confidence interval for the true proportion of patients with a shunt infection in the $<=1$ year age group is

$$0.170 \pm 1.96\sqrt{\frac{0.170 \times (1-0.170)}{47}} = 0.170 \pm 0.107$$

or 0.063 to 0.278. The investigators may therefore be 95% confident that the interval 0.063 to 0.278 contains the true proportion of subjects ≤ 1 year old with an infection after a CSF shunt placement.

Find the values of the z distribution used for the 90% and 99% confidence intervals and calculate the resulting confidence intervals. What happens to the width of the confidence interval as the confidence level changes decreases? Increases?

The z Distribution to Test a Hypothesis About a Proportion

Recall that we can draw conclusions from samples using two methods: finding confidence intervals or testing hypotheses. We have already stated our preference for confidence intervals, but we also illustrate a statistical test. If the investigators want to know if the sample mean infection rate of 17.1%, for the ≤ 1 year age group was greater than 5%. We use the six-step procedure to test the hypotheses that this infection rate exceeds 5%.

Step 1: State the research question in terms of statistical hypotheses. Suppose the investigators wanted to know whether the observed proportion of 0.170 was significantly greater than 0.05. The z distribution can be used to test the hypothesis for this research question. The Greek letter π stands for the hypothesized population proportion because the null hypothesis refers to the population:

H_0: The proportion of subjects in the ≤ 1 year age group with a CSF shunt infection is 0.05 or less, or $\pi \leq 0.05$.

H_1: The proportion of subjects in the ≤ 1 year age group with a CSF shunt infection is more than 0.05, or $\pi > 0.05$.

In this example, we are interested in concluding that the infection rate is greater than 5%; therefore, a one-tailed test to detect only a positive difference is appropriate. A two-tailed test would be appropriate to test whether the success rate is either $>$ or $<5\%$.

Step 2: Decide on the appropriate test statistic. The sample size (47) times the proportion (0.170) is 8, and the sample size times 1 minus the proportion (0.830) is 39. Because both are greater than 5, we can use the z test. The z test, just like the t test, takes the common form of the observed value of the statistic minus its hypothesized value divided by its standard error.

$$z = \frac{p - \pi}{\sqrt{\pi(1-\pi)/n}}$$

Step 3: Select the level of significance for the statistical test. For this one-tailed test, we use $\alpha = 0.05$.
Step 4: Determine the value the test statistic must attain to be declared significant. A one-tailed test with the alternative hypothesis in the positive direction places the entire rejection area in the upper part of the probability distribution. The value of z that divides the normal distribution into the lower 95% and upper 5% is 1.645 (Table A–2). The null hypothesis that the true population proportion is less than or equal to 0.05 will be rejected if the observed value of z is greater than 1.645 (see Figure 5–5).
Step 5: Perform the calculations. The null hypothesis says the proportion is 0.05 or less, so this is the value we use in the standard error, not the observed proportion of 0.170. Substituting these values in the z test gives

$$\frac{0.170 - 0.05}{\sqrt{0.05 \times (1-0.05)/47}} = \frac{0.120}{0.032} = 3.75$$

Step 6: Draw and state the conclusion. Because the observed value of z (3.75) is greater than the critical value, 1.645, the decision is to reject the null hypothesis and conclude that the alternative hypothesis, that

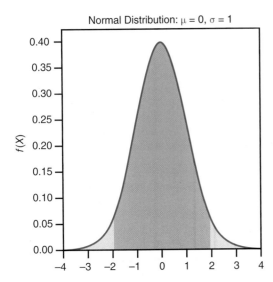

Figure 5–5. Defining areas of acceptance and rejection in the standard normal distribution (z) using $\alpha = 0.05$.

the proportion of patients with an infection rate is >5%, is correct. The conclusion is that the infection rate is greater than 5% with $p < 0.05$.

Continuity Correction

The z distribution is continuous and the binomial distribution is discrete, and many statisticians recommend making a small correction to the test statistic to create a more accurate approximation. One **continuity correction** involves subtracting $z/(2n)$ from the **absolute value** of the numerator of the z statistic. (Recall that the absolute value of a number is positive, regardless of whether the number is positive or negative.) The test statistic is

$$z = \frac{|\, p - \pi \,| - [1 / (2n)]}{\sqrt{\pi(1 - \pi) / n}}$$

Newcombe (1998) compared seven confidence interval procedures and found that the Wilson score was more accurate than all others for confidence intervals. This statistic is

$$z = \frac{(2np + z_{\alpha/2}^2) \pm \sqrt{z_{\alpha/2}^2 + 4np(1 - p)}}{2(n + z_{\alpha/2}^2)}$$

The continuity correction has minimal effect with large sample sizes. Should a continuity correction be used? To be honest, even statisticians do not agree on the answer to this.

MEANS WHEN THE SAME GROUP IS MEASURED TWICE

Earlier in this chapter, we found confidence intervals for means and proportions. We also illustrated research questions that investigators ask when they want to compare one group of subjects to a known or assumed population mean or proportion. In actuality, these latter situations do not occur very often in medicine (or, indeed, in most other fields). We discussed the methods because they are relatively simple statistics, and, more importantly, minor modifications of these tests can be used for research questions that do occur with great frequency.

In the next two sections, we concentrate on studies in which the same group of subjects is observed twice using **paired designs** or **repeated-measures designs.** Typically, in these studies, subjects are measured to establish a baseline (sometimes called the *before* measurement); then, after some intervention or at a later time, the same subjects are measured again (called the *after* measurement). The research question asks whether the intervention makes a difference—whether there is a change. In this design, each subject serves as their own control. The observations in these studies are called *paired* observations because the before-and-after measurements made on the same people (or on matched pairs) are paired in the analysis. We sometimes call these *dependent* observations as well, because, if we know the first measurement, we have some idea of what the second measurement will be (as we will see later in this chapter).

Sometimes, the second measurement is made shortly after the first. In other studies, a considerable time passes before the second measurement.

Why Researchers Use Repeated-Measures Studies

Suppose a researcher wants to evaluate the effect of a new diet on weight loss. Furthermore, suppose the population consists of only six people who have used the diet for 2 months; their weights before and after the diet are given in Table 5–4. To estimate the amount of weight loss, the researcher selects a random sample of three patients (patients 2, 3, and 6) to determine their mean weight before the diet and finds a mean weight of $(89 + 83 + 95)/3 = 89$ kg. Two months later, the researcher selects an independent random sample of three patients (patients 1, 4, and 5) to determine their mean weight after the diet and finds a

Table 5–4. Illustration of observations in a paired design (before and after measurements).

Patient	Weight Before (kg)	Weight After (kg)
1	100	95
2	89	84
3	83	78
4	98	93
5	108	103
6	95	90

mean weight of (95 + 93 + 103)/3 = 97 kg. The researcher would conclude that the patients gained an average of 8 kg on the diet. What is the problem here?

The means for the two independent samples indicate that the patients gained weight, while, in fact, they each lost 5 kg on the diet. In this case, the conclusion based on these samples is incorrect because the population is presented in the table. Therefore, the value can be examined for the entire population and the actual differences may be determined; however, in real life the population can rarely be observed. The problem is that the characteristic being studied (weight) is quite *variable* from one patient to another; in this small population of six patients, weight varied from 83 to 108 kg before the diet program began. Furthermore, the amount of change, 5 kg, is relatively small compared with the variability among patients and is obscured by this variability. The researcher needs a way to control for variability among patients.

The solution, as you may have guessed, is to select a single random sample of patients and measure their weights both before and after the diet. Because the measurements are taken on the same patients, a better estimate of the true change is more likely. The goal of paired designs is to control for extraneous factors or confounders that might influence the result; then, any differences caused by the intervention will not be masked by the differences among the subjects themselves.

The paired design allows researchers to detect change more easily by controlling for extraneous variation among the observations. Many biologic measurements exhibit wide variation among individuals, and the use of the paired design is thus especially appropriate in the health field.

The statistical test that researchers use when the same subjects are measured on a numerical (interval) variable before and after an intervention is called the **paired *t*** test, because the observations on the same subject are paired with one another to find the difference. This test is also called the **matched groups *t*** test and the dependent groups *t* test.

The good news is that paired, or before-and-after, designs are easy to analyze. Instead of having to find the mean and standard deviation of both the before and the after measurements, we need find only the mean and standard deviation of the *differences* between the before-and-after measurements. Then, the *t* distribution we used for a single mean (described in the sections titled, "What to Do When Observations Are Not Normally Distributed" and "Hypothesis Testing") can be used to analyze the differences themselves.

To illustrate, examine the mean weights of the six subjects in the weight-loss example presented in Table 5–4. Before the diet, the mean weight was 95.5 kg; after the diet, the mean was 90.5 kg. The difference between the means, 95.5 − 90.5 = 5 kg, is exactly the same as the mean weight loss, 5 kg, for each subject. The standard deviation of the differences, however, is not equal to the difference between the standard deviations in the before-and-after measurements. The differences between each before-and-after measurement must be analyzed to obtain the standard deviation of the differences. Actually, the standard deviation of the differences is frequently smaller than the standard deviation in the before measurements and in the after measurements. This is because the two sets of measurements are generally correlated, meaning that the lower values in the before measurements are associated with the lower values in the after measurements and similarly for the higher values. In this illustration, the standard deviations of the weights both before and after the diet program are 8.74, whereas the standard deviation of the differences is zero. Why is this the case? Because we made the before-and-after measurements perfectly correlated. Of course, as with the *t* distribution used with one mean, we must assume that the differences are normally distributed.

Confidence Intervals for the Mean Difference in Paired Designs

One way to evaluate the effect of an intervention in a before-and-after study is to form a confidence interval (CI) for the mean difference. To illustrate, we use data from the Dittrich and colleagues' (2018) study investigating the impact of hypnotic suggestion on knee neuromuscular activity. Some descriptive information on the patients and muscle response pathway (M-wave) values are given in Table 5–5.

The value of M-wave is a numerical variable, so means and standard deviations are appropriate. We see that the mean M-wave value for the vastus medialis (thigh muscle that extends the knee) in the 13 patients was 15.1 mV pre-exercise (SD 7.5). After exercise, the mean decreased to 14.4 mV (SD 6.9). We want to

Table 5–5. M-wave peak to peak amplitude from vastus lateralus (VL), vastus medealis (VM), and rectus femoris (RF) muscles measured before and after exercise.

Muscle	Control Pre	Control Post	Hypnosis Pre	Hypnosis Post
VL	14.7±7.9	14.5±7.5	12.2±7.9	10.9±7.4
VM	15.1±7.2	14.4±6.6	14.8±7.2	12.9±6.6
RF	9.7±5.6	7.9±3.6	6.9±5.6	6.1±3.6

Data from Dittrich N, Agostino D, Antonini Philippe R, etal: Dataset Effect of hypnotic suggestion on knee extensor neuromuscular properties in resting and fatigued states, April 6, 2018. Available at https://doi.org/10.5281/zenodo.1213604.

Table 5–6. Difference between before and after exercise for controls M-wave amplitude – vastus medialis (mV).

Subject	Controls Pre	Controls Post	Controls Difference
1	14.9	13.4	−1.5
2	7.5	7.2	−0.3
3	24.7	23.9	−0.8
4	15.3	13.5	−1.8
5	14.2	13.8	−0.4
6	10.0	13.5	3.4
7	13.3	13.0	−0.3
8	23.0	21.4	−1.6
9	23.7	24.2	0.5
10	7.1	5.6	−1.5
11	2.4	3.1	0.6
12	26.7	22.6	−4.1
13	13.0	12.0	−0.9
Mean	15.1	14.4	−0.7
SD	7.5	6.9	1.7

know whether this decrease could happen by chance. To examine the mean difference in a paired study, we need the raw data so we can find the mean and standard deviation of the differences between the before-and-after scores. The before, after, and difference scores are given in Table 5–6.

For patients in this study, the mean of the 13 differences is −0.7 (indicating that, on average, M-wave decreased after exercise), and the standard deviation of the differences is 1.7. The calculations for the mean and the standard deviation of the differences use the same formulas as in Chapter 3, except that we replace the symbol X (used for an observation on a single subject) with the symbol d to stand for the difference in the measurements for a single subject. Then, the mean difference is the sum of the differences divided by the number of subjects. Using the differences d's instead of X's and the mean difference instead, the standard deviation is:

$$SD_d = \sqrt{\frac{\sum(d - \bar{d})^2}{n - 1}} = 1.7$$

Just as in one group of observations and find the standard error of the mean by dividing the standard deviation SD by the square root of the sample size, the standard error of the mean differences is calculated by dividing the standard deviation of the differences SD_d by the square root of n,

$$\frac{SD_d}{\sqrt{n}} = \frac{1.7}{\sqrt{13}} = 0.47$$

Finding a 95% confidence interval for the mean difference is just like finding a 95% confidence interval for the mean of one group, except again the mean difference and the standard error of the mean differences are used instead of the mean and standard error of the mean. The t distribution with $n - 1$ degrees of freedom is used to evaluate research hypotheses about mean differences. To illustrate, a 95% confidence interval for the mean difference in M-wave, the value of t for $n - 1 = 13 - 1 = 12$ df, which is 2.179 from Appendix A–3. Using these values in the formula for a 95% confidence interval for the true population difference gives

Difference $\pm$ Confidence factor $\times$ Standard error

of the difference

or

$$\bar{d} \pm t_{n-1}\frac{SD_d}{\sqrt{n}}$$

$$-0.7 \pm 2.179\frac{1.7}{\sqrt{13}} = -0.7 \pm 2.179 \times 0.47$$

$$= -0.7 \pm 1.02$$

This confidence interval can be interpreted as follows. We are 95% sure that the *true mean difference* in M-wave is between −1.72 and 0.32. Logically, because the interval includes zero, we can be 95% sure that the mean difference includes zero. In plain words, we cannot conclude that M-wave signal changed following exercise.

The Paired t Test for the Mean Difference

The t distribution is used for both confidence intervals and hypothesis tests about mean differences. Again, we use data from Presenting Problem 3, in which researchers examined changes in muscle response pathway (Dittrich et al 2018).

Step 1: State the research question in terms of statistical hypotheses. The statistical hypothesis for a paired design is usually stated as follows, where the Greek letter delta (δ) stands for the difference in the population:

H_0: The true difference in the M-wave is zero, or, in symbols, $\delta = 0$.

H_1: The true difference in the M-wave is not zero, or, in symbols, $\delta \neq 0$.

We are interested in rejecting the null hypothesis of no difference in two situations: when M-wave significantly increases, and when it significantly decreases; it is a two-sided test.

Step 2: Decide on the appropriate test statistic. When the purpose is to see if a difference exists between before and after measurements in a paired design, and the observations are measured on a numerical (either interval or ratio) scale, the test statistic is the t statistic, assuming the differences are normally distributed. We almost always want to know if a change occurs, or, in other words, if the difference is zero. If we wanted to test the hypothesis that the mean difference is equal to some value other than zero, we would need to subtract that value (instead of zero) from the mean difference in the numerator of the following formula:

$$t = \frac{\bar{d} - 0}{SD_d / \sqrt{n}}$$

with $n - 1$ df, where $\bar{d}$ stands for the mean difference and $SD_d / \sqrt{n}$ for the standard error of the mean differences as explained earlier.

Step 3: Select the level of significance for the statistical test. Let us use $\alpha = 0.1$.

Step 4: Determine the value the test statistic must attain to be declared significant. The value of t that divides the distribution into the central 90% is 1.782, with 5% of the area in each tail with $n - 1 = 12$ df. We therefore reject the null hypothesis that the program does not make a difference if the value of the t statistic is less than -1.782 or greater than $+1.782$.

Step 5: Perform the calculations. Substituting our numbers (mean difference of -0.7, hypothesized difference of 0, standard deviation of 1.7, and a sample size of 13), the observed value of the t statistic is

$$t = \frac{\bar{d} - \delta}{SD_d / \sqrt{n}} = \frac{-0.7 - 0}{1.7 / \sqrt{13}} = 1.49$$

Step 6: Draw and state the conclusion. Because the observed value of the t statistic is 1.49, not larger than the critical value 1.782, we do not reject the null hypothesis that means we cannot say that the M-wave signal decreases after exercise (p > 0.10).

PROPORTIONS WHEN THE SAME GROUP IS MEASURED TWICE

Researchers might want to ask two types of questions when a measurement has been repeated on the same group of subjects. Sometimes they are interested in knowing how much the first and second measurements agree with each other; other times they want to know only whether a change has occurred following an intervention or the passage of time. We discuss the first situation in detail in this section and then cover the second situation briefly.

Measuring Agreement Between Two People or Methods

Frequently in the health field, a practitioner must interpret a procedure as indicating the presence or the absence of a disease or abnormality; that is, the observation is a yes-or-no outcome, a nominal measure. A common strategy to show that measurements are reliable is to repeat the measurements and see how much they agree with each other. When one person observes the same subject or specimen twice and the observations are compared, the degree of agreement is called **intrarater reliability** (*intra-* meaning within). When two or more people observe the same subject or specimen, their agreement is called **interrater reliability** (*inter-* meaning between). A common way to measure interrater reliability when the measurements are nominal is to use the **kappa (κ)** statistic. If the measurements are on a numerical scale, the correlation between the measurements is found. We discussed the correlation coefficient in Chapter 3 and will return to it in Chapter 8.

In other similar situations, two different procedures are used to measure the same characteristic. If one can be assumed to be the "gold standard," then **sensitivity** and **specificity**, discussed in Chapter 12, are appropriate. When neither is the gold standard, the kappa statistic is used to measure the agreement between the two procedures. In Presenting Problem 4, Leone and colleagues (2013) evaluated the interrater reliability of using color-Doppler to evaluate five criteria in diagnosing multiple sclerosis (MS). The kappa statistic can be used to estimate the level of agreement between the two raters' findings. Information regarding the evaluation of Criterion 1, reflux in the internal jugular veins (IJVs) and/or vertebral veins (VV) has been reproduced in Table 5–7 and rearranged in

Table 5–7 Reviewer performance using color-Doppler to diagnose reflux in the internal jugular and/or vertebral veins.

Subject	Criterion 1 - Rater 1	Criterion 1 - Rater 2	Subject	Criterion 1 - Rater 1	Criterion 1 - Rater 2	Subject	Criterion 1 - Rater 1	Criterion 1 - Rater 2
	−	−	59	−	−	101	−	−
5	+	+	60	−	−	102	−	−
9	−	−	61	−	−	104	−	+
13	−	−	62	−	+	105	+	−
24	+	−	63	+	−	108	+	+
32	−	−	64	+	+	109	−	+
33	+	+	65	−	+	112	−	−
34	+	+	66	−	−	113	−	−
35	−	−	68	−	−	114	−	−
36	−	−	69	+	+	118	+	+
37	−	−	70	−	+	119	−	−
38	−	−	71	−	−	120	+	−
39	−	−	72	−	−	121	−	−
40	+	−	73	−	−	122	−	−
41	−	−	74	−	+	126	−	−
42	+	−	75	−	−	127	−	−
43	+	−	76	−	−	129	−	−
44	+	+	77	+	−	132	+	−
45	+	−	78	+	+	134	+	−
46	−	−	79	−	−	144	+	−
47	+	−	87	−	−	145	−	−
48	−	−	90	+	+	147	−	+
49	−	+	91	−	−	148	+	−
50	−	+	92	−	−	150	−	−
51	−	−	93	+	+	151	−	−
52	−	+	95	−	−	154	−	−
54	−	−	96	−	−	161	+	−
55	−	−	97	−	−	168	−	−
56	−	−	98	−	−	169	−	−
57	+	+	99	−	−	181	−	−
58	−	−	100	−	−	182	−	−

+positive; −negative

Data from Leone MA, Raymkulova O, Lucenti A, et al: A reliability study of colour-Doppler sonography for the diagnosis of chronic cerebrospinal venous insufficiency shows low inter-rater agreement, *BMJ Open*. 2013 Nov 15;3(11):e003508.

Table 5–8 to make the analysis simpler. The results of the two reviewers agreed that 12 of 93 were positive and 56 were negative.

We can describe the degree of agreement between the two raters as follows. The total observed agreement [(12+56)/93 = 73%] is an overestimate, because it ignores the fact that, with only two categories (positive and negative), they would agree by chance part of the time. We need to adjust the observed agreement and see how much they agree beyond the level of chance.

To find the percentage of specimens on which they would agree by chance we use a straightforward application of one of the probability rules from Chapter 4.

Because the two raters were blinded as to the other's findings, the two measurements are independent, and we can use the multiplication rule for two independent events to see how likely it is that they agree merely by chance.

The statistic most often used to measure agreement between two observers on a binary variable is **kappa (κ),** defined as the agreement beyond chance divided by the amount of possible agreement beyond chance. Reviewing the data in Table 5–9, Rater 1 indicated that 27, or 29%, were positive, and Rater 2 indicated that 22, or 24%, were positive. Using the multiplication rule, they would agree that by chance 29% × 24%, or 7%, of the specimens were positive. By chance alone the

Table 5–8. Observed agreement between Rater 1 and Rater 2 findings.

Observed Counts

		Rater 1		
		Positive	Negative	Total
Rater 2	Positive	12	10	22
	Negative	15	56	71
	Total	27	66	93

Expected Counts Assuming Independence

		Rater 1		
		Positive	Negative	Total
Rater 2	Positive	6.4	15.6	22.0
	Negative	20.6	50.4	71.0
	Total	27.0	66.0	93.0

Data from Leone MA, Raymkulova O, Lucenti A, et al: A reliability study of colour-Doppler sonography for the diagnosis of chronic cerebrospinal venous insufficiency shows low inter-rater agreement, *BMJ Open.* 2013 Nov 15;3(11):e003508.

Table 5–9. Kappa test output from R.

```
Kappa.test(Rater_1,Rater_2)
$`Result`

	Estimate Cohen's kappa statistics and test the null-
hypothesis that the extent of agreement is same as
random (kappa=0)

data:  Rater_1 and Rater_2
Z = 2.3871, p-value = 0.00849
95 percent confidence interval:
 0.07856433 0.54120415
sample estimates:
[1] 0.3098842


$Judgement
[1] "Fair agreement"
```

The potential agreement beyond chance is 100% minus the chance agreement of 61%, or, using proportions, $1 - 0.61 = 0.39$. Kappa in this example is therefore $0.12/0.39 = 0.30$. The formula for kappa and our calculations are as follows:

$$\kappa = \left(\frac{\text{Observed} - \text{Expected agreement}}{1 - \text{Expected agreement}} \right) = \left(\frac{0 - E}{1 - E} \right)$$

$$= \left(\frac{0.73 - 0.61}{1 - 0.61} \right) = \left(\frac{0.12}{0.39} \right) = 0.30$$

Sackett and associates (1991) point out that the level of agreement varies considerably depending on the clinical task, ranging from 57% agreement with a κ of 0.30 for two cardiologists examining the same electrocardiograms from different patients, to 97% agreement with a κ of 0.67 for two radiologists examining the same set of mammograms. Byrt (1996) proposed the following guidelines for interpreting κ:

raters would agree that 76% × 71%, or another 54%, were negative. The two procedures would therefore agree by chance on 7% + 54%, or 61%, of the images. In actuality, the procedures agreed on (12+56)/93, or 73%, of the 93 specimens, so the level of agreement beyond chance was 0.73 − 0.61, or 0.12, the numerator of κ.

0.93–1.00	Excellent agreement
0.81–0.92	Very good agreement
0.61–0.80	Good agreement
0.41–0.60	Fair agreement
0.21–0.40	Slight agreement
0.01–0.20	Poor agreement
≤0.00	No agreement

Based on these guidelines, the agreement been the two raters was slight. When κ is zero, agreement is only at the level expected by chance. When κ is negative, the observed level of agreement is *less* than we would expect by chance alone.

Most of the time, we are interested in the kappa statistic as a descriptive measure and not whether it is statistically significant. The R statistical program reports the value of z for the kappa statistic; the output of the R Kappa test function is presented in Table 5–9.

Proportions in Studies with Repeated Measurements and the McNemar Test

In studies in which the outcome is a binary (yes/no) variable, researchers may want to know whether the proportion of subjects with (or without) the characteristic of interest changes after an intervention or the passage of time. In these types of studies, we need a statistical test that is similar to the paired *t* test and appropriate with nominal data. The McNemar test can be used for comparing paired proportions.

He and colleagues (2015) wanted to know whether the sleep quality of patients with thyroid cancer could be improved with I-131 radioiodine therapy. They collected information on the number of patients who had A Pittsburgh Sleep Quality Index (PSQI) of 5 or less and those with a PSQI of more than 5 before and after I-131 treatment. The results are displayed in a 2 × 2 table in Table 5–10. Before treatment, 88, or 54.3%, of the patients had a PSQI score of greater than 5, but after I-131 treatment, the number increased to 115, or 71.0%.

The null hypothesis is that the proportions of patients with a PSQI of more than 5 are the same at the two different time periods. The alternative hypothesis is that the paired proportions are not equal. The McNemar test for paired proportions is very easy to calculate; it uses only the numbers in the cells where before-and-after scores change; that is, the upper right and lower left cells. For the numerator we find the absolute value of the difference between the top right and the bottom left cells in the 2 × 2 table and square the number. In our example this is the absolute value of $|-115-74| = 41^2 = 1,681$. For the denominator we take the sum of the top right and bottom left cells: $115+74 = 189$. Dividing gives 8.89; in symbols, the equation is

$$\text{McNemar} = \frac{(|\, b - c\, |)}{b + c} = \frac{(|\, 115 - 74\, |)}{115 + 74} = \frac{41^2}{189}$$

$$= \frac{1681}{189} = 8.89$$

If we want to use $\alpha = 0.05$, we compare the value of the McNemar test to the critical value of 3.84 to decide if we can reject the null hypothesis that the paired proportions are equal. (We explain more about how we determined this value when we discuss chi-square in the next chapter.) Because 8.89 is larger than 3.84, we can reject the null hypothesis and conclude that there is a difference, increase in this situation, in the proportion of patients having PSQI scores greater than 5 before and after I-131 therapy.

As with the z statistic, it is possible to use a continuity correction with the McNemar test. The correction involves subtracting 1 from the absolute value in the numerator before squaring it.

WHAT TO DO WHEN OBSERVATIONS ARE NOT NORMALLY DISTRIBUTED

If observations are quite skewed, the *t* distribution should not be used, because the values that are supposed to separate the upper and lower 2.5% of the area of the central 95% of the distribution do not really do so. In this situation, we can **transform** or rescale the observations or we can use nonparametric methods.

Transforming or Rescaling Observations

Transforming observations expresses their values on another scale. To take a simple example, if weight is measured in pounds, we can multiply by 2.2 to get weight in kilograms. The main reason for knowing about **transformations** is that they sometimes make it possible to use statistical tests that otherwise would be inappropriate. You already know about several transformations. For example, the standard normal, or z, distribution introduced in Chapter 4 is obtained by subtracting the mean from each observation and then dividing by the standard deviation. The

Table 5–10. Analysis using the McNemar statistic for the number of patients having more analysis of sleep quality before and after therapy.

	DTC patients before I therapy	DTC patients after I therapy	Total
PSQI > 5	88	115	203
PSQI ≤ 5	74	47	121
Total	162	162	
% with PSQI > 5	54.3%	71.0%	

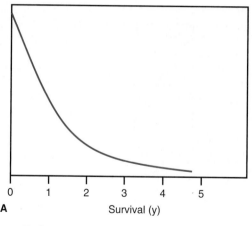

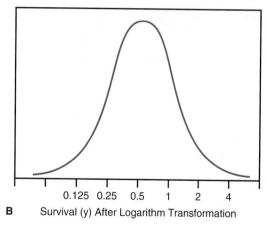

A Survival (y)

B Survival (y) After Logarithm Transformation

Figure 5–6. Example of logarithm transformation for survival of patients with cancer of the prostate metastatic to bone.

z transformation is a linear transformation; it rescales a distribution with a given mean and standard deviation to a distribution in which the mean is 0 and the standard deviation is 1. The basic bell shape of the distribution itself is not changed by this transformation.

Nonlinear transformations change the shape of the distribution. We also talked about rank ordering observations when we discussed ordinal scales in Chapter 3. This transformation ranks observations from lowest to highest (or vice versa). The rank transformation can be very useful in analyzing observations that are skewed, and many of the **nonparametric** methods we discuss in this book use ranks as their basis.

Other nonlinear transformations can be used to straighten out the relationship between two variables by changing the shape of the skewed distribution to one that more closely resembles the normal distribution. Consider the survival time of patients who are diagnosed with cancer of the prostate. A graph of possible values of survival time (in years) for a group of patients with prostate cancer metastatic to the bone is given in Figure 5–6A. The distribution has a substantial positive skew, so methods that assume a normal distribution would not be appropriate. Figure 5–6B illustrates the distribution if the logarithm[†] of survival time is used instead, that is, $Y = \log(X)$, where Y is the transformed value (or exponent) related to a given value of X. This is the log to base 10.

Another log transformation uses the transcendental number *e* as the base and is called the *natural log,* abbreviated ln. Log transformations are frequently used with laboratory values that have a skewed distribution. Another transformation is the square root transformation. Although this transformation is not used as frequently in medicine as the log transformation, it can be very useful when a log transformation overcorrects. In the study regarding patient activation presented in Chapter 3, one of the variables used in the study was the total score of support (SUPP_Total_Score) was skewed. Both a square root and squared transformation are presented in Figures 5–7B and C. You can see that neither transformation is very close to a normal distribution. In this situation, the investigators might well choose a **nonparametric** procedure that does not make any assumptions about the shape of the distribution.

The Sign Test for Hypotheses About the Median in One Group

An alternative to transforming data is to use statistical procedures called **nonparametric,** or **distribution-free,** methods. Nonparametric methods are based on weaker assumptions than the *z* and *t* tests, and they do not require the observations to follow any particular distribution.

Figure 5–8 is a histogram of step length as reported in the Rabago study. Can we assume they are normally distributed? How would you describe the distribution? It is somewhat positively skewed, or skewed to the right? Should we have used the *t* test to compare the mean step length with the norm reported in the Sekiya study? Let us see the conclusion if we use a method that does not require assuming a normal distribution.

[†]Remember from your high school or college math courses that the log of a number is the power of 10 that gives the number. For example, the log of 100 is 2 because 10 raised to the second power (10^2) is 100, the log of 1,000 is 3 because 10 is raised to the third power (10^3) to obtain 1,000, and so on. We can also think about logs as being exponents of 10 that must be used to get the number.

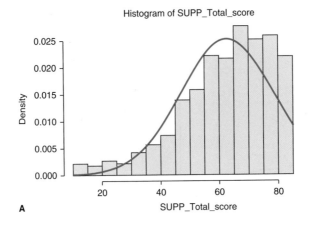

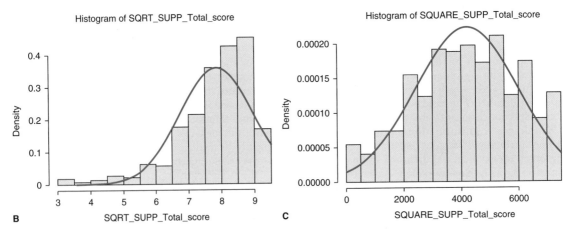

Figure 5–7. Original observations and two transformations of the social support score. (Data from Bos-Touwen I, Schuurmans M, Monninkhof EM, et al: Patient and disease characteristics associated with activation for self-management in patients with diabetes, chronic obstructive pulmonary disease, chronic heart failure and chronic renal disease: a cross-sectional survey study, *PLoS One.* 2015 May 7;10(5):e0126400.)

The **sign test** is a nonparametric test that can be used with a single group using the median rather than the mean. For example, we can ask: Did male subjects in the study by Rabago and colleagues have the same median step length as the 0.66 m normative value, (Because the median step length is not reported in the Sekiya data, the mean and median values are assumed to be the same for this example.)

The logic behind the sign test is as follows: If the median step length in the population of a male subject is 0.66 m, the probability is 0.50 that any observation is less than 0.66. The probability is also 0.50 that any observation is greater than 0.66. We count the number of observations less than 0.66 and can use the binomial distribution (Chapter 4) with $\pi = 0.50$.

Table 5–11 contains the data on the step length of male subjects ranked from lowest to highest. Four subjects have step lengths less than or equal to 0.66 and 11 have longer step lengths. The probability of observing $X = 4$ out of $n = 15$ values less than or equal to 0.66 using the binomial distribution is

$$P(X) = \frac{n!}{x!(n-x)!}(\pi)^x(1-\pi)^{n-x}$$

$$P(X) = \frac{15!}{4!(15-4)!}(0.5)^4(0.5)^{15-4}$$

Rather than trying to calculate this probability, we use this example as an opportunity to use the z approximation to the binomial distribution to illustrate the

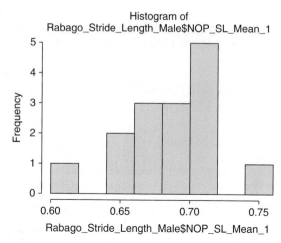

Histogram of
Rabago_Stride_Length_Male$NOP_SL_Mean_1

Figure 5–8. A histogram of step length for male subjects. (Data from Rábago CA, Dingwell JB, Wilken JM: Reliability and Minimum Detectable Change of Temporal-Spatial, Kinematic, and Dynamic Stability Measures during Perturbed Gait, *PLoS One.* 2015 Nov 4;10(11):e0142083.)

Table 5–11. Step length for male subjects.

Subjects	Sex	Stride Length
17	M	0.61
8	M	0.64
19	M	0.65
13	M	0.66
11	M	0.67
7	M	0.67
20	M	0.69
3	M	0.70
9	M	0.70
6	M	0.71
18	M	0.71
2	M	0.71
10	M	0.71
4	M	0.71
12	M	0.74

Data from Rabago CA, Dingwell JB, Wilken JM: Reliability and minimum detectable change of temporalspatial, kinematic, and dynamic stability measures during perturbed gait, *BPLoS One.* 2015 Nov 4;10(11):e0142083.

sign test. We use the same level of α and use a two-tailed test so we can directly compare the results to the *t* test in the section titled, "Steps in Hypothesis Testing."

Step 1: The null and alternative hypotheses are

H_0: The population median step length for adult males is 0.66 m.

H_1: The population median step length for adult males is not 0.66 m.

Step 2: Assuming step length is not normally distributed, the appropriate test is the sign test; and because the π is 0.5, we can use the z distribution. In the sign test, we deal with frequencies instead of proportions, so the z test is rewritten in terms of frequencies.

$$z = \frac{|X - n\pi| - (1/2)}{\sqrt{n\pi(1-\pi)}}$$

where X is the number of men with step length less than or equal to 0.66 (4 in our example), or we could use the number with step lengths greater than 0.66; it does not matter. The total number of subjects n is 15, and the probability π is 0.5, to reflect the 50% chance that any observation is less than (or greater than) the median. Note that ½ is subtracted from the absolute value in the numerator; this is the continuity correction for frequencies.

Step 3: We use $\alpha = 0.05$ so we can compare the results with those found with the *t* test.

Step 4: The critical value of the z distribution for $\alpha = 0.05$ is ± 1.96. So, if the z test statistic is less than -1.96 or greater than $+1.96$, we will reject the null hypothesis of no difference in median levels of energy intake.

Step 5: The calculations are

$$z \frac{|4 - 15(0.5)| - 0.5}{\sqrt{15(0.5)(1 - 0.5)}} = \frac{|-35| - 0.5}{\sqrt{3.75}} = \frac{3.00}{1.94} = 1.55$$

Step 6: The value of the sign test is 1.55 and is less than $+1.96$. The null hypothesis is not rejected because the value of the test statistic is less than the critical value. Two points are interesting. First, the value of the test statistic using the *t* test was 2.00. Looking at the formula tells us that the critical value of the sign test is positive because we use the absolute value in the numerator. Second, we drew the same conclusion when we used the *t* test.

MEAN DIFFERENCES WHEN OBSERVATIONS ARE NOT NORMALLY DISTRIBUTED

Using the *t* test requires that we assume the differences are normally distributed, and this is especially important with small sample sizes, $(n < 30)$. If the distribution of the differences is skewed, several other methods are more appropriate. First, one of the transformations we discussed earlier can be used. More often, however, researchers in the health sciences use a nonparametric statistical test that does not require the normal distribution. For paired designs, we can use the sign test that we used with a single group, applying it to the differences. Alternatively, we can use a

Table 5–12. Wilcoxon signed rank test for difference in M-wave signal.

Wilcoxon signed rank test

data: PRE and POST
V = 70, p-value = 0.09424

alternative hypothesis: true location shift is not equal to 0

---

nonparametric procedure called the **Wilcoxon signed rank test** (also called the Mann–Whitney U test). In fact, there is absolutely no disadvantage in using the Wilcoxon signed rank test in any situation, even when observations are normally distributed. The Wilcoxon test is almost as powerful (correctly rejecting the null hypothesis when it is false) as the *t* test. For paired comparisons, we recommend the Wilcoxon test over the sign test because it is more powerful. In the past, the Wilcoxon signed rank test required either exhaustive calculations or employing extensive statistical tables. Today, however, nonparametric tests are easy to do with computerized routines.

Using the study by Dittrich and colleagues (2018), we can compare the conclusion using the Wilcoxon signed rank test with that found with the paired *t* test. Figure 5–9 is a box plot of the change in M-wave before and after exercise; there is some evidence of negative skewness, so using a nonparametric procedure is justified. The results of the Wilcoxon test using the R nonparametric procedure is shown in Table 5–12. Note that the significance level is given as 0.094. Since the *p* value of 0.094 is greater than our alpha level of 0.05, we do not reject the null hypothesis. Note that this is same conclusion as the *t* test. Use the study data file

found here: https://zenodo.org/record/1213604#.XB5n-1xKiUl to calculate the Wilcoxon test for the difference in pre- and post-M-wave before-and-after exercise for the hypnosis trials.

FINDING THE APPROPRIATE SAMPLE SIZE FOR RESEARCH

Researchers must learn how large a sample is needed before beginning their research because they may not otherwise be able to determine significance when it occurs. Earlier in this chapter, we talked about type I (α) errors and type II (β) errors, and we defined power ($1 - \beta$) as the probability of finding significance when there really is a difference. Low power can occur because the difference is small or because the sample size is too small.

Readers of research reports also need to know what sample size was needed in a study. This is especially true when the results of a study are not statistically significant (a negative study), because the results would possibly have been significant if the sample size had been larger. Increasingly, we see examples of sample size information in the method section of published articles. Institutional review boards (IRB) examine proposals before giving approval for research involving human and animal subjects and require sample size estimates before approving a study. Granting agencies require this information as well.

Many researchers report a variable called effect size. Effect size was introduced by Jacob Cohen (1962) and later summarized in his 1992 article titled "A Power Primer." It is a measure of how far the researcher believes the alternative hypothesis is from the null hypothesis. It is an important concept to use in sample size determination because if the researcher believes that the null and alternative hypotheses are relatively close together, then the sample size required to be powerful enough to detect a small difference is larger than that required if the hypotheses are believed to be very different.

The effect size is used in the G*Power computer program to calculate sample size. The program also provides a calculator to derive the effect size for various scenarios. The effect size is related to the difference in means that the researcher would like to detect (see Exercise 3). A variety of formulas can determine what size sample is needed, and several computer programs can estimate sample sizes for a wide range of study designs and statistical methods. Many people prefer to use a computer program to calculate sample sizes. The manuals that come with these programs are very helpful. We present typical computer output from some of these programs in this section and in following chapters.

We also give formulas that protect against both type I and type II errors for two common situations: a study

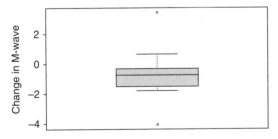

Figure 5–9. Box-and-whisker (boxplot) of change in M-wave activation (Data from Dittrich N, Agostino D, Antonini Philippe R: Effect of hypnotic suggestion on knee extensor neuromuscular properties in resting and fatigued states, *PLoS One.* 2018 Apr 23;13(4):e0195437.)

that involves one mean or one proportion, and a study that measures a group twice and compares the difference before and after an intervention.

Finding the Sample Size for Studies with One Mean

 To estimate sample size for a research study involving a single mean, we must answer the following four questions:

1. What level of significance (α level or p value) related to the null hypothesis is wanted?
2. What is the desired level of power (equal to $1 - \beta$)?
3. How large should the difference be between the mean and the standard value or norm ($\mu_1 - \mu_0$) in order to be clinical importance?
4. What is an estimate of the standard deviation σ?

Specifications of α for a null hypothesis and β for an alternative hypothesis permit us to solve for the sample size. These specifications lead to the following two critical ratios, where z_α is the two-tailed value (for a two-sided test) of z related to α, generally 0.05, and $z\beta$ is the lower one-tailed value of z related to β, generally 0.20. We use the lower one-sided value for β because we want power to be equal to $(1 - \beta)$ or more.

$$z_\alpha = \frac{\bar{X} - \mu_0}{\sigma / \sqrt{n}} \text{ and } z_\beta = \frac{\bar{X} - \mu_1}{\sigma / \sqrt{n}}$$

Solving these two critical ratios for the sample size gives

$$n = \left[\frac{(z_\alpha - z_\beta)\sigma}{\mu_1 - \mu_0} \right]^2$$

Suppose that prior to beginning their study, Rabago and colleagues (2015) wanted to know whether the mean step length for males was different from 0.66 m—either more or less. Researchers generally choose a type I error of 0.05, and power of 0.80. We assume the standard deviation is about 0.03. From the given information, what is the sample size needed to detect a difference of 0.02 m or more?

The two-tailed z value for α of 0.05 is ± 1.96 (from Table A–2); refer to Table 5–5. The lower one-tailed z value related to β is approximately -0.84 (the critical value that separates the lower 20% of the z distribution from the upper 80%). With a standard deviation of 0.03 and the 0.02 difference the investigators want to be able to detect (consumption of ≤ 0.66 m or ≥ 0.70 m), the sample size is

$$n = \left[\frac{(z_\alpha - z_\beta)\sigma}{\mu_1 - \mu_0} \right]^2$$

$$= \left[\frac{(1.96 - (-0.84)) \times 0.03}{0.68 - 0.66} \right]^2$$

$$= \left[\frac{0.084}{0.02} \right]^2 = 17.64 \text{ or } 18$$

To conclude that mean step length of ≤ 0.66 m or ≥ 0.70 m is a significant departure from an assumed 0.68 m (with standard deviation of 0.03), investigators need a sample of 18. (The sample size is 18 instead of 17 because we always round up to the next whole number.) In Exercise 3, you are asked to calculate how large a sample would be needed if they wanted to detect a difference of 0.04 or more meters.

The Sample Size for Studies with One Proportion

Just as in estimating the sample size for a mean, the researcher must answer the same four questions to estimate the sample size needed for a single proportion.

1. What is the desired level of significance (the α level) related to the null hypothesis, π_0?
2. What level of power ($1 - \beta$) is desired associated with the alternative hypothesis, π_1?
3. How large should the difference between the proportions ($\pi_1 - \pi_0$) be for it to be clinically significant?
4. What is a good estimate of the standard deviation in the population? For a proportion, it is easy: the proportion itself, π, determines the estimated standard deviation. It is $\pi(1 - \pi)$.

The formula to determine the sample size is

$$n = \left[\frac{z_\alpha \sqrt{\pi_0(1 - \pi_0)} - z_\beta \sqrt{\pi_1(1 - \pi_1)}}{\pi_0 - \pi_1} \right]^2$$

where, using the same logic as with the sample size for a mean, z_α is the *two-tailed* z value related to the null hypothesis and $z\beta$ is the lower *one-tailed* z value related to the alternative hypothesis.

To illustrate, we consider the study by van Lindert and colleagues (2018) regarding the infection rate for shunt placements. The proportion of people with an infection after shunt placement in the ≤ 1 year age group was 0.170. In the methods section of their article, the investigators do not document their sample size determination, but the example may still be used to demonstrate the concept. Suppose we want to be sure to detect a change in the shunt infection rate by at least 5% from the baseline rate of 17.0% for subjects less than 1 year old. As with finding sample sizes or means, the two-tailed z value related to $\alpha = 0.05$ is ± 1.96, and the lower one-tailed z value related to β is approximately -0.84. Then, the estimated sample size is

$$
n = \left[\frac{z_\alpha \sqrt{\pi_0 \times (1 - \pi_0)} - z_\beta \sqrt{\pi_1 \times (1 - \pi_1)}}{\pi_0 - \pi_1} \right]^2
$$

$$
= \left[\frac{1.96\sqrt{0.17 \times 0.83} - (-0.84)\sqrt{0.12 \times 0.88}}{0.17 - 0.12} \right]^2
$$

$$
= \left[\frac{1.0092}{0.05} \right]^2 = 407.40 \; or \; 408
$$

Exercise 4 calculates the sample size needed if we use 15% instead of 12% as the infection rate we want to detect.

Sample Sizes for Before-and-After Studies

When studies involve the mean in a group measured twice, the research question focuses on whether there has been a change, or stated another way, whether the mean difference varies from zero. As we saw in the section titled, "Means When the Same Group Is Measured Twice," we can use the same approach to finding confidence intervals and doing hypothesis tests for determining a change in the mean in one group measured twice as for a mean in one group. We can also use the same formulas to find the desired sample size. The only difference from the previous illustration is that we test the change (or difference between the means) against a population value of zero. If you have access to one of the power computer programs such as G*Power, you can compare the result from the procedure to calculate the sample size for one mean with the result from the procedure to calculate the sample size for a mean difference, generally referred to as the paired t test. If you assume the standard deviations are the same in both situations, you will get the same number. Unfortunately, the situation is not as simple when the focus is on proportions. In this situation, we need to use different

formulas to determine sample sizes for before-and-after studies. Because paired studies involving proportions occur less often than paired studies involving means, we refer you to the power programs for calculating sample sizes for paired proportions.

Computer Programs for Finding Sample Sizes

Using data from Rabago and colleagues (2015), we use the G*Power program to calculate the sample size for a study involving one mean. Output from the program is given in Figure 5–10. (If you use this program, you must click on the [Determine] button to input the two hypothesis means and the standard deviation.) G*Power indicates we need n of 20, close to the value we calculated of 18.

G*Power may also be used to find the sample size for a proportion as demonstrated by the van Lindert. Output from this procedure is given in Figure 5–11 and states that 381 patients will provide 80% power.

SUMMARY

This chapter illustrated several methods for estimating and testing hypotheses about means and proportions. Methods to use in paired or before-and-after designs in which the same subjects are measured twice were also discussed. These studies are typically called repeated-measures designs.

Observations on gait parameters under various perturbations studied by Rabago and colleagues (2015) were used to form a 95% confidence interval for the mean step length by males and found it to be 0.66 to 0.70 m. Hypothesis testing for the mean in one group was demonstrated by asking whether the mean step length for males was different from the norm found in a national study and showed the equivalence of conclusions when using confidence intervals and hypothesis tests.

In the study published by van Lindert and colleagues (2018), the investigators found that the infection rate for shunt placement for subjects less than 1 year of age was 17%. Data from this study was used to illustrate statistical methods for a proportion. The authors concluded that the addition of vancomycin to the protocol reduced the infection rate.

To illustrate the usefulness of paired or before-and-after studies, we used data from the study by Dittrich and colleagues (2018) in which knee neuromuscular activity was observed before and after hypnotic suggestion. There was no statistically significant change in M-wave signal before and after treatment in this study.

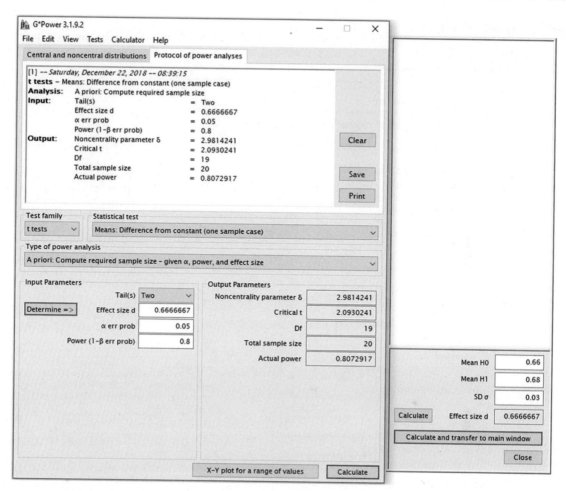

Figure 5–10. Computer output from the G*Power program estimating a sample size for the mean step length in adult males. (Data from Rábago CA, Dingwell JB, Wilken JM: Reliability and Minimum Detectable Change of Temporal-Spatial, Kinematic, and Dynamic Stability Measures during Perturbed Gait, *PLoS One.* 2015 Nov 4;10(11):e0142083.)

Leone and colleagues (2013) evaluated the interrater reliability of using color-Doppler to evaluated five criteria in diagnosing multiple sclerosis (MS). This data was used to illustrate agreement between two evaluators with the κ statistic and found a good level of agreement. On occasion, investigators want to know whether the proportion of subjects changes after an intervention. In this situation, the McNemar test is used, as with changes in sleep quality studied by He and colleagues (2015).

Alternative methods to use when observations are not normally distributed were presented. Among these are several kinds of transformations, with the log (logarithmic transformation) being fairly common, and

nonparametric tests. These tests make no assumptions about the distribution of the data. The sign test is a nonparametric test used for testing hypotheses about the median in one group and the Wilcoxon signed rank test for paired observations, which has power almost as great as that of the *t* test.

The chapter was concluded with a discussion of the important concept of power. The procedures for estimating the sample size for research questions involving one group and illustrated the use of three statistical programs that make the process much easier were outlined.

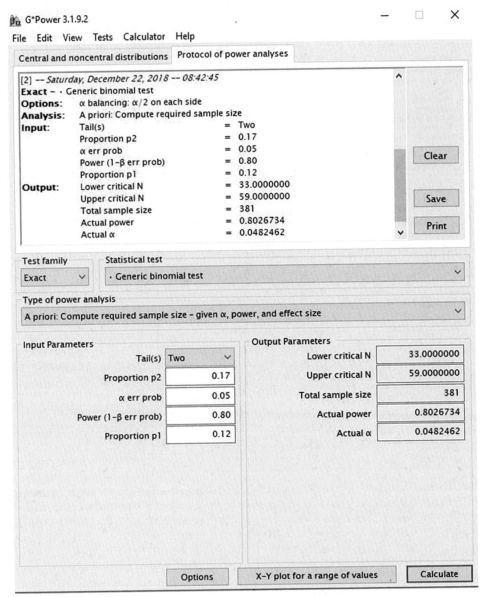

Figure 5–11. Computer output from the G*Power program estimating the sample size for a proportion. (Data from van Lindert EJ, Bilsen MV, Flier MV: Topical vancomycin reduces the cerebrospinal fluid shunt infection rate: A retrospective cohort study, *PLoS One*. 2018 Jan 9;13(1):e0190249.)

The next chapter will explore research questions that involve two independent groups. The methods you learned in this chapter are not only important for their use with one group of subjects, but they also serve as the basis for the methods in the next chapter.

A summary of the statistical methods discussed in this chapter is given in Appendix C. These flowcharts can help both readers and researchers determine which statistical procedure is appropriate for comparing means.

EXERCISES

1. Using the study by Rabago and coworkers (2015), find the 99% confidence interval for the mean step length for men and compare the result with the 95% confidence interval we found (0.66 to 0.70).

   a. Is it wider or narrower than the confidence interval corresponding to 95% confidence?

   b. How could Rabago and coworkers increase the precision with which the mean step length for men is measured?

   c. Recalculate the 99% confidence interval assuming the number of men is 200. Is it wider or narrower than the confidence interval corresponding to 95% confidence?

2. Using the study by Rabago and coworkers, test whether the mean step length for men is different from 0.76. What is the p value? Find the 95% confidence interval for the mean and compare the results to the hypothesis test.

3. Using the Rabago and coworkers study, determine the sample size needed if the researchers wanted 80% power to detect a difference of >0.01 m (assuming the standard deviation is .03 m). Compare the results with the sample size needed for a difference of 0.02 m.

4. What sample size is needed if van Lindert and coworkers (2018) wanted to know if an observed 17% of patients with an initial success to vaccination is different from an assumed norm of 10%? How does this number compare with the number we found assuming a rate of 12%?

5. Our calculations indicated that a sample size of 18 is needed to detect a difference of ≥0.02 m from an assumed mean of 0.66 m in the Rabago and coworkers' study, assuming a standard deviation of 0.03 m. Rabago and coworkers had 20 men in their study and found a step length of 0.68 m. Because 20 is larger than 18, we expect that a 95% CI for the mean would not contain 0.66 m. The CI we found was 0.66–0.70, however, and because this CI contains 0.66, we cannot reject a null hypothesis that the true mean is 0.66. What is the most likely explanation for this seeming contradiction?

6. Using the data from the Dittrich and colleague's study (2018), how large would the mean difference need to be to be considered significant at the 0.05 level if only ten patients were in the study? Hint: Use the formula for one mean and solve for the difference, using 1.7 as an estimate of the standard deviation.

7. Two physicians evaluated a sample of 50 mammograms and classified them as negative (needing no follow-up) versus positive (needing follow-up). Physician 1 determined that 30 mammograms were negative and 20 were positive, and physician 2 found 35 negative and 15 positive. They agreed that 25 were negative. What is the agreement beyond chance?

8. Use the data from the Dittrich and colleagues' study to determine if a change occurs in M-wave amplitude—rectus femoris pre- and post-exercise under the hypnosis condition.

   a. First, examine the distribution of the changes in M-wave. Is the distribution normal so we can use the paired t test, or is the Wilcoxon test more appropriate?

   b. Second, use the paired t test to compare the before-and-after measures of M-wave; then, Wilcoxon test. Compare the answers from the two procedures.

9. Rabago and coworkers also studied stride width under a number of conditions. Use the stride width for men under no perturbation to answer the following questions:

   a. Are the observations normally distributed?

   b. Perform the t test and sign test for one group with a null hypothesis value of 0.15 m. Do these two tests lead to the same conclusion? If not, which is the more appropriate?

10. **Group Exercise.** Congenital or developmental dysplasia of the hip (DDH) is a common pediatric affliction that may precede arthritic deformities of the hip in adult patients. Among patients undergoing total hip arthroplasty, the prevalence of DDH is 3–10%. Ömeroglu and colleagues (2002) analyzed a previously devised radiographic classification system for the shape of the acetabular roof. The study design required that four orthopedic surgeons independently evaluate the radiographs of 33 patients who had previously been operated on to treat unilateral or bilateral DDH. They recorded their measurements independently on two separate occasions during a period of 1 month. You may find it helpful to obtain a copy of the article to help answer the following questions.

   a. What was the study design? Was it appropriate for the research question?

b. How did the investigators analyze the agreement among the orthopedic surgeons? What is this type of agreement called?

c. How did the investigators analyze the agreement between the measurements made on two separate occasions by a given orthopedic surgeon?

d. Based on the guidelines presented in this chapter, how valuable is the classification system?

 DISCUSSION QUESTIONS

1. What do you think about the idea of giving polls as intervals rather than as specific percentages? Would this help also in weather predictions?

2. Do you agree that weather predictions of the temperature are understood better than poll estimates? For example, what confidence interval would you put on a weather predictor's 60% chance for rain?

Research Questions About Two Separate or Independent Groups

KEY CONCEPTS

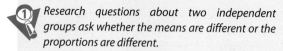 Research questions about two independent groups ask whether the means are different or the proportions are different.

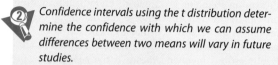 Confidence intervals using the t distribution determine the confidence with which we can assume differences between two means will vary in future studies.

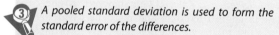 A pooled standard deviation is used to form the standard error of the differences.

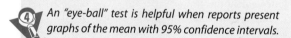 An "eye-ball" test is helpful when reports present graphs of the mean with 95% confidence intervals.

Using the t distribution requires the two groups to be independent from each other as well as the assumptions of normality and equal variances in the two groups.

Tests of hypothesis are another way to test the difference between two means.

The assumption of equal variances can be tested with several procedures.

The nonparametric Wilcoxon rank sum test is an excellent alternative to the t test when the assumptions of normality or equal variances are not met.

Both confidence intervals and statistical tests can be used to compare two proportions using the z test, again using a pooled standard deviation to form the standard error.

The chi-square test is a very versatile statistical procedure used to test for differences in proportions as well as an association between two variables.

Fisher's exact test is preferred to chi-square when two characteristics are being compared, each at two levels (i.e., 2 × 2 tables) because it provides the exact probability.

The relative risk, or odds ratio, is appropriate if the purpose is to estimate the strength of a relationship between two nominal measures.

When two groups are compared on a numerical variable, the numerical variable should not be turned into categories to use the chi-square test; it is better to use the t test.

It is possible to estimate sample sizes needed to compare the means or proportions in two groups, but it is much more efficient to use one of the statistical power packages, such as G*Power.

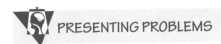

PRESENTING PROBLEMS

Presenting Problem 1

See Chapter 3, Presenting Problem 1 (Davids et al, 2014)

Presenting Problem 2

Ström and colleagues (2013) studied the effectiveness of an Internet-delivered therapist-guided physical activity to treat mild to moderate depression. They used a randomized design to assign 48 participants to the Internet-delivered therapy and standard care.

The article may be accessed at this link:
Ström M, Uckelstam C, Andersson G, Hassmén P, Umefjord G, Carlbring P: Internet-delivered therapist-guided physical activity for mild to moderate depression: a randomized controlled trial.

https://doi.org/10.7717/peerj.178

The data used in the study may be downloaded from this link:
Ström M, Uckelstam C, Andersson G, Hassmén P, Umefjord G, Carlbring P: Internet-delivered therapist-guided physical activity for mild to moderate depression: a randomized controlled trial. Dryad Digital Repository 2013.

https://doi.org/10.5061/dryad.c6q65

Presenting Problem 3

See Chapter 3, Presenting Problem 3 (Anderson et al, 2018).

PURPOSE OF THE CHAPTER

In the previous chapter, statistical methods to use when the research question involves the following situations were reviewed:

1. A single group of subjects and the goal is to compare a proportion or mean to a norm or standard.
2. A single group measured twice and the goal is to estimate how much the proportion or mean changes between measurements.

The procedures in this chapter are used to examine differences between two **independent groups** (when knowledge of the observations for one group does not provide any information about the observations in the second group). In all instances, the groups represented are assumed to be random samples from the larger population to which researchers want to apply the conclusions.

When the research question asks whether the means of two groups are equal (numerical observations), either the two-sample (independent-groups) *t* **test** or the **Wilcoxon rank sum** test may be used. When the research question asks whether proportions in two independent groups are equal, several methods may apply: the *z* distribution to form a confidence interval and the *z* distribution, chi-square, or Fisher's exact test to test hypotheses.

DECISIONS ABOUT MEANS IN TWO INDEPENDENT GROUPS

Investigators often want to know if the means are equal or if one mean is larger than the other mean. For example, Bos-Touwen and colleagues (2015) in Presenting Problem 1 wanted to know if information on a patient's comorbid disease and demographics are related to the level of self-management activation. We noted in Chapter 5 that the *z* test can be used to analyze questions involving means if the *population standard deviation is known*. This, however, is rarely the case in applied research, and researchers typically use the *t* test to analyze research questions involving two independent means.

Surveys of statistical methods used in the medical literature consistently indicate that *t* tests and chi-square tests are among the most commonly used. Furthermore, Greenland and coworkers (2016) noted a number of problems in using confidence intervals and hypothesis tests including citing of assumptions. Thus, being able to evaluate the use of tests comparing means and proportions—whether they are used properly and how to interpret the results—is an important skill for medical practitioners.

Comparing Two Means Using Confidence Intervals

The means and standard deviations from selected variables from the Bos-Touwen study are given in Table 6–1. In this chapter, we analyze the patient activation measure (PAM) for patients who had chronic renal disease (CRD) and those who did not. The average PAM score for these two groups of patients will be compared. PAM is a numerical variable; therefore, the mean provides an appropriate way to describe the average with numerical variables. We can find the mean PAM for each set of patients and form a confidence interval for the difference.

Table 6–1. Summary statistics for patient activation measure variables for subjects with and without chronic renal disease (CRD), [n/mean±sd].

	No CRD	**CRD**
Age	732/70.6±10.9	422/68.0±10.8
BMI	707/26.9±4.6	421/28.6±4.3
Patient Activation Measure	732/53.4±10.6	422/55.3±11.0
SF12 Total Score	719/53.5±24.1	413/65.8±24.0
IPQ Total Score	715/39.6±12.0	419/30.6±11.6
Social Support Total Score	725/63.0±16.2	412/62.6±15.0

Data from Bos-Touwen I, Schuurmans M, Monninkhof EM, et al: Patient and disease characteristics associated with activation for self-management in patients with diabetes, chronic obstructive pulmonary disease, chronic heart failure and chronic renal disease: a cross-sectional survey study, *PLoS One*. 2015 May 7; 10(5):e0126400.

The form for a confidence interval for the difference between two means is

Confidence interval = Mean difference ± Number

related to confidence level (often 95%)

× Standard error of the difference

If we use symbols to illustrate a confidence interval for the difference between two means and let $\bar{X}_1$ stand for the mean of the first group and $\bar{X}_2$ for the mean of the second group, then we can write the difference between the two means as $\bar{X}_1 - \bar{X}_2$.

As you know from the previous chapter, the number related to the level of confidence is the critical value from the t distribution. For two means, we use the t distribution with $(n_1 - 1)$ degrees of freedom corresponding to the number of subjects in group 1, plus $(n_2 - 1)$ degrees of freedom corresponding to the number of subjects in group 2, for a total of $(n_1 + n_2 - 2)$ degrees of freedom.

With two groups, there are also two standard deviations. One assumption for the t test, however, is that the standard deviations are equal (the section titled, "Assumptions for the t Distribution"). A more stable estimate of the true standard deviation in the population is achieved if the two separate standard deviations are averaged to obtain a **pooled standard deviation** based on a larger sample size. The pooled standard deviation is a weighted average of the two variances (squared standard deviations) with weights based on the sample sizes. Once we have

the pooled standard deviation, we use it in the formula for the standard error of the difference between two means, the last term in the preceding equation for a confidence interval.

The standard error of the mean difference measures how much the differences between two means tend to vary if a study is repeated many times.

The formula for the pooled standard deviation looks complicated, but remember that the calculations are for illustration only, and we generally use a computer to do the computation. We first square the standard deviation in each group (SD_1 and SD_2) to obtain the variance, multiply each variance by the number in that group minus 1, and add to get $(n_1 - 1)\,SD_1^2 + (n_2 - 1)\,SD_2^2$. The standard deviations are based on the samples because we do not know the true population standard deviations. Next, we divide by the sum of the number of subjects in each group minus 2.

$$\frac{(n + 1)SD_1^2 + (n_2 - 1)SD_2^2}{n_1 + n_2 - 2}$$

Finally, we take the square root to find the pooled standard deviation.

$$SD_p = \sqrt{\frac{(n_1 - 1)SD_1^2 + (n_2 - 1)SD_2^2}{n_1 + n_2 - 2}}$$

The pooled standard deviation is used to calculate the standard error of the difference. In words, the standard error of the difference between two means is the pooled standard deviation, SD_p, multiplied by the square root of the sum of the reciprocals of the sample sizes. In symbols, the standard error of the mean difference is

$$SE_{(\bar{X}_1 - \bar{X}_2)} = SD_p\sqrt{\frac{1}{n_1} + \frac{1}{n_2}}$$

Based on the study by Bos-Touwen and colleagues (2015), 422 patients with CRD and 732 patients without CRD had values for PAM (see Table 6–1). Substituting 422 and 732 for the two sample sizes and 11.0 and 10.6 for the two standard deviations, we have

$$\text{Pooled } SD = SD_p = \sqrt{\frac{(422 - 1)11.0^2 + (732 - 1)10.6^2}{422 + 732 - 2}}$$

$$= 10.75$$

Does it make sense that the value of the pooled standard deviation is always between the two sample standard deviations? In fact, if the sample sizes are equal, it is the mean of the two standard deviations (see Exercise 4).

Finally, to find the standard error of the difference, we substitute 10.75 for the pooled standard deviation and 422 and 732 for the sample sizes and obtain

$$SE_{(\bar{X}_1 - \bar{X}_2)} = 10.75\sqrt{\frac{1}{422} + \frac{1}{732}} = 10.75 \times 0.06 = 0.66$$

The standard error of the difference in PAM measured in the two groups is 0.66. The standard error is simply the standard deviation of the differences in means if we repeated the study many times. It indicates that we can expect the *mean differences* in a large number of similar studies to have a standard deviation of about 0.66.

The means of the two groups and the standard error of the difference in the means is all the information needed to find a confidence interval for the mean difference in PAM. From Table 6–1, the mean PAM scores were 55.3 for patients having CRD and 53.4 for patients without CRD. To find the 95% confidence limits for the difference between these means (55.3 − 53.4 = 1.9), we use the two-tailed value from the *t* distribution for 422 + 732 − 2 = 1,152 degrees of freedom (Appendix A–3) that separates the central 95% of the *t* distribution from the 5% in the tails. The value is 1.96; note that the value *z* is also 1.96, demonstrating once more that the *t* distribution approaches the shape of the *z* distribution with large samples.

Using these numbers in the formula for 95% confidence limits, 1.9 ± (1.96) (0.66) = 1.9 ± 1.29, or 0.61

to 3.28. Interpreting this confidence interval, we can be 95% confident that the interval from 0.61 to 3.28 contains the true mean difference in PAM. Because the interval does not contain the value 0, it is not likely that the mean difference is 0. Table 6–2 illustrates the output of the R command (*t* test) for comparing two means and determining a confidence interval. The confidence interval found by R is 0.66 to 3.24, slightly different from ours due to rounding. Use the dataset from the study and replicate this analysis.

Recall in Chapter 3, we used box plots to examine the distribution of PAM for male and female subjects (Figure 3–6). Do you think the difference is statistically significant? R gives the 95% confidence interval as −0.39 to 2.16. What can we conclude about the difference in PAM?

An "Eyeball" Test Using Error Bar Graphs

Readers of the literature and those attending presentations of research findings find it helpful if information is presented in graphs and tables, and most researchers use them whenever possible.

We introduced error bar plots in Chapter 3 when we talked about different graphs that can be used to display data for two or more groups, and error bar plots can be used for an "eyeball" test of the mean in two (or more) groups. Using error bar charts with 95% confidence limits, one of the following three results always occurs:

1. The top of one error bar does not overlap with the bottom of the other error bar, as illustrated in

Table 6–2. Two sample *t*-test comparing patient activation management score for subjects with and without chronic renal disease.

```
> t.test(activation_score~DMII, alternative='two.sided', conf.level=.95,
+    var.equal=FALSE, data=activation)

        Welch Two Sample t-test

data:  activation_score by DMII
t = 2.9429, df = 856.71, p-value = 0.003339
alternative hypothesis: true difference in means is not equal to 0
95 percent confidence interval:
 0.6500697 3.2534279
sample estimates:
    mean in group DMII mean in group No DMII
            55.33768              53.38593
```

Data from Bos-Touwen I, Schuurmans M, Monninkhof EM, et al: Patient and disease characteristics associated with activation for self-management in patients with diabetes, chronic obstructive pulmonary disease, chronic heart failure and chronic renal disease: a cross-sectional survey study, *PLoS One.* 2015 May 7;10(5):e0126400.

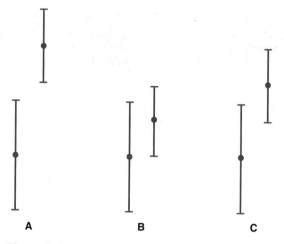

Figure 6–1. Visual assessment of differences between two independent groups, using 95% confidence limits.

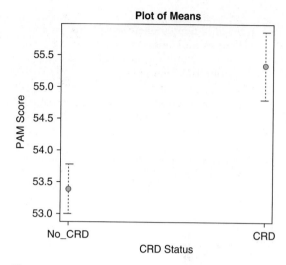

Figure 6–2. Illustration of error bars. (Data from Bos-Touwen I, Schuurmans M, Monninkhof EM, et al: Patient and disease characteristics associated with activation for self-management in patients with diabetes, chronic obstructive pulmonary disease, chronic heart failure and chronic renal disease: a cross-sectional survey study, *PLoS One.* 2015 May 7;10(5):e0126400.)

Figure 6–1A. When this occurs, we can be 95% sure that the means in two groups are significantly different.

2. The top of one 95% error bar overlaps the bottom of the other so much that the mean value for one group is contained within the limits for the other group (see Figure 6–1B). This indicates that the two means are not statistically significant.

3. If 95% error bars overlap some but not as much as in situation 2, as in Figure 6–1C, we do not know if the difference is significant unless we form a confidence interval or do a statistical test for the difference between the two means.

To use the eyeball method for the mean PAM, we find the 95% confidence interval for the mean in each individual group. The 95% confidence interval for PAM in patients without CRD is 52.6 to 54.1 and 54.3 to 56.4 in patients with DMII.

These two confidence intervals are shown in Figure 6–2. This example illustrates the situation in Figure 6–1A: The graphs do not overlap, so we can conclude that mean pulse oximetry in the two groups is different.

A word of caution is needed. When the sample size in each group is greater than ten, the 95% confidence intervals are approximately equal to the mean ± 2 standard errors (SE), so graphs of the mean ± 2 standard errors can be used for the eyeball test. Some authors, however, instead of using the mean ± 2 standard errors, present a graph of the mean ± 1 standard error or the mean ± 2 standard deviations (SD). Plus or minus 1 standard error gives only a 68% confidence interval for the mean. Plus or minus 2 standard deviations results

in the 95% interval in which the *individual* measurements are found *if the observations are normally distributed*. Although nothing is inherently wrong with these graphs, they cannot be interpreted as indicating differences between means. Readers need to check graph legends very carefully before using the eyeball test to interpret published graphs.

Assumptions for the *t* Distribution

Three assumptions are needed to use the *t* distribution for either determining confidence intervals or testing hypotheses. We briefly mention them here and outline some options to use if observations do not meet the assumptions.

1. As is true with one group, the *t* test assumes that the observations in *each group* follow a normal distribution. Violating the assumption of normality gives *p* values that are lower than they should be, making it easier to reject the null hypothesis and conclude a difference when none really exists. At the same time, confidence intervals are narrower than they should be, so conclusions based on them may be wrong. What is the solution to the problem? Fortunately, this issue is of less concern if the sample sizes are at least 30 in each group.

With smaller samples that are not normally distributed, a **nonparametric** procedure called the **Wilcoxon rank sum** test is a better choice (see the section titled, "Comparing Means with the Wilcoxon Rank Sum Test").

2. The standard deviations (or variances) in the two samples are assumed to be equal (statisticians call them homogeneous variances). Equal variances are assumed because the null hypothesis states that the two means are equal, which is actually another way of saying that the observations in the two groups are from the same population. In the population from which they are hypothesized to come, there is only one standard deviation; therefore, the standard deviations in the two groups must be equal if the null hypothesis is true. What is the solution when the standard deviations are not equal? Fortunately, this assumption can be ignored when the sample sizes are equal (Box, 1953). This is one of several reasons many researchers try to have fairly equal numbers in each group. (Statisticians say the *t* test is **robust** with equal sample sizes.) Statistical tests can be used to decide whether standard deviations are equal before doing a *t* test (see the section titled, "Comparing Variation in Independent Groups").

3. The final assumption is one of independence, meaning that knowing the values of the observations in one group tells us nothing about the observations in the other group. In contrast, consider the paired group design discussed in Chapter 5, in which knowledge of the value of an observation at the time of the first measurement does tell us something about the value at the time of the second measurement. For example, we would expect a subject who has a relatively low value at the first measurement to have a relatively low second measurement as well. For that reason, the paired *t* test is sometimes referred to as the dependent groups *t* test. No statistical test can determine whether independence has been violated, however, so the best way to ensure two groups are independent is to design and carry out the study properly.

Comparing Means in Two Groups with the *t* Test

In a study assessing Internet administered treatment for depression, Ström et al (2013) wanted to compare the efficacy of the treatment approaches by measuring the impact of the Beck Depression Inventory-II (BDI-II). Means and standard deviations for the total BDI-II and subscales are reported in Table 6–3.

The research questions in this study is whether or not Internet-administered treatment resulted in a lower BDI-II. Stating the research question in this way implies that the researcher is interested in a directional or one-tailed test, testing only whether the severity of depression is less in the group with the predicted optimal treatment. From Table 6–3, the mean change in BDI score for subjects participating in Internet-based treatment was −9.00 versus −5.79 for those in the control group. This difference could occur by chance, however, and we need to know the probability that a difference this large would occur by chance before we can conclude that these results can generalize to similar populations of individuals with depression.

The sample sizes are smaller than 30, but a test of normality shows no concerns. Since the sample sizes are equal the assumption of equal variances is not a concern, and the *t* test for two independent groups can be used to answer this question. Let us designate subjects participating in the Internet-administered treatment as

Table 6–3. Means and standard deviations on variables from the study on Internet-administered treatment for depression.

Variable	Group	N	Mean	Standard Deviation	Standard Error of Mean
BDI – Pre-Treatment	Control	24	28.25	7.08	1.44
	Treatment	24	26.92	9.30	1.90
BDI – Post-Treatment	Control	24	22.46	6.75	1.38
	Treatment	24	17.92	12.24	2.50
BDI – Post – Pre	Control	24	(5.79)	6.55	1.34
	Treatment	24	(9.00)	9.33	1.90

Data from Ström M, Uckelstam CJ, Andersson G: Internet-delivered therapist-guided physical activity for mild to moderate depression: a randomized controlled trial, *PeerJ*. 2013 Oct 3;1:e178.

group 1 and the controls as group 2. The six steps in testing the hypothesis are as follows:

Step 1: H_0: Subjects who participated in Internet-administered treatment had a mean BDI change at least as those as large as subjects who had no treatment. Note that a negative change in BDI is considered a good result, so we want the change for the treament group to be less than or more negative than the control group. In symbols, we express it as

$$\bar{X}_1 \leq \bar{X}_2 \quad \text{or} \quad \bar{X}_1 - \bar{X}_2 \leq 0$$

H_1: Subjects who participated in Internet-administered treatment had a mean BDI change lower than subjects who had no treatment. In symbols, we express it as

$$\bar{X}_1 > \bar{X}_2 \quad \text{or} \quad \bar{X}_1 - \bar{X}_2 > 0$$

Step 2: The t test can be used for this research question (assuming the observations follow a normal distribution, the standard deviations in the population are equal, and the observations are independent). The t statistic for testing the mean difference in two independent groups has the difference between the means in the numerator and the standard error of the mean difference in the denominator; in symbols it is

$$t_{(n_1 + n_1 - 2)} = \frac{(\bar{X}_1 - \bar{X}_2)}{SD_p \sqrt{[(1 / n_1) + (1 / n_2)]}}$$

where there are $(n_1 - 1) + (n_2 - 1) = (n_1 + n_2 - 2)$ degrees of freedom and SD_p is the pooled standard deviation. (See section titled, "Comparing Two Means Using Confidence Intervals" for details on how to calculate SD_p.)

Step 3: Let us use $\alpha = 0.01$ so there will be only 1 chance in 100 that we will incorrectly conclude that BDI is less after therapy when it really is not.

Step 4: The degrees of freedom are $(n_1 + n_2 - 2) = 24 + 24 - 2 = 46$. For a one-tailed test, the critical value separating the lower 1% of the t distribution from the upper 99% is approximately -2.42 (using the more conservative value for 40 degrees of freedom in Table A-3). So, the decision is to reject the null hypothesis if the observed value of t is less than -2.42 (Figure 6-3).

Step 5: The calculations for the t statistic follow. First, the pooled standard deviation is 28.27 (see Exercise 2). Then the observed value for t is

$$t_{(24 + 24 - 2)} = \frac{(-9.00 - [-5.79])}{8.06\sqrt{\frac{1}{24} + \frac{1}{24}}} = \frac{-3.21}{8.06 \times 0.29} = -1.37$$

Please check the calculations using the downloaded dataset.

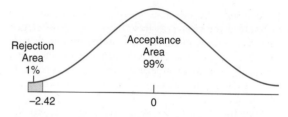

Figure 6-3. Area of rejection for testing hypothesis on mean BDI change for subjects with and without Internet-administered treatment ($\alpha = 0.01$, one-tailed).

Step 6: The observed value of t, -1.37, is not less than the critical value of -2.42, so we cannot reject the null hypothesis. In plain words, there is not enough evidence in this study to conclude that, on the average, patients with depression receiving Internet-administered therapy may not experience a larger decrease in depression symptoms as measured by BDI score change.

Comparing Variation in Independent Groups

The t test for independent groups assumes equal standard deviations or variances, called homogeneous variances, as do the analysis of variance procedures to compare more than two groups discussed in Chapter 7. We can ignore this assumption if the sample sizes are approximately equal. If not, many statisticians recommend testing to see if the standard deviations are equal. If they are not equal, the degrees of freedom for the t test can be adjusted downward, making it more difficult to reject the null hypothesis; otherwise, a nonparametric method, such as the Wilcoxon rank sum test (illustrated in the next section), can be used.

The F Test for Equal Variances: A common statistical test for the equality of two variances is called the F test. This test can be used to determine if two standard deviations are equal, because the standard deviation is the square root of the variance, and if the variances are equal, so are the standard deviations. Many computer programs calculate the F test. This test has some major shortcomings, as we discuss later on; however, an illustration is worthwhile because the F test is the statistic used to compare more than two groups (analysis of variance, the topic of Chapter 7).

To calculate the F test, the *larger* variance is divided by the *smaller* variance to obtain a ratio, and this ratio is then compared with the critical value from the F distribution (corresponding to the desired significance level). If two variances are about equal, their ratio will be about 1. If their ratio is significantly greater than 1, we conclude the variances are unequal. Note that we guaranteed the ratio is at least 1 by putting the larger variance in the numerator. How much greater than 1 does F need to be to conclude that the variances are unequal? As you might expect, the significance of F depends partly on the sample sizes, as is true with most statistical tests.

Sometimes, common sense indicates no test of homogeneous variances is needed. For example, the standard deviations of the PAM scores in the study by Bos-Touwen et al (2015) are approximately 11.0 for the CRD group and 10.6 for the group without CRD, so the variances are 121.0 and 112.4. The practical significance of this difference is nil, so a statistical test for equal variances is unnecessary, and the t test is an appropriate choice. As another example, consider the standard deviations of post-treatment BDI scores from the study by Ström and colleagues (2013) given in Table 6–3: 6.75 for the control group and 12.24 for the treatment group. The relative difference is such that a statistical test will be helpful in deciding the best approach to analysis. The null hypothesis for the test of equal variances is that the variances are equal. Using the BDI variances to illustrate the F test, $12.24^2 = 149.82$ and $6.75^2 = 45.56$, and the F ratio is (putting the larger value in the numerator) $149.82/45.56 = 3.29$.

Although this ratio is greater than 1, you know by now that we must ask whether a value this large could happen by chance, assuming the variances are equal. The F distribution has two values for degrees of freedom (df): one for the numerator and one for the denominator, each equal to the sample size minus 1. The F distribution for our example has $24 - 1 = 23$ df for the numerator and $24 - 1 = 23$ df for the denominator. Using $\alpha = 0.05$, the critical value of the F distribution from Table A–4 is approximately 2.03. (Because of limitations of the table, we used 20 df for the numerator and 20 df for the denominator, resulting in a conservative value.) Because the result of the F test is 3.29, greater than 2.03, we reject the null hypothesis of equal variances. Recall that in this particular case, the sample sizes are equal and we can use the robustness of the two-sample t test under the equal sample size case, but in cases where the sample sizes are not equal, a different approach to the two-sample t test must be used.

If the F test is significant and the hypothesis of equal variances is rejected, the standard deviations from the two samples cannot be pooled for the t test because pooling assumes they are equal. When this happens, one approach is to use separate variances and decrease the degrees of freedom for the t test. Reducing the degrees of freedom requires a larger observed value for t in order to reject the null hypothesis; in other words, a larger difference between the means is required. We can think of this correction as a penalty for violating the assumption of equal standard deviations when we

have unequal sample sizes. Alternatively, a nonparametric procedure may be used.

The Levene Test for Equal Variances: The major problem with using the F test is that it is very sensitive to data that are not normal. Statisticians say the F test is not **robust** to departures from normality—it may appear significant because the data are not normally distributed and not because the variances are unequal.

Several other procedures can be used to test the equality of standard deviations, and most computer programs provide options to the F statistic. A good alternative is the Levene test. For two groups, the Levene test is a t test of the absolute value of the distance each observation is from the mean in that group (not a t test of the original observations). So, in essence, it tests the hypothesis that the average deviations (of observations from the mean in each group) are the same in the two groups. If the value of the Levene test is significant, the conclusion is that, on average, the deviations from the mean in one group exceed those in the other. It is a good approach, whether or not the data are normally distributed.

The Levene test can also be used for testing the equality of variances when more than two groups are being compared. Most commercial statistical packages include the Levene test in their array of hypothesis tests.

Table 6–4 shows computer output when R is used to test the equality of variances. Note that R provides the test based on both the deviations from mean and median. Because the p value of the Levene test is less than 0.05, 0.0198 in this example, we reject the hypothesis of equal variances. Note that this is the same result derived from the F test.

Comparing Means with the Wilcoxon Rank Sum Test

Sometimes, researchers want to compare two independent groups, for which one or more of the assumptions for the t test is seriously violated. The following options are available. In Chapter 5, we discussed transformations when observations are not normally distributed; this approach may also be used when two groups are being analyzed. In particular, transformations can be effective when standard deviations are not equal. More often, however, researchers in the health field use a nonparametric test. The test goes by various names: Wilcoxon rank sum test, Mann–Whitney U Test, or Mann–Whitney–Wilcoxon rank sum test.[*] The test

---

[*] As an aside, the different names for this statistic occurred when a statistician, Wilcoxon, developed the test at about the same time as a pair of statisticians, Mann and Whitney. Unfortunately for readers of the medical literature, there is still no agreement on which name to use for this test.

Table 6–4. Computer listing from R on testing the quality of variances.

```
> leveneTest(BDI_post ~ Group, data=depression, center="median")
Levene's Test for Homogeneity of Variance (center = "median")
      Df F value Pr(>F)
group  1  5.8288 0.0198 *
      46
---
Signif. codes:  0 '***' 0.001 '**' 0.01 '*' 0.05 '.' 0.1 ' ' 1

> with(depression, tapply(BDI_post, Group, var, na.rm=TRUE))
  Control Treatment
45.56341 149.90580

> leveneTest(BDI_post ~ Group, data=depression, center="mean")
Levene's Test for Homogeneity of Variance (center = "mean")
      Df F value  Pr(>F)
group  1  6.4197 0.01476 *
      46
---
Signif. codes:  0 '***' 0.001 '**' 0.01 '*' 0.05 '.' 0.1 ' ' 1
```

Data from Ström M, Uckelstam CJ, Andersson G: Internet-delivered therapist-guided physical activity for mild to moderate depression: a randomized controlled trial, *PeerJ*. 2013 Oct 3;1:e178.

Table 6–5. Rank of BDI scores from the study on Internet-administered treatment for depression.

		Treatment Group						Control Group			
ID	Group	BDI_pre	BDI_post	BDI Change	Rank	ID	Group	BDI_pre	BDI_post	BDI Change	Rank
2	Trmt	27	19	−8	23	1	Cnrtl	23	21	−2	38
5	Trmt	45	30	−15	6	3	Cnrtl	21	12	−9	22
7	Trmt	29	17	−12	11	4	Cnrtl	19	15	−4	33
9	Trmt	18	3	−15	6	6	Cnrtl	27	31	4	46
10	Trmt	38	28	−10	18	8	Cnrtl	33	23	−10	18
11	Trmt	27	9	−18	3	15	Cnrtl	31	23	−8	23
12	Trmt	14	8	−6	26	16	Cnrtl	39	34	−5	29
13	Trmt	22	11	−11	14	17	Cnrtl	37	11	−26	2
14	Trmt	22	4	−18	3	18	Cnrtl	38	26	−12	11
21	Trmt	10	6	−4	33	19	Cnrtl	24	27	3	44
25	Trmt	33	20	−13	10	20	Cnrtl	22	20	−2	38
27	Trmt	15	5	−10	18	22	Cnrtl	29	26	−3	36
29	Trmt	20	9	−11	14	23	Cnrtl	25	26	1	42
31	Trmt	34	29	−5	29	24	Cnrtl	20	15	−5	29
32	Trmt	32	49	17	48	26	Cnrtl	33	31	−2	38
33	Trmt	32	21	−11	14	28	Cnrtl	29	32	3	44
34	Trmt	32	3	−29	1	30	Cnrtl	29	21	−8	23
35	Trmt	40	30	−10	18	36	Cnrtl	27	16	−11	14
37	Trmt	16	13	−3	36	38	Cnrtl	29	17	−12	11
39	Trmt	20	30	10	47	41	Cnrtl	20	16	−4	33
40	Trmt	30	16	−14	8	42	Cnrtl	20	18	−2	38
43	Trmt	34	18	−16	5	44	Cnrtl	31	25	−6	26
45	Trmt	38	40	2	43	47	Cnrtl	47	33	−14	8
46	Trmt	18	12	−6	26	48	Cnrtl	25	20	−5	29
Mean		26.92	17.92	(9.00)	19.17	Mean		28.25	22.46	(5.79)	28.13
Standard Deviation		9.30	12.24	9.33	14.16	Standard Deviation		7.08	6.75	6.55	12.49

Data from Ström M, Uckelstam CJ, Andersson G: Internet-delivered therapist-guided physical activity for mild to moderate depression: a randomized controlled trial, *PeerJ*. 2013 Oct 3;1:e178.

Table 6-6. Illustration of *t* test of BDI change to obtain Wilcoxon rank sum and *t* test of ranks of BDI change.

```
> with(depression, tapply(BDI.Change, Group, median, na.rm=TRUE))
  Control Treatment
    -5.0    -10.5

> wilcox.test(BDI.Change ~ Group, alternative="greater", data=depression)

        Wilcoxon rank sum test with continuity correction

data:  BDI.Change by Group
W = 397.5, p-value = 0.01218
alternative hypothesis: true location shift is greater than 0


> t.test(Rank~Group, alternative='greater', conf.level=.99, var.equal=TRUE, data=depression)

        Two Sample t-test

data:  Rank by Group
t = 2.4021, df = 46, p-value = 0.0102
alternative hypothesis: true difference in means is greater than 0
99 percent confidence interval:
 -0.03105556        Inf
sample estimates:
  mean in group Control mean in group Treatment
                29.125                  19.875
```

Data from Ström M, Uckelstam CJ, Andersson G: Internet-delivered therapist-guided physical activity for mild to moderate depression: a randomized controlled trial, *PeerJ*. 2013 Oct 3;1:e178.

by Hollander and Wolfe (1998) provides information on many nonparametric tests, as does the text by Conover (1999).

In essence, this test tells us whether medians (as opposed to means) are different. The Wilcoxon rank sum test is available in most statistical computer packages, so our goal will be only to acquaint you with the procedure.

To illustrate the Wilcoxon rank sum test, we use the change in BDI scores from the Ström and colleagues' study (2013). The first step is to rank *all* the scores from lowest to highest (or vice versa), ignoring the group they are in. Table 6–5 lists the scores and their rankings. In this example, the lowest score is −29, given by subject 34. Note that subjects 7, 18, and 38 all have scores of −12. Ordinarily, these three subjects would be assigned ranks 1, 12, and 13. When subjects have the same or tied scores, however, the practice is to assign the average rank, so each of these three subjects is given the rank of 12. This process continues until all scores have been ranked, with the highest score, 17 by subject 32, receiving the rank of 48 because there are 48 subjects.

After the observations are ranked, the ranks are analyzed just as though they were the original observations. The mean and standard deviation of the ranks are calculated for each group, and these are used to calculate the pooled standard deviation of the ranks and the *t* test.

The Wilcoxon rank sum method tests the hypothesis that the means of the ranks are equal. Conceptually, the test proceeds as follows: If there is no significant difference between the two groups, some low ranks and some high ranks will occur in each group, that is, the ranks will be distributed across the two groups more or less evenly. In this situation, the mean ranks will be similar as well. On the other hand, if a large difference occurs between the two groups, one group will have more subjects with higher ranks than the other group, and the mean of the ranks will be higher in that group.

Use R to do the *t* test on the rank variable in the Ström dataset. To be consistent with the *t* test on the original observations reported in the section titled, "Comparing Means in Two Groups with the *t* Test," use $\alpha = 0.01$ and do a one-tailed test to see if the Internet-administered treatment results in a larger decrease in BDI scores.

Using R, the *t* test on the rank of cramping scores is 2.40, not greater than the critical value of 2.41, so again we cannot reject the null hypothesis and conclude the Internet-based treatment did not have a beneficial result. The output from R on both the Wilcoxon rank sum test on the original observations and the *t* test using the ranked data is given in Table 6–6. Note from Table 6–6 that the *p* value for the differences is 0.01218 when the Wilcoxon rank sum test is used and 0.0102

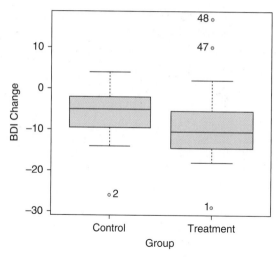

Figure 6–4. Illustration of box plots to compare distributions of cramping scores.

when the *t* test on the ranks is done instead. As we see, using the *t* test on ranks is a good alternative if a computer program for the Wilcoxon test is not available.

We used box-and-whisker plots to evaluate the distribution of the observations (Figure 6–4). What do you conclude about the distributions? The medians (denoted by heavy horizontal lines) fall close midway in the boxes that enclose the 25th to 75th percentile of scores in both groups, indicating a symmetric distribution. The positive tail for the scores for the subjects receiving the treatment is a little longer than the negative tail, indicating a slightly positive skew, but overall, the distributions are fairly normal. So, it appears that the assumptions for the *t* test are adequately met in this example, and, as we would expect, the *t* test and the nonparametric Wilcoxon rank sum test lead to the same conclusion.

The Wilcoxon rank sum test illustrated earlier and the signed rank test discussed in Chapter 5 are excellent alternatives to the *t* test. When assumptions are met for the *t* test and the null hypothesis is not true, the Wilcoxon test is almost as likely to reject the null hypothesis. Statisticians say the Wilcoxon test is as powerful as the *t* test. Furthermore, when the assumptions are not met, the Wilcoxon tests are more powerful than the *t* test.

DECISIONS ABOUT PROPORTIONS IN TWO INDEPENDENT GROUPS

We now turn to research questions in which the outcome is a counted or categorical variable. As discussed in Chapter 3, proportions or percentages are commonly used to summarize counted data. When the research question involves two independent groups, we can learn whether the proportions are different using any of three different methods:

1. Form a confidence interval for the difference in proportions using the *z* distribution.
2. Test the hypothesis of equal proportions using the *z* test.
3. Test the hypothesis of expected frequencies using a chi-square test.

The first two methods are extensions of the way we formed confidence intervals and used the *z* test for one proportion in Chapter 5. The chi-square method is new in this chapter, but we like this test because it is very versatile and easy to use. Although each approach gives a different numerical result, they all lead to the same conclusion about differences between two independent groups. The method that investigators decide to use depends primarily on how they think about and state their research question.

Confidence Interval for Comparing Two Independent Proportions

We discussed the survey by Anderson and colleagues (2018) about clinical and laboratory predictors of flu diagnosis. Table 3–9 gives information from the study. The investigators may want to know if the proportion of patients with confirmed flu diagnoses was different between those vaccinated and not. To find a confidence interval for the difference in proportions, we first need to convert the numbers to proportions. In this example, the proportion of vaccinated patients with confirmed flu diagnosis was $210/959 = 0.219$, and the proportion of not vaccinated patients with confirmed flu diagnosis was $1283/3610 = 0.355$. See Table 3–17 for data

Recall that the general form for a confidence interval is

$$CI = Statistic \pm Number\ related\ to\ the\ confidence$$
$$level\ desired\ (often\ 95\%) \times Standard\ error$$
$$of\ statistic$$

In Chapter 5, we saw that the *z* test provides a good approximation to the binomial when the product of the proportion and the sample size is 5 or more. We illustrated this method for research questions about one proportion in Chapter 5, and we can use a similar approach for research questions about two proportions, except that the product of the proportion and the sample size must be at least 5 in each group. To do this we let p_1 stand for the proportion of vaccinated patients with confirmed flu diagnosis and p_2 not vaccinated patients with confirmed flu diagnosis. These proportions are estimates of the proportions in the population, and the difference between the two proportions ($\pi_1 - \pi_2$ in the population) is estimated by $p_1 - p_2$

or $0.219 - 0.355 = -0.136$. This difference is the statistic about which we want to form a confidence interval (the first term in the formula for a confidence interval).

Generally, we form 95% confidence intervals, so referring to the z distribution in Table A–2 and locating the value that defines the central 95% of the z distribution, we find 1.96, a value that is probably becoming familiar by now.

The third term is the standard error of the difference between two proportions. Just as with the difference in two means, it is quite a chore to calculate the standard error of the difference in two proportions, so again we will illustrate the calculations to show the logic of the statistic but expect that you will always use a computer to calculate this value.

Recall from Chapter 5 that the standard error of one proportion is $\sqrt{p(1-p)\,|\,n}$. With two proportions, there are two standard errors and the standard error of the difference $p_1 - p_2$ is a combination of them.

$$SE_{(p_1-p_2)} = \sqrt{\left\{\left[\frac{p_1(1-p_1)}{n_1}\right] + \left[\frac{p_2(1-p_2)}{n_2}\right]\right\}}$$

Similar to the way two sample standard deviations are pooled when two means are compared, the two sample proportions are pooled to form a weighted average using the sample sizes as weights. The pooled proportion provides a better estimate to use in the standard error; it is designated simply as p without any subscripts and is calculated by adding the observed frequencies ($n_1 p_1 + n_2 p_2$) and dividing by the sum of the sample sizes, $n_1 + n_2$. When we substitute $p = (n_1 p_1 + n_2 p_2) \div (n_1 + n_2)$ for each of p_1 and p_2 in the preceding formula, we have the formula for the standard error of the difference which is the square root of the product of three values: the pooled proportion p, 1 minus the pooled proportion $(1 - p)$, and the sum of the reciprocals of the sample sizes $(1/n_1) + (1/n_2)$. In symbols, the standard error for the difference in two proportions is

$$SE_{(p_1-p_2)} = \sqrt{p(1-p)\left(\frac{1}{n_1} + \frac{1}{n_2}\right)}$$

The formula for the standard error of the difference between two proportions can be thought of as an average of the standard errors in each group. Putting all these pieces together, a 95% confidence interval for the difference in two proportions is $(p_1 - p_2) \pm 1.96 \times SE_{(p_1 - p_2)}$. To illustrate, first find the standard error of the difference between the proportions of patients diagnosed with the flu. The two proportions are 0.218 and 0.355. The pooled, or average, proportion is therefore

$$p = \frac{n_1 p_1 + n_2 p_2}{n_1 + n_2}$$

$$= \frac{(959 \times 0.219) + (3610 \times 0.355)}{959 + 3610}$$

$$= 0.327$$

As you might expect, the value of the pooled proportion, like the pooled standard deviation, always lies between the two proportions.

Next, we substitute 0.327 for the pooled proportion, p, and use the sample sizes from this study to find the standard error of the difference between the two proportions.

$$SE_{(p_1-p_2)} = \sqrt{p(1-p)\left(\frac{1}{n_1} + \frac{1}{n_2}\right)}$$

$$= \sqrt{0.327(1 - 0.327)\left(\frac{1}{959} + \frac{1}{3610}\right)}$$

$$= 0.017$$

So, the 95% confidence interval for the difference in the two proportions is

$$95\%\,CI = (p_1 - p_2) \pm 1.96 \times SE(p_1 - p_2)$$

$$= (0.219 - 0.355) \pm 0.033$$

$$= -0.136 \pm 0.033$$

The interpretation of this confidence interval is similar to that for other confidence intervals: Although we observed a difference of -0.136, we have 95% confidence that the interval from -0.169 to -0.103 contains the true difference in the proportion of patients with a confirmed flu diagnosis that did and did not have a flu vaccine.

Because the entire confidence interval is less than zero (i.e., zero is *not* within the interval), we can conclude that the proportions are significantly different from each other at $P < 0.05$ (i.e., because it is a 95% confidence interval). If, however, a confidence interval contains zero, there is not sufficient evidence to conclude a difference exists between the proportions. Please confirm these calculations using the R, and obtain a 99% confidence interval as well. Are the two proportions also significantly different at $P < 0.01$?

The z Test and Two Independent Proportions

Recall that confidence intervals and hypothesis tests lead to the same conclusion. We use the same data on patients diagnosed with the flu from the study by

Anderson and colleagues (2018) to illustrate the z test[†] for the difference between two independent proportions. The six-step process for testing a statistical hypothesis follows. The symbols π_1 and π_2 stand for the proportion in the population of patients.

Step 1: H_0: The proportion of patients with a flu vaccine with a confirmed flu diagnosis is the same as the proportion of patients without a flu vaccine with a confirmed flu diagnosis, or $\pi_1 = \pi_2$.

H_1: The proportion of patients with a flu vaccine with a confirmed flu diagnosis is not the same as the proportion of patients without a flu vaccine with a confirmed flu diagnosis, or $\pi_1 \neq \pi_2$.

Here, a two-tailed or nondirectional test is used because the researcher is interested in knowing whether a difference exists in either direction; that is, whether the receipt of a vaccine results in more or less patients being diagnosed with the flu.

Step 2: The z test for one proportion, introduced in Chapter 5, can be modified to compare two independent proportions as long as the observed frequencies are ≥ 5 in each group. The test statistic, in words, is the difference between the observed proportions divided by the standard error of the difference. In terms of sample values,

$$z = \frac{p_1 - p_2}{\sqrt{p(1 - p)[(1/n_1) + (1/n_2)]}}$$

where p_1 is the proportion in one group, p_2 is the proportion in the second group, and p (with no subscript) stands for the pooled, or average, proportion (defined in the section titled, "Confidence Interval for Comparing Two Independent Proportions").

Step 3: Choose the level for a type I error (concluding there is a difference in the screening when there really is no difference). We use $\alpha = 0.05$ so the findings will be consistent with those based on the 95% confidence interval in the previous section.

Step 4: Determining the critical value for a two-tailed test at $\alpha = 0.05$, the value of the z distribution that separates the upper and lower 2.5% of the area under the curve from the central 95% is ± 1.96 (from Table A–2). Therefore, we reject the null hypothesis of equal proportions if the observed value of the z statistic is less than the critical value of -1.96 or greater than $+1.96$. (Before continuing, based on the confidence interval in the previous section, do you expect

the value of z to be greater or less than either of these critical values?)

Step 5: Calculations are

$$z = \frac{(0.219 - 0.355)}{\sqrt{0.327(1 - 0.327)\left(\dfrac{1}{959} + \dfrac{1}{3610}\right)}}$$

$$= \frac{-0.136}{0.017}$$

$$= -8.00$$

Step 6: The observed value of z, -8.00, is less than -1.96, so the null hypothesis—that the proportion of patients diagnosed with the flu is the same regardless of whether the patient was vaccinated—is rejected. And we conclude that different proportions of patients were diagnosed. In this situation, patients presenting with flu-like symptoms were less likely to actually be diagnosed with the flu if they received a vaccine in the previous 12 months. Note the consistency of this conclusion with the 95% confidence interval in the previous section.

To report results in terms of the p value, we find the area of the z distribution closest to -8.00 in Table A–2 and see that no probabilities are given for a z value this large. In this situation, we recommend reporting $P < 0.001$. The actual probability can be found in R Commander under the Distributions menu item: go to Continuous Distributions > Normal Distribution > Normal Probabilities and then enter -8 as the Variable value. The p value reported is 6.22E-16. Few computer programs give procedures for the z test for two proportions. Instead, they produce an alternative method to compare two proportions: the chi-square test, the subject of the next section.

Using Chi-Square to Compare Frequencies or Proportions in Two Groups

We can use the chi-square test to compare frequencies or proportions in two or more groups and in many other applications as well. Used in this manner, the test is referred to as the chi-square test for independence. This versatility is one of the reasons researchers so commonly use chi-square. In addition, the calculations are relatively easy to apply to data presented in tables. Like the z approximation, the chi-square test is an approximate test, and using it should be guided by some general principles we will mention shortly.

Anderson and colleagues (2018) wanted to know whether the proportion of patients arriving with flu symptoms tested positive for the flu virus, regardless of their receipt of a flu vaccine in the previous 12 months

---

[†]The z test for the difference between two independent proportions is actually an approximate test. That is why we must assume the proportion times the sample size is ≥ 5 in each group. If not, we must use the binomial distribution or, if np is really small, we might use the Poisson distribution (both introduced in Chapter 4).

Table 6–7. Hypothetical data for chi-square.

A. Observed Frequencies			
	Treatment	Control	Total
Positive	40	10	50
Negative	60	90	150
Total	100	100	200
B. Expected Frequencies			
	Treatment	Control	Total
Positive	25	25	50
Negative	75	75	150
Total	100	100	200

(see Table 3–17). Actually, we can state this research question in two different ways:

1. Is there a difference in the proportions of patients who were diagnosed and were not diagnosed with the flu? Stated this way, the chi-square test can be used to test the equality of two proportions.

2. Is there an association (or relationship or dependency) between a patient's vaccine history and whether the patient has a confirmed flu diagnosis? Stated this way, the chi-square test can be used to test whether one of the variables is associated with the other. When we state the research hypothesis in terms of independence, the chi-square test is generally (and appropriately) called the chi-square test for independence.

In fact, we use the same chi-square test regardless of how we state the research question—an illustration of the test's versatility.

An Overview of the Chi-Square Test: Before using the chi-square test with the data from Anderson and colleagues, it is useful to have an intuitive understanding of the logic of the test. Table 6-7A contains data from a hypothetical study in which 100 patients are given an experimental treatment and 100 patients receive a control treatment. Fifty patients, or 25%, respond positively; the remaining 150 patients respond negatively. The numbers in the four cells are the observed frequencies in this hypothetical study.

Now, if no relationship exists between treatment and outcome, meaning that treatment and outcome are **independent,** we would expect approximately 25% of the patients in the treatment group and 25% of the patients in the control group to respond positively. Similarly, we would expect approximately 75% of the patients in the treatment group and approximately 75% in the control group to respond negatively. Thus, if no relationship exists between treatment and outcome, the frequencies should be as listed in Table 7B. The numbers in the cells of Table 7B are called **expected frequencies.**

The logic of the chi-square test follows:

1. The total number of observations in each column (treatment or control) and the total number of observations in each row (positive or negative) are considered to be given or fixed. (These column and row totals are also called **marginal frequencies.**)

2. If we assume that columns and rows are independent, we can calculate the number of observations expected to occur by chance—the **expected frequencies.** We find the expected frequencies by multiplying the column total by the row total and dividing by the grand total. For instance, in Table 6–7 the number of treated patients expected to be positive by chance is $(100 \times 50)/200 = 25$. We put this expected value in cell (1, 1) where the first 1 refers to the first row and the second 1 refers to the first column.

3. The chi-square test compares the observed frequency in each cell with the expected frequency. If no relationship exists between the column and row variables (i.e., treatment and response), the observed frequencies will be very close to the expected frequencies; they will differ only by small amounts.[‡] In this instance, the value of the chi-square statistic will be small. On the other hand, if a relationship (or dependency) does occur, the observed frequencies will vary quite a bit from the expected frequencies, and the value of the chi-square statistic will be large.

Putting these ideas into symbols, O stands for the observed frequency in a cell and E for the expected frequency in a cell. In each cell, we find the difference and square it (just as we did to find the standard deviation—so, when we add them, the differences do not cancel each other—see Chapter 3). Next, we divide the squared difference by the expected value. At this point we have the following term corresponding to each cell:

$$\frac{(O - E)^2}{E}$$

Finally, we add the terms from each cell to get the chi-square statistic:

$$\chi_{(df)} = \sum \frac{(\text{Observed frequency} - \text{Expected frequency})^2}{\text{Expected frequency}}$$

$$= \sum \frac{(O - E)^2}{E}$$

where χ^2 stands for the chi-square statistic, and (df) stands for the degrees of freedom.

[‡] We say small amounts because of what is called sampling variability—variation among different samples of patients who could be randomly selected for the study.

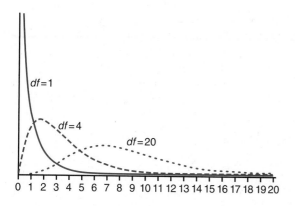

Figure 6–5. Chi-square distribution corresponding to 1, 4, and 20 degrees of freedom.

The Chi-Square Distribution: The chi-square distribution, χ^2 (lowercase Greek letter chi, pronounced like the "ki" in *kite*), like the t distribution, has degrees of freedom. In the chi-square test for independence, the number of degrees of freedom is equal to the number of rows minus 1 times the number of columns minus 1, or $df = (r - 1)(c - 1)$, where r is the number of rows and c the number of columns. Figure 6–5 shows the chi-square distribution for 1, 4 and 20 degrees of freedom. As you can see, the chi-square distribution has no negative values. The mean of the chi-square distribution is equal to the degrees of freedom; therefore, as the degrees of freedom increase, the mean moves more to the right. In addition, the standard deviation increases as degrees of freedom increase, so the chi-square curve spreads out more as the degrees of freedom increase. In fact, as the degrees of freedom become very large, the shape of the chi-square distribution becomes more like the normal distribution.

To use the chi-square distribution for hypothesis testing, we find the critical value in Table A–5 that separates the area defined by α from that defined by $1 - \alpha$. Table A–5 contains only upper-tailed values for χ^2 because they are the values generally used in hypothesis testing. Because the chi-square distribution is different for each value of the degrees of freedom, different critical values correspond to degrees of freedom. For example, the critical value for $\chi^2_{(1)}$ with $\alpha = 0.05$ is 3.841.

Use R Commander to graph chi-square distributions for various degrees of freedom (Distributions > Continuous distributions > Chi-square distribution > Plot chi-square distribution). Note how the curve changes as the degrees of freedom change.

The Chi-Square Test for Independence

Now we apply the chi-square test to the observations in Table 3–9.

Step 1: H_0: Flu vaccination and subsequent flu diagnosis (i.e., rows and columns) are independent.

H_1: Flu vaccination and subsequent flu diagnosis (i.e., rows and columns) are not independent.

Step 2: The chi-square test is appropriate for this research question because the observations are nominal data (frequencies).

Step 3: We use the traditional α of 0.05.

Step 4: The contingency table has two rows and two columns, so $df = (2 - 1)(2 - 1) = 1$. The critical value in Table A–5 that separates the upper 5% of the χ^2 distribution from the remaining 95% is 3.841. The chi-square test for independence is almost always a one-tailed test to see whether the observed frequencies vary from the expected frequencies by more than the amount expected by chance. We will reject the null hypothesis of independence if the observed value of χ^2 is greater than 3.841.

Step 5: The first step in calculating the chi-square statistic is to find the expected frequencies for each cell. The illustration using hypothetical data (see Table 6–7) showed that expected frequencies are found by multiplying the column total by the row total and dividing by the grand total:

$$\text{Expected frequency} = \frac{\text{Row total} \times \text{Column total}}{\text{Grand total}}$$

See Exercise 7 to learn why expected values are found this way.

As an illustration, multiplying the number of patients with flu vaccines, 959, by the number who were diagnosed with the flu, 1493, and then dividing by the total number of patients, 4569, gives $(959 \times 1493)/(4569) = 313.4$, the expected frequency for cell $(1, 1)$, abbreviated $E(1, 1)$. The expected frequencies for the remaining cells in Table 3–17 are listed in Table 6–8. None of the expected frequencies is <5, so we can proceed with the chi-square test. (We explain why expected frequencies should not be too small in the next section.) Then, squaring the difference between the observed and expected frequencies in each cell, dividing by the expected frequency, and then adding them all to find χ^2 gives the following:

$$\chi^2 = \frac{(210 - 313.4)^2}{313.4} + \frac{(749 - 645.6)^2}{645.6}$$

$$+ \frac{(1283 - 1179.6)^2}{1179.6} + \frac{(2327 - 2430.4)^2}{2430.4}$$

$$\chi^2 = 34.10 + 16.55 + 9.06 + 4.40 = 64.10$$

Table 6–8. A 2 × 2 table for study on flu vaccine and diagnosis.

```
Frequency table:
              Flu_final_posneg
Vaccine12mo_yn    No   Yes
           No   2327  1283
           Yes   749   210


        Pearson's Chi-squared test

data:  .Table
X-squared = 64.103, df = 1, p-value = 1.181e-15



Expected counts:
              Flu_final_posneg
Vaccine12mo_yn        No        Yes
           No   2430.3699  1179.6301
           Yes   645.6301   313.3699

Chi-square components:
              Flu_final_posneg
Vaccine12mo_yn    No    Yes
           No   4.40   9.06
           Yes 16.55  34.10




        Fisher's Exact Test for Count Data

data:  .Table
p-value = 2.314e-16
alternative hypothesis: true odds ratio is not equal to 1
95 percent confidence interval:
 0.4279606 0.6026591
sample estimates:
odds ratio
 0.5085904
```

Data from Anderson KB, Simasathien S, Watanaveeradej V, et al: Clinical and laboratory predictors of influenza infection among individuals with influenza-like illness presenting to an urban Thai hospital over a five-year period, *PLoS One.* 2018 Mar 7;13(3):e0193050.

Step 6: The observed value of $\chi^2_{(1)}$, 64.10, is greater than 3.841, so we easily reject the null hypothesis of independence and conclude that a dependency or relationship exists between flu vaccination and confirmed flu diagnosis. Because this study is not an experimental study, it is not possible to conclude that a flu vaccine *causes* a patient to be less likely to be diagnosed with the flu. We can only say that vaccination status and confirmed diagnosis are associated. Use R to confirm these calculations and compare the value of χ^2 with that in Table 6–8.

Using Chi-Square Tests

Because of widespread use of chi-square tests in the literature, it is worthwhile to discuss several aspects of these tests.

Shortcut Chi-Square Formula for 2 × 2 Tables: A shortcut formula simplifies the calculation of χ^2 for 2 × 2 tables, eliminating the need to calculate expected frequencies. Table 6–9 gives the setup of the table for the shortcut formula. Note that the output of computer

Table 6–9. Standard notation for chi-square 2×2 table.

	Disease	No Disease	Total
Treatment	a	b	$a + b$
Control	c	d	$c + d$
Total	$a + c$	$b + d$	$a + b + c + d = n$

Shortcut formula for chi-square

$$\chi^2_{(1)} = \frac{n(ad - bc)^2}{(a + c)(b + d)(a + b)(c + d)}$$

Fisher's exact test

$$P = \frac{(a + b)!(c + d)!(a + c)!(b + d)!}{a!\,b!\,c!\,d!\,n!}$$

programs, such as R, may not arrange the cells in this way. Always review the output of any computer program carefully before applying this method. Table 3–17 is arranged according to this standard and will be the data source for this example.

The shortcut formula for calculating χ^2 from a 2×2 contingency table is

$$\chi^2 = \frac{n(ad - bc)^2}{(a + c)(b + d)(a + b)(c + d)}$$

Using this formula with data gives

$$\chi^2 = \frac{4569[(210 \times 2327) - (749 \times 1283)]^2}{(210 + 1283)(749 + 2327)(210 + 749)(1283 + 2327)}$$

$$= 64.10$$

This value for χ^2 agrees with the value obtained in the previous section. In fact, the two approaches are equivalent for 2×2 tables.

Small Expected Frequencies & Fisher's Exact Test: The chi-square procedure, like the test based on the z approximation, is an approximate method. Just as the z test should not be used unless np in both groups is ≥ 5, the chi-square test should not be used when the *expected frequencies* are small. Look at the formula for chi-square.

$$\chi^2 = \sum \frac{(O - E)^2}{E}$$

It is easy to see that a small expected frequency in the denominator of one of the terms in the equation causes that term to be large, which, in turn, inflates the value of chi-square.

How small can expected frequencies be before we must worry about them? Although there is no absolute rule, most statisticians agree that an expected frequency of 2 or less means that the chi-square test should not be used; and many argue that chi-square should not be used if an expected frequency is less than 5. We suggest that if any expected frequency is less than 2 or if more than 20% of the expected frequencies are less than 5, then an alternative procedure called **Fisher's exact test** should be used for 2×2 tables. (We emphasize that the *expected* values are of concern here, not the *observed* values.) If the contingency table of observations is larger than 2×2, categories should be combined to eliminate most of the expected values <5.

Fisher's exact test gives the exact probability of the occurrence of the observed frequencies, given the assumption of independence and the size of the marginal frequencies (row and column totals). For example, using the notation in Table 6–9, the probability P of obtaining the observed frequencies in the table is

$$P = \frac{(a + b)!(c + d)!(b + d)!}{a!\,b!\,c!\,d!\,n!}$$

Recall that ! is the symbol for factorial; that is, $n! = n(n - 1)(n - 2) \dots (3)(2)(1)$.

The null hypothesis tested with both the chi-square test and Fisher's exact test is that the observed frequencies or *frequencies more extreme* could occur by chance, given the fixed values of the row and column totals. For Fisher's exact test, the probability for each distribution of frequencies more extreme than those observed must, therefore, also be calculated, and the probabilities of all the more extreme sets are added to the probability of the observed set. Fisher's exact test is especially appropriate with small sample sizes, and most statistical programs automatically provide it as an alternative to chi-square for 2×2 tables; see the output from R in Table 6–8.

Readers of medical journals need a basic understanding of the purpose of this statistic and not how to calculate it, that is, you need only remember that Fisher's exact test is more appropriate than the chi-square test in 2×2 tables when expected frequencies are small.

Continuity Correction: Some investigators report corrected chi-square values, called chi-square with **continuity correction** or chi-square with **Yates' correction.** This correction is similar to the one for the z test for one proportion discussed in Chapter 5; it involves subtracting ½ from the difference between observed and expected frequencies in the numerator of χ^2 before squaring; it has the effect of making the value for χ^2 smaller. (In the shortcut formula, $n/2$ is subtracted from the absolute value of $ad - bc$ prior to squaring.)

A smaller value for χ^2 means that the null hypothesis will not be rejected as often as it is with the larger, uncorrected chi-square; that is, it is more conservative. Thus, the risk of a type I error (rejecting the null hypothesis when it is true) is smaller; however, the risk of a type II error (not rejecting the null hypothesis when it is false and should be rejected) then increases. Some statisticians recommend the use of the continuity correction for all 2×2 tables but others caution against its use. Both corrected and uncorrected chi-square statistics are commonly encountered in the medical literature.

Risk Ratios versus Chi-Square: Both the chi-square test and the z approximation test allow investigators to test a hypothesis about equal proportions or about a relationship between two nominal measures, depending on how the research hypothesis is articulated. It may have occurred to you that the risk ratios (**relative risk** or **odds ratio**) introduced in Chapter 3 could also be used with 2×2 tables when the question is about an association. Note that R displays the odds ratio along with the Fisher's Exact Test results in Table 6–8. The statistic selected depends on the purpose of the analysis. If the objective is to estimate the relationship between two nominal measures, then the relative risk or the odds ratio is appropriate. Furthermore, confidence intervals can be found for relative risks and odds ratios (illustrated in Chapter 8), which, for all practical purposes, accomplish the same end as a significance test. Confidence intervals for risk ratios are being used with increasing frequency in medical journals.

Overuse of Chi-Square: Because the chi-square test is so easy to understand and calculate, it is sometimes used when another method is more appropriate. A common misuse of chi-square tests occurs when two groups are being analyzed and the characteristic of interest is measured on a numerical scale. Instead of correctly using the t test, researchers convert the numerical scale to an ordinal or even binary scale and then use chi-square. As an example, investigators brought the following problem to one of us.

Some patients who undergo a surgical procedure are more likely to have complications than other patients. The investigators collected data on one group of patients who had complications following surgery and on another group of patients who did not have complications, and they wanted to know whether a relationship existed between the patient's age and the patient's likelihood of having a complication. The investigators had formed a 2×2 contingency table, with the columns being complication versus no complication, and the rows being patient age ≥ 45 years versus age < 45 years. The investigators had performed a chi-square test for independence. The results, much to their surprise, indicated no relationship between age and complication.

The problem was the arbitrary selection of 45 years as a cutoff point for age. When a t test was performed, the mean age of patients who had complications was significantly greater than the mean age of patients who did not. Forty-five years of age, although meaningful perhaps from a clinical perspective related to other factors, was not the age sensitive to the occurrence of complications.

When numerical variables are analyzed with methods designed for ordinal or categorical variables, the greater specificity or detail of the numerical measurement is wasted. Investigators may opt to categorize a numerical variable, such as age, for graphic or tabular presentation or for use in logistic regression (Chapter 10), but only after investigating whether the categories are appropriate.

FINDING SAMPLE SIZES FOR MEANS AND PROPORTIONS IN TWO GROUPS

In Chapter 5, we discussed the importance of having enough subjects in a study to find significance if a difference really occurs. We saw that a relationship exists between sample size and being able to conclude that a difference exists: As the sample size increases, the power to detect an actual difference also increases. The process of estimating the number of subjects for a study is called finding the **power** of the study. Knowing the sample sizes needed is helpful in determining whether a negative study is negative because the sample size was too small. More and more journal editors now require authors to provide this key information as do all funding agencies.

Just as with studies involving only one group, a variety of formulas can be used to estimate how large a sample is needed, and several computer programs are available for this purpose as well. The formulas given in the following section protect against both type I and type II errors for two common situations: when a study involves two means or two proportions.

Finding the Sample Size for Studies About Means in Two Groups

This section presents the process to estimate the approximate sample size for a study comparing the means in two independent groups of subjects. The researcher needs to answer four questions, the first two of which are the same as those presented in Chapter 5 for one group:

1. What level of significance (α level or p value) related to the null hypothesis is wanted?

2. How great should the chances be of detecting an actual difference; that is, what is the desired level of power (equal to $1 - \beta$)?

3. How large should the difference between the mean in one group and the mean in the other group be for the difference to have clinical importance?

4. What is a good estimate of the standard deviations? To simplify this process, we assume that the standard deviations in the two populations are equal.

To summarize, if $\mu_1 - \mu_2$ is the magnitude of the difference to be detected between the two groups, σ is the estimate of the standard deviation in each group, z_α is the two-tailed value of z related to α, and z_β is the lower one-tailed value of z related to β, then the sample size needed in *each* group is

$$n = 2\left[\frac{(z_\alpha - z_\beta)\sigma}{\mu_1 - \mu_2}\right]^2$$

To illustrate this formula, recall that Bos-Touwen and his colleagues (2015) in Presenting Problem 1 compared patient activation measures (PAM) for 422 patients who had chronic renal disease with 732 patients who did not. We found the 95% confidence interval for the difference in PAM (1.9) in the section titled, "Comparing Two Means Using Confidence Intervals." The 95% CI, 0.61 to 3.28, does not contain 0, so we conclude that a difference exists between PAM in the two groups. Suppose the investigators, prior to beginning their study, wished to have a large enough sample of patients to be able to detect a mean difference of 2 or more. Assume they were willing to accept a type I error of 0.05 and wanted to be able to detect a true difference with 0.80 probability ($\beta = 0.20$). Based on their clinical experience, they estimated the standard deviation as 10. Using these values, what sample size is needed?

The two-tailed z value for α of 0.05 is 1.96 and the lower one-tailed z value for β of 0.20 is −0.84 (the critical value separating the lower 20% of the z distribution from the upper 80%). From the given estimates, the sample size for each group is

$$n = 2\left[\frac{(z_\alpha - z_\beta)\sigma}{\mu_1 - \mu_2}\right]^2$$

$$= 2\left[\frac{[1.96 - (-0.84)10]}{2}\right]^2$$

$$= 2\left(\frac{28.0}{2}\right)^2$$

$$= 392$$

Thus, 392 patients are needed in each group if the investigators want to have an 80% chance (or 80% power) of detecting a mean difference of 2 or more in patient activation. One advantage of using computer programs for power analysis is that they permit different sample sizes. The output from the G*Power program for two means, assuming there are approximately two times as many patients without CRD as with CRD, is given in Box 6–1. The plot makes it easy to see the relationship between the sample size (N_1) and power.

Shortcut Estimate of Sample Size: We developed a rule of thumb for quickly estimating the sample sizes needed to compare the means of two groups. First, determine the ratio of the standard deviation to the difference to be detected between the means $[\sigma/(\mu_1 - \mu_2)]$; then, square this ratio. For a study with a p value of 0.05, an experiment will have a 90% chance of detecting an actual difference between the two groups if the sample size in each group is approximately 20 times the squared ratio. For a study with the same p value but only an 80% chance of detecting an actual difference, a sample size of approximately 15 times the squared ratio is required. In the previous example, we would have $15 \times (10/2)^2$, or 375 subjects, a slight underestimate. Exercise 8 allows you to learn how this rule of thumb was obtained.

Note that the estimates we calculated assume that the sample sizes are equal in the two groups. As illustrated in Box 6–1, many computer programs, including G*Power, provide estimates for unequal sample sizes.

Finding the Sample Size for Studies About Proportions in Two Groups

This section presents the formula for estimating the approximate sample size needed in a study with two groups when the outcome is expressed in terms of proportions. Just as with studies involving two means, the researcher must answer four questions.

1. What is the desired level of significance (the α level) related to the null hypothesis?

2. What should be the chance of detecting an actual difference, that is, what the desired power ($1 - \beta$) to be associated with the alternative hypothesis?

3. How large should the difference be between the two proportions for it to be clinically significant?

4. What is a good estimate of the standard deviation in the population? For a proportion, it is easy: The null hypothesis assumes the proportions are equal, and the proportion itself determines the estimated standard deviation: $\pi (1 - \pi)$.

To simplify matters, we again assume that the sample sizes are the same in the two groups. The symbol π_1

BOX 1. TWO-SAMPLE *t* TEST POWER ANALYSIS FOR PULSE OXIMETRY.

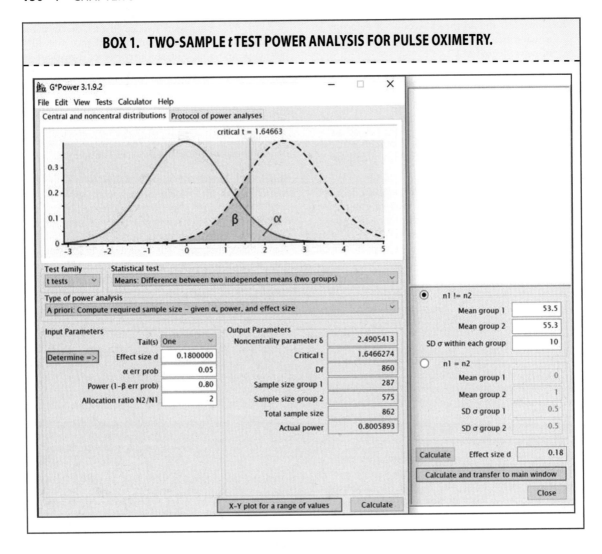

denotes the proportion in one group, and π_2 the proportion in the other group. Then, the formula for n is

$$n = \left[\frac{z_\alpha \sqrt{2\pi_1(1-\pi_1)} - z_+\sqrt{\pi_1(1-\pi_1) + \pi_2(1-\pi_2)}}{\pi_1 - \pi_2} \right]$$

where z_α is the two-tailed z value related to the null hypothesis and z_β is the lower one-tailed z value related to the alternative hypothesis.

To illustrate, we use the study by Anderson and colleagues (2018) of diagnosing the flu. Among patients with a flu vaccine in the last 12 months and flu-like symptoms, 210 of 959 were diagnosed with the flu (0.219), compared with 1,283 of 3,610 patients without training flu vaccine (0.355). We found that the 95%

confidence interval for the difference in proportions was -0.169 to -0.103, and because the interval does not contain 0, we concluded a difference existed in the proportion who are diagnosed with the flu. Suppose that the investigators, prior to doing the study, wanted to estimate the sample size needed to detect a significant difference if the proportions diagnosed were 0.22 and 0.36. They are willing to accept a type I error (or falsely concluding that a difference exists when none really occurred) of 0.05, and they wanted a 0.90 probability of detecting a true difference (i.e., 90% power).

The two-tailed z value related to α is $+1.96$, and the lower one-tailed z value related to β is -1.645, the value that separates the lower 10% of the z distribution from the upper 90%. Then, the estimated sample size is

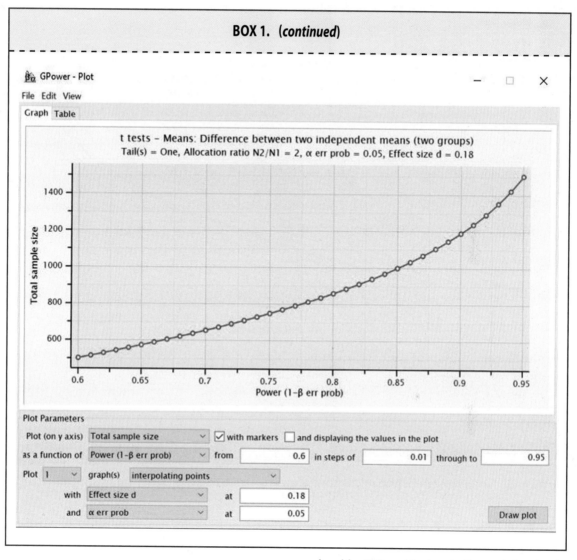

BOX 1. (continued)

$$n = \left[\frac{1.96\sqrt{2 \times 0.22 \times 0.88} - (-1.645)}{\sqrt{0.22 \times 0.88 + 0.36 \times 0.72}} \over 0.36 - 0.22 \right]^2$$

$$= \left(\frac{2.26}{0.14} \right)^2$$

$$= 260.2 \text{ or } 261 \text{ in each group}$$

We use the G*Power program with data from Anderson and colleagues to illustrate finding the sample size for the difference in two proportions. The plot

produced by G*Power is given in Figure 6–6 and indicate that the total sample size should be approximatley 460 or 230 per group for power of 0.9. This is slightly smaller than our estimate.

SUMMARY

This chapter has focused on statistical methods that are useful in determining whether two independent groups differ on an outcome measure. In the next chapter, we extend the discussion to studies that involve more than two groups.

The *t* test is used when the outcome is measured on a numerical scale. If the distribution of the observations is skewed or if the standard deviations in the two groups are different, the Wilcoxon rank sum test is the

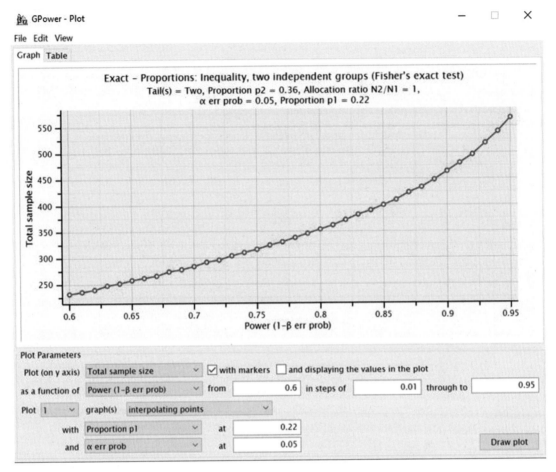

Figure 6–6. Two-sample test for proportions power analysis using G*Power.

procedure of choice. In fact, it is such a good substitute for the *t* test that some statisticians recommend it for almost all situations.

The chi-square test is used with counts or frequencies when two groups are being analyzed. We discussed what to do when sample sizes are small, commonly referred to as small expected frequencies. We recommend Fisher's exact test with a 2 × 2 table. We briefly touched on some other issues related to the use of chi-square in medical studies.

In Presenting Problem 1, Bos-Touwen and his colleagues (2015) wanted to know if patients with chronic renal disease differed from those who did not, and they looked at patient activation measures. The researchers found a difference in patient activation between the two groups. We used the study by Ström and colleagues (2013) to illustrate the *t* test for two independent groups. Ström wanted to know whether patients diagnosed with depression would experience

symptom relief after Internet-administered treatment. We compared the BDI score changes before and after treatment for those that participated in the Internet-administered treatment. The difference in the BDI score changes was not statistically significant. We used the same data to illustrate the Wilcoxon rank sum test and came to the same conclusion. The Wilcoxon test is recommended when assumptions for the *t* test (normal distribution, equal variances) are not met. Turning to research questions involving nominal or categorical outcomes, we introduced the *z* statistic for comparing two proportions and the chi-square test.

In Anderson and colleagues' (2018) study, investigators were interested in learning whether receipt of a flu vaccine and confirmed flu diagnosis after presenting with symptoms were related. We used the same data to illustrate the construction of confidence intervals and the *z* test for two proportions and came to the same conclusion, illustrating once more the equivalence between the conclusions reached using confidence intervals and statistical tests.

The chi-square test uses observed frequencies and compares them to the frequencies that would be expected if no differences existed in proportions. We again used the data from Anderson and colleagues (2018) to illustrate the chi-square test for two groups, that is, for observations that can be displayed in a 2 × 2 table. Once more, the results of the statistical test indicated that a difference existed in proportions of patients diagnosed with the flu based on whether or not the received a vaccine in the last 12 months.

The importance of sample size calculations was again stressed. We illustrated formulas and computer programs that estimate the sample sizes needed when two independent groups of subjects are being compared.

A summary of the statistical methods discussed in this chapter is given in Appendix C.

EXERCISES

1. How does a decrease in sample size affect the confidence interval? Recalculate the confidence interval for PAM score in the section titled, "Decisions About Means in Two Independent Groups," assuming that the means and standard deviations were the same but only 50 patients were in each group. Recalculate the pooled standard deviation and standard error and repeat the confidence interval. Is the conclusion the same?

2. Calculate the pooled standard deviation for the BDI Pre-treatment from Table 6–3.

3. Show that the pooled standard deviation for two means is the average of the two standard deviations when the sample sizes are equal.

4. Use the data from Bos-Touwen and colleagues (2015) to compare PAM in patients who did and those who did not have CRD. Compare the conclusion with the confidence interval in the section titled, "Decisions About Means in Two Independent Groups."

5. Use the rules for finding the probability of independent events to show why the expected frequency in the chi-square statistic is found by the following formula:

$$\text{Expected frequency} = \frac{\text{Row total} \times \text{Column total}}{\text{Grand total}}$$

6. How was the rule of thumb for calculating the sample size for two independent groups found?

7. How large a sample is needed to detect a difference of 0.85 versus 0.55 in the proportions of patients discharged home after a stroke with 80% power? Use $\alpha=0.05$ and assume a two-sided test is desired.

8. Compute the 90% and 99% confidence intervals for the difference in PAM for the patients with and without CRD (Bos-Touwen et al, 2015). Compare these intervals with the 95% interval obtained in the section titled, "Comparing Two Means Using Confidence Intervals." What is the effect of lower confidence on the width of the interval? Of higher confidence?

9. Suppose investigators compared the number of cardiac procedures performed by 60 cardiologists in large health centers during one year to the number of procedures done by 25 cardiologists in midsized health centers. They found no significant difference between the number of procedures performed by the average cardiologist in large centers and those performed in mid-sized centers using the t test. When they reanalyzed the data using the Wilcoxon rank sum test, the investigators noted a difference. What is the most likely explanation for the different findings?

10. **Group Exercise.** Many older patients use numerous medications, and, as patients age, the chances for medication errors increases. Gurwitz and colleagues (2003) undertook a study of all Medicare patients seen by a group of physicians (multispecialty) during one year. The primary outcomes were number of adverse drug events, seriousness of the events, and whether they could have been prevented. Obtain a copy of the article to answer the following questions.

    a. What was the study design? Why was this design particularly appropriate?

    b. What methods did the investigators use to learn the outcomes? Were they sufficient?

    c. What statistical approach was used to evaluate the outcome rates?

    d. What statistical methods were used to analyze the characteristics in Table 6–1 in the Gurwitz study?

    e. What was the major conclusion from the study? Was this conclusion justified? Would additional information help readers decide whether the conclusion was appropriate?

11. *Group Exercise. Physicians and dentists may be at risk for exposure to blood-borne diseases during invasive surgical procedures. In a study that is still relevant, Serrano and coworkers (1991) wanted to determine the incidence of glove perforation during obstetric procedures and identify risk factors. The latex gloves of all members of the surgical teams performing cesarean deliveries, postpartum tubal ligations, and vaginal deliveries were collected for study; 100 unused gloves served as controls. Each glove was tested by inflating it with a pressurized air hose to 1.5–2 times the normal volume and submerging it in water. Perforations were detected by the presence of air bubbles when gentle pressure was applied to the palmar surface. Among the 754 study gloves, 100 had holes; none of the 100 unused control gloves had holes. In analyzing the data, the investigators found that 19 of the gloves with holes were among the 64 gloves worn by scrub technicians. Obtain a copy of this paper from your medical library and use it to help answer the following questions:*

a. *What is your explanation for the high perforation rate in gloves worn by scrub technicians? What should be done about these gloves in the analysis?*

b. *Are there other possible sources of bias in the way this study was designed?*

c. *An analysis reported by the investigators was based on 462 gloves used by house staff. The levels of training, number of gloves used, and number of gloves with holes were as follows: Interns used 262 gloves, 30 with holes; year 2 residents used 71 gloves, 9 with holes; year 3 residents used 58 gloves, 4 with holes; and year 4 residents used 71 gloves, 17 with holes. Confirm that a relationship exists between training level and proportion of perforation, and explain the differences in proportions of perforations.*

d. *What conclusions do you draw from this study? Do your conclusions agree with those of the investigators?*

Research Questions About Means in Three or More Groups

7

KEY CONCEPTS

 Special statistical tests are needed when more than two groups are studied or when a group is measured on several variables.

 Analysis of variance, or ANOVA, is a statistical method that divides the variance in an observation into the variance among groups and the rest of the variance, called the within-group or error variance.

 The F test used to compare two variances in Chapter 6 is used to compare the variance among groups to the error.

 An example of the way ANOVA is calculated from the definitional formulas is helpful in understanding the logic behind the test.

 The terms used in ANOVA are important, but the details of the computations are given for illustration only, and computer programs are used for all ANOVA procedures.

 One-way ANOVA is the appropriate method when more than two groups are studied on one variable.

 As with the t test, certain assumptions must be made to use ANOVA, and equal variances is one of the most important.

 Making many comparisons among groups increases the chances of a type I error, that a difference is concluded when there is none.

 Investigators can decide ahead of time what specific comparisons they want to make.

 The Bonferroni procedure is a common way to compensate for making many comparisons among groups; it works by reducing the size of α for each comparison, essentially increasing the difference needed to be significant.

 Some multiple comparison methods, called post hoc, are done only if the ANOVA results are statistically significant.

 Tukey's test is one of the most highly recommended post hoc tests for comparing mean differences.

 The Scheffé post hoc procedure is the most conservative (requiring a larger difference to be significant), but it is also the most versatile.

 The Newman–Kuels post hoc procedure is used frequently in basic science research.

 Dunnett's procedure is the test of choice if the only comparisons being made are between the mean in a control group and the means in other groups.

 Two-way ANOVA analyzes two factors instead of just one, as in one-way ANOVA. It also permits the analysis of the interaction between two factors.

 ANOVA designs involving more than two factors are possible, generally called factorial designs.

 Confounding variables can be accommodated by the ANOVA randomized block design.

 Repeated-measures ANOVA is a common procedure in medical research; it is analogous to the paired t test with more than two groups and is also called the split-plot design.

Nonparametric ANOVA methods include Kruskal-Wallis for one-way designs and Friedman two-way ANOVA for repeated measures. These methods are analogous to the Wilcoxon procedures and are used when the assumptions for ANOVA are not met.

 The chi-square test can be used to compare more than two proportions and to determine if there is an association between two factors, each of which can have two or more levels. It is a simple extension of the chi-square test we discussed in Chapter 6.

 As with research questions involving one or two groups, power analysis is important for studies that use ANOVA. The calculations become increasingly complex, but statistical power programs are available to cover many of the designs.

 PRESENTING PROBLEMS

Presenting Problem 1

Patients with HIV infections have increased cardiovascular disease risk. Dysangco and colleagues (2017) compared a number of biomarkers for three groups: 28 HIV infected patients on antiretroviral therapy (ART), 44 patients with HIV infection and not on ART, and 39 healthy controls.

Citation: Dysangco A, Liu Z, Stein JH, Dubé MP, Gupta SK: HIV infection, antiretroviral therapy, and measures of endothelial function, inflammation, metabolism, and oxidative stress. PLoS ONE 2017;12(8):e0183511.

The article may be accessed here:

https://doi.org/10.1371/journal.pone.0183511

The data file may be accessed here:

https://figshare.com/articles/PLOS_ONE_-_Gupta_2017_-_data_pub_csv/5226166

Presenting Problem 2

Cornelis et al (2017) created a new scale to measure the ability of subjects with cognitive impairment to perform activities of daily living (ADL). They created a scale called i-ADL-CDI and tested in on three groups of subjects: 79 healthy controls, 73 subjects with mild cognitive impairment (MCI), and 71 patients with Alzheimer Disease.

Citation: Cornelis E, Gorus E, Beyer I, Bautmans I, De Vriendt P: Early diagnosis of mild cognitive impairment and mild dementia through basic and instrumental activities of daily living: Development of a new evaluation tool. PLoS Med 2017;14(3):e1002250.

The article may be found here:

https://doi.org/10.1371/journal.pmed.1002250

The data file is linked at the end of the article or may also be downloaded here:

https://doi.org/10.1371/journal.pmed.1002250.s001

Presenting Problem 3

Durand et al (2015) studied the blood flow in paretic and nonparetic lower limbs in subjects with chronic stroke (n = 10) and healthy controls (n = 10). The blood flow was measured using ultrasound under the following maximum voluntary contraction (MVC) levels: 20%, 40%, 60%, and 80%. They found that blood flow after 80% MVC was the best predictor of which limb was paretic.

Citation: Durand MJ, Murphy SA, Schaefer KK, et al: Impaired Hyperemic Response to Exercise Post Stroke. PLOS ONE 2015;10(12):e0144023.

The article may be found here:

https://doi.org/10.1371/journal.pone.0144023

The data may be downloaded from here:

https://journals.plos.org/plosone/article/file?type=supplementary&id=info:doi/10.1371/journal.pone.0144023.s002

PURPOSE OF THE CHAPTER

Many research projects in medicine employ more than two groups, and the chi-square tests discussed in Chapter 6 can be extended for three or more groups when the outcome is a categorical (or counted) measure. When the outcome is numerical, means are used, and the t tests discussed in Chapters 5 and 6 are applicable only for the comparison of two groups. Other studies examine the influence of more than one factor. These situations call for a global, or omnibus, test to see whether any differences exist in the data prior to testing various combinations of means to determine individual group differences.

If a global test is not performed, multiple tests between different pairs of means will alter the significance or α level for the experiment as a whole rather than for each comparison. For example, Marwick and colleagues (1999) studied the relationship between myocardial profusion imaging and cardiac mortality in men and women. Factors included the number of involved coronary vessels (zero to three) and whether the profusion defect was fixed or could be reversed. Had these investigators not properly used multivariate methods to analyze the data, methods we discuss in Chapter 10, comparing men and women on the 4×2 different combinations of these factors would produce eight p values. If each comparison is made by using $\alpha = 0.05$, the chance that each comparison will falsely be called significant is 5%; that is, a type I error may occur eight different times. Overall, therefore, the chance ($8 \times 5\%$) of declaring one of the comparisons incorrectly significant is 40%.[*]

One approach for analyzing data that include multiple observations is called the **analysis of variance,** abbreviated **ANOVA** or **anova.** This method protects against error "inflation" by first asking if any differences exist at all among means of the groups. If the result of the ANOVA is significant, the answer is yes, and the investigator then makes comparisons among pairs or combinations of groups.

The topic of analysis of variance is complex, and many textbooks are devoted to the subject. Its use in the medical literature is somewhat limited, however, because regression methods (see Chapter 10) can be used to answer the same research questions. Our goal is to provide enough discussion so that you can identify situations in which ANOVA is appropriate and interpret the results. If you are interested in learning more about analysis of variance, consult Berry and coworkers (2001) or the still classic text by Dunn and Clark (1987). Except for simple study designs, our advice to researchers conducting a study that involves more than two groups or two or more variables is to consult a statistician to determine how best to analyze the data.

INTUITIVE OVERVIEW OF ANOVA

The Logic of ANOVA

In Presenting Problem 1, high density lipoprotein cholesterol (HDL-C) levels were measured in three groups of subjects: group A (39 control individuals without HIV) and groups B and C (HIV-infected patients who were or were not on antiretroviral therapy [ART]). Summary statistics for three of the biomarkers (ADMA, asymmetric dimethyl arginine; IL-6, interleukin 6; and HDL-C) studied in the Dysangco et al (2017) study are displayed in Table 7–1. ANOVA provides a way to divide the total variation in HDL-C of each subject into two parts. Suppose we denote a given subject's HDL-C as X and consider how much X differs from the mean HDL-C for all the subjects in the study, abbreviated $\overline{\overline{X}}$. This difference (symbolized $X - \overline{\overline{X}}$) can be divided into two parts: the difference between X and the mean of the group this subject is in, $\overline{X}_j$, and the difference between the group mean and the grand mean. In symbols, we write

$$(X - \overline{\overline{X}}) = (X - \overline{X}_j) + (\overline{X}_j - \overline{\overline{X}})$$

Table 7–2 contains the original observations for the subjects in the study. Subject 1 in the control group has a HDL-C of 78 mg/dL. The grand mean for all subjects is 42.48, so subject 1 differs from the grand mean by $78 - 42.48$, or 35.52. This difference can be divided into two parts: the difference between 78 and the mean for the control group, 49.84; and the

Table 7–1. HIV CVD study biomarker values.

Group	ADMA	IL-6	HCL-C
A (HIV-)	0.59 ± 0.11 (n =38)	3.29 ± 9.52 (n =35)	49.84 ± 18.68 (n =38)
B (HIV+ ART-)	0.62 ± 0.17 (n =44)	2.82 ± 2.55 (n =44)	37.02 ± 10.27[a] (n =44)
C (HIV+ ART+)	0.47 ± 0.09[b] (n =28)	1.64 ± 1.16 (n =28)	41.07 ± 10.77[a] (n =28)

ADMA, μmol/L asymmetric dimethyl arginine
IL-6, pg/mL, interleukin 6
HDL-C, mg/dL, high density lipoprotein cholesterol
[a]$P < 0.05$ vs. A
[b]$P < 0.05$ vs. A and B
Data from Dysangco A, Liu Z, Stein JH, et al: HIV infection, antiretroviral therapy, and measures of endothelial function, inflammation, metabolism, and oxidative stress, *PLoS One.* 2017 Aug 17;12(8):e0183511.

---

[*]Actually, 40% is only approximately correct; it does not reflect the fact that some of the comparisons are not independent.

Table 7–2. Biomarker levels.

Group A	ADMA	IL6	HDLC	Group B	ADMA	IL6	HDLC	Group C	ADMA	IL6	HDLC
HIV−	0.629	0.832	78	HIV+ART−	0.897	1.2754	30	HIV+ART+	0.565	2.069	44
HIV−	0.489	1.611	26	HIV+ART−	0.577	0.3934	30	HIV+ART+	0.643	1.127	38
HIV−	0.61	2.653	73	HIV+ART−	0.615	2.2164	32	HIV+ART+	0.564	2.43	27
HIV−	0.664	3	32	HIV+ART−	0.636	2.3795	38	HIV+ART+	0.623	0.583	39
HIV−	0.461	1.117	57	HIV+ART−	0.612	1.141	23	HIV+ART+	0.59	1.658	30
HIV−	0.511	2.703	48	HIV+ART−	0.526	0.6803	61	HIV+ART+	0.403	0.48	65
HIV−	0.59	1.116	39	HIV+ART−	0.587	2.2574	29	HIV+ART+	0.257	1.752	28
HIV−	0.591	0.622	118	HIV+ART−	0.629	0.9139	43	HIV+ART+	0.438	0.852	40
HIV−	0.486	57.738	42	HIV+ART−	0.453	1.5525	29	HIV+ART+	0.51	0.785	62
HIV−	0.691	2.13	35	HIV+ART−	0.742	1.8025	32	HIV+ART+	0.421	0.819	39
HIV−	0.559	1.878	56	HIV+ART−	0.722	0.9902	35	HIV+ART+	0.503	0.885	42
HIV−	0.91	2.2	44	HIV+ART−	0.518	2.0082	32	HIV+ART+	0.422	2.031	38
HIV−	0.52	2.31	47	HIV+ART−	0.518	3.8902	54	HIV+ART+	0.458	5.037	50
HIV−	0.534	0.716	46	HIV+ART−	0.676	2.0082	55	HIV+ART+	0.422	4.489	33
HIV−	0.531	1.173	35	HIV+ART−	0.536	5.9828	48	HIV+ART+	0.511	1.489	43
HIV−	0.506	1.285	59	HIV+ART−	0.548	2.2549	36	HIV+ART+	0.449		45
HIV−	0.724	1.731	69	HIV+ART−	0.589	1.5533	33	HIV+ART+	0.402		24
HIV−	0.783	1.855	28	HIV+ART−	0.35	1.8852	38	HIV+ART+	0.514	1.643	34
HIV−	0.613	2.549	33	HIV+ART−	0.444	0.9459	26	HIV+ART+	0.54	0.887	62
HIV−	0.457	1.512	42	HIV+ART−	0.611	7.4926	27	HIV+ART+	0.587	3.34	43
HIV−	0.525	0.929	31	HIV+ART−	0.409	0.7648	37	HIV+ART+	0.496	1.961	41
HIV−	0.71	1.824	51	HIV+ART−	0.496	2.0885	49	HIV+ART+	0.441	0.988	34
HIV−	0.632	1.512	24	HIV+ART−	0.373	1.0787	48	HIV+ART+	0.384	2.4	52
HIV−	0.572	0.726	40	HIV+ART−	0.499	0.6689	43	HIV+ART+	0.398	0.854	40
HIV−	0.682		69	HIV+ART−	0.832	1.5049	34	HIV+ART+	0.471	0.48	54
HIV−	0.477		38	HIV+ART−	0.368	9.0369	59	HIV+ART+	0.409	0.854	28
HIV−	0.558		45	HIV+ART−	0.634	2.038	31	HIV+ART+	0.384	1.803	30
HIV−	0.672	0.996	48	HIV+ART−	0.564	3.578	34	HIV+ART+	0.537	0.954	45
HIV−	0.587	2.608	60	HIV+ART−	1.024	2.901	30				
HIV−	0.525	2.31	42	HIV+ART−	0.785	2.552	28				
HIV−	0.507	1.062	63	HIV+ART−	0.664	1.34	28				
HIV−	0.527	1.354	78	HIV+ART−	0.614	2.038	64				
HIV−	0.781	5.16	39	HIV+ART−	1.204	3.999	24				
HIV−	0.618	1.062	42	HIV+ART−	0.61	11.768	36				
HIV−	0.589	0.76	81	HIV+ART−	0.52	5.736	47				
HIV−	0.504	0.587	47	HIV+ART−	0.456	3.146	42				
HIV−	0.529	1.257	44	HIV+ART−	0.736	1.395	27				
HIV−	0.81	2.19	45	HIV+ART−	0.581	2.901	31				
				HIV+ART−	0.501	1.985	37				
				HIV+ART−	0.735	10.57	30				
				HIV+ART−	0.623	3.435	33				
				HIV+ART−	0.956	2.038	45				
				HIV+ART−	0.778	1.505	34				
				HIV+ART−	0.728	2.603	27				

Data from Dysangco A, Liu Z, Stein JH, et al: HIV infection, antiretroviral therapy, and measures of endothelial function, inflammation, metabolism, and oxidative stress, *PLoS One.* 2017 Aug 17;12(8):e0183511.

difference between the mean for the normal group and the grand mean. Thus,

$$(78 - 49.84) + (49.84 - 42.48) = 28.16 + 7.36$$
$$= 35.52$$

Although our example does not show exactly how ANOVA works, it illustrates the concept of dividing the variation into different parts. Here, we were looking at simple differences related to just one observation; ANOVA considers the variation in all observations and divides it into (1) the variation between each subject and the subject's group mean and (2) the variation between each group mean and the grand mean. If the group means are quite different from one another, considerable variation will occur between them and the grand mean, compared with the variation within each group. If the group means are not very different, the variation between them and the grand mean will not be much more than the variation among the subjects within each group. The **F test** for two variances (Chapter 6) can be used to test the ratio of the variance among means to the variance among subjects within each group.

The null hypothesis for the F test is that the two variances are equal; if they are, the variation among means is not much greater than the variation among individual observations within any given group. In this situation, we cannot conclude that the means are different from one another. Thus, we think of ANOVA as a test of the equality of means, even though the variances are being tested in the process. If the null hypothesis is rejected, we conclude that not all the means are equal; however, we do not know which ones are not equal, which is why post hoc comparison procedures are necessary.

Illustration of Intuitive Calculations for ANOVA

Recall that the formula for the variance of the observations (or squared standard deviation; see Chapter 3) involves the sum of the squared deviations of each X from the mean $\bar{X}$:

$$SD^2 = \frac{\sum(X - \bar{X})}{n - 1}$$

A similar formula can be used to find the variance of means from the grand mean:

$$\text{Estimate of variance of means} = \frac{\sum n_j(\bar{X}_j - \bar{\bar{X}})^2}{j - 1}$$

where n_j is the number of observations in each group and j is the number of groups. This estimate is called

the **mean square among groups,** abbreviated MS_A, and it has $j - 1$ degrees of freedom.

To obtain the variance within groups, we use a pooled variance like the one for the t test for two independent groups:

$$\text{Estimate of variance within groups} = \frac{\sum(n_j - 1)SD_j^2}{\sum(n_j - 1)}$$

This estimate is called the **error mean square** (or mean square within), abbreviated MS_E. It has $\sum(n_j - 1)$ degrees of freedom, or, if the sum of the number of observations is denoted by N, $N - j$ degrees of freedom. The F ratio is formed by dividing the estimate of the variance of means (mean square among groups) by the estimate of the variance within groups (error mean square), and it has $j - 1$ and $N - j$ degrees of freedom.

We will use the data from the study by Dysangco et al (2017) to illustrate the calculations. In this example, the outcome of interest (HDL-C) is the **dependent variable,** and the grouping variable (control subjects and two sets of HIV patients) is the **independent variable.** The data in Table 7–1 indicate that the mean HDL-C for groups B and C, the patients with HIV, is higher than the mean for the control groups. If these three groups of subjects are viewed as coming from a larger population, then the question is whether HDL-C levels differ in the population. Although differences exist in the means in Table 7–1, some differences in the samples would occur simply by chance, even when no variation exists in the population. So, the question is reduced to whether the observed differences are large enough to convince us that they did not occur merely by chance but reflect real distinctions in the population.

The statistical hypothesis being tested, the null hypothesis, is that the mean HDL-C is equal among the three groups. The alternative hypothesis is that a difference does exist; that is, not all the means are equal. The steps in testing the null hypothesis follow.

Step 1: H_0: The mean HDL-C is equal in the three groups, or, in symbols, $\mu_1 = \mu_2 = \mu_3$

H_1: The means are not equal, or, in symbols, $\mu_1 \neq \mu_2$ or $\mu_2 \neq \mu_3$ or $\mu_1 \neq \mu_3$

Step 2: The test statistic in the test of equality of means in ANOVA is the F ratio, $F = MS_A/MS_E$, with $j - 1$ and $\sum(n_j - 1)$ degrees of freedom.

Step 3: We use $\alpha = 0.05$ for this statistical test.

Step 4: The value of the F distribution from Table A–4 with $j - 1 = 2$ degrees of freedom in the numerator and $\sum(n_j - 1) = 107$ in the denominator is between 3.15 and 3.07; exact value from Excel function (=F.INV.RT(0.05,2,107)) is 3.08. The decision is to reject the null hypothesis of equal means if the observed value of F is greater than 3.08 and falls in the rejection area (Figure 7–1).

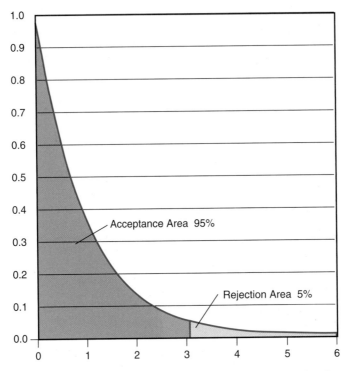

Figure 7–1. Illustration of critical value for F distribution with 2 and 107 degrees of freedom.

Step 5: First we calculate the grand mean. Because we already know the means for the three groups, we can form a weighted average of these means to find the grand mean:

$$\overline{\overline{X}} = \frac{38 \times 49.84 + 44 \times 37.02 + 28 \times 41.07}{38 + 44 + 28}$$

$$= 42.48$$

The numerator of the MS_A is:

$$38(49.84 - 42.48)^2 + 44(37.02 - 42.48)^2$$

$$+ 28(41.07 - 42.48)^2 = 3426.6$$

The term MS_A, found by dividing the numerator by the number of groups minus 1, $(j - 1)$—which is 2 in this example, is:

$$MS_A = \frac{3426.6}{2} = 1712.8$$

The individual group variances are used to calculate the pooled estimate of the MS_E:

$$MS_E = \frac{\Sigma(n_j - 1)SD_j^2}{\Sigma(n_j - 1)}$$

$$= \frac{37 \times 18.68^2 + 43 \times 10.27^2 + 27 + 10.77^2}{37 + 43 + 27}$$

$$= \frac{20576.1}{107} = 192.3$$

Finally, the F ratio is found by dividing the mean square among groups by the error mean square:

$$F = \frac{MS_A}{MS_E}$$

$$= \frac{1712.8}{192.3} = 8.91$$

Step 6: The observed value of the F ratio is 8.91, which is larger than 3.08 (the critical value from Step 4). The null hypothesis of equal means is therefore rejected. We conclude that a difference does exist in HDL-C levels among normal control subjects, HIV+ patients not on ART, and HIV+ patients on ART. Note that rejecting the null hypothesis does not tell us *which* group means differ, only that a difference exists; in the section titled, "Multiple-Comparison Procedures," we illustrate different methods that can be used to learn which specific groups differ.

TRADITIONAL APPROACH TO ANOVA

In the preceding section, we presented a simple illustration of ANOVA by using formulas to estimate the variance among individual group means and the grand mean, called the mean square *among groups* (MS_A), and the variance *within* groups, called the mean square error or mean square *within groups* (MS_E). Traditionally in ANOVA, formulas are given for **sums of squares,** which are generally equivalent to the numerators of the formulas used in the preceding section; then, sums of squares are divided by appropriate degrees of freedom to obtain mean squares. Before illustrating the calculations for the data on HDL-C levels, we define some terms and give the traditional formulas.

Terms & Formulas for ANOVA

In ANOVA, the term **factor** refers to the variable by which groups are formed, the **independent variable.** For example, in Presenting Problem 1, subjects were divided into groups based on their HIV and ART status; therefore, this study is an example of a one-factor ANOVA, called a one-way ANOVA. The number of groups defined by a given factor is referred to as the number of *levels* of the factor; the factor in Presenting Problem 1 has three groups, or we say that the group factor has three levels. In experimental studies in medicine, levels are frequently referred to as *treatments*.

Some textbooks approach analysis of variance from the perspective of models. The **model** for one-way ANOVA states that an individual observation can be divided into three components related to (1) the grand mean, (2) the group to which the individual belongs, and (3) the individual observation itself. To write this model in symbols, we let i stand for a given individual observation and j stand for the group to which this individual belongs. Then, X_{ij} denotes the observation of individual i in group j; for example, X_{11} is the first observation in the first group, and X_{53} is the fifth observation in the third group. The grand mean in the model is denoted by μ. The *effect* of being a member of group j may be thought of as the difference between the mean of group j and the grand mean; the effect associated with being in group j is written α_j. Finally, the difference between the individual observation and the mean of the group to which the observation belongs

is written e_{ij} and is called the **error term, or residual.** Putting these symbols together, we can write the model for one-way ANOVA as

$$X_{ij} = \mu + \alpha_j + e_{ij}$$

which states that the ith observation in the jth group, X_{ij}, is the sum of three components: the grand mean, μ; the effect associated with group j, α_j; and an error (residual), e_{ij}.

The size of an effect is, of course, related to the size of the difference between a given group mean and the grand mean. When inferences involve only specific levels of the factor included in the study, the model is called a *fixed-effects model*. The fixed-effects model assumes we are interested in making inferences only to the populations represented in the study. For example, if investigators wish to draw conclusions about three dosage levels of a drug. If, in contrast, the dosage levels included in the study are viewed as being randomly selected from all different possible dosage levels of the drug, the model is called a *random-effects model*, and inferences can be made to other levels of the factor not represented in the study.[†] Both models are used to test hypotheses about the equality of group means. The random-effects model, however, can also be used to test hypotheses and form confidence intervals about group variances, and it is also referred to as the components-of-variance model for this reason.

Definitional Formulas: In the section titled, "The Logic of ANOVA," we showed that the variation of 35.22 of HDL-C from the grand mean of 42.48 (subject 1 in the control group) can be expressed as a sum of two differences: (1) the difference between the observation and the mean of the group it is in, plus (2) the difference between its group mean and the grand mean. This result is also true when the differences are squared and the squared deviations are added to form the sum of squares.

To illustrate, for one factor with j groups, we use the following definitions:

X_{ij} is the ith observation in the jth group.

$\bar{X}_j$ is the mean of all observations in the jth group.

$\bar{\bar{X}}$ is the grand mean of the observations.

Then, $\Sigma(X_{ij} - \bar{\bar{X}})^2$, the total sum of squares, or SS_T, can be expressed as the sum of $\Sigma(X_{ij} - \bar{X})^2$, the error sum of squares (SS_E) and $\Sigma(\bar{X}_j - \bar{\bar{X}})^2$, the sum of squares among groups (SS_A).

[†]The calculations of sums of squares and mean squares are the same in both models, but the type of model determines the way the F ratio is formed when two or more factors are included in a study.

That is,

$$\Sigma(X_{ij} - \overline{\overline{X}})^2 = \Sigma(X_{ij} - \overline{X}_j)^2 + \Sigma(\overline{X}_i - \overline{\overline{X}})^2$$

$$\text{or } SS_T = SS_E + SS_A$$

We do not provide the proof of this equality here, but interested readers can consult any standard statistical reference for more details (e.g., Berry et al, 2001; Daniel and Cross, 2018; Hays, 1997).

Computational Formulas: Computational formulas are more convenient than definitional formulas when sums of squares are calculated manually or when using calculators, as was the situation before computers were so readily available. Computational formulas are also preferred because they reduce round-off errors. They can be derived from definitional ones, but because the algebra is complex, we do not explain it here. If you are interested in the details, consult the previously mentioned texts.

The symbols in ANOVA vary somewhat from one text to another; the following formulas are similar to those used in many books and are the ones we will use to illustrate calculations for ANOVA. Let N be the total number of observations in all the groups, that is, $N = \Sigma n_j$. Then, the computational formulas for the sums of squares are

$$SS_T = \Sigma(X_{ij} - \overline{\overline{X}})^2 = \Sigma X_{ij}^2 - \frac{(\Sigma X_{ij})^2}{N}$$

$$SS_A = \Sigma(\overline{X}_j - \overline{\overline{X}})^2 = \Sigma n_j \overline{X}_j^2 - \frac{(\Sigma X_{ij})^2}{N}$$

and SS_E is found by subtraction: $SS_E = SS_T - SS_A$.

The sums of squares are divided by the degrees of freedom to obtain the mean squares:

$$MS_A = \frac{SS_A}{j-1}$$

where j is the number of groups or levels of the factor, and

$$MS_E = \frac{SS_E}{N-j}$$

where j is the number of groups or levels of the factor, and N is the total sample size.

One-Way ANOVA

Presenting Problem 1 is an example of a one-way ANOVA model in which there is a numerical dependent variable: level of HDL-C. There are three groups of patients that serve as the independent variable:

controls, and HIV+ patients who are taking or not taking ART. The mean level of HDL-C is examined for subjects in each group (see Table 7–1.)

Illustration of Traditional Calculations: To calculate sums of squares by using traditional ANOVA formulas, we must obtain three terms:

1. We square each observation (X_{ij}) and add, to obtain ΣX_{ij}^2.
2. We add the observations, square the sum, and divide by N, to obtain $(\Sigma X_{ij})^2/N$.
3. We square each mean ($\overline{X}_j$), multiply by the number of subjects in that group (n_j), and add, to obtain $\Sigma n_j \overline{X}_j^2$.

These three terms using the data in Table 7–2 are

$$\Sigma X_{ij}^2 = 17^2 + 26^2 + \cdots + 30^2 + 45^2$$
$$= 222517$$

$$\frac{(\Sigma X_{ij})^2}{N} = \frac{(17 + 26 + \cdots + 30 + 45)^2}{N}$$
$$= 198517.54$$

and

$$\Sigma n_j \overline{X}_{ij}^2 = 38 \times 49.84^2 + 44 \times 37.02^2$$
$$+28 \times 41.07^2$$
$$= 201943.11$$

Then, the sums of squares are

$$SS_T = \Sigma X_{ij}^2 - \frac{(\Sigma X_{ij})^2}{N}$$
$$= 222517.00 - 198517.54$$
$$= 23999.46$$

$$SS_A = \Sigma n_j \overline{X}_j^2 - \frac{(\Sigma X_{ij})^2}{N}$$
$$= 201943.11 - 198517.54$$
$$= 3425.58$$

$$SS_E = SS_T - SS_A$$
$$= 23999.46 - 3425.58$$
$$= 20573.46$$

Next, the mean squares are calculated.

$$MS_A = \frac{SS_A}{j-1} = \frac{3425.58}{2} = 1712.8$$

$$MS_E = \frac{SS_E}{N-j} = \frac{20573.46}{107} = 192.8$$

Slight differences between these results and the results for the mean squares calculated in the section titled, "Illustration of Intuitive Calculations for ANOVA," are due to round-off error. Otherwise, the results are the same regardless of which formulas are used.

Finally, the F ratio is determined.

$$F = \frac{MS_A}{MS_E} = \frac{1712.8}{192.3} = 8.91$$

The calculated F ratio is compared with the value from the F distribution with 2 and 107 degrees of freedom at the desired level of significance. As we found in the section titled, "Illustration of Intuitive Calculations for ANOVA," for $\alpha = 0.05$, the value of F (2, 107) is 3.08. Because 8.91 is greater than 3.08, the null hypothesis is rejected; and we conclude that mean HDL-C levels are not the same for patients who are HIV− (controls), and those who are HIV+ and either are or are not on ART. The formulas for one-way ANOVA are summarized in Table 7–3.

Assumptions in ANOVA: Analysis of variance uses information about the means and standard deviations in each group. Like the t test, ANOVA is a parametric method, and some important assumptions are made.

1. The values of the dependent or outcome variable are assumed to be normally distributed within each group or level of the factor. In our example, this assumption requires that HDL-C levels be normally distributed in each of the three groups.

2. The population variance is the same in each group, that is, $\sigma_1^2 = \sigma_2^2 = \sigma_3^2$. In our example, this means that the variance (or squared standard deviation) of HDL-C levels should be the same in each of the three groups.

3. The observations are a random sample, and they are independent in that the value of one observation is not related in any way to the value of another observation. In our example, the value of one subject's HDL-C level must have no influence on that of any other subject.

Not all these assumptions are equally important. The results of the F test are not affected by moderate departures from normality, especially for a large number of observations in each group or sample. In other words, the F test is **robust** with respect to violation of the assumption of normality. If the observations are extremely skewed, however, especially for small samples, the Kruskal–Wallis nonparametric procedure, discussed later in this chapter, should be used.

The F test is more sensitive to the second assumption of equal variances, also called **homogeneity** of variances. Concern about this assumption is eliminated, however, if sample sizes are equal (or close to equal) in each group (Box, 1953, 1954). For this reason, it's a good idea to design studies with similar sample sizes. If they cannot, as is sometimes the situation in observational studies, two other solutions are possible. The first is to transform data within each group to obtain equal variances, using one of the transformations discussed in Chapter 5. The second solution is to select samples of equal sizes randomly from each group, although many investigators do not like this solution because perfectly good observations are thrown away. Investigators should consult a statistician for studies with greatly unequal variances and unequal sample sizes.

The last assumption is particularly important. In general, investigators should be certain that they have **independent observations.** Independence is a

Table 7–3. Formulas for one-way ANOVA.

Source of Variation	Sums of Squares	Degrees of Freedom	Mean Squares	F Ratio
Among groups	$SS_A = \Sigma n_j \bar{X}_1^2 - \dfrac{(\Sigma X_{ij})^2}{N}$	$j-1$	$MS_A = \dfrac{SS_A}{j-1}$	$F = \dfrac{MS_A}{MS_E}$
Error	$SS_E = SS_T - SS_A$	$N-j$	$MS_E = \dfrac{SS_E}{N-j}$	
Total	$SS_T = \Sigma X_{ij}^2 - \dfrac{(\Sigma X_{ij})^2}{N}$	$N-1$		

problem primarily with studies involving repeated measurements of the same subjects, and they must be handled in a special way, as we discuss later in this chapter.

As a final comment, recall that the fixed-effects model assumes that each observation is really a sum, consisting of the grand mean, the effect of being a member of the particular group, and the error (residual) representing any unexplained variation. Some studies involve observations that are proportions, rates, or ratios; and for these data, the assumption about sums does not hold.

Interpretation of Presenting Problem 1

The analysis of variance table for HCL-C activity using R is shown in Table 7–4. The among-group factor is designated by A (group) in the first row of the table. We see that the value for the sum of squares for the among factor, 3,426, is close to the value we obtained in the section titled, "One-Way ANOVA" (3,425.58). Similarly, the mean squares and the F ratio are close to those we calculated.

Thus, the probability of observing a difference this large merely by chance (i.e., if no difference exists between the three groups) is less than 3 in 10,000. The author used the Bonferroni comparison procedure and reported that the groups B and C (HIV+ patients with and without ART) differed significantly from the control group. We discuss the Bonferroni statistic in the next section.

The investigators controlled for possible **confounding variables** in follow-up analyses that we will review later. Graphs help readers appreciate the magnitude of results from a study. A box plot of HDL-C levels using R is given in Figure 7–2. The analysis of variance indicates that at least one difference exists among the groups. Based on the box plot, what is your best guess as to which groups differ? In the next section, we examine statistical tests that help answer this question.

MULTIPLE-COMPARISON PROCEDURES

Sometimes, investigators have a limited number of specific comparisons—planned, or a priori, comparisons—in mind prior to designing the study. In this special situation, comparisons can be made without performing an ANOVA first, although in actual practice, most investigators prefer to perform an ANOVA anyway. Typically, investigators want the freedom and flexibility of making comparisons afforded by the posteriori, or post hoc, methods. Before discussing these types of comparisons, however, we need two definitions.

A *comparison* or *contrast* between two means is the difference between the means, such as $\mu_1 - \mu_2$. Comparisons can also involve more than two means. For example, in a study to compare a new drug with a placebo, investigators may wish to compare the mean response for dosage 1 with the mean response for

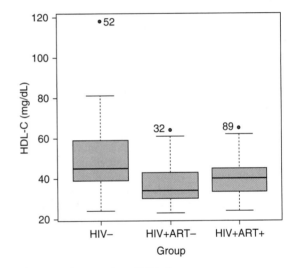

Figure 7–2. Box plot of HDL-C.

Table 7–4. Analysis of variance table for HDL-C (mg/dL).

Source Term	df	Sum of Squares	Mean Square	F-Ratio	Probability Level
A: Group	2	3,426	1,712.8	8.908	0.000264
S: Error	107	20,574	192.3		
Total	109				

Data from Dysangco A, Liu Z, Stein JH, et al: HIV infection, antiretroviral therapy, and measures of endothelial function, inflammation, metabolism, and oxidative stress, *PLoS One*. 2017 Aug 17;12(8):e0183511.

placebo, $\mu_1 - \mu_P$, as well as the mean response for dosage 2 with the mean response for placebo, $\mu_2 - \mu_P$. In addition, they may wish to compare the overall effect of the drug with the effect of placebo $[(\mu_1 + \mu_2)/2] - \mu_P$. Note that in all examples, the *coefficients* of the means add to 0; that is, rewriting the first comparison slightly gives $(1)\mu_1 + (-1)\mu_2$ and $(1) + (-1) = 0$; rewriting the last comparison gives $(\frac{1}{2})\mu_1 + (\frac{1}{2})\mu_2 + (-1)\mu_P$ and $(\frac{1}{2}) + (\frac{1}{2}) + (-1)$ again is 0.

The second definition involves the distinction between two different kinds of comparisons or contrasts. Two comparisons are *orthogonal* if they do not use the same information. For example, suppose a study involves four different therapies: 1, 2, 3, and 4. Then, comparisons between $\mu_1 - \mu_2$ and between $\mu_3 - \mu_4$ are orthogonal because the information used to compare groups 1 and 2 is not the same information used to compare groups 3 and 4. In a sense, the questions asked by two orthogonal comparisons may be considered independent from each other. Conversely, comparisons of $\mu_1 - \mu_2$ and $\mu_1 - \mu_3$ are not orthogonal because they use redundant information; that is, observations in group 1 are used in both comparisons.

A Priori, or Planned, Comparisons

When comparisons are planned, they may be undertaken without first performing ANOVA. When the comparisons are all orthogonal, the t test for independent groups (see Chapter 6) may be used to compare two groups with the following modification: Instead of using the pooled standard deviation SD_p in the denominator of the t ratio, we use the error mean square MS_E. When sample sizes are equal, denoted by n, the t ratio becomes

$$t = \frac{(\bar{X}_i - \bar{X}_j)}{\sqrt{2MS_E / n}}$$

with $N - j$ degrees of freedom, where N is the total number of observations, $n_1 + n_2$, in the two groups.

Adjusting the α Level Downward: When several planned comparisons are made, the probability of obtaining significance by chance is increased; namely, the probability of a type I error increases. For example, for four independent comparisons, all at $\alpha = 0.05$, the probability of one or more significant results is $4 \times 0.05 = 0.20$. One way to compensate for multiple (orthogonal) comparisons is to decrease the α level, and this can be done by dividing α by the number of comparisons made. For example, if four independent comparisons are made, α is divided by 4 to obtain a comparison-wise α of $0.05/4 = 0.0125$ to maintain the overall probability of a type I error at 0.05. Using this method, each orthogonal comparison must be significant at the 0.0125 level to be statistically significant.

The Bonferroni t Procedure: Another approach for planned comparisons is the **Bonferroni t method,** also called Dunn's multiple-comparison procedure. This approach is more versatile because it is applicable for both orthogonal and nonorthogonal comparisons. The Bonferroni t method increases the critical F value needed for the comparison to be declared significant. The amount of increase depends on the number of comparisons and the sample size.

To illustrate, consider the three groups in Presenting Problem 1. We will use the pairwise differences for HDL-C levels listed in Table 7–5 to illustrate all multiple comparisons in this section so we can compare results of the different procedures. To simplify our illustrations, we assume the number of subjects is 40 in each group (computer programs make adjustments for different sample sizes).

In the Bonferroni t procedure, $\sqrt{2MS_E / n}$ is multiplied by a factor related to the number of comparisons made and the degrees of freedom for the error mean square. In this example, three pairwise comparisons are possible; for $\alpha = 0.05$ and assuming approximately 120 degrees of freedom, the multiplier is 2.43 (see Table 7–6). Therefore,

$$2.43 \times \sqrt{\frac{2MS_E}{n}} = 2.43 \times \sqrt{\frac{2 \times 192.3}{40}}$$
$$= 2.43 \times 3.10$$
$$= 7.53$$

where the value for MS_E comes from the results of the ANOVA (Table 7–4). The mean difference between groups B and C is compared with 7.53. The mean difference between groups B and C is only -4.05 and not statistically different. However, both of the mean differences between groups A and C and groups A and B are statistically significant: both 12.82 and 8.77 exceed 7.53. We conclude that HIV+ patients both on and not on ART have different HDL-C levels than the control subjects. Is this conclusion consistent with your best guess after looking at the box plots in Figure 7–2?

Table 7–5. Differences between means of HDL-C (mg/dL) groups.

	$\bar{X}_A$	$\bar{X}_B$	$\bar{X}_C$
$\bar{X}_A$	—	12.82	8.77
$\bar{X}_B$		—	−4.05
$\bar{X}_C$			—

Table 7–6. Excerpts from tables for use with multiple-comparison procedures for $\alpha = 0.05$.

Error df	Number of Means/Steps for Studentized Range			Number of Means for Dunnett's Test			Number of Comparisons for Bonferroni t				
	2	**3**	**4**	**2**	**3**	**4**	**2**	**3**	**4**	**5**	**6**
10	3.15	3.88	4.33	1.81	2.15	2.34	2.64	2.87	3.04	3.17	3.28
20	2.95	3.58	3.96	1.73	2.03	2.19	2.42	2.61	2.75	2.85	2.93
30	2.89	3.49	3.85	1.70	1.99	2.15	2.36	2.54	2.66	2.75	2.83
60	2.83	3.40	3.74	1.67	1.95	2.10	2.30	2.47	2.58	2.66	2.73
120	2.80	3.36	3.68	1.66	1.93	2.08	2.27	2.43	2.54	2.62	2.68

Data from Kirk RE: *Experimental Design: Procedures for the Behavioral Sciences*, 4th ed. Los Angeles, CA: Sage Publications, Inc; 2013.

 A Posteriori, or Post Hoc, Comparisons

Post hoc comparisons (the Latin term means "after this") are made after an ANOVA has resulted in a significant F test. The *t* test introduced in Chapter 5 should *not* be used for these comparisons because it does not take into consideration the number of comparisons being made, the possible lack of independence of the comparisons, and the unplanned nature of the comparisons.

Several procedures are available for making post hoc comparisons. Four of them are recommended by statisticians, depending on the particular research design, and two others are not recommended but are commonly used nonetheless. The data from Presenting Problem 1, as summarized in Table 7–5, are again used to illustrate these six procedures. As with the Bonferroni *t* method, special tables are needed to find appropriate multipliers for these tests when computer programs are not used for the analysis; excerpts from the tables are reproduced in Table 7–6 corresponding to $\alpha = 0.05$.

Tukey's HSD Procedure: The first procedure we discuss is the Tukey test, or **Tukey's HSD** (honestly significant difference) test, so named because some post hoc procedures make significance too easy to obtain. It was developed by the same statistician who invented stem-and-leaf plots and box-and-whisker plots, and he obviously had a sense of humor. Tukey's HSD test can be used only for pairwise comparisons, but it permits the researcher to compare all pairs of means. A study by Stoline (1981) found it to be the most accurate and powerful procedure to use in this situation. (Recall that power is the ability to detect a difference if one actually exists, and the null hypothesis is correctly rejected more often.)

The HSD statistic, like the Bonferroni *t*, has a multiplier that is based on the number of treatment levels and the degrees of freedom for error mean square

(3 and approximately 120 in this example). In Table 7–6, under column 3 and for the studentized range,[‡] we find the multiplier 3.36. The HSD statistic is

$$HSD = \text{Multiplier} \times \sqrt{\frac{MS_E}{n}}$$

where *n* is the sample size in each group. Thus,

$$HSD = 3.36 \times \sqrt{\frac{192.3}{40}} = 7.37$$

The differences in Table 7–5 are now compared with 7.37 and are significantly different if they exceed this value. The differences between groups A and B and groups A and C are greater than 7.37. The conclusion is the same as with the Bonferroni *t*—that HIV+ patients both on and not on ART have different HDL-C values than the controls; no differences exist, however, between the two HIV+ groups. Tukey's procedure can also be used to form confidence intervals about the mean difference (as can the Bonferroni *t* method). For instance, the 95% confidence interval for the mean difference between HIV+ patients not on ART versus controls

$$(\bar{X}_1 - \bar{X}_2) \pm 7.37 = 12.82 \pm 7.37 \text{ or } 5.45 \text{ to } 20.19$$

Scheffé's Procedure: Scheffé's procedure is the most versatile of all the post hoc methods because it permits the researcher to make all types of comparisons, not simply pairwise ones. For example, Scheffé's procedure allows us to compare the overall mean of two or more dosage levels with a placebo.

[‡]The studentized range distribution was developed for a test of the largest observed difference in a set of means, essentially a test of significance of the range of the means. It is used as the basis for several post hoc comparisons.

A price is extracted for this flexibility, however: a higher critical value is used to determine significance, making Scheffé's procedure the most conservative of the multiple-comparison procedures.

The formula, which looks complicated, is

$$S = \sqrt{(j-1)F_{\alpha,df}} \sqrt{MS_E \sum \frac{C_j^2}{n_j}}$$

where j is the number of groups, $F_{\alpha,df}$ is the critical value of F used in ANOVA, MS_E is the error mean square, and $\sum(C_j^2 / n_j)$ is the sum of squared coefficients divided by sample sizes in the contrast of interest. For example, in the contrast defined by comparing the patients taking versus not taking ART (still assuming 40 patients in each group),

$$\sum C_j^2 / n_j = \frac{(1)^2}{40} + \frac{(-1)^2}{40} = 0.05.$$

The critical value for F was found to be 3.08 in the section titled, "Intuitive Overview of ANOVA." Substituting values in S yields

$$S = \sqrt{(j-1)F_{\alpha,df}} \sqrt{MS_E \sum \frac{C_j^2}{n_j}}$$

$$= \sqrt{2 \times 3.08} \sqrt{192.3 \times 0.05}$$

$$= 2.48 \times 3.10$$

$$= 7.69$$

Therefore, any contrast greater than 7.69 is significant. As we see from Table 7–5, the difference in means HIV+ patients both on and not on ART have different HDL-C values and the controls are both greater than 7.69 and are significant by the Scheffé's procedure. Because the Scheffé's procedure is the most conservative of all post hoc tests, 7.69 is the largest critical value required by any of the multiple-comparison procedures. Confidence intervals can also be formed by using the Scheffé's procedure.

The Newman–Keuls Procedure: Next, we examine the **Newman–Keuls procedure.** Commonly used in basic science research, Newman–Keuls uses a stepwise approach to testing differences between means and can be used only to make pairwise comparisons. The procedure ranks means from lowest to highest, and the number of steps that separate pairs of means is noted. For our example, the rank orders and the number of steps are given in Figure 7–3. The mean differences are compared with a critical value that

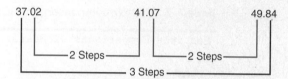

Figure 7–3. Ranking of means and steps for Newman–Keuls procedure.

depends on the number of steps between the two means, the sample size, and the number of groups being compared. In addition, the testing must be done in a prescribed sequence.

The critical value uses the studentized range, but the value corresponds to the number of *steps* between the means (instead of the number of means, as in the Tukey test); this value is multiplied by $\sqrt{2MS_E / n}$ as in the Tukey test. The value from Table 7–6 corresponding to two steps with 120 degrees of freedom is 2.80; the value for three steps is 3.36. The critical values for this example are therefore

$$Newman - Keuls = Multiplier \times \sqrt{\frac{MS_E}{n}}$$

$$= 2.80 \times \sqrt{\frac{192.3}{40}}$$

$$= 6.13$$

$$Newman - Keuls = Multiplier \times \sqrt{\frac{MS_E}{n}}$$

$$= 3.36 \times \sqrt{\frac{192.3}{40}}$$

$$= 7.37$$

As with the other procedures, the conclusion is that control subjects and HIV+ patients both on and not on ART have different HDL-C levels than controls; no differences exist, however, between the HIV+ patients on and not on ART. Although the conclusions are the same as in Tukey's test in this example, using the Newman–Keuls procedure with several groups may permit the investigator to declare a difference between two steps to be significant when it would not be significant in Tukey's HSD test. The primary disadvantage of the Newman–Keuls procedure is that confidence intervals for mean differences cannot be formed.

Dunnett's Procedure: The fourth procedure recommended by statisticians is called **Dunnett's procedure,** and it is applicable *only* in situations in which several treatment means are

Table 7–7. Multiple comparisons for HDL-C (mg/dL) using R.

```
Multiple Comparisons of Means: Tukey Contrasts


Fit: aov(formula = HDLC ~ group, data = HIV_CVD)

Linear Hypotheses:
                         Estimate Std. Error t value Pr(>|t|)
HIV+ART- - HIV- == 0      -12.819      3.071  -4.175 0.000197 ***
HIV+ART+ - HIV- == 0       -8.771      3.454  -2.540 0.033166 *
HIV+ART+ - HIV+ART- == 0    4.049      3.352   1.208 0.450512
---
Signif. codes:  0 '***' 0.001 '**' 0.01 '*' 0.05 '.' 0.1 ' ' 1
(Adjusted p values reported -- single-step method)
```

Data from Dysangco A, Liu Z, Stein JH, et al: HIV infection, antiretroviral therapy, and measures of endothelial function, inflammation, metabolism, and oxidative stress, *PLoS One*. 2017 Aug 17;12(8):e0183511.

compared with a single control mean. No comparisons are permitted between the treatment means themselves, so this test has a very specialized application. When applicable, however, Dunnett's procedure is convenient because it has a relatively low critical value. The size of the multiplier depends on the number of groups, including the control group, and the degrees of freedom for error mean square. The formula is

$$\text{Dunnett's procedure} = \text{Multiplier} \times \sqrt{\frac{2MS_E}{n}}$$

Even though Dunnett's procedure is not applicable to our example, we will determine the critical value for the sake of comparison. From Table 7–6, under the column for Dunnett's procedure and three groups, we find the multiplier 1.95. Multiplying it by $\sqrt{2MS_E / n}$ gives 1.95×3.10, or 6.04, a value much lower than either the Tukey or Scheffé value.

Other Tests: Two procedures that appear in the medical literature but that are *not* recommended by statisticians are Duncan's new multiple-range test and the least significant difference test. Duncan's new multiple-range test uses the same principle as the Newman–Keuls procedure; however, the multipliers in the formula are smaller, so statistically significant differences are found with smaller mean differences. Duncan contended that the likelihood of finding differences is greater with a larger number of groups, and he increased the power of the test by using smaller multipliers. But his test, as a result, is too liberal and rejects the null hypothesis too often. Thus, it is not recommended by statisticians.

The least significant difference (LSD) test is one of the oldest multiple-comparison procedures. As with the other post hoc procedures, it requires a significant F ratio from the ANOVA to make pairwise comparisons. Instead of using an adjustment to make the critical value larger, however, as the other tests have done, the LSD test uses the t distribution corresponding to the number of degrees of freedom for error mean square. Statisticians do not recommend this test because, with a large number of comparisons, differences that are too small may be incorrectly declared significant.

As we just illustrated, the multiple-comparison procedures are tedious to calculate; fortunately, they are available in most statistical software programs. Output from Tukey's multiple-comparison test using the R program is reproduced in Table 7–7. R also creates a set of familywise confidence intervals for the pairwise differences as displayed in Figure 7–4. This allows the reader to easily tell which differences are significant by noting which confidence intervals do not cross the value 0. Do the conclusions from the graph agree with our findings?

ADDITIONAL ILLUSTRATIONS OF THE USE OF ANOVA

In this section, we extend the use of analysis of variance to several other important designs used in the health field. Most ANOVA designs are combinations of a relatively small number of designs: randomized factorial designs, randomized block designs, and Latin square designs. The principle of randomized assignment resulted from the work of two statisticians in the early twentieth

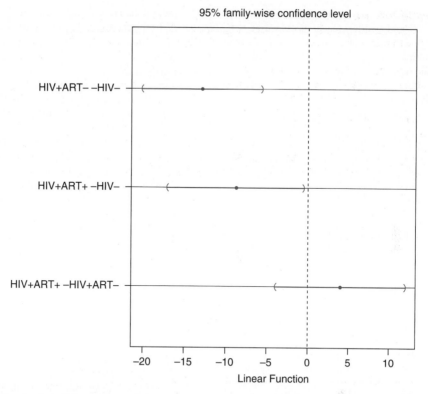

95% family-wise confidence level

Figure 7–4. Graph of confidence intervals for pairwise difference in HDL-C.

century, Ronald Fisher and Karl Pearson, who had considerable influence on the development and the direction of modern statistical methods. For this reason, the term "randomized" occurs in the names of many designs; recall that one of the assumptions is that a random sample has been assigned to the different treatment levels.

Two-Way ANOVA: Factorial Design

Two-way ANOVA is similar to one-way ANOVA except that two factors (or two independent variables) are analyzed. For example, in the study described in Presenting Problem 2, Cornelis and colleagues (2017) wanted to know if a difference existed in a global activities of daily living (ADL) measure for subjects with various levels of cognitive impairment. For this example, we will expand the study to compare the effect of gender and include only two of the impairment groups: minor cognitive impairment (MCI) and subjects with Alzheimer's disease (AD). They created a new scale to measure ADL functionality impairment (i-ADL-CDI). Summarized data are given in Table 7–8. In this example, both factors are measured at two levels on all subjects and are said to be *crossed*.

Table 7–8. Activities of Daily Living scores for subjects in different groups.

Group Statistics	n	Mean i-ADL-CDI	SD i-ADL-CDI
Mild Cognitive Impairment	**73**	**0.19**	**0.19**
Female	31	0.20	0.18
Male	42	0.19	0.20
Alzheimer's Disease	**71**	**0.43**	**0.22**
Female	23	0.53	0.22
Male	48	0.39	0.20
Overall	**144**	**0.31**	**0.24**

Gender Group Statistics	n	Mean i-ADL-CDI	SD i-ADL-CDI
Female	54	0.34	0.25
Male	90	0.29	0.22

Data from Cornelis E, Gorus E, Beyer I, et al: Early diagnosis of mild cognitive impairment and mild dementia through basic and instrumental activities of daily living: Development of a new evaluation tool, *PLoS Med.* 2017 Mar 14;14(3): e1002250.

Because two factors are analyzed in this study (impairment level and gender), each measured at two levels (AD vs. MCI and male vs. female), $2 \times 2 = 4$ treatment combinations are possible: female subjects with AD, female subjects with MCI, male subjects with AD, and male subjects with MCI. Three questions may be asked in this two-way ANOVA:

1. Do differences exist between AD and MCI subjects? If so, the means for each treatment combination might resemble the hypothetical values given in Table 7–9A, and we say a difference exists in the *main effect* for cognitive status. The null hypothesis for this question is that i-ADL-CDI is the same in AD subjects and in MCI subjects ($\mu_A = \mu_M$).

2. Do differences exist between male and female subjects? If so, the means for each treatment combination might be similar to those in Table 7–9B, and we say a difference occurs in the *main effect* for gender. The null hypothesis for this question is that i-ADL-CDI is the same in male subjects and in female subjects ($\mu_M = \mu_F$).

3. Do differences exist owing to neither cognitive status nor gender alone but to the combination of factors? If so, the means for each treatment combination might resemble those in Table 7–9C, and we say an **interaction** effect occurs between the two factors. The null hypothesis for this question is that any difference in ADL between male subjects with AD and male subjects with MCI the same as the difference between female subjects with AD and female subjects with MCI ($\mu_{MA} - \mu_{MM} = \mu_{FA} - \mu_{FM}$).

This study can be viewed as two separate experiments on the same set of subjects for each of the first two questions. The third question can be answered, however, only in a single experiment in which both factors are measured and more than one observation is made at each treatment combination of the factors (i.e., in each cell).

The topic of interactions is important and worth pursuing a bit further. Figure 7–5A is a graph of *hypothetical* mean i-ADL-CDI levels from Table 7–9A for AD and MCI, men and women. When lines connecting means are parallel, no interaction exists between the factors of cognitive status and gender status, and the effects are said to be *additive*. If the interaction is significant, however, as in Table 7–9C, the lines intersect and the effects are called *multiplicative*. Figure 7–5B illustrates this situation and shows that main effects, such as

Table 7–9. Possible results for hypothetical data in two-way ANOVA: Means for each treatment combination.

	Gender	
Subjects	**Male**	**Female**
A. Difference between Patients and Controls		
Alzheimer's Disease	1.00	1.00
Controls	0.50	0.50
B. Difference between Over and Normal Weight Subjects		
Alzheimer's Disease	0.50	1.00
Controls	0.50	1.00
C. Differences Owing Only to Combination of Factors		
Alzheimer's Disease	0.50	1.00
Controls	1.00	0.50

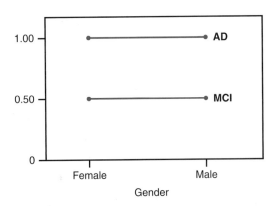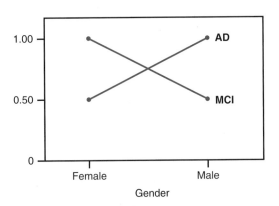

Figure 7–5. Graphs of interaction. **A:** No interaction; effects are additive. **B:** Significant interaction; effects are multiplicative.

cognitive status and gender status, are difficult to interpret when significant interactions occur. For example, if the interaction is significant, any conclusions regarding differences in i-ADL-CDI depend on both cognitive status and gender; any comparison between subjects with AD and MCI depends on the gender of the subject. Although this example illustrates an extreme interaction, many statisticians recommend that the interaction be tested first and, if it is significant, main effects *not* be tested.

The calculations in two-way ANOVA are tedious and will not be illustrated in this book. They are conceptually similar to the calculations in the simpler one-way situation; however, the total variation in observations is divided, and sums of squares are determined for the first factor, the second factor, the interaction of the factors, and the error (residual), which is analogous to the within-group sums of squares in one-way ANOVA.

Refer again to Table 7–8 for the means and standard deviations for each of the four individual groups of subjects and for the two cognitive groups and two genders as well. The mean i-ADL-CDI is 0.19 for subjects with MCI and 0.43 for subjects with AD. For women, mean i-ADL-CDI is 0.34, compared with 0.29 for men. When the means are examined for each individual group, AD women have the highest i-ADL-CDI score, and male MCI subjects have the lowest scores. Two-way analysis of variance can help us make sense of all these means and see which are significantly different. The results are given in Table 7–10.

The computer output produced by R lists a great deal of information, but we focus on the rows containing the *main effects* (DIAGNOSISGROUP and GENDER) and *two-way interactions* (DIAGNOSISGROUP:GENDER). We first examine the interaction effect; the mean square

is 0.1395 (MS = SS/df = 0.1395/1), the *F* statistic is 3.5292, and the *p* value is 0.06238 (in the column labeled Pr(>F)). Because the *p* value is greater than 0.05, the null hypothesis of no interaction is not rejected, so we conclude there is no evidence of significant interaction between level of cognitive impairment and gender. A graph of the interaction is given in Figure 7–6. If the interaction were significant, we would stop at this point and not proceed to interpret the main effects of impairment and gender. The lines in Figure 7–6 do not cross, however, so we are able to consider the main effects. Note that the graph in Figure 7–6 is simply the mean values given in Table 7–8 for the four individual groups.

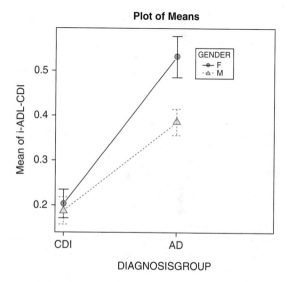

Figure 7–6. Graph of interaction for study of HDL-C.

Table 7–10. Analysis of variance for study of i-ADL-CDI.

```
> Anova(AnovaModel.2)
Anova Table (Type II tests)

Response: IADL_CDI
                       Sum Sq  Df F value     Pr(>F)
DIAGNOSISGROUP         2.1666   1 54.7947 1.134e-11 ***
GENDER                 0.1960   1  4.9563   0.02759 *
DIAGNOSISGROUP:GENDER  0.1395   1  3.5292   0.06238 .
Residuals              5.5357 140
---
Signif. codes:  0 '***' 0.001 '**' 0.01 '*' 0.05 '.' 0.1 ' ' 1
```

Data from Cornelis E, Gorus E, Beyer I, et al: Early diagnosis of mild cognitive impairment and mild dementia through basic and instrumental activities of daily living: Development of a new evaluation tool, *PLoS Med.* 2017 Mar 14;14(3):e1002250.

Table 7–11. Latin square design with three dosage levels (D1, D2, D3).

Body Weight (kg)		Age level (years)		
		<50	**50–70**	**>70**
	< 60	D1	D2	D3
	60–90	D2	D3	D1
	>90	D3	D1	D2

The cognitive impairment (DIAGNOSISGROUP) main effect has 1 degree of freedom (because two impairment groups are being analyzed), so the mean square is the same as the sum of squares, 2.1666 in Table 7–10. The F statistic for this effect is 54.7947, and the p value is <0.0001 (1.134E-11 in scientific notation). Therefore, we reject the null hypothesis of equal mean i-ADL-CDI for the two groups defined by cognitive impairment status and conclude that subjects with AD have a higher i-ADL-CDI score than those with MCI. Similarly, the gender main effect is significant, with a p value of 0.02, so we conclude that gender has an impact on i-ADL-CDI score as well. Note that a higher i-ADL-CDI score denotes more impairment.

Randomized Factorial Designs

The studies discussed in this chapter thus far are examples of randomized **factorial designs** with one or two factors. Randomized factorial designs with three or more factors are possible as well, and the ideas introduced in the section titled, "Two-Way ANOVA: Factorial Design" generalize in a logical way. For example, a study examining cognitive impairment level, gender, and weight (with more than one observation per treatment combination) has sums of squares and mean squares for cognitive impairment level, weight, and gender; for the interactions between cognitive impairment level and weight, between weight and gender, and between cognitive impairment level and gender; and, finally, for the three-way interaction among all three factors. Studies that employ more than three or four factors are rare in medicine because of the large number of subjects needed. For example, a study with three factors, each with two levels as we just described, has $2 \times 2 \times 2 = 8$ treatment combinations; if one factor has two levels, another has three levels, and the third has four levels, then $2 \times 3 \times 4 = 24$ different treatment combinations are possible. Finding equal numbers of subjects for each treatment combination can be difficult.

Randomized Block Designs

A factor is said to be **confounded** with another factor if it is impossible to determine which factor is responsible for the observed effect. Age is frequently a confounding factor in medical studies, so investigators often age-match control subjects with treatment subjects. Randomized **block designs** are useful when a confounding factor contributes to variation.

In the *randomized block design,* subjects are first subdivided into homogeneous blocks; subjects from each block are then randomly assigned to each level of the experimental factor. This type of study is especially useful in laboratory experiments in which investigators are concerned about genetic variation and its effect on the outcome being studied. Litters of animals are defined as the blocks, and littermates are then randomly assigned to the different levels of treatment. In this experiment, blocking is said to control for genetic differences. In studies involving humans, blocking on age or severity of a condition is often useful. Sometimes, investigators cannot control for possible confounding factors in the design of a study. The procedure called **analysis of covariance,** discussed in Chapter 10, allows investigators to control statistically for such factors in the analysis.

Latin Square Designs

Latin square designs employ the blocking principle for two confounding (or nuisance) factors. The levels of the confounding factors are assigned to the rows and the columns of a square; then, the cells of the square identify treatment levels. For example, suppose that both age and body weight are important blocking factors in an experiment that has three dosage levels of a drug as the treatment. Then, three blocks of age and three blocks of body weight form a Latin square with nine cells, and each dosage level appears one or more times for each age-weight combination. Table 7–11 illustrates this design. The Latin square design can be powerful, because only nine subjects are needed and yet two possible confounding factors have been controlled.

Nested Designs

In the factorial designs described previously, the factors are *crossed,* meaning that all levels of one factor occur within all levels of the other factors. Thus, all possible combinations are included in the experiment.

In some situations, however, crossed factors cannot be employed; so *hierarchical,* or *nested,* designs are used instead. In hierarchical designs, one or more of the treatments is nested within levels of another factor. Nesting is often an artifact of organizational structure.

For example, a hospital medical director may want to compare outcomes for patients undergoing cardiac surgery. A given patient is typically operated on by a single physician, so any comparison of outcomes depends on both patient characteristics and physician proficiency. Patients are said to be nested within physicians, and it is impossible to determine interaction effects between patient characteristics and physician proficiency unless special methods, sometimes called generalized estimating equations and discussed in Chapter 10, are used.

Repeated-Measures Designs

Recall from Chapter 5 that the paired *t* test is used when the same group of subjects is observed on two occasions. This design is powerful because it controls for individual variation, which can be large in studies involving human subjects. The counterpart to the paired *t* test in ANOVA is the **repeated-measures** (or split-plot) **design.** In this design, subjects serve as their own controls, so that the variability due to individual differences is eliminated from the error (residual) term, increasing the chances of observing significant differences between levels of treatment. Repeated measures designs are useful in three distinct situations. First, one group of subjects is measured more than twice, generally over time, such as patients weighed at baseline and every month after a weight loss program. Second, one group of subjects is measured on several levels of the same treatment, such as patients who are given three different dosages of a medication. Third, two or more groups of subjects are measured more than once, such as the study of the blood flow in stroke subjects by Durand et al (2015). In this study, the paretic and nonparetic legs for ten post-stroke subjects were tested for blood flow under five muscle contraction conditions of the knee extensor (Resting, 20% maximal voluntary contraction (MVC), 40% MVC, 60% MVC, and 80% MVC). The means and standard deviations of the blood flow for each limb at each of the MVC levels are given in Table 7–12. The raw data on all of the measurements are published with the article.

The results of a repeated-measures analysis of femoral blood flow are given in Table 7–14. The measure that is repeated, the MVC, is called the *within-subjects measure*; and the variable that defines different groups (paretic vs. non-paretic) is called the *between-subjects measure.* The R repeated measures procedure is very versatile because it can use any analysis of variance design, but it is also fairly complicated.

The portion of Table 7–13 labeled "Univariate Type II Repeated-Measures ANOVA Assuming Sphericity" shows that there is a significant difference in the MVC, meaning that the blood flow changes with level of MVC. Although a *p* value of 0.000 is shown,

Table 7–12. Summary statistics for femoral artery blood flow for paretic and nonparetic limb for each MVC level.

	Limb (Group Variable)		
Variable	Nonparetic	Paretic	Overall
n	10	10	20
Average of Resting	109.51	79.65	94.58
StdDev of Resting	68.68	39.69	56.70
Average of 20% MVC	160.45	100.81	130.63
StdDev of 20% MVC	92.12	48.58	77.93
Average of 40% MVC	206.77	140.40	173.59
StdDev of 40% MVC	110.13	76.04	98.20
Average of 60% MVC	237.23	137.06	187.14
StdDev of 60% MVC	118.12	70.39	107.69
Average of 80% MVC	264.18	162.96	213.57
StdDev of 80% MVC	135.18	85.18	121.61

Data from Durand MJ, Murphy SA, Schaefer KK, et al: Impaired Hyperemic Response to Exercise Post Stroke, *PLoS One.* 2015 Dec 2;10(12):e0144023.

the authors correctly reported it as <0.001, because it is always remotely possible that the conclusion is incorrect.

The set of numbers in Table 7–13 in the row labeled Side:MVC shows the result of the test of the interaction between the MVC and side shows a *p* value of 0.01917, but this is under the assumption of sphericity. The test of sphericity in a repeated measures ANOVA is analogous to the test of equality of variances in the two-sample *t*-test. The portion in same table labeled Mauchly Tests for Sphericity states that the null *p* value is <0.05 and, therefore, we must use a slightly different test for the MVC main effect and interaction of side and MVC using an adjustment called Greenhouse-Geisser. The final section in Table 7–13 shows that the main effect for MVC is still significant (*p* < 0.0001), but the *p* value for testing for interaction is now 0.05086 which is larger than 0.05. Because this interaction is not significant at 0.05, we conclude that the pattern of changes in the femoral blood flow is not different for the two sides.

Recall that another assumption in ANOVA is that the observations be independent of one another. This assumption is frequently not met in repeated-measures ANOVA; therefore, certain other assumptions concerning the dependent nature of the observations must be made and tested. Although we do not discuss these assumptions here, readers of the medical literature need to know that repeated-measures ANOVA should be used in studies that repeat measurements on the same subjects.

Table 7–13. Repeated-measures ANOVA of femoral blood flow.

```
> summary(.myAnova, multivariate=FALSE)

Univariate Type II Repeated-Measures ANOVA Assuming Sphericity

                 Sum Sq num Df Error SS den Df F value    Pr(>F)
(Intercept) 2556862      1  612311     18 75.1637 7.657e-08 ***
Side         127631      1  612311     18  3.7519   0.06860 .
MVC          178652      4  103064     72 31.2014 4.526e-15 ***
Side:MVC      18032      4  103064     72  3.1493   0.01917 *
---
Signif. codes:  0 '***' 0.001 '**' 0.01 '*' 0.05 '.' 0.1 ' ' 1


Mauchly Tests for Sphericity

          Test statistic     p-value
MVC              0.10348 0.000026334
Side:MVC         0.10348 0.000026334


Greenhouse-Geisser and Huynh-Feldt Corrections
   for Departure from Sphericity

           GG eps     Pr(>F[GG])
MVC       0.53582 0.000000004699 ***
Side:MVC  0.53582        0.05086 .
---
```

NONPARAMETRIC ANOVA

Nonparametric ANOVA is not a different design but a different method of analysis. Recall from Chapters 5 and 6 that nonparametric methods, such as the Wilcoxon rank sum test for two independent groups or the signed rank test for paired designs, are used if the assumptions for the t tests are seriously violated. A similar situation holds in ANOVA. Even though the F test is robust with respect to violating the assumption of normality and, if the sample sizes are equal, the assumption of equal variances, it is sometimes advisable to transform observations to a logarithm scale or use nonparametric procedures.

Like the nonparametric procedures discussed in Chapters 5 and 6, the nonparametric methods in ANOVA are based on the analysis of ranks of observations rather than on original observations. For one-way ANOVA, the nonparametric procedure is the Kruskal–Wallis one-way ANOVA by ranks. Post hoc comparisons between pairs of means may be made by using the Wilcoxon rank sum test, with a downward adjustment of the α level to compensate for multiple comparisons, as described in the section titled, "A Priori, or Planned, Comparisons." When more than two related samples are of interest, as in repeated measures, the nonparametric procedure of choice is the Friedman two-way ANOVA by ranks. The term "two" in Friedman two-way ANOVA refers to (1) levels of the factor (or treatment) and (2) the repeated occasions on which the subjects were observed. As a follow-up procedure to make pairwise comparisons, the Wilcoxon signed rank test with adjusted degrees of freedom can be used.

COMPARING FREQUENCIES OR PROPORTIONS IN MORE THAN TWO GROUPS

Recall the problem from Chapter 5 that sought to determine the efficacy of a new protocol to reduce infections for the insertion of CSF shunts by van Lindert and colleagues (2018). We can use either the

Table 7–14. Illustration of chi-square for comparing more than two proportions.

```
Frequency table:
         infection
agegroup  No Yes
    <1    47   5
  1-17   141   5
 >=17    296   5

Row percentages:
          infection
agegroup   No  Yes  Total  Count
    <1    90.4  9.6   100     52
  1-17    96.6  3.4   100    146
 >=17     98.3  1.7   100    301
```

Data from van Lindert EJ, van Bilsen M, van der Flier M, et al: Topical vancomycin reduces the cerebrospinal fluid shunt infection rate: a retrospective cohort study, *PLoS One*. 2018 Jan 9;13(1):e0190249.

z test or the chi-square test when only two groups are being analyzed, but with frequency tables having more than two rows and two columns, the z test is no longer applicable. We can still use chi-square, however, regardless of the number of levels or categories within each variable. Table 7–14 gives the results in a 2 × 3 contingency table with the response to the protocol (No = no infection, Yes = infection) as columns and age group of the subject combination as the rows.

We use the chi-square statistic regardless of whether we state the research question in terms of proportions or frequencies. For example, van Lindert and colleagues could ask whether the proportion of subjects who avoided infections were the same for each age group. Alternatively, van Lindert could ask whether age group is associated with the infection outcome.

The chi-square statistic for the van Lindert data in Table 7–14 is exactly the same formula as used earlier:

$$\chi^2_{(df)} = \Sigma \frac{(O - E)^2}{E}$$

except that the degrees of freedom are different. There are six terms in the formula for χ^2 in this example, one for each of the six cells of the 2 × 3 table, so the degrees of freedom are $(r - 1)(c - 1) = (3 - 1)(2 - 1) = 2$.

The following are abbreviated steps for the chi-square hypothesis test. Be sure and confirm these calculations using R and the raw data file.

Step 1: H_0: The response to the protocol is independent of age group.

H_1: The response to the new protocol is not independent of age group.

Step 2: The chi-square test is appropriate for this research question because the observations are nominal data (frequencies).

Step 3: For this test, we use an α of 0.05.

Step 4: The contingency table has three rows and two columns, so $df = (3 - 1)(2 - 1) = 2$. The critical value separating the upper 1% of the χ^2 distribution from the remaining 99% with 2 df is 9.210 (Table A–5). So, χ^2 must be greater than 9.210 in order to reject the null hypothesis of independence.

Step 5: After calculating the expected frequencies for the cells (see Table 7–16), we calculate χ^2:

$$\chi^2 = \frac{(47 - 50.44)^2}{50.44} + \frac{(141 - 141.61)^2}{141.61} + \frac{(296 - 291.95)^2}{291.95}$$
$$+ \frac{(5 - 1.56)^2}{1.56} + \frac{(5 - 4.39)^2}{4.39} + \frac{(5 - 9.05)^2}{90.5}$$

Step 6: The observed value of χ^2 with $2df$, 9.7459, is larger than the critical value of 9.210, so we reject the null hypothesis. We can conclude that response to the new protocol is associated with the age group. The output from R is given in Table 7–15.

The astute reader has probably wondered about the number of small expected values in Table 7–15: Two of the six cells have an expected value less than 5, and one has an expected value less than 2. Therefore, chi-square should be used with caution because small expected values make the value of chi-square too large. In this example, the Fisher's Exact Test may be applied as a conservative approach. Note that the p value for the Fisher's exact test is 0.01354—the null hypothesis of the independence of protocol response and age group would not be rejected at the 0.01 level using this test, but would be rejected at the 0.05 level.

The previous illustration of chi-square had only three rows and two columns, but contingency tables can have any number of rows and columns. Of course, the sample size needs to increase as the number of categories increases to keep the expected values of an acceptable size.

The chi-square test provides a nice illustration of the concept of degrees of freedom. Suppose we have a contingency table with three rows and four columns and marginal frequencies, such as Table 7–16. How many cells in the table are "free to vary" (within the constraints imposed by the marginal frequencies)?

In column 1, the frequencies for rows 1 and 2 can be of any value at all, as long as neither is greater than their row total and their sum does not exceed 100, the column 1 total. The frequency for row 3, however, is

Table 7–15. Results of chi-square test on data in Table 7–14.

```
          Pearson's Chi-squared test

data:  .Table
X-squared = 9.7459, df = 2, p-value = 0.007651


Expected counts:
         infection
agegroup      No       Yes
    <1    50.43687  1.563126
   1-17  141.61122  4.388778
   >=17  291.95190  9.048096

Chi-square components:
         infection
agegroup   No   Yes
    <1    0.23  7.56
   1-17   0.00  0.09
   >=17   0.06  1.81


       Fisher's Exact Test for Count Data

data:  .Table
p-value = 0.01354
alternative hypothesis: two.sided
```

Data from van Lindert EJ, van Bilsen M, van der Flier M, et al: Topical vancomycin reduces the cerebrospinal fluid shunt infection rate: a retrospective cohort study, *PLoS One.* 2018 Jan 9;13(1): e0190249.

Table 7–16. Illustration of degrees of freedom in chi-square.

	Columns				
Rows	**1**	**2**	**3**	**4**	**Total**
1	*	*	*		75
2	*	*	*		100
3					225
Total	100	100	100	100	

determined once the frequencies for rows 1 and 2 are known; that is, it is 100 minus the values in rows 1 and 2. The same reasoning applies for columns 2 and 3. At this point, however, the frequencies in row 3 as well as all the frequencies in column 4 are determined. Thus, there are $(3 - 1) \times (4 - 1) = 2 \times 3 = 6$ degrees of freedom. In general, the degrees of freedom for a contingency table are equal to the number of rows minus 1 times the number of columns minus 1, or, symbolically, $df = (r - 1) \times (c - 1)$.

SAMPLE SIZES FOR ANOVA

It is just as important to look at the sample size needed for ANOVA as it is when studying only one or two groups. Unfortunately, the procedures in the power analysis programs are not as simple to use as the ones for means and proportions. As noted several times in this chapter, if you are planning a study in which an ANOVA is appropriate, it is a good idea to see a statistician prior to beginning.

We used the G*Power program to find the estimated sample size for the study by Dysangco et al (2017). We used the observed results for HCL-C (mg/dL) to determine the number in each group required for 80% power. G*Power requires the desired effect size to determine the sample size. In this case, we assume that we would like to detect a medium effect size (0.25) with three groups, 80% power and alpha of 0.05. The required total sample size is 159. See Figure 7–7 for the resulting power calculation.

SUMMARY

In the study described in Presenting Problem 1, van Lindert analyzed data for the HDL-C using a one-way analysis of variance and followed up the significant findings with the Bonferroni/Dunn correction for multiple comparisons.

His study evaluated the effect HIV and ART on the level of HDL-C. He performed a retrospective analysis of three groups of patients with: HIV+ without ART, HIV+ with ART and HIV– controls. Van Lindert found that the HDL-C levels were higher in both HIV+ groups versus the controls.

Cornelis and colleagues (2017) found significant differences in a composite measure of activities of daily living in subjects with Alzheimer's disease and subjects with minor cognitive impairment. We confirmed the findings for i-ADL-CDI using two-way analysis of variance. The investigators also reported that, there was no significant interaction between subject gender and their level of impairment with respect to their level ADL functionality.

Data from the study by Durand and colleagues (2015) were used to illustrate repeated-measures analysis of variance. They found significant changes in femoral artery flow as muscular contraction level varied. There was also a significant group effect—paretic versus nonparetic side.

Determining which ANOVA study design is most appropriate for a given investigation is often difficult. Making this decision requires knowledge of the area being investigated and of experimental design methods. Considerations must include the kind of data to be collected (nominal, ordinal, interval), the number of treatments to be included and whether obtaining

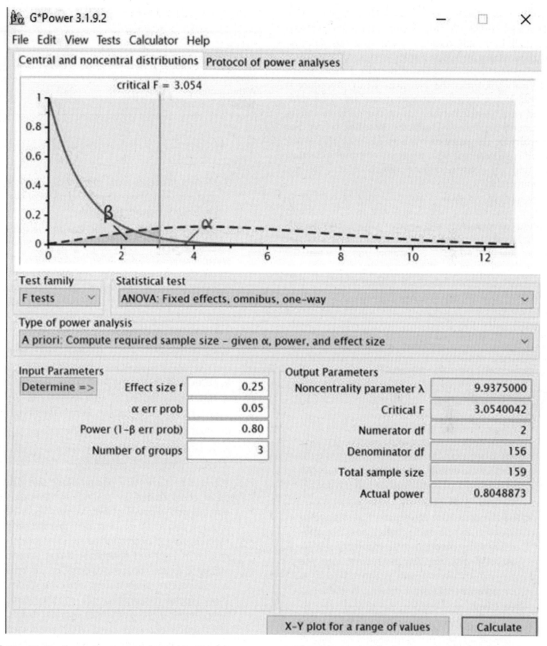

Figure 7–7. Computer output from the G*Power program estimating the sample size for one-way analysis of variance.

estimates of interaction effects is important, the number of treatment levels to be included and whether they should be fixed or random, the possibility of blocking on confounding factors, the number of subjects needed and whether that number is adequate for the proposed designs, and the ramifications of violating assumptions in ANOVA. Although Flowchart C–2 in Appendix C gives some guidelines for elementary designs, selecting the best design requires communication between investigators and statisticians, and the best design may be impossible because of one or more of the considerations just listed.

Although all the post hoc procedures described in the section titled, "Multiple-Comparison Procedures," are used in health research, some methods are better than others for specific study designs. For pairwise comparisons (between pairs of means), Tukey's test is the first choice and the Newman–Keuls procedure is second. When several treatment means are to be compared with a single control but no comparisons among treatments are desired, Dunnett's procedure is best. For nonpairwise comparisons, such as $[(\mu_1 + \mu_2)/2] - \mu_3$, Scheffé's procedure is best. Duncan's new multiple-range test and the least significant difference test are not recommended.

Readers of the medical literature may have difficulty judging whether the best design was used in a study. Authors of journal articles do not always provide sufficient detail on experimental design, and it may not be possible to know the constraints present when the study was designed. In these situations, the reader can only judge the reputation of the authors and their affiliations and evaluate the scholarly practices of the journal in which the study is published. Journals are increasingly requiring authors to specify their study designs and methods of analysis, and we hope they will continue their efforts.

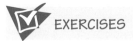

EXERCISES

1. Use the data from Dysangco et al (2017) to perform a one-way ANOVA of IL-6, using $\alpha = 0.05$. Interpret the results of your analysis. You can use either the shortcut formula and the data in Table 7–1 or the raw data.

2. Use the data from Dysangco et al to perform Tukey's HSD test and Scheffé's post hoc procedure for comparing three means of ADMA; you may also run this procedure with the one-way ANOVA program in either SPSS or R. Compare the conclusions drawn with these two procedures.

3. A study was undertaken comparing drug use by physicians, pharmacists, medical students, and pharmacy students. Are the following sets of comparisons independent or dependent?

   a. Physicians with pharmacists and medical students with pharmacy students

   b. Medical students with physicians and physicians with pharmacists

   c. Medical students with physicians and pharmacists with pharmacy students

Table 7–17. ANOVA on mean blood pressures.

Source of Variation	Sums of Squares	df	Mean Squares	F
Among groups	800	3	—	—
Within groups	1,200	36	33.3	
Total	—			

   d. Medical students with physicians, medical students with pharmacists, and medical students with pharmacy students.

4. Medical researchers are interested in the relationship between alcohol use along with other life-style characteristics and the development of diseases, such as cancer and hypertension. The hypothetical data in Table 7–17 could result from an ANOVA in a study comparing the mean blood pressures of patients who consume different amounts of alcohol.

   a. What type of ANOVA is represented in Table 7–17?

   b. What is the total variation?

   c. How many groups of patients were in the study? How many patients were in the study?

   d. What is the value of the F ratio?

   e. What is the critical value at 0.01?

   f. What conclusion is appropriate?

5. Psoriasis is a chronic, inflammatory skin disorder characterized by scaling erythematous patches and plaques of skin. It can begin at any age, frequently involves the fingernails and toenails, and is accompanied by joint inflammation in 5–10% of patients. A strong genetic influence exists—about one-third of patients have a positive family history, and twin studies show a higher concordance rate in monozygotic twins than in dizygotic twins or siblings (70% vs. 23%). Stuart and colleagues (2002) conducted a study to determine whether any differences in clinical manifestations exist between patients with positive and negative family histories of psoriasis and with early-onset vs. late-onset disease. The study group consisted of 537 individuals selected randomly from a population of people with psoriasis evaluated at the University of Michigan. In 227 individuals, there was no known family history of psoriasis and these

Table 7–18. Analysis of variance table.

Source of Variation	Sum of Squares	Degrees of Freedom	Mean Square	F	F-Distribution p	Randomization p
Onset	0.472	1	0.472	0.37	0.545	0.547
Familial	25.99	1	25.99	20.22	8.49×10^{-6}	1.00×10^{-5}
Interaction	26.96	1	26.96	20.98	5.80×10^{-6}	1.00×10^{-5}
Error	685.1	533	1.285			

Reproduced with permission from Stuart P, Malick F, Nair RP, et al: Analysis of phenotypic variation in psoriasis as a function of age at onset and family history, Arch Dermatol Res. 2002 Jul;294(5):207–213.

represented the sporadic psoriasis group. The familial psoriasis group consisted of 310 individuals in whom psoriasis was reported in at least one first-degree relative. Early-onset psoriasis was defined as age at diagnosis of 40 years or younger. Measures of disease severity included percent of total body surface area affected (%TBSA), nail changes, and presence or absence of joint symptoms.

The results of ANOVA are given in Table 7–18.
a. Is there a difference in %TBSA related to age at onset?
b. Is there a difference in %TBSA related to type of psoriasis (familial vs. sporadic)?
c. Is the interaction significant?
d. What is your conclusion?

Research Questions About Relationships Among Variables

KEY CONCEPTS

 Correlation and regression are statistical methods to examine the linear relationship between two numerical variables measured on the same subjects. Correlation describes a relationship, and regression describes both a relationship and predicts an outcome.

 Correlation coefficients range from −1 to +1, both indicating a perfect relationship between two variables. A correlation equal to 0 indicates no relationship.

 Scatterplots provide a visual display of the relationship between two numerical variables and are recommended to check for a linear relationship and extreme values.

 The coefficient of determination, or r^2, is simply the squared correlation; it is the preferred statistic to describe the strength between two numerical variables.

 The t test can be used to test the hypothesis that the population correlation is zero.

 The Fisher z transformation is used to form confidence intervals for the correlation or to test any hypotheses about the value of the correlation.

 The Fisher z transformation can also be used to form confidence intervals for the difference between correlations in two independent groups.

 It is possible to test whether the correlation between one variable and a second is the same as the correlation between a third variable and a second variable.

 When one or both of the variables in correlation is skewed, the Spearman rho nonparametric correlation is advised.

 Linear regression is called linear because it measures only straight-line relationships.

 The least squares method is the one used in almost all regression examples in medicine. With one independent and one dependent variable, the regression equation can be given as a straight line.

 The standard error of the estimate is a statistic that can be used to test hypotheses or form confidence intervals about both the intercept and the regression coefficient (slope).

 One important use of regression is to be able to predict outcomes in a future group of subjects.

 When predicting outcomes, the confidence limits are called confidence bands about the regression line. The most accurate predictions are for outcomes close to the mean of the independent variable X, and they become less precise as the outcome departs from the mean.

 It is possible to test whether the regression line is the same (i.e., has the same slope and intercept) in two different groups.

 A residual is the difference between the actual and the predicted outcome; looking at the distribution of residuals helps statisticians decide if the linear regression model is the best approach to analyzing the data.

17 Regression toward the mean can result in a treatment or procedure appearing to be of value when it has had no actual effect; having a control group helps to guard against this problem.

 18 Correlation and regression should not be used unless observations are independent; it is not appropriate to include multiple measurements of the same subjects.

 19 Mixing two populations can also cause the correlation and regression coefficient to be larger than they should.

 20 The use of correlation versus regression should be dictated by the purpose of the research—whether it is to establish a relationship or to predict an outcome.

 21 The regression model can be extended to accommodate two or more independent variables; this model is called multiple regression.

 22 Determining the needed sample size for correlation and regression is not difficult using one of the power analysis statistical programs.

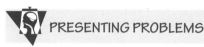 PRESENTING PROBLEMS

Presenting Problem 1

Neidert and colleagues (2016) studied the relationship between body composition measurements: plasma DPP-IV activity, gynoid fat, BMI and lean mass. They recruited 111 subjects from Auburn University (40 men and 71 women) and collected the body composition variables for the study.

The full article may be found here:

Neidert LE, Wainright KS, Zheng C, Babu JR, Kluess HA: Plasma dipeptidyl peptidase IV activity and measures of body composition in apparently healthy people. Heliyon 2016;2:e00097.

https://doi.org/10.1016/j.heliyon.2016.e00097

The data file may be downloaded from this link:
Neidert LE, Wainright KS, Zheng C, Babu JR, Kluess HA: Plasma dipeptidyl peptidase IV activity and measures of body composition in apparently healthy people. Dryad Digital Repository 2016.

https://doi.org/10.5061/dryad.2680t

Presenting Problem 2

Pereira et al (2015) collected data from 145 patients in an adult mixed-ICU to study the accuracy of devices used to measure blood glucose levels at the bedside. They tested: Precision PCx, Accu-chek Advantage II (arterial), Accu-check Advantage II (fingerstick), and Accu-chek

Advantage II (venous). They used regression methods to evaluate the accuracy of each compared to the gold standard arterial blood test from the central lab.

The full article may be found here:

Pereira AJ, Corrêa TD, de Almeida FP, et al: Inaccuracy of venous point-of-care glucose measurements in critically ill patients: a cross-sectional study. PLOS ONE 2015;10(6):e0129568.

https://doi.org/10.1371/journal.pone.0129568

The data file for the study may be accessed here:

Pereira AJ, Corrêa TD, de Almeida FP, et al: Inaccuracy of venous point-of-care glucose measurements in critically ill patients: a cross-sectional study. Dryad Digital Repository 2015.

https://doi.org/10.5061/dryad.sr7c7

AN OVERVIEW OF CORRELATION & REGRESSION

In Chapter 3, we introduced methods to describe the association or relationship between two variables. In this chapter, we review these concepts and extend the idea to predicting the value of one characteristic from the other. We also present the statistical procedures used to test whether a relationship between two characteristics is significant. Two probability distributions introduced previously, the t distribution and the chi-square distribution, can be used for statistical tests in correlation and regression. As a result, you will be pleased to learn that much of the material in this chapter will be familiar to you.

When the goal is merely to establish a relationship (or association) between two measures, as in these studies, the correlation coefficient (introduced in Chapter 3) is the statistic most often used. Recall that correlation is a measure of the *linear* relationship between two variables measured on a numerical scale.

In addition to establishing a relationship, investigators sometimes want to predict an **outcome, dependent,** or **response,** variable from an **independent,** or **explanatory, variable.** Generally, the explanatory characteristic is the one that occurs first or is easier or less costly to measure. The statistical method of **linear regression** is used; this technique involves determining an equation for predicting the value of the outcome from values of the explanatory variable. One of the major differences between correlation and regression is the purpose of the analysis—whether it is merely to describe a relationship or to predict a value. Several important similarities also occur as well, including the direct relationship between the correlation coefficient and the regression coefficient. Many of the same assumptions are required for correlation and regression, and both measure the extent of a linear relationship between the two characteristics.

CORRELATION

Figure 8–1 illustrates several hypothetical **scatterplots** of data to demonstrate the relationship between the size of the correlation coefficient r and the shape of the scatterplot. When the correlation is near zero, as in Figure 8–1E, the pattern of plotted points is somewhat circular. When the degree of relationship is small, the pattern is more like an oval, as in Figures 8–1D and 8–1B. As the value of the correlation gets closer to either $+1$ or -1, as in Figure 8–1C, the plot has a long, narrow shape; at $+1$ and -1, the observations fall directly on a line, as for $r = +1.0$ in Figure 8–1A.

The scatterplot in Figure 8–1F illustrates a situation in which a strong but nonlinear relationship exists. For example, with temperatures less than 10°C to 15°C, a cold nerve fiber discharges few impulses; as the temperature increases, so do numbers of impulses per second until the temperature reaches about 25°C. As the temperature increases beyond 25°C, the numbers of impulses per second decrease once again, until they cease at 40°C to 45°C. The correlation coefficient, however, measures only a linear relationship, and it has a value close to zero in this situation.

One of the reasons for producing scatterplots of data as part of the initial analysis is to identify nonlinear relationships when they occur. Otherwise, if researchers calculate the correlation coefficient without

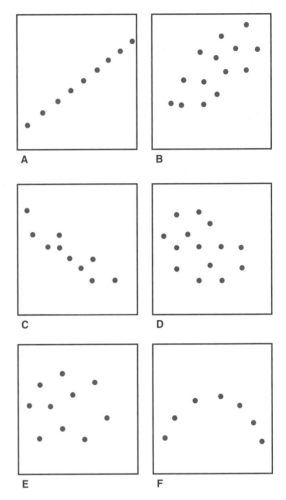

Figure 8–1. Scatterplots and correlations.
A: $r = +1.0$; **B:** $r = 0.7$; **C:** $r = -0.9$; **D:** $r = -0.4$;
E: $r = 0.0$; **F:** $r = 0.0$.

examining the data, they can miss a strong, but nonlinear, relationship, such as the one between temperature and number of cold nerve fiber impulses.

Calculating the Correlation Coefficient

We use the study by Neidert and colleagues (2016) to extend our understanding of correlation. We assume that anyone interested in actually calculating the **correlation coefficient** will use a computer program, as we do in this chapter. If you are interested in a detailed illustration of the calculations, refer to Chapter 3, in the section titled, "Describing the Relationship between Two Characteristics," and the study by Bos-Touwen and associates (2015).

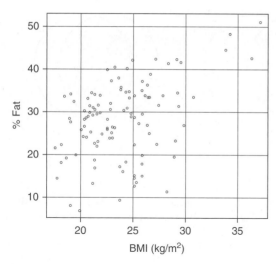

Figure 8–2. Scatterplot of body mass index and percent body fat. (Adapted with permission from Neidert LE, Wainright KS, Zheng C, et al: Plasma dipeptidyl peptidase IV activity and measures of body composition in apparently healthy people, *Heliyon*. 2016 Apr 18;2(4):e00097.)

Recall that the formula for the Pearson product moment correlation coefficient, symbolized by r, is

$$r = \frac{\sum(X - \bar{X})(Y - \bar{Y})}{\sqrt{\sum(X - \bar{X})^2 \sum(Y - \bar{Y})^2}}$$

where X stands for the independent variable and Y for the outcome variable.

A highly recommended first step in looking at the relationship between two numerical characteristics is to examine the relationship graphically. Figure 8–2 is a scatterplot of the data, with body mass index (BMI) on the X-axis and percent body fat (X..Fat) on the Y-axis. We see from Figure 8–2 that a positive relationship exists between these two characteristics: Small values for BMI are associated with small values for percent body fat. The question of interest is whether the observed relationship is statistically significant.

The extent of the relationship can be found by calculating the correlation coefficient. Using a statistical program, the correlation between BMI and percent body fat is 0.42, indicating a strong relationship between these two measures. Use R to confirm our calculations. Also, see Chapter 3, in the section titled, "Describing the Relationship between Two Characteristics," for a review of the properties of the correlation coefficient.

Interpreting the Size of *r*

The size of the correlation required for statistical significance is related to the sample size. With a very large sample of subjects, such as 2,000, even small correlations, such as 0.06, are significant. A better way to interpret the size of the correlation is to consider what it tells us about the strength of the relationship.

The Coefficient of Determination: The correlation coefficient can be squared to form the statistic called the **coefficient of determination.** For the subjects in the study by Neidert et al (2016), the coefficient of determination is $(0.42)^2$, or 0.18. This means that 18% of the variation in the values for one of the measures, such as percent body fat, may be accounted for by knowing the BMI. This concept is demonstrated by the Venn diagrams in Figure 8–3. For the left diagram, $r^2 = 0.25$; so 25% of the variation in A is accounted for by knowing B (or vice versa). The middle diagram illustrates $r^2 = 0.50$, and the diagram on the right represents $r^2 = 0.80$.

The coefficient of determination tells us how strong the relationship really is. In the health literature, confidence limits or results of a statistical test for significance of the correlation coefficient are also commonly presented.

The *t* Test for Correlation: The symbol for the correlation coefficient in the population (the population parameter) is ρ (lowercase Greek letter rho). In a random sample, ρ is estimated by r. If several random samples of the same size are selected from a given population and the correlation coefficient r is calculated for each, we expect r to vary from one sample to another but to follow some sort of distribution about the population value ρ. Unfortunately, the sampling distribution of the correlation does not behave as nicely as the sampling distribution of the mean, which is normally distributed for large samples.

Part of the problem is a ceiling effect when the correlation approaches either –1 or +1. If the value of the population parameter is, say, 0.8, the sample values can exceed 0.8 only up to 1.0, but they can be less than 0.8 all the way to –1.0. The maximum value of 1.0 acts like a ceiling, keeping the sample values from varying as much above 0.8 as below it, and the result is a **skewed distribution.** However, when the population parameter is hypothesized to be zero, the ceiling effects at +1 and –1 are equal, and the sample values are approximately distributed according to the t distribution, which can be used to test the hypothesis that the true value of the population parameter ρ is equal to zero. The following mathematical expression involving the correlation coefficient, often called the t ratio, has

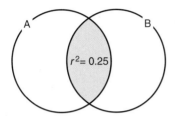 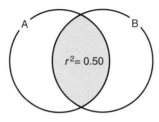 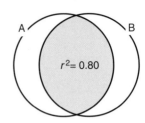

Figure 8–3. Illustration of r^2, proportion of explained variance.

been found to have a ***t distribution*** with $n - 2$ degrees of freedom:

$$t = \frac{r\sqrt{n-2}}{\sqrt{1-r^2}}$$

Let us use this t ratio to test whether the observed value of $r = 0.42$ is sufficient evidence with 109 observations to conclude that the true population value of the correlation ρ is different from zero.

Step 1: H_0: No relationship exists between BMI and percent body fat; or, the true correlation is zero: $\rho = 0$.

H_1: A relationship does exist between BMI and percent body fat; or, the true correlation is not zero: $\rho \neq 0$.

Step 2: Because the null hypothesis is a test of whether ρ is zero, the t ratio may be used when the assumptions for correlation (see the section titled, "Assumptions in Correlation") are met.

Step 3: Let us use $\alpha = 0.01$ for this example.

Step 4: The degrees of freedom are $n - 2 = 111 - 2 = 109$. The value of a t distribution with 109 degrees of freedom that divides the area into the central 99% and the upper and lower 1% is approximately 2.617 (using the value for 120 df in Table A–3). Therefore, we reject the null hypothesis of zero correlation if (the absolute value of) the observed value of t is greater than 2.617.

Step 5: The calculation is

$$t = \frac{0.42\sqrt{107}}{\sqrt{1-0.42^2}} = 4.79$$

Step 6: The observed value of the t ratio with 109 degrees of freedom is 4.79, which is greater than the critical value of 2.617. The null hypothesis of zero correlation is therefore rejected, and we conclude that the relationship between BMI and percent body fat is large enough to conclude that these two variables are associated.

Fisher's z Transformation to Test the Correlation: Investigators generally want to know whether $\rho = 0$, and this test can easily be done with computer programs. Occasionally, however, interest lies in whether the correlation is equal to a specific value other than zero. For example, consider a diagnostic test that gives accurate numerical values but is invasive and somewhat risky for the patient. If someone develops an alternative testing procedure, it is important to show that the new procedure is as accurate as the test in current use. The approach is to select a sample of patients and perform both the current test and the new procedure on each patient and then calculate the correlation coefficient between the two testing procedures.

Either a test of hypothesis can be performed to show that the correlation is greater than a given value, or a confidence interval about the observed correlation can be calculated. In either case, we use a procedure called **Fisher's z transformation** to test any null hypothesis about the correlation as well as to form confidence intervals.

To use Fisher's exact test, we first transform the correlation and then use the standard normal (z) distribution. We need to transform the correlation because, as we mentioned earlier, the distribution of sample values of the correlation is skewed when $\rho \neq 0$. Although this method is a bit complicated, it is actually more flexible than the t test, because it permits us to test any null hypothesis, not simply that the correlation is zero. Fisher's z transformation was proposed by the same statistician (Ronald Fisher) who developed Fisher's exact test for 2×2 contingency tables (discussed in Chapter 6).

Fisher's z transformation is

$$z(r) = \frac{1}{2}\ln\left(\frac{1+r}{1-r}\right)$$

where ln represents the natural logarithm. Table A–6 gives the z transformation for different values of r, so we do not actually need to use the formula. With moderate-sized samples, this transformation follows a normal distribution, and the following expression for the z test can be used:

$$z = \frac{z(r) - z(\pi)}{\sqrt{1 / (n - 3)}}$$

To illustrate Fisher's z transformation for testing the significance of ρ, we evaluate the relationship between BMI and percent body fat (Neidert et al, 2016). The observed correlation between these two measures was 0.42. Neidert and colleagues (2016) may have expected a sizable correlation between these two measures; let us suppose they want to know whether the correlation is significantly greater than 0.25. A one-tailed test of the null hypothesis that $\rho \leq 0.25$, which they hope to reject, may be carried out as follows.

Step 1: H_0: The relationship between BMI and percent body fat is ≤ 0.25; or, the true correlation $\rho \leq 0.25$.

H_1: The relationship between BMI and percent body fat is > 0.25; or, the true correlation $\rho > 0.25$.

Step 2: Fisher's z transformation may be used with the correlation coefficient to test any hypothesis.

Step 3: Let us again use $\alpha = 0.01$ for this example.

Step 4: The alternative hypothesis specifies a one-tailed test. The value of the z distribution that divides the area into the lower 99% and the upper 1% is approximately 2.326 (from Table A–2). We therefore reject the null hypothesis that the correlation is ≤ 0.25 if the observed value of z is > 2.326.

Step 5: The first step is to find the transformed values for $r = 0.42$ and $\rho = 0.25$ from Table A–6; these values are 0.448 and 0.255, respectively. Then, the calculation for the z test is

$$z = \frac{z(0.42) - z(0.25)}{\sqrt{1 / (111 - 3)}}$$

$$= \frac{0.448 - 0.255}{0.096}$$

$$= 2.01$$

Step 6: The observed value of the z statistic, 2.01, does not exceed 2.358. The null hypothesis that the correlation is 0.25 or less is not rejected.

Confidence Interval for the Correlation: A major advantage of Fisher's z transformation is that **confidence intervals** can be formed. The transformed value of the correlation is used to calculate confidence limits in the usual manner, and then they are transformed back to values corresponding to the correlation coefficient.

To illustrate, we calculate a 95% confidence interval for the correlation coefficient 0.42 in Neidert and colleagues (2016). We use Fisher's z transformation of $0.42 = 0.448$ and the z distribution in Table A–2 to find the critical value for 95%. The confidence interval is

z Transform of $r \pm$ confidence coefficient $\times$ standard error

z Transform of $r \pm 1.96 \times \sqrt{1 / (n - 3)}$

$0.448 \pm (1.96)(0.096)$

0.448 ± 0.188

Transforming the limits 0.260 and 0.636 back to correlations using Table A–6 in reverse gives approximately $r = 0.25$ and $r = 0.56$ (using conservative values). Therefore, we are 95% confident that the true value of the correlation in the population is contained within this interval. R has a function that calculates a confidence interval for the correlation coefficient. The function results in the range 0.26 to 0.56, which is very close to the approximation calculated using Table A–6.

Assumptions in Correlation

The assumptions needed to draw valid conclusions about the correlation coefficient are that the sample was randomly selected and the two variables, X and Y, vary together in a joint distribution that is normally distributed, called the bivariate normal distribution. Just because each variable is normally distributed when examined separately, however, does not guarantee that, jointly, they have a bivariate normal distribution. Some guidance is available: If either of the two variables is *not* normally distributed, Pearson's product moment correlation coefficient is *not* the most appropriate method. Instead, either one or both of the variables may be transformed so that they more closely follow a normal distribution, as discussed in Chapter 5, or the Spearman rank correlation may be calculated. This topic is discussed in the section titled, "Other Measures of Correlation."

COMPARING TWO CORRELATION COEFFICIENTS

On occasion, investigators want to know if a difference exists between two correlation coefficients. Here are two specific instances: (1) comparing the correlations between the same two variables that have been measured in two independent groups of subjects and (2) comparing two correlations that involve a variable in common in the same group of individuals. These situations are not extremely common and not always contained in statistical programs.

Comparing Correlations in Two Independent Groups

Fisher's z transformation can be used to test hypotheses or form confidence intervals about the difference between the correlations between the same two variables in two independent groups. The results of such tests are also called *independent correlations*. For example, revisiting the data from the study by Neidert et al (2016), we can compare the correlation between BMI and percent body fat by gender, see Figure 8–4.

The correlation between BMI and percent body fat is 0.737 for the 71 female subjects and 0.508 for the 40 male subjects. In this situation, the value for the second group replaces $z(\rho)$ in the numerator for the z test shown in the previous section, and $1/(n-3)$ is found for each group and added before taking the square root in the denominator. The test statistic is

$$z = \frac{(z_{r1} - z_{r2})}{\sqrt{[1/(n_1 - 3)] + [1/(n_2 - 3)]}}$$

To illustrate, the values of z from Fisher's z transformation tables (A–6) for 0.737 and 0.508 are approximately 0.951 and 0.563 (with rounding), respectively.

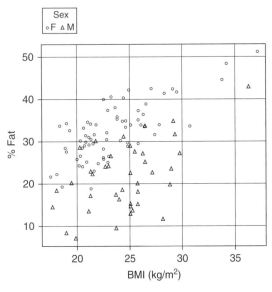

Figure 8–4. Scatterplot of body mass index and percent body fat by gender. (Adapted with permission from Neidert LE, Wainright KS, Zheng C, et al: Plasma dipeptidyl peptidase IV activity and measures of body composition in apparently healthy people, *Heliyon*. 2016 Apr 18;2(4):e00097.)

Note that Fisher's z transformation is the same, regardless of whether the correlation is positive or negative. Using these values, we obtain

$$z = \frac{0.951 - 0.563}{\sqrt{1/(71 - 3) + 1/(40 - 3)}}$$

$$= \frac{0.388}{\sqrt{0.042}}$$

$$= 1.89$$

Assuming we choose the traditional significance level of 0.05, the value of the test statistic, 1.89, is less than the critical value, 1.96, so we do not reject the null hypothesis of equal correlations. We decide that the evidence is insufficient to conclude that the relationship between BMI and body fat percentage is different for men and women. What is a possible explanation for the lack of statistical significance? It is possible that there is no difference in the relationships between these two variables in the population. When sample sizes are small, however, as they are in this study, it is always advisable to keep in mind that the study may have low power.

Comparing Correlations with Variables in Common in the Same Group

The second situation occurs when the research question involves correlations that contain the same variable (also called *dependent correlations*). For example, a very natural question for Pereira and colleagues (2015) was whether one of the bedside glucose devices was more highly correlated with the arterial central lab value—considered to be the gold standard—than the other two. If so, this would be a product they might wish to recommend for patients to use at home. To illustrate, we compare the blood glucose with Accu-chek arterial measure and the arterial central lab value ($r_{xy} = 0.57$) to the blood glucose with the Accu-chek finger stick and the arterial central lab value ($r_{xz} = 0.87$).

There are several formulas for testing the difference between two dependent correlations. We present the simplest one, developed by Hotelling (1940) and described by Glass and Stanley (1970). We will show the calculations for this example but, as always, suggest that you use a computer program. The formula follows the t distribution with $n - 3$ degrees of freedom; it looks rather forbidding and requires the calculation of several correlations:

$$t = (r_{xy} - r_{xz})\sqrt{\frac{(n-3)(1 + r_{yz})}{2(1 - r_{xy}^2 - r_{xz}^2 - r_{yz}^2 + 2r_{xy}r_{xz}r_{yz})}}$$

Table 8–1. Correlation matrix of blood glucose measurements for 145 subjects.

	Arterial Central Lab (mg/dL)	Accu-chek Arterial (mg/dL)	Accu-chek Fingerstick (mg/dL)	Accu-chek Central Venous Catheter (mg/dL)
Arterial central lab (mg/dL)	1.000			
Accu-chek arterial (mg/dL)	0.570	1.000		
Accu-chek fingerstick (mg/dL)	0.867	0.666	1.000	
Accu-chek central venous catheter (mg/dL)	0.780	0.710	0.696	1.000

Data from Pereira AJ, Corrêa TD, de Almeida FP, et al: Inaccuracy of venous point-of-care glucose measurements in critically ill patients: a cross-sectional study, *PLoS One.* 2015 Jun 12;10(6): e0129568.

We designate the arterial central lab value as X, Accu-chek arterial as Y, and Accu-chek fingerstick as Z. Therefore, we want to compare r_{xy} with r_{xz}. Both correlations involve the X, or arterial central lab value, so these correlations are dependent. To use the formula, we also need to calculate the correlation between Accu-chek arterial and Accu-chek fingerstick, which is $r_{yz} = 0.67$. Table 8–1 shows the correlations needed for this formula.

The calculations are

$$t = (0.57 - 0.87) \sqrt{\frac{(145 - 3)(1 + 0.67)}{2 \left[\begin{array}{c} (1 - 0.57^2 - 0.87^2 + 0.67^2) \\ + 2(0.57)(0.87)(0.67) \end{array} \right]}}$$

$$= -0.30 \sqrt{\frac{237.14}{2.06}} = -3.22$$

You know by now that the difference between these two correlations is statistically significant because the observed value of t is -3.22, and $|-3.22| = 3.22$ is greater than the critical value of t with 142 degrees of freedom, 1.97.

OTHER MEASURES OF CORRELATION

Several other measures of correlation are often found in the medical literature. Spearman's rho, the rank correlation introduced in Chapter 3, is used with ordinal data or in situations in which the numerical variables are not normally distributed. When a research question involves one numerical and one nominal variable, a correlation called the point–biserial correlation is used. With nominal data, the risk ratio, or kappa (κ), discussed in Chapter 5, can be used.

Spearman's Rho

Recall that the value of the correlation coefficient is markedly influenced by extreme values and thus does not provide a good description of the relationship between two variables when their distributions are skewed or contain outlying values. For example, consider the relationships among the various blood glucose measurement devices from Presenting Problem 2. To illustrate, we use the first 25 subjects from this study, listed in Table 8–2.

Table 8–2. Data on blood glucose for the first 25 subjects.

Subject	Arterial Central Lab (mg/dL)	Accu-chek Arterial (mg/dL)	Accu-chek Fingerstick (mg/dL)	Accu-chek Central Venous Catheter (mg/dL)
1	186	198	207	195
2	202	227	221	221
3	115	127	125	135
4	155	152	161	142
5	124	137	130	119
6	193	182	196	190
7	165	192	175	188
8	130	136	128	331
9	92	83	92	84
10	129	125	111	129
11	259	258	257	274
12	89	78	84	95
13	168	181	210	193
14	137	132	128	119
15	137	131	150	138
16	161	182	175	203
17	974	90	600	600
18	84	72	80	78
19	134	108	125	111
20	192	217	196	221
21	194	200	226	217
22	242	242	255	235
23	118	127	137	120
24	104	104	89	94
25	126	119	115	600

Data from Pereira AJ, Corrêa TD, de Almeida FP, et al: Inaccuracy of venous point-of-care glucose measurements in critically ill patients: a cross-sectional study, *PLoS One.* 2015 Jun 12;10(6): e0129568.

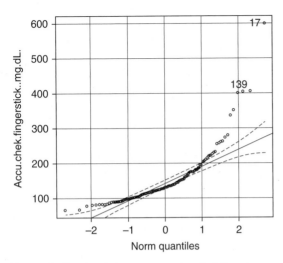

Figure 8–5. Blood glucose normal probability plot. (Data from Pereira AJ, Corrêa TD, de Almeida FP, et al: Inaccuracy of venous point-of-care glucose measurements in critically ill patients: a cross-sectional study, *PLoS One*. 2015 Jun 12;10(6):e0129568.)

It is difficult to tell if the observations are normally distributed without looking at graphs of the data. Some statistical programs have routines to plot values against a normal distribution to help researchers decide whether a nonparametric procedure should be used. A normal probability plot for the Accu-chek fingerstick measurement is given in Figure 8–5. Use R to produce similar plots for other device measurements.

When the observations are plotted on a graph, as in Figure 8–5, it appears that the data are indeed somewhat skewed. As we indicated in Chapter 3, a simple method for dealing with the problem of extreme observations in correlation is to rank order the data and then recalculate the correlation on ranks to obtain the nonparametric correlation called **Spearman's rho,** or **rank correlation.** To illustrate this procedure, we continue to use data on the first 25 subjects in the study on blood glucose devices (Presenting Problem 2). Let us focus on the correlation between the arterial central lab value and the Accu-chek fingerstick device, which we learned was 0.87 in the section titled, "Comparing Correlations with Variables in Common in the Same Group."

Table 8–3 illustrates the ranks of the diastolic readings on the first 25 subjects. Note that each variable is ranked separately; when ties occur, the average of the ranks of the tied values is used.

The ranks of the variables are used in the equation for the correlation coefficient, and the resulting

Table 8–3. Rank order of the blood glucose for the first 25 subjects.

Subject	Rank Arterial Central Lab (mg/dL)	Rank Accu-chek Arterial (mg/dL)	Rank Accu-chek Fingerstick (mg/dL)	Rank Accu-chek Central Venous Catheter (mg/dL)
1	8	6	7	10
2	4	3	5	6.5
3	21	16.5	18.5	16
4	12	11	12	14
5	19	12	15	19.5
6	6	8.5	8.5	12
7	10	7	10.5	13
8	16	13	16.5	3
9	23	23	22	24
10	17	18	21	17
11	2	1	2	4
12	24	24	24	22
13	9	10	6	11
14	13.5	14	16.5	19.5
15	13.5	15	13	15
16	11	8.5	10.5	9
17	1	22	1	1.5
18	25	25	25	25
19	15	20	18.5	21
20	7	4	8.5	6.5
21	5	5	4	8
22	3	2	3	5
23	20	16.5	14	18
24	22	21	23	23
25	18	19	20	1.5

Data from Pereira AJ, Corrêa TD, de Almeida FP, et al: Inaccuracy of venous point-of-care glucose measurements in critically ill patients: a cross-sectional study, *PLoS One*. 2015 Jun 12;10(6): e0129568.

calculation gives Spearman's rank correlation (r_S), also called Spearman's rho:

$$r_s = \frac{\Sigma(R_x - \bar{R}_x)(R_y - \bar{R}_y)}{\sqrt{\Sigma(R_x - \bar{R}_x)^2} \sqrt{\Sigma(R_y - \bar{R}_y)^2}}$$

where R_X is the rank of the X variable, R_Y is the rank of the Y variable, and $\bar{R}_X$ and $\bar{R}_Y$ are the mean ranks for the X and Y variables, respectively. The rank correlation r_S may also be calculated by using other formulas, but this approximate procedure is quite good (Conover and Iman, 1981).

Calculating r_S for the ranked observations in Table 8–3 gives

$$r_s = \frac{998.5}{\sqrt{1299.5}\sqrt{1299.0}}$$

$$= 0.77$$

The value of r_S is smaller than the value of Pearson's correlation; this may occur when the bivariate distribution of the two variables is not normal. The t test, as illustrated for the Pearson correlation, can be used to determine whether the Spearman rank correlation is significantly different from zero. For example, the following procedure tests whether the value of Spearman's rho in the population, symbolized ρ_S (Greek letter rho with subscript S denoting Spearman), differs from zero.

Step 1: H_0: The population value of Spearman's rho is zero; that is, $\rho_S = 0$.

H_1: The population value of Spearman's rho is not zero; that is, $\rho_S \neq 0$.

Step 2: Because the null hypothesis is a test of whether ρ_S is zero, the t ratio may be used.

Step 3: Let us use $\alpha = 0.05$ for this example.

Step 4: The degrees of freedom are $n - 2 = 25 - 2 = 23$. The value of the t distribution with 23 degrees of freedom that divides the area into the central 95% and the upper and lower 2½% is 2.069 (Table A–3), so we will reject the null hypothesis if (the absolute value of) the observed value of t is greater than 2.069.

Step 5: The calculation is

$$t = \frac{r\sqrt{(n-2)}}{\sqrt{1-r^2}}$$

$$= \frac{0.77\sqrt{23-2}}{\sqrt{1-0.77^2}}$$

$$= 5.53$$

Step 6: The observed value of the t ratio with 23 degrees of freedom is 5.53, greater than 2.069, so we reject the null hypothesis and conclude there is sufficient evidence that a nonparametric correlation exists between the blood glucose measurements made by the lab test and the fingerstick device.

Of course, if investigators want to test only whether Spearman's rho is greater than zero—that there is a significantly positive relationship—they can use a one-tailed test. For a one-tailed test with $\alpha = 0.05$ and 23 degrees of freedom, the critical value is 1.714, and the conclusion is the same.

To summarize, Spearman's rho is appropriate when investigators want to measure the relationship between: (1) two ordinal variables, or (2) two numerical variables when one or both are not normally distributed and investigators choose not to use a data transformation (such as taking the logarithm). Spearman's rank correlation is especially appropriate when outlying values occur among the observations.

Confidence Interval for the Odds Ratio & the Relative Risk

Chapter 3 introduced the **relative risk** (or risk ratio) and the **odds ratio** as measures of relationship between two nominal characteristics. Developed by epidemiologists, these statistics are used for studies examining risks that may result in disease. To discuss the odds ratio, recall the study discussed in Chapter 3 by Billioti de Gage and colleagues (2014) that examined the use of benzodiazepine. Data from this study were given in Chapter 3, Table 3–21. We calculated the odds ratio as 1.5, meaning that a subject in the benzodiazepine group is 1.5 times more likely to develop Alzheimer's disease than a subject in with no exposure. It is important to learn if the increased risk is statistically significant.

Significance can be determined in several ways. For instance, to test the significance of the relationship between treatment (benzodiazepine exposure) and the development of Alzheimer's disease, investigators may use the chi-square test discussed in Chapter 6. The chi-square test for this example is left as an exercise (see Exercise 2). An alternative chi-square test, based on the natural logarithm of the odds ratio, is also available, and it results in values close to the chi-square test illustrated in Chapter 6 (Fleiss, 1999).

More often, articles in the medical literature use confidence intervals for risk ratios or odds ratios. Billioti de Gage and colleagues reported a 95% confidence interval for the odds ratio as (1.36–1.69). Let us see how they found this confidence interval.

Finding confidence intervals for odds ratios is a bit more complicated than usual because these ratios are not normally distributed, so calculations require finding natural logarithms and antilogarithms. The formula for a 95% confidence interval for the odds ratio is

$$\exp\left[\ln(OR) \pm 1.96\sqrt{\frac{1}{a} + \frac{1}{b} + \frac{1}{c} + \frac{1}{d}}\right]$$

where exp denotes the exponential function, or antilogarithm, of the natural logarithm, ln, and a, b, c, d are the cells in a 2×2 table (see Table 6–9 in Chapter 6). The confidence interval for the odds ratio for risk of Alzheimer's disease for subjects exposed to benzodiazepine from Table 3–19 is

$$\exp\left[\ln(1.51) \pm 1.96\sqrt{\frac{1}{894} + \frac{1}{2873} + \frac{1}{902} + \frac{1}{4311}}\right]$$

$$\exp(0.412 \pm 1.96\sqrt{0.003})$$

$$1.36 \text{ to } 1.68$$

This interval contains the value of the true odds ratio with 95% confidence. If the odds are the same in each group, the value of the odds ratio is approximately 1, indicating similar risks in each group. Because the interval does not contain 1, we may conclude that there is sufficient evidence to conclude that the risk of Alzheimer's disease increases with exposure to benzodiazepine

To illustrate the confidence interval for the relative risk, we refer to the study on flu symptoms by Anderson et al (2018) summarized in Chapter 3 and Table 3–17. Recall that the relative risk for a flu diagnosis in patients with a flu vaccine in the last 12 months was 0.616. The 95% confidence interval for the true value of the relative risk also involves logarithms:

$$\exp\left[\ln(RR) \pm 1.96\sqrt{\frac{1 - [a/(a+b)]}{a} + \frac{1 - [c/(c+d)]}{c}}\right]$$

Again, the values for a, b, c, d are the cells in the 2×2 table illustrated in Table 6–9. Although it is possible to include a continuity correction for the relative risk or odds ratio, it is not commonly done. Substituting values from Table 3–19, the 95% confidence interval for a relative risk of 0.616 is

$$\exp[\ln(0.616)$$
$$\pm 1.96\sqrt{\frac{1 - [210/(210+749)]}{210} + \frac{1 - [1283/(1283+2327)]}{1283}}$$
$$= \exp[-0.484 \pm 0.127]$$
$$= 0.54 \text{ to } 0.70$$

The 95% confidence interval does *not* contain 1, so the evidence indicates that the use of a flu vaccine resulted in a reduced risk for a flu diagnosis for patients exhibiting flu symptoms. For a detailed and insightful discussion of the odds ratio and its advantages and disadvantages, see Feinstein (1985, Chapter 20) and Fleiss (1999, Chapter 5); for a discussion of the odds ratio and the risk ratio, see Greenberg and coworkers (2015, Chapter 2).

LINEAR REGRESSION

Remember that when the goal is to predict the value of one characteristic from knowledge of another, the statistical method used is **regression** analysis. This method is also called linear regression, simple linear regression, or least squares regression. A brief review of the history of these terms is interesting and sheds some light on the nature of regression analysis.

The concepts of correlation and regression were developed by Sir Francis Galton, a cousin of Charles Darwin, who studied both mathematics and medicine in the mid-nineteenth century (Walker, 1931). Galton was interested in heredity and wanted to understand why a population remains more or less the same over many generations with the "average" offspring resembling their parents; that is, why do successive generations not become more diverse. By growing sweet peas and observing the average size of seeds from parent plants of different sizes, he discovered regression, which he termed the "tendency of the ideal mean filial type to depart from the parental type, reverting to what may be roughly and perhaps fairly described as the average ancestral type." This phenomenon is more typically known as regression toward the mean. The term "correlation" was used by Galton in his work on inheritance in terms of the "co-relation" between such characteristics as heights of fathers and sons. The mathematician Karl Pearson went on to work out the theory of correlation and regression, and the correlation coefficient is named after him for this reason.

The term **linear regression** refers to the fact that correlation and regression measure only a straight-line, or linear, relationship between two variables. The term "simple regression" means that only one explanatory (independent) variable is used to predict an outcome. In **multiple regression,** more than one independent variable is included in the prediction equation.

Least squares regression describes the mathematical method for obtaining the regression equation. The important thing to remember is that when the term "regression" is used alone, it generally means linear regression based on the least squares method. The concept behind least squares regression is described in the next section and its application is discussed in the section after that.

Least Squares Method

Several times previously in this chapter, we mentioned the linear nature of the pattern of points in a scatterplot. For example, in Figure 8–2, a straight line can be drawn through the points representing the values of BMI and percent body fat to indicate the direction of the relationship. The **least squares method** is a way to determine the equation of the line that provides a good fit to the points.

To illustrate the method, consider the straight line in Figure 8–6. Elementary geometry can be used to determine the equation for any straight line. If the point where the line crosses, or *intercepts*, the Y-axis is denoted by a and the **slope** of the line by b, then the equation is

$$Y = a + bX$$

The slope of the line measures the amount Y changes each time X changes by 1 unit. If the slope is positive, Y increases as X increases; if the slope is negative, Y decreases as X increases; and vice versa. In the regression model, the slope in the population is generally

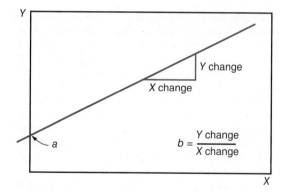

Figure 8–6. Geometric interpretation of a regression line.

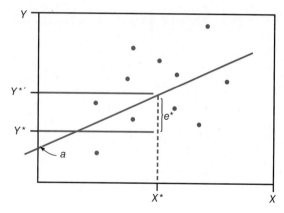

Figure 8–7. Least squares regression line.

symbolized by β_1, called the **regression coefficient;** and β_0 denotes the **intercept** of the regression line, that is, β_1 and β_0 are the population parameters in regression. In most applications, the points do not fall exactly along a straight line. For this reason, the regression model contains an *error term, e,* which is the distance the actual values of Y depart from the regression line. Putting all this together, the regression equation is given by

$$Y = \beta_0 + \beta_1 X + \varepsilon$$

When the regression equation is used to describe the relationship in the sample, it is often written as

$$Y' = b_0 + b_1 X \text{ or } Y' = a + bX$$

Where Y' is the symbol for the predicted value of Y based on an observed value X. For a given value of X, say X^*, the predicted value of Y^* is found by extending a horizontal line from the regression line to the Y-axis as in Figure 8–7. The difference between the actual value for Y^* and the predicted value, $e^* = Y^* - Y^{*\prime}$, can be used to judge how well the line fits the data points. The least squares method determines the line that minimizes the sum of the squared vertical differences between the actual and predicted values of the Y variable; that is, β_0 and β_1 are determined so that $\Sigma(Y - Y')^2$ is minimized. The formulas for β_0 and β_1 are found,* and in terms of the sample estimates b and a, these formulas are

$$b = \frac{\Sigma(X - \bar{X})(Y - \bar{Y})}{\Sigma(X - \bar{X})^2}$$
$$a = \bar{Y} - b\bar{X}$$

---

*The procedure for finding β_0 and β_1 involves the use of differential calculus. The partial derivatives of the preceding equations are found with respect to β_0 and β_1; the two resulting equations are set equal to zero to locate the minimum values; these two equations in two unknowns, β_0 and β_1, are solved simultaneously to obtain the formulas for β_0 and β_1.

Calculating the Regression Equation

Suppose we wish to fit a regression line to the data displayed in Figure 8–2. This model could be used to predict the percentage of body fat if the subject's BMI was known.

Before calculating the regression equation for these data, let us revise the scatterplot in Figure 8–2 and practice "guesstimating" the value of the correlation coefficient from the plot (although it is difficult to estimate the size of r accurately when the sample size is small). Figure 8–2 is a scatterplot with BMI score as the explanatory X variable and percentage of body fat as the response Y variable. From previous calculations, we know that the correlation is 0.42.

Since we know the correlation between BMI and percent body fat is positive, we know that the slope of the regression line is also positive. Here are the terms that are required to calculate the slope and intercept of the regression line:

$$\Sigma(X - \bar{X})(Y - \bar{Y}) = 1523.32$$
$$\Sigma(X - \bar{X})^2 = 1577.02$$
$$\bar{X} = 23.08 \text{ and } \bar{Y} = 28.34$$

Then,

$$b = \frac{\Sigma(X - \bar{X})(Y - \bar{Y})}{\Sigma(X - \bar{X})^2}$$
$$= \frac{1523.32}{1577.02} = 0.97$$
$$a = \bar{Y} - b\bar{X} = 28.34 - 0.97 \times 23.08 = 5.15$$

In this example, the percent body fat percentage are said to be regressed on BMI scores, and the regression

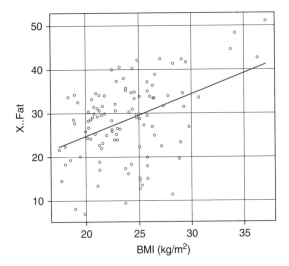

Figure 8–8. Regression of observations on body mass index and percent body fat. (Adapted with permission from Neidert LE, Wainright KS, Zheng C, et al: Plasma dipeptidyl peptidase IV activity and measures of body composition in apparently healthy people, *Heliyon.* 2016 Apr 18;2(4):e00097.)

equation is written as $Y' = 5.15 + 0.97X$, where Y' is the predicted body fat percentage, and X is the observed BMI.

Figure 8–8 illustrates the regression line drawn through the observations. The regression equation has a positive intercept of +5.15, so that theoretically a patient with zero BMI would have an insulin sensitivity of 5.15, even though, in the present example, a zero BMI is not possible. The slope of +0.97 indicates that each time BMI increases by 1, the predicted percent body fat increases by approximately 0.97. For example, as the BMI increases from 20 to 30, predicted percent body fat increases from about 24.55 to about 34.25. Whether the relationship between BMI and percent body fat is significant is discussed in the next section.

Assumptions & Inferences in Regression

In the previous section, we worked with a sample of observations instead of the population of observations. Just as the sample mean $\bar{X}$ is an estimate of the population mean μ, the regression line determined from the formulas for a and b in the previous section is an estimate of the regression equation for the underlying population.

As in Chapters 6 and 7, in which we used statistical tests to determine how likely it was that the observed differences between two means occurred by chance, in regression analysis we must perform statistical tests to

determine the likelihood of any observed relationship between X and Y variables. Again, the question can be approached in two ways: using hypothesis tests or forming confidence intervals. Before discussing these approaches, however, we briefly discuss the assumptions required in regression analysis.

If we are to use a regression equation, the observations must have certain properties. Thus, for each value of the X variable, the Y variable is assumed to have a normal distribution, and the mean of the distribution is assumed to be the predicted value, Y' In addition, no matter the value of the X variable, the standard deviation of Y is assumed to be the same. These assumptions are rather like imagining a large number of individual normal distributions of the Y variable, all of the same size, one for each value of X. The assumption of this equal variation in the Y's across the entire range of the X's is called **homogeneity,** or **homoscedasticity**. It is analogous to the assumption of equal variances (homogeneous variances) in the t test for independent groups, as discussed in Chapter 6.

The straight-line, or linear, assumption requires that the mean values of Y corresponding to various values of X fall on a straight line. The values of Y are assumed to be independent of one another. This assumption is not met when repeated measurements are made on the same subjects; that is, a subject's measure at one time is not independent from the measure of that same subject at another time. Finally, as with other statistical procedures, we assume the observations constitute a random sample from the population of interest.

Regression is a robust procedure and may be used in many situations in which the assumptions are not met, as long as the measurements are fairly reliable and the correct regression model is used. (Other regression models are discussed in Chapter 10.) Meeting the regression assumptions generally causes fewer problems in experiments or clinical trials than in observational studies because reliability of the measurements tends to be greater in experimental studies. Special procedures can be used when the assumptions are seriously violated, however; and as in ANOVA, researchers should seek a statistician's advice before using regression if questions arise about its applicability.

The Standard Error of the Estimate: Regression lines, like other statistics, can vary. After all, the regression equation computed for any one sample of observations is only an estimate of the true population regression equation. If other samples are chosen from the population and a regression equation is calculated for each sample, these equations will vary from one sample to another with respect to both their slopes and their intercepts. An estimate of this variation is symbolized $S_{Y \cdot X}$ (read s of y given x) and is called the standard error of regression, or the **standard**

error of the estimate. It is based on the squared deviations of the predicted Y's from the actual Ys and is found as follows:

$$S_{Y \cdot X} = \sqrt{\frac{\Sigma(Y - Y')^2}{n - 2}}$$

The computation of this formula is quite tedious; and although more user-friendly computational forms exist, we assume that you will use a computer program to calculate the standard error of the estimate. In testing both the slope and the intercept, a t test can be used, and the standard error of the estimate is part of the formula. It is also used in determining confidence limits. To present these formulas and the logic involved in testing the slope and the intercept, we illustrate the test of hypothesis for the intercept and the calculation of a confidence interval for the slope, using the BMI–percent body fat regression equation.

Inference about the Intercept: To test the hypothesis that the intercept departs significantly from zero, we use the following procedure:

Step 1: $H_0: \beta_0 = 0$ (The intercept is zero)

$H_1: \beta_0 \neq 0$ (The intercept is not zero)

Step 2: Because the null hypothesis is a test of whether the intercept is zero, the t ratio may be used if the assumptions are met. The t ratio uses the standard error of the estimate to calculate the standard error of the intercept (the denominator of the t ratio):

$$t = \frac{a - \beta_0}{\sqrt{S_{Y \cdot X}^2 \{(1 / n) + [\bar{X}^2 / \Sigma(X - \bar{X})^2]\}}}$$

Step 3: Let us use α equal to 0.05.

Step 4: The degrees of freedom are $n - 2 = 111 - 2 = 109$. The value of the t distribution with 109 degrees of freedom that divides the area into the central 95% and the combined upper and lower 5% is approximately 1.98 (from Table A–3). Therefore, we reject the null hypothesis of a zero intercept if (the absolute value of) the observed value of t is greater than 1.98.

Step 5: The calculation follows; we used a spreadsheet (Microsoft Excel) to calculate $S_{YX} = 7.98$ and $\Sigma(X - \bar{X})^2 = 1577.02$.

$$t = \frac{5.15 - 0}{\sqrt{7.98^2(1 / 111 + [23.08^2 / 1577.02])}}$$

$$= \frac{5.15}{\sqrt{23.47}}$$

$$= 1.06$$

Step 6: The absolute value of the observed t ratio is 1.06, which is not greater than 1.98. The null hypothesis of a zero intercept is therefore not rejected. We conclude that the evidence is insufficient to show that the intercept is significantly different from zero for the regression of percent body fat on BMI.

As you know by now, it is also possible to form confidence limits for the intercept using the observed value and adding or subtracting the critical value from the t distribution multiplied by the standard error of the intercept.

Inferences about the Regression Coefficient: Instead of illustrating the hypothesis test for the population regression coefficient, let us find a 95% confidence interval for β_1. The interval is given by

$$b \pm t_{n-2} \sqrt{S_{Y \cdot X}^2 \left[\frac{1}{\Sigma(X - \bar{X})^2} \right]}$$

$$= 0.97 \pm 1.98 \sqrt{7.98^2 \left(\frac{1}{1577.02} \right)}$$

$$= 0.97 \pm 0.40 \text{ or } 0.57 \text{ to } 1.37$$

Because the interval excludes zero, we can be 95% confident that the regression coefficient is not zero but that it is between 0.57 and 1.37. Because the regression coefficient is significantly greater than zero, can the correlation coefficient be equal to zero? (See Exercise 2.) The relationship between b and r illustrated earlier and Exercise 2 should convince you of the equivalence of the results obtained with testing the significance of correlation and the regression coefficient. In fact, authors in the medical literature often perform a regression analysis and then report the P values to indicate a significant correlation coefficient.

The output from the R regression program is given in Table 8–4. The program produces the value of t and the associated P value, as well as 95% confidence limits. Do the results agree with those we found earlier? To become familiar with using regression, we suggest you replicate these results using the data file and R.

Predicting with the Regression Equation: Individual and Mean Values: One of the important reasons for obtaining a regression equation is to predict future values for a group of subjects (or for individual subjects). For example, a clinician may want to predict percent body fat from BMI for a group of participants in a new fitness regimen. Or the clinician may wish to predict the percent body fat for a particular patient. In either case, the variability associated with the regression line must be reflected in the prediction.

Table 8–4. Computer output of regression of percent body fat on body mass index.

```
Call:
lm(formula = X..Fat ~ BMI..kg.m2., data = BMI)

Residuals:
    Min      1Q   Median      3Q      Max
-21.126  -3.875   1.262    5.564   12.927

Coefficients:
             Estimate Std. Error t value   Pr(>|t|)
(Intercept)    5.1539     4.8438   1.064       0.29
BMI..kg.m2.    0.9742     0.2010   4.847 0.00000418 ***
---
Signif. codes:  0 '***' 0.001 '**' 0.01 '*' 0.05 '.' 0.1 ' ' 1

Residual standard error: 7.982 on 109 degrees of freedom
Multiple R-squared:  0.1773, Adjusted R-squared:  0.1698
F-statistic: 23.49 on 1 and 109 DF,  p-value: 0.000004181


> Confint(RegModel.7, level=0.95)
              Estimate      2.5 %     97.5 %
(Intercept) 5.1539051 -4.4463707  14.754181
BMI..kg.m2. 0.9741944  0.5758458   1.372543
```

The 95% confidence interval for a *predicted mean Y* in a group of subjects is

$$\text{Mean } Y' \pm t_{(n-2)}\sqrt{S_{Y\cdot X}^2\left[\frac{1}{n}+\frac{(X-\bar{X})^2}{\Sigma(X-\bar{X})^2}\right]}$$

The 95% confidence interval for predicting a *single observation* is

$$Y'' \pm t_{(n-2)}\sqrt{S_{Y\cdot X}^2\left[1+\frac{1}{n}+\frac{(X-\bar{X})^2}{\Sigma(X-\bar{X})^2}\right]}$$

Comparing these two formulas, we see that the confidence interval predicting a single observation is wider than the interval for the mean of a group of individuals; 1 is added to the standard error term for the individual case. This result makes sense, because for a given value of X, the variation in the scores of individuals is greater than that in the mean scores of groups of individuals. Note also that the numerator of the third term in the standard error is the squared deviation of X from $\bar{X}$. The size of the standard error therefore depends on how close the observation is to the mean; the closer X is to its mean, the more accurate is the prediction of Y. For values of X quite far from the mean, the variability in predicting the Y score is considerable. You can appreciate why it is difficult for economists and others who wish to predict future events to be very accurate!

Table 8–5 gives 95% confidence intervals associated with predicted mean percent body fat and predicted percent body fat for an individual corresponding to several different BMI values. Several insights about regression analysis can be gained by examining this table. First, note the differences in magnitude between the standard errors associated with the predicted mean percent body fat and those associated with individual percent body fat: The standard errors are much larger when we predict individual values than when we predict the mean value. In fact, the standard error for individuals is always larger than the standard error for means because of the additional 1 in the formula. Also note that the standard errors take on their smallest values when the observation of interest is close the mean (BMI of 23.80 in our example). As the observation departs in either direction from the mean, the standard errors and confidence intervals become increasingly larger, reflecting the squared difference between the observation and the mean. If the confidence intervals are plotted as **confidence bands** about

Table 8–5. 95% confidence intervals for predicted mean percent body fat and predicted individual percent body fat.

BMI	Percent Bodyfat	Predicted	Predicting Means			Predicting Individuals	
			SE[a]	Confidence Interval		SE[b]	Confidence Interval
19.30	32.60	23.87	1.180	21.53 to 26.21		8.069	7.89 to 39.85
20.00	25.90	24.55	1.076	22.42 to 26.68		8.054	8.6 to 40.5
20.80	30.00	25.33	0.969	23.41 to 27.24		8.041	9.41 to 41.25
21.00	34.60	25.52	0.944	23.65 to 27.39		8.038	9.61 to 41.43
23.00	26.60	27.46	0.775	25.93 to 28.99		8.020	11.58 to 43.34
23.20	40.60	27.65	0.767	26.13 to 29.17		8.019	11.78 to 43.53
25.80	37.30	30.18	0.857	28.48 to 31.87		8.028	14.28 to 46.07
26.60	38.90	30.95	0.943	29.08 to 32.82		8.038	15.04 to 46.87
27.80	34.00	32.12	1.104	29.93 to 34.3		8.058	16.16 to 48.07
30.70	33.60	34.93	1.580	31.8 to 38.06		8.137	18.82 to 51.04
23.80	**35.30**	**28.24**	**0.758**	**26.74 to 29.74**		**8.018**	**12.36 to 44.11**

BMI, body mass index.
[a]Standard error for means.
[b]Standard error for individuals.

the regression line, they are closest to the line at the mean of X and curve away from it in both directions on each side of $\bar{X}$. Figure 8–9 shows the graph of the confidence bands.

Table 8–5 illustrates another interesting feature of the regression equation (the bolded row). When the mean of X is used in the regression equation, the predicted Y' is the mean of Y. The regression line therefore goes through the mean of X and the mean of Y.

Now we can see why confidence bands about the regression line are curved. The error in the intercept means that the true regression line can be either above or below the line calculated for the sample observations, although it maintains the same orientation (slope). The error in measuring the slope therefore means that the true regression line can rotate about the point $(\bar{X}, \bar{Y})$ to a certain degree. The combination of these two errors results in the *concave* confidence bands illustrated in Figure 8–9. Sometimes journal articles have regression lines with confidence bands that are parallel rather than curved. These confidence bands are incorrect, although they may correspond to standard errors or to confidence intervals at their narrowest distance from the regression line.

Comparing Two Regression Lines

Sometimes investigators wish to compare two regression lines to see whether they are the same. For example, the investigators in the previous problem may be interested in the relationship between BMI and percent body fat for men and

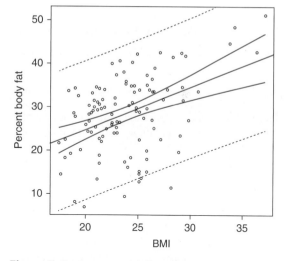

Figure 8–9. Regression of observations on body mass index and percent body fat with confidence bands (heavy lines for means, light lines for individuals). (Adapted with permission from Neidert LE, Wainright KS, Zheng C, et al: Plasma dipeptidyl peptidase IV activity and measures of body composition in apparently healthy people, *Heliyon.* 2016 Apr 18;2(4):e00097.)

women. The regression lines for each gender are displayed in Figure 8–10.

As you might guess, researchers are often interested in comparing regression lines to learn whether the relationships are the same in different groups of

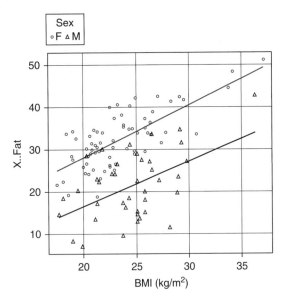

Figure 8–10. Separate regression lines for males (*triangles*) and females (*circles*). (Adapted with permission from Neidert LE, Wainright KS, Zheng C, et al: Plasma dipeptidyl peptidase IV activity and measures of body composition in apparently healthy people, *Heliyon.* 2016 Apr 18;2(4):e00097.)

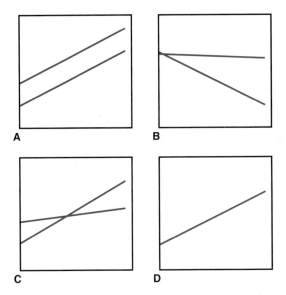

Figure 8–11. Illustration of ways regression lines can differ. **A:** Equal slopes and different intercepts. **B:** Equal intercepts and different slopes. **C:** Different slopes and different intercepts. **D:** Equal slopes and equal intercepts.

subjects. When we compare two regression lines, four situations can occur, as illustrated in Figure 8–11. In Figure 8–11A, the slopes of the regression lines are the same, but the intercepts differ. This situation occurs, for instance, in Figure 8–10 when percent body fat regressed on BMI in men and women; that is, the relationship between percent body fat and BMI is similar for men and women (equal slopes), but men tend to have lower percent body fat levels at all BMIs than women (lower intercept for men).

In Figure 8–11B, the intercepts are equal, but the slopes differ. This pattern may describe, say, the regression of platelet count on number of days following bone marrow transplantation in two groups of patients: those for whom adjuvant therapy results in remission of the underlying disease and those for whom the disease remains active. In other words, prior to and immediately after transplantation, the platelet count is similar for both groups (equal intercepts), but at some time after transplantation, the platelet count remains steady for patients in remission and begins to decrease for patients not in remission (more negative slope for patients with active disease).

In Figure 8–11C, both the intercepts and the slopes of the regression lines differ. Although they did not specifically address any difference in intercepts, the

relationship between BMI and percent body fat resembles the situation in Figure 8–11A.

If no differences exist in the relationships between the predictor and outcome variables, the regression lines are similar to Figure 8–11D, in which the lines are coincident: Both intercepts and slopes are equal. This situation occurs in many situations in medicine and is considered to be the expected pattern (the null hypothesis) until it is shown not to apply by testing hypotheses or forming confidence limits for the intercept and or slope (or both intercept and slope).

From the four situations illustrated in Figure 8–11, we can see that three statistical questions need to be asked:

1. Are the slopes equal?
2. Are the intercepts equal?
3. Are both the slopes and the intercepts equal?

Statistical tests based on the *t* distribution can be used to answer the first two questions; these tests are illustrated in Kleinbaum and Klein (2010). The authors point out, however, that the preferred approach is to use regression models for more than one independent variable—a procedure called multiple regression—to answer these questions. The procedure consists of pooling observations from both samples of subjects (e.g., observations

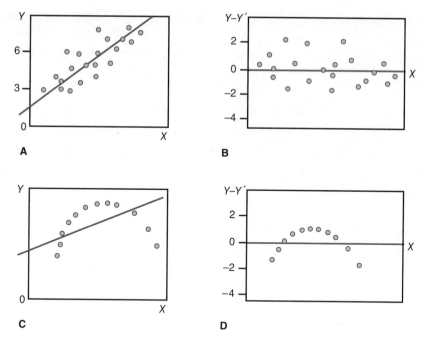

Figure 8–12. Illustration of analysis of residuals. **A:** Linear relationship between X and Y. **B:** Residuals versus values of X for relation in part **A**. **C:** Curvilinear relationship between X and Y. **D:** Residuals versus values of X for relation in part **C**.

on both men and women) and computing one regression line for the combined data. Other regression coefficients indicate whether it matters to which group the observations belong. The simplest model is then selected.

USE OF CORRELATION & REGRESSION

Some of the characteristics of correlation and regression have been noted throughout the discussions in this chapter, and we recapitulate them here as well as mention other features. An important point to reemphasize is that correlation and regression describe *only* linear relationships. If correlation coefficients or regression equations are calculated blindly, without examining plots of the data, investigators can miss very strong, but nonlinear relationships.

Analysis of Residuals

A procedure useful in evaluating the fit of the regression equation is the analysis of residuals (Pedhazur, 1997). We calculated *residuals* when we found the difference between the actual value of Y and the predicted value of Y', or $Y - Y'$, although we did not use the term. A residual is the part of Y that is not predicted by X (the part left over, or the residual). The residual values on the Y-axis are plotted against the X

values on the X-axis. The mean of the residuals is zero, and, because the slope has been subtracted in the process of calculating the residuals, the correlation between them and the X values should be zero.

Stated another way, if the regression model provides a good fit to the data, as in Figure 8–12A, the values of the residuals are not related to the values of X. A plot of the residuals and the X values in this situation should resemble a scatter of points corresponding to Figure 8–12B in which no correlation exists between the residuals and the values of X. If, in contrast, a curvilinear relationship occurs between Y and X, such as in Figure 8–12C, the residuals are negative for both small values and large values of X, because the corresponding values of Y fall below a regression line drawn through the data. They are positive, however, for midsized values of X because the corresponding values of Y fall above the regression line. In this case, instead of obtaining a random scatter, we get a plot like the curve in Figure 8–12D, with the values of the residuals being related to the values of X. Other patterns can be used by statisticians to help diagnose problems, such as a lack of equal variances or various types of nonlinearity.

Use the data file and R to produce a graph of residuals for the data in Neidert et al (2016). Which of the four situations in Figure 8–12 is most likely? See Exercise 8.

Dealing with Nonlinear Observations

Several alternative actions can be taken if serious problems arise with nonlinearity of data. As we discussed previously, a *transformation* may make the relationship linear, and regular regression methods can then be used on the transformed data. Another possibility, especially for a curve, is to fit a straight line to one part of the curve and a second straight line to another part of the curve, a procedure called *piecewise linear regression*. In this situation, one regression equation is used with all values of X less than a given value, and the second equation is used with all values of X greater than the given value. A third strategy, also useful for curves, is to perform polynomial regression; this technique is discussed in Chapter 10. Finally, more complex approaches called nonlinear regression may be used (Snedecor and Cochran, 1989).

Regression Toward the Mean

The phenomenon called **regression toward the mean** often occurs in applied research and may go unrecognized. A good illustration of regression toward the mean occurred in the MRFIT study (Multiple Risk Factor Intervention Trial Research Group; Gotto, 1997), which was designed to evaluate the effect of diet and exercise on blood pressure in men with mild hypertension. To be eligible to participate in the study, men had to have a diastolic blood pressure of ≥90 mm Hg. The eligible subjects were then assigned to either the treatment arm of the study, consisting of programs to encourage appropriate diet and exercise, or the control arm, consisting of typical care.

To illustrate the concept of regression toward the mean, we consider the hypothetical data in Table 8–6 for diastolic blood pressure in 12 men. If these men were being screened for the MRFIT study, only subjects 7 through 12 would be accepted; subjects 1 through 6 would not be eligible because their baseline diastolic pressure is <90 mm Hg. Suppose all subjects had another blood pressure measurement some time later. Because a person's blood pressure varies considerably from one reading to another, about half the men can be expected to have higher blood pressures and about half to have lower blood pressures, owing to random variation. Regression toward the mean tells us that those men who had lower pressures on the first reading are more likely to have higher pressures on the second reading. Similarly, men who had a diastolic blood pressure ≥90 on the first reading are more likely to have lower pressures on the second reading. If the entire sample of men is remeasured, the increases and decreases tend to cancel each other. If, however, only a subset of the subjects is examined again, for example, the men with initial diastolic pressures >90, the blood pressures will appear to have dropped, when in fact they have not.

Regression toward the mean can result in a treatment or procedure appearing to be of value when it has had no actual effect; the use of a control group helps to guard against this effect. The investigators in the MRFIT study were aware of the problem of regression toward the mean and discussed precautions they took to reduce its effect.

Common Errors in Regression

One error in regression analysis occurs when multiple observations on the same subject are treated as though they were independent. For example, consider ten patients who have their weight and skinfold measurements recorded prior to beginning a low-calorie diet. We may reasonably expect a moderately positive relationship between weight and skinfold thickness. Now suppose that the same ten patients are weighed and measured again after 6 weeks on the diet. If all 20 pairs of weight and skinfold measurements are treated as though they were independent, several problems occur. First, the sample size will appear to be 20 instead of 10, and we are more likely to conclude significance due to the increased power. Second, because the relationship between weight and skinfold thickness in the same person is somewhat stable across minor shifts in weight, using both before

Table 8–6. Hypothetical data on diastolic blood pressure to illustrate regression toward the mean.

Subject	Baseline	Repeat
1	78	80
2	80	81
3	82	82
4	84	86
5	86	85
6	88	90
7	90	88
8	92	91
9	94	95
10	96	95
11	98	97
12	100	98

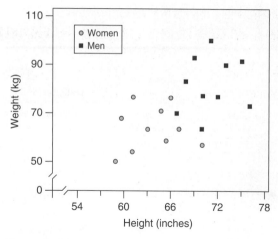

Figure 8–13. Hypothetical data illustrating spurious correlation.

and after diet observations has the same effect as using duplicate measures, and this results in a correlation larger than it should be.

The magnitude of the correlation can also be erroneously increased by combining two different groups. For example, consider the relationship between height and weight. Suppose the heights and weights of ten men and ten women are recorded, and the correlation between height and weight is calculated for the combined samples. Figure 8–13 illustrates how the scatterplot might look and indicates the problem that results from combining men and women in one sample. The relationship between height and weight appears to be more significant in the combined sample than it is when measured in men and women separately. Much of the apparent significance results because men tend both to weigh more and to be taller than women. Inappropriate conclusions may result from mixing two different populations—a rather common error to watch for in the medical literature.

Comparing Correlation & Regression

Correlation and regression have some similarities and some differences. First, correlation is scale-independent, but regression is not; that is, the correlation between two characteristics, such as height and weight, is the same whether height is measured in centimeters or inches and weight in kilograms or pounds. The regression equation predicting

weight from height, however, depends on which scales are being used; that is, predicting weight measured in kilograms from height measured in centimeters gives different values for the intercept (a) and slope (b) than if predicting weight in pounds from height in inches.

An important consequence of scale independence in correlation is that the correlation between X and Y is the same as the correlation between Y' and Y. They are equal because the regression equation itself, $Y' = a + bX$, is a simple rescaling of the X variable; that is, each value of X is multiplied by a constant value b and then the constant a is added. The fact that the correlation between the original variables X and Y is equal to the correlation between Y and Y' provides a useful alternative for testing the significance of the regression, as we will see in Chapter 10. Finally, the slope of the regression line has the same sign (+ or −) as the correlation coefficient (see Exercise 10). If the correlation is zero, the regression line is horizontal with a slope of zero. Thus, the formulas for the correlation coefficient and the regression coefficient are closely related. If r has already been calculated, it can be multiplied by the ratio of the standard deviation of Y to the standard deviation of X, SD_Y/SD_X to obtain b (see Exercise 9). Thus,

$$b = r \frac{SD_Y}{SD_X}$$

Similarly, if the regression coefficient is known, r can be found by

$$r = b \frac{SD_X}{SD_Y}$$

Multiple Regression

Multiple regression analysis is a straightforward generalization of simple regression for applications in which two or more independent (explanatory) variables are used to predict an outcome. For example, in the simple regression example, we related BMI and percent body fat. We can also control for the age of the subject, however. The results from two analyses are given in Table 8–7. First, regression was done using the BMI to predict

Table 8–7. Regression equations for percent body fat for normal subjects BMI versus BMI and age as predictor variables.

Regression Equation Section

Independent Variable	Regression Coefficient	Standard Error	t Value (H_0: B=0)	Probability Level	Decision (5%)
Intercept	5.1539	4.8438	1.064	0.29	Do Not Reject H_0
BMI	0.9742	0.2010	4.847	<0.0001	Reject H_0
R^2	0.177				

Regression Equation Section

Independent Variable	Regression Coefficient	Standard Error	t Value (H_0: B=0)	Probability Level	Decision (5%)
Intercept	5.13122	0.461	1.064	0.294	Do Not Reject H_0
Age	0.01020	0.08602	0.119	0.906	Do Not Reject H_0
BMI	0.96420	0.21880	4.407	<0.0001	Reject H_0
R^2	0.177				

BMI, body mass index.
Data from Neidert LE, Wainright KS, Zheng C, et al: Plasma dipeptidyl peptidase IV activity and measures of body composition in apparently healthy people, *Heliyon.* 2016 Apr 18;2(4):e00097.

insulin sensitivity among hyperthyroid women; the resulting equation was

$$\text{Predicted percent body fat} = 5.15 + 0.97 \times \text{BMI}$$

Next, the regression was repeated using both BMI and age as independent variables. The results were

$$\text{Predicted percent body fat} = 5.13 + 0.96 \times \text{BMI}$$
$$+ 0.01 \times \text{Age}$$

As you can see, the addition of the age variable has relatively little effect; in fact, the P value for age is 0.91, indicating that age is not significantly associated with percent body fat in this group of normal subjects.

As an additional point, note that R^2 (called *R*-squared) is 0.177 for both regression equations in Table 8–7. R^2 is interpreted in the same manner as the coefficient of determination, r^2, discussed in the section titled, "Interpreting the Size of *r*." This topic, along with multiple regression and other statistical

methods based on regression, is discussed in detail in Chapter 10.

SAMPLE SIZES FOR CORRELATION & REGRESSION

As with other statistical procedures, it is important to have an adequate number of subjects in any study that involves correlation or regression. Complex formulas are required to estimate sample sizes for these procedures, but fortunately we can use statistical power programs to do the calculations.

Suppose that Neidert and colleagues (2016) wanted to know what sample size would be necessary to determine if the correlation between BMI and percent body fat was greater than 0.3 with 80% power? We used the G*Power program to illustrate the sample size needed in this situation; the output is given in Figure 8–15. A sample of 326 patients would be necessary. We could have used the null hypothesis of 0.25 instead of 0.3. Do you think the sample size would be the same? Try it and see.

To illustrate the power analysis for regression, consider the regression equation to predict percent body fat from BMI (Neidert et al, 2016). Recall that we found that a 95% confidence interval for the regression coefficient was between 0.57 and 1.37 in the entire sample of

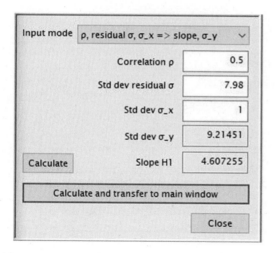

Figure 8–14. Data input for G*Power results in Figure 8-15. (Data from Neidert LE, Wainright KS, Zheng C, et al: Plasma dipeptidyl peptidase IV activity and measures of body composition in apparently healthy people, *Heliyon.* 2016 Apr 18;2(4):e00097.)

111 subjects. Suppose Neidert and colleagues wanted to know how many subjects would be needed for the regression. The power program G*Power finds the sample size by estimating the number needed to obtain a given value for R^2 (or r^2 when only one independent variable is used) and the standard deviation of the residuals. We assume they want the correlation between the actual insulin sensitivity and the predicted sensitivity to be at least 0.50, producing an r^2 of 0.25 and used the actual value of the standard deviation of the residuals ($S_{Y \cdot X} = 7.98$). The setup and output from the G*Power program are given in Figures 8–14 and 8–15. From Figure 8–15, we see that a sample size of about 21 is needed in each group for which a regression equation is to be determined.

SUMMARY

Two presenting problems were used in this chapter to illustrate the application of correlation and regression in medical studies. The findings from the study described in Presenting Problem 1 demonstrate the relationship between BMI and percent body fat, a correlation equal to 0.42. Several factors other than BMI affected the relationship.

In Presenting Problem 2, Pereira and colleagues (2015) evaluated four bedside blood glucose devices marketed as being accurate devices for blood glucose. We examined the relationship among these devices and the standard method using an arterial lab test. The observed correlations were quite high, ranging from

0.57 to 0.87. We compared these two correlation coefficients and concluded that statistical differences exist between them.

Data from Neidert and colleagues (2016) was also used to illustrate regression, specifically the relationship between percent body fat and BMI for normal men and women. We found separate regression lines for men and for women and observed that the relationships between percent body fat and BMI are different in these two groups of subjects.

The flowcharts for Appendix C summarize the methods for measuring an association between two characteristics measured on the same subjects. Flowchart C–4 indicates how the methods depend on the scale of measurement for the variables, and flowchart C–5 shows applicable methods for testing differences in correlations and in regression lines.

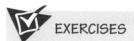

EXERCISES

1. a. Perform a chi-square test of the significance of the relationship between benzodiazepine use and the subsequent development of Alzheimer's disease using the data in Chapter 3, Table 3–19.

   b. Determine 95% confidence limits for the relative risk of Alzheimer's disease among subjects with a daily dose of benzodiazepine using the data from Table 3-19. What is your conclusion?

2. Calculate the correlation between BMI and body fat percentage for the entire sample of 71 women from Neidert et al (2016), using the results in the section titled, "Calculating the Regression Equation," for b. The standard deviation of BMI is 3.80 and of body fat percentage is 6.54.

3. Helmrich and coworkers (1987) conducted a study to assess the risk of deep vein thrombosis and pulmonary embolism in relation to the use of oral contraceptives. They were especially interested in the risk associated with low dosage (<50 μg estrogen) and confined their study to women under the age of 50 years. They administered standard questionnaires to women admitted to the hospital for deep vein thrombosis or pulmonary embolism as well as to a control set of women admitted for trauma and upper respiratory infections to determine their history and current use of oral contraceptives. Twenty of the

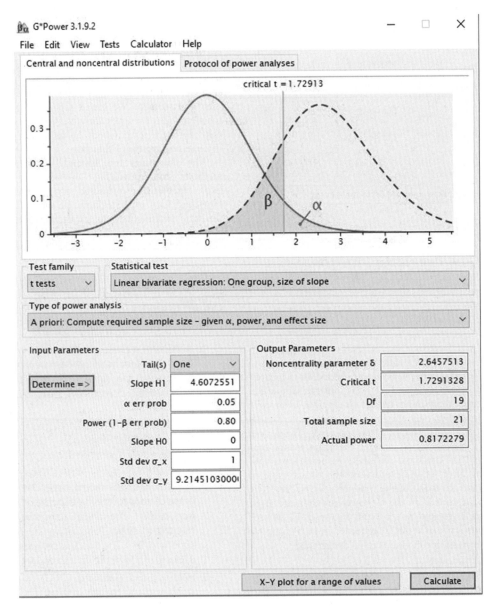

Figure 8–15. Illustration of setup for using the G*Power sample size program for multiple regression using the data on percent body fat. (Data from Neidert LE, Wainright KS, Zheng C, et al: Plasma dipeptidyl peptidase IV activity and measures of body composition in apparently healthy people, *Heliyon*. 2016 Apr 18;2(4):e00097.)

61 cases and 121 of the 1,278 controls had used oral contraceptives in the previous month.

a. What research design was used in this study?

b. Find 95% confidence limits for the odds ratio for these data.

c. The authors reported an age-adjusted odds ratio of 8.1 with 95% confidence limits of 3.7 and 18. Interpret these results.

4. Presenting Problem 2 in Chapter 3 by Bos-Touwen and colleagues (2015) measured

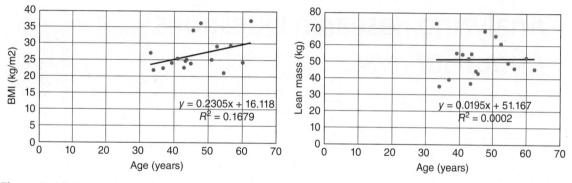

Figure 8–16. Scatterplots and regression lines for the relationship between age and BMI; age and Lean Mass. (Data from Neidert LE, Wainright KS, Zheng C, et al: Plasma dipeptidyl peptidase IV activity and measures of body composition in apparently healthy people, *Heliyon*. 2016 Apr 18;2(4):e00097.)

patient activation scores, demographic and psychosocial variables. Use the data from this study and select or filter those subjects with sex = 1 (men) and disease = 2 (COPD; 184 subjects should remain for the analysis.

a. Calculate the correlation between the illness perception score (IPQ_Total_score) and the SF-12 score (SF12_total_score) for men with COPD.

b. Form a 95% confidence interval for this correlation.

5. The graphs in Figure 8–16 were were created in Excel using the data from Neidert and colleagues (2016).

a. Which graph exhibits the strongest relationship with age?

b. Which variable would be best predicted from a patient's age?

6. Explain why the mean of the predicted values, $\overline{Y'}$, is equal to $\overline{Y}$.

7. Develop an intuitive argument to explain why the sign of the correlation coefficient and the sign of the slope of the regression line are the same.

8. Group Exercise. The MRFIT study (Multiple Risk Factor Intervention Trial Research Group, 1982), has been called a landmark trial; it was the first large-scale clinical trial, and it is rare to have a study that follows more than 300,000 men who were screened for the trial for a number of years. The Journal of the American Medical Association reprinted this article in 1997. In addition, the journal published a comment in the Landmark Perspective section by Gotto (1997). Obtain a copy of both articles.

a. What research design was used in the study?

b. Discuss the eligibility criteria. Are these criteria still relevant today?

c. What were the treatment arms? Are these treatments still relevant today?

d. What statistical methods were used? Were they appropriate? One method, the Kaplan–Meier product-limit method, is discussed in Chapter 9.

e. Refer to Figure 1 in the original study. What do the lines in the figure indicate?

f. Examine the distribution of deaths given in the article's Table 4. What statistical method is relevant to analyzing these results?

g. The perspective by Gotto discusses the issue of power in the MRFIT study. How was the power of the study affected by the initial assumptions made in the study design?

Analyzing Research Questions About Survival

9

KEY CONCEPTS

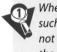 When research involves time-related variables, such as survival and recurrence, we generally do not know the outcome for all patients at the time the study is published, so these outcomes are called censored.

 Observations are doubly censored when not all patients enter the study at the same time.

 An example of why special methods are needed to analyze survival data helps illustrate the logic behind them.

 Life table or actuarial methods were developed to show survival curves; although generally surpassed by Kaplan–Meier curves, they occasionally appear in the literature.

 Survival analysis gives patients credit for how long they have been in the study, even if the outcome has not yet occurred.

 The Kaplan–Meier procedure is the most commonly used method to illustrate survival curves.

 Estimates of survival are less precise as the time from entry into the study becomes longer, because the number of patients in the study decreases.

 Survival curves can also be used to compare survival in two or more groups.

 The logrank statistic is one of the most commonly used methods to learn if two curves are significantly different.

 The hazard ratio is similar to the odds ratio; the difference is that the hazard ratio compares risk over time, while the odds ratio examines risk at a given time.

 The Mantel–Haenszel statistic is also used to compare curves, not just survival curves.

 Several versions of the logrank statistic exist. The logrank statistic assumes that the risk of the outcome is the constant over time.

 The Mantel–Haenszel statistic essentially combines a number of 2×2 tables for an overall measure of difference.

 The hazard function gives the probability that an outcome will occur in a given period, assuming that the outcome has not occurred during previous periods.

 The intention-to-treat principle states that subjects are analyzed in the group to which they were assigned. It minimizes bias when there are treatment crossovers or dropouts.

PRESENTING PROBLEMS

Presenting Problem

Metastatic colorectal cancer may be treated by regorafenib alone or regorafenib in combination with chemotherapy. Lin et al (2018) studied the survival curves for patients on each treatment. They analyzed data from 61 patients that completed the study: 34 on regorafenib combined with chemotherapy and 27 received regorafenib alone.

The full article may be accessed here:

Lin C-Y, Lin T-H, Chen C-C, Chen M-C, Chen C-P: Combination chemotherapy with Regorafenib in metastatic colorectal cancer treatment: A single center, retrospective study. PLoS ONE 2018;13(1):e0190497.

https://doi.org/10.1371/journal.pone.0190497

The accompanying data file may be accessed here:

https://ndownloader.figshare.com/files/10158633

PURPOSE OF THE CHAPTER

Many studies in medicine are designed to determine whether a new medication, a new treatment, or a new procedure will perform better than the one in current use. Although measures of short-term effects are of interest with efforts to provide more efficient health care, long-term outcomes, including mortality and major morbidity, are also important. Often, studies focus on comparing survival times for two or more groups of patients.

The methods of data analysis discussed in previous chapters are not appropriate for measuring length of survival for two reasons.

First, investigators frequently must analyze data before all patients have died; otherwise, it may be many years before they know which treatment is better. When analysis of survival is done while some patients in the study are still living, the observations on these patients are called **censored observations,** because we do not know how long these patients will remain alive. Figure 9–1 illustrates a situation in which observations on patients B and E are censored.

The second reason special methods are needed to analyze survival data is that patients do not typically begin treatment or enter the study at

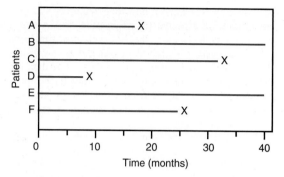

Figure 9–1. Example of censored observations (X means patient died).

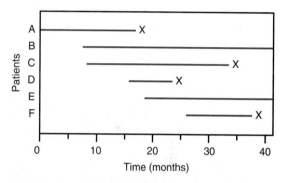

Figure 9–2. Example of progressively censored observations (X means patient died).

the same time, as they did for Figure 9–1. When the entry time for patients is not simultaneous and some patients are still in the study when the analysis is done, the data are said to be **progressively censored.** Figure 9–2 shows results for a study with progressively censored observations. The study began at time 0 months with patient A; then, patient B entered the study at time 7 months; patient C entered at time 8 months; and so on. Patients B and E were still alive at the time the data were analyzed at 40 months.

Analysis of survival times is sometimes called **actuarial,** or **life table, analysis.** Historically, astronomer Edmund Halley (of Halley's Comet fame) first used life tables in the seventeenth century to describe survival times of residents of a town. Since then, these methods have been used in various ways. Life insurance companies use them to determine the life expectancy of individuals, and this information is subsequently used to establish premium schedules. Insurers generally use cross-sectional data about how long people of different age groups are expected to live in order to develop a *current* life table. In medicine, however, most studies of survival use *cohort* life tables, in which the same group of subjects is followed for a given period. The data for life tables may come from cohort studies (either prospective or historical) or from clinical trials; the key feature is that the same group of subjects is followed for a prescribed time.

In this chapter, we examine two methods to determine survival curves. Actually, it is more accurate to describe them as methods to examine curves with censored data, because many times the outcome is something other than survival.

WHY SPECIALIZED METHODS ARE NEEDED TO ANALYZE SURVIVAL DATA

Before illustrating the methods for analyzing survival data, let us consider briefly why some intuitive methods are not very useful or appropriate. To illustrate these points, we selected a sample of 28 patients being treated for metastatic colon cancer: 14 patients taking regorafenib alone (R) and 14 taking regorafenib in combination with chemotherapy (Table 9–1).

Colton (1974, pp. 238–241) gives a creative presentation of some simple methods to analyze survival data; the arguments presented in this section are modeled on his discussion. Some

Table 9–1. Data report on a sample of 28 patients.

Case	Sex	Age	Treatment	Months Progression Free Survival	Months Survival	Survive
1	F	67	R	1.61	10.28	1
2	M	81	R	2.99	5.55	1
3	M	73	R	4.34	5.82	1
4	M	58	R	4.07	8.90	1
5	F	54	R	2.53	10.41	1
6	M	43	R	2.63	10.68	1
8	M	60	R	1.58	3.71	1
9	F	54	R	5.78	20.01	0
11	F	40	R	2.04	9.00	1
13	M	55	R	0.92	5.09	1
14	M	48	R	0.69	10.55	1
15	F	57	R	2.66	12.16	0
16	M	60	R	2.76	13.17	1
18	M	60	R	7.82	10.55	1
7	F	67	C	5.06	17.71	0
10	F	66	C	0.92	11.30	1
12	M	75	C	2.53	9.43	1
17	F	67	C	6.21	14.95	0
19	M	62	C	8.74	20.90	1
30	F	61	C	2.79	11.20	1
21	M	58	C	7.59	21.19	0
22	M	80	C	1.84	4.44	1
23	M	47	C	4.83	19.81	0
24	M	76	C	16.59	18.56	0
25	M	56	C	2.96	10.61	1
26	F	59	C	2.63	4.99	1
27	M	61	C	4.86	19.55	0
28	F	61	C	0.92	7.13	1

Data from Lin C-Y, Lin T-H, Chen C-C, et al: Combination chemotherapy with Regorafenib in metastatic colorectal cancer treatment: A single center, retrospective study, *PLoS One*. 2018 Jan 5;13(1):e0190497.

methods appear at first glance to be appropriate for analyzing survival data, but closer inspection shows they are incorrect.

Suppose someone suggests calculating the mean length of time patients survive with metastatic colon cancer. Using the data on 28 patients in Table 9–1, the mean survival time for patients on regorafenib combination treatment is 13.70 months, and for patients on regorafenib only 9.70 months. The problem is that mean survival time depends on when the data are analyzed; it will change with each passing month until the point when all the subjects have died. Therefore, mean survival estimates calculated in this way are useful only when all the subjects have died or the event being analyzed has occurred. Almost always, however, investigators wish to analyze their data prior to that time.

An estimate of median length of survival time is also possible, and it can be calculated after only half of the subjects have died. Again, however, investigators often wish to evaluate the outcome prior to that time.

A concept sometimes used in epidemiology is the number of deaths per each 100 **person-years of observation.** To illustrate, we use the observations in Table 9–1 to determine the number of person-months of survival. Regardless of whether patients are alive or dead at the end of the study, they contribute to the calculation for however long they have been in the study. Patient 1, therefore, contributes 10.28 months, patient 2 is in the study for 5.55 months, and so on. The total number of months patients have been observed is 327.65 months; converting to years by dividing by 12 gives 27.3 person-years.

One problem with using person-years of observation is that the same number is obtained by observing 1,000 patients for 1 year or by observing 100 patients for 10 years. Although the number of subjects is involved in the calculation of person-years, it is not evident as an explicit part of the result; and no statistical methods are available to compare these numbers. Another problem is the inherent assumption that the risk of an event, such as death or rejection, during any one unit of time is constant throughout the study (although several other survival methods also make this assumption).

Mortality rates (see Chapter 3) are a familiar way to deal with survival data, and they are used (especially in oncology) to estimate 3- and 5-year survival with various types of medical conditions. We cannot determine a mortality rate using data on *all* patients until the specified length of time has passed.

Suppose we have a study with 20 patients: 10 lived at least 1 year, and 4 died prior to 1 year, and 6 had been in the study less than a year (i.e., they were censored). We have to decide what to do with the six censored patients in order to calculate a 1-year survival rate. One solution is to divide the number who died in the first year, 4, by the total number in the study, 20, for an estimate of 0.20, or 20%. This estimate, however, is probably too low, because it assumes that none of the six patients in the study less than 1 year will die before the year is up.

An alternative solution is to ignore the patients who were not in the study for 1 year to obtain $4/(20 - 6) = 0.286$, or 28.6%. This technique is similar to the approach used in cancer research in which 3- and 5-year mortality rates are based on only those patients who were in the study at least 3 or 5 years. The shortcoming of this approach is that it completely ignores the contribution of the six patients who were in the study for part of a year. We need a way to use information gained from all patients who entered the study. A reasonable approach should produce an estimate between 20% and 28.6%, which is exactly what actuarial life table analysis and Kaplan–Meier product limit methods do. They give credit for the amounts of time subjects survived up to the time when the data are analyzed.

ACTUARIAL, OR LIFE TABLE, ANALYSIS

Actuarial, or life table, analysis is also sometimes referred to in the medical literature as the Cutler–Ederer method (Cutler and Ederer, 1958). The actuarial method is not computationally overwhelming and, at one time, was the predominant method used in medicine. However, the availability of computers makes it used far less often today than the Kaplan–Meier product limit method discussed in the next section.

We briefly illustrate the calculations involved in actuarial analysis by arranging the 14 patients on the regorafenib only therapy according to the length of time they survived (Table 9–2). We use the observations in Table 9–2 to produce Table 9–3. The time intervals are arbitrary but should be selected so that the number of censored observations in any interval is small; we group by 5-month intervals for this example.

The column heading n_i in Table 9–3 is the number of patients in the study at the beginning of the interval; all patients (14) began the study, so n_1 is 14. One patient did not complete the first time interval: patient 8. Patient 8 died, referred to as a terminal event (d_1); there are no withdrawals in this period (w_1).

The actuarial method assumes that patients withdraw randomly throughout the interval; therefore, on the average, they withdraw halfway through the time represented by the interval. In a sense, this method gives patients who withdraw credit for being in the study for half of the period. One-half of the number of patients withdrawing is subtracted from the number beginning the interval, so the denominator used to calculate the proportion having a terminal event is reduced by half of the number who

Table 9–2. Survival of a sample of patients in the regorafenib only arm.

Case	Sex	Age	Treatment	Months Progression Free Survival	Months Overall Survival	Status
8	M	60	R	1.58	3.71	Dead
13	M	55	R	0.92	5.09	Dead
2	M	81	R	2.99	5.55	Dead
3	M	73	R	4.34	5.82	Dead
4	M	58	R	4.07	8.90	Dead
11	F	40	R	2.04	9.00	Dead
1	F	67	R	1.61	10.28	Dead
5	F	54	R	2.53	10.41	Dead
14	M	48	R	0.69	10.55	Dead
18	M	60	R	7.82	10.55	Dead
6	M	43	R	2.63	10.68	Dead
15	F	57	R	2.66	12.16	Alive
16	M	60	R	2.76	13.17	Dead
9	F	54	R	5.78	20.01	Alive

Data from Lin C-Y, Lin T-H, Chen C-C, et al: Combination chemotherapy with Regorafenib in metastatic colorectal cancer treatment: A single center, retrospective study, *PLoS One*. 2018 Jan 5;13(1):e0190497.

Table 9–3. Life table for sample of 14 patients treated with regorafenib combination treatment.

Life Table Survival Variable: Overall Survival

	n_i	w_i		d_i	$q_i = d_i/$ $[n_i-(w_i/2)]$	$p_i = 1-q_i$	$s_i = p_ip_{i-1} \cdot$ $p_{i-2} \cdots p_1$
Interval Start Time	Number Entering This Interval	Number Withdrawn During Interval	Number Exposed to Risk	Number of Terminal Events	Proportion Terminating	Proportion Surviving	Cumulative Proportion Survival at End
0	14	0	14.0	1	0.071	0.929	0.929
5	13	0	13.0	5	0.385	0.615	0.571
10	8	1	7.5	6	0.800	0.200	0.114
15	1	0	1.0	0	0.000	1.000	0.114
20	1	1	1.0	0	0.000	1.000	0.114

Data from Lin C-Y, Lin T-H, Chen C-C, et al: Combination chemotherapy with Regorafenib in metastatic colorectal cancer treatment: A single center, retrospective study, *PLoS One*. 2018 Jan 5;13(1):e0190497.

withdraw during the period. In period starting with 10, there is one withdrawal (case 15). Eight subjects started the interval, so 8 − (½ × 1), or 7.5 is the number of subjects exposed to risk in our example. The proportion terminating is 6/7.5 = 0.8. The proportion surviving is 1 − 0.800 = 0.200, and the cumulative survival is 0.929 × 0.615 × 0.200 = 0.114. This computation procedure continues until the table is completed.

Note that p_i is the probability of surviving interval i only; and to survive interval i, a patient must have survived all previous intervals as well. Thus, p_i is an example of a conditional probability because the probability of surviving interval i is dependent, or conditional, on

surviving until that point. This probability is sometimes called the *survival function*. Recall from Chapter 4 that if one event is conditional on a previous event, the probability of their joint occurrence is found by multiplying the probability of the conditional event by the probability of the previous event. The cumulative probability of surviving interval i plus all previous intervals is, therefore, found by multiplying p_i by $p_{i-1}, p_{i-2} \cdots p_1$.

The results from an actuarial analysis can help answer questions that may help clinicians counsel patients or their families. For example, we might ask, If X is the length of time survived by a patient selected at random from the population represented by these patients, what is the probability that X is 5 months or greater? From Table 9–3, the probability is about 0.57, that a patient will live for at least 5 months.

Journal articles rarely present the results from life table analysis as we have in Table 9–3; rather, the results are usually presented in a survival curve. The line in Figure 9–3 is a survival curve for the sample of 14 patients on regorafenib only.

The actuarial method involves two assumptions about the data. The first is that all withdrawals during a given interval occur, on average, at the midpoint of the interval. This assumption is of less consequence when short time intervals are analyzed; however, considerable bias can occur if the intervals are large, if many withdrawals occur, and if withdrawals do not occur midway in the interval. The Kaplan–Meier method introduced in the next section overcomes this problem. The second assumption is that, although survival in a given period depends on survival in all previous periods, the probability of survival at one period is treated as though it is independent of the probability of survival at others. This condition, although probably violated somewhat in much medical research, does not appear to cause major concern to biostatisticians.

KAPLAN–MEIER PRODUCT LIMIT METHOD

The Kaplan–Meier method of estimating survival is similar to actuarial analysis except that time since entry in the study is not divided into intervals for analysis. Depending on the number of patients who died, the **Kaplan–Meier product limit method,** commonly called Kaplan–Meier curves, may involve fewer calculations than the actuarial method, primarily because survival is estimated each time a patient dies, so withdrawals are ignored. We will illustrate with data from Lin and colleagues (2018) using the same subset of patients as with life table analysis, patients on regorafenib only.

The first step is to list the times when a death or dropout occurs, as in the column "Event Time" in Table 9–4. One patient died at 3.71 months and another at 5.09

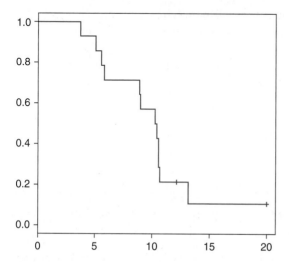

Figure 9–3. Life table survival plot of a sample of patients in the regorafenib arm.

Table 9–4. Kaplan–Meier survival curve in detail for patients on regorafenib only.

Event Time (T)	Number at Risk	Number of Events	Mortality	Survival	Cumulative Survival
3.710	14	1	0.071	0.929	0.929
5.090	13	1	0.077	0.923	0.857
5.550	12	1	0.083	0.917	0.786
5.820	11	1	0.091	0.909	0.714
8.900	10	1	0.100	0.900	0.643
9.000	9	1	0.111	0.889	0.571
10.280	8	1	0.125	0.875	0.500
10.410	7	1	0.143	0.857	0.429
10.550	6	1	0.167	0.833	0.357
10.550	5	1	0.200	0.800	0.286
10.680	4	1	0.250	0.750	0.214
12.160	3	0			
13.170	2	1	0.500	0.500	0.107
20.010	1	0			

Data from Lin C-Y, Lin T-H, Chen C-C, et al: Combination chemotherapy with Regorafenib in metastatic colorectal cancer treatment: A single center, retrospective study, *PLoS One.* 2018 Jan 5;13(1):e0190497.

months, and they are listed under the column "Number of Events." Then, each time an event or outcome occurs, the mortality, survival, and cumulative survival are calculated in the same manner as with the life table method. If the table is published in an article, it is often formatted in an abbreviated form, such as in Table 9–5.

Note that the Kaplan–Meier procedure gives exact survival proportions because it uses exact survival times; the actuarial method gives approximations because

it groups survival times into intervals. Prior to the widespread use of computers, the actuarial method was much easier to use for a very large number of observations.

Typically, as the interval from entry into the study becomes longer, the number of patients who remain in the study becomes increasingly smaller. This means that the standard deviation of the estimate of the proportion surviving gets

Table 9–5. Survival analysis for OSM (months of survival) in both treatment arms.

Treatment=C

time	n.risk	n.event	survival	std.err	lower 95% CI	upper 95% CI
3.52	34	1	0.971	0.0290	0.915	1.000
3.98	33	1	0.941	0.0404	0.865	1.000
4.04	32	1	0.912	0.0486	0.821	1.000
4.30	31	1	0.882	0.0553	0.780	0.998
4.44	30	1	0.853	0.0607	0.742	0.981
4.99	28	1	0.822	0.0658	0.703	0.962
6.83	23	1	0.787	0.0720	0.658	0.941
7.13	22	1	0.751	0.0771	0.614	0.918
9.43	19	1	0.711	0.0825	0.567	0.893
10.61	17	1	0.670	0.0876	0.518	0.865
11.20	16	1	0.628	0.0916	0.472	0.836
11.30	14	1	0.583	0.0954	0.423	0.803
13.54	8	1	0.510	0.1078	0.337	0.772
20.90	2	1	0.255	0.1882	0.060	1.000

Treatment=R

time	n.risk	n.event	survival	std.err	lower 95% CI	upper 95% CI
2.89	27	1	0.963	0.0363	0.8943	1.000
3.71	26	1	0.926	0.0504	0.8322	1.000
4.37	25	1	0.889	0.0605	0.7779	1.000
4.96	24	2	0.815	0.0748	0.6807	0.975
5.09	22	1	0.778	0.0800	0.6358	0.952
5.55	18	1	0.735	0.0864	0.5833	0.925
5.82	16	1	0.689	0.0924	0.5294	0.896
6.14	15	1	0.643	0.0970	0.4782	0.864
8.90	12	1	0.589	0.1027	0.4187	0.829
9.00	11	1	0.536	0.1064	0.3629	0.791
10.28	10	1	0.482	0.1084	0.3102	0.749
10.41	9	1	0.428	0.1088	0.2605	0.705
10.55	8	2	0.321	0.1047	0.1697	0.609
10.68	6	1	0.268	0.1000	0.1288	0.557
13.17	2	1	0.134	0.1071	0.0279	0.642

Treatment:
C, combination treatment
R, regorafenib only
Data from Lin C-Y, Lin T-H, Chen C-C, et al: Combination chemotherapy with Regorafenib in metastatic colorectal cancer treatment: A single center, retrospective study, *PLoS One*. 2018 Jan 5;13(1):e0190497.

increasingly larger over time. Sometimes, the number of patients remaining in the study is printed under the timeline. Some authors provide graphs with dashed lines on either side of the survival curve that represent 95% **confidence bands** for the curve. The confidence limits become wider as time progresses, reflecting decreased confidence in the estimate of the proportion as the sample size decreases. These practices are desirable, but not all computer programs provide them.

To illustrate confidence bands, we analyze actual survival for all patients in both treatment arms. The procedure for obtaining confidence bands uses the **standard error** of the cumulative survival estimate S_i:

$$SE(S_i) = S_i \sqrt{\sum \frac{d_i}{n_i(n_i - d_i)}}$$

For example, at month 4, 13 patients taking combination therapy are still in the study and 1 patient died, so

$$\frac{d_i}{n_i(n_i - d_i)} = \frac{1}{14(14 - 1)} = 0.0055$$

and the standard error is

$$SE(S_i) = S_i \sqrt{\sum \frac{d_i}{n_i(n_i - d_i)}}$$

$$= 0.929\sqrt{0.0055}$$

$$= 0.069$$

The remaining calculations for both treatment arms are given in Table 9–5.

Figure 9–4 is a graph of the Kaplan–Meier product limit curve for all patients on regorafenib alone illustrating 95% confidence bands. In this graph, the curve is step-like because the proportion of patients surviving changes precisely at the points when a subject dies.

COMPARING TWO SURVIVAL CURVES

Although some journal articles report survival for only one group, more often investigators wish to compare two or more samples of patients. Table 9–6 contains the analysis of survival for the entire sample of 61 patients, separately by each treatment arm (Lin et al, 2018).

The Kaplan–Meier survival curves for both treatment arms are given in Figure 9–5. It is difficult to tell by looking whether the two curves are significantly different. We cannot make judgments simply on the basis of the amount of separation between two lines; a small

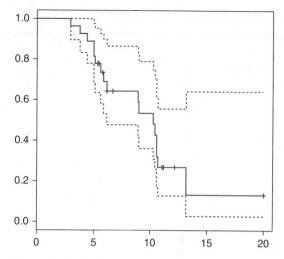

Figure 9–4. Kaplan–Meier curve with 95% confidence limits for patients on regorafenib alone.

difference may be statistically significant if the sample size is large, and a large difference may not if the sample size is small. As you might suspect, we need to perform a statistical test to evaluate the degree of any differences. Use the R and replicate our analysis to produce the survival curves.

We need special methods to compare survival distributions. If no censored observations occur, the **Wilcoxon rank sum test** introduced in Chapter 6 is appropriate for comparing the ranks of survival time. The independent-groups t test is not appropriate because survival times are not normally distributed and tend to be positively skewed (extremely so, in some cases).

If some observations are censored, several methods may be used to compare survival curves. Most articles in the medical literature report a comparison of survival curves using the logrank statistic or the Mantel–Haenszel chi-square statistic. The computations for all of the methods are very time-consuming, and computer programs are readily available. We illustrate the logrank and Mantel-Haenszel methods; both methods are straightforward, if computationally onerous, and are useful in helping us understand the logic behind the method. Within the context of the logrank statistic, we illustrate the hazard ratio, a useful descriptive statistic for comparing two groups at risk.

The Logrank Test

Several forms of the logrank statistic have been published by different biostatisticians, so it is called by several different names in the literature: the Mantel logrank statistic, the Cox–Mantel logrank

Table 9–6. Logrank statistic for survival.

	Number at Risk			Observed Deaths			Expected Deaths		
Month	C	R	Total	C	R	Total	C	R	Total
2.89	34	27	61	0	1	1	0.557	0.443	1
3.52	34	26	60	1	0	1	0.567	0.433	1
3.71	33	26	59	0	1	1	0.559	0.441	1
3.98	33	25	58	1	0	1	0.569	0.431	1
4.04	32	25	57	1	0	1	0.561	0.439	1
4.30	31	25	56	1	0	1	0.554	0.446	1
4.37	30	25	55	0	1	1	0.545	0.455	1
4.44	30	24	54	1	0	1	0.556	0.444	1
4.96	29	24	53	0	2	2	1.094	0.906	2
4.99	28	22	50	1	0	1	0.560	0.440	1
5.09	27	22	49	0	1	1	0.551	0.449	1
5.55	26	18	44	0	1	1	0.591	0.409	1
5.82	26	16	42	0	1	1	0.619	0.381	1
6.14	25	15	40	0	1	1	0.625	0.375	1
6.83	23	12	35	1	0	1	0.657	0.343	1
7.13	22	12	34	1	0	1	0.647	0.353	1
8.90	21	12	33	0	1	1	0.636	0.364	1
9.00	21	11	32	0	1	1	0.656	0.344	1
9.43	19	10	29	1	0	1	0.655	0.345	1
10.28	17	10	27	0	1	1	0.630	0.370	1
10.41	17	9	26	0	1	1	0.654	0.346	1
10.55	17	8	25	0	2	2	1.360	0.640	2
10.61	17	6	23	1	0	1	0.739	0.261	1
10.68	16	6	22	0	1	1	0.727	0.273	1
11.20	16	3	19	1	0	1	0.842	0.158	1
11.30	14	3	17	1	0	1	0.824	0.176	1
13.17	8	2	10	0	1	1	0.800	0.200	1
13.54	8	1	9	1	0	1	0.889	0.111	1
20.90	2	0	2	1	0	1	1.000	–	1
Grand Total				14	17	31	20.225	10.775	

Calculation of logrank statistic

	O-E	(O-E)²	(O-E)²/E	Sum	*p* value
C	(6.23)	38.75	1.92	5.51	0.018882
R	6.23	38.75	3.60		

Data from Lin C-Y, Lin T-H, Chen C-C, et al: Combination chemotherapy with Regorafenib in metastatic colorectal cancer treatment: A single center, retrospective study, *PLoS One.* 2018 Jan 5;13(1):e0190497.

statistic, and simply the logrank statistic. The **logrank test** compares the number of observed deaths in each group with the number of deaths that would be expected based on the number of deaths in the combined groups, that is, if group membership did not matter. An approximate **chi-square test** is used to test the significance of a mathematical expression involving the observed and expected number of deaths.

To illustrate the logrank test, we continue use the data from Lin and colleagues (2018). We grouped the data for the entire sample of 61 patients in the study using the same groupings previously presented in the life table in Table 9–3; the steps for calculating the logrank statistic follow.

1. Create rows for each time increment where a patient dies for either treatment. The second and third columns contain the number of patients in each group who were at risk of dying during the time interval. Each row should be decreased by the number of subjects that die as well as the number that are withdrawn or censored.

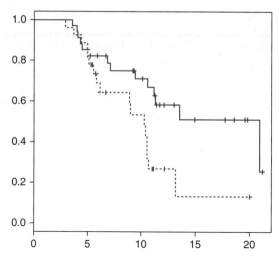

Figure 9–5. Kaplan–Meier survival curve patients in both treatment arms.

$$\chi^2 = \frac{(14 - 20.225)^2}{20.225} + \frac{(17 - 10.775)^2}{10.775}$$

$$= 1.92 + 3.60 = 5.51$$

The chi-square distribution with 1 degree of freedom in Table A–5 indicates that a critical value of 3.841 is required for significance at 0.05. Therefore, we conclude that a statistically significant difference exists in the distributions of overall survival time for the patients undergoing the two treatment protocols.

Use the R and find the value of the logrank statistic for this sample. Is it in close agreement with our calculations?

The Hazard Ratio

One benefit of calculating the logrank statistic is that the **hazard ratio** can easily be calculated from the information given in Table 9–6. It is estimated by O_1/E_1 divided by O_2/E_2. In our example, the hazard ratio, or risk of mortality in patients treated with regorafenib only versus the combination treatment is

$$\text{Hazard Ratio} = \frac{O_1 / E_1}{O_2 / E_2} = \frac{17 / 10.775}{14 / 20.225} = \frac{1.578}{0.692} = 2.28$$

The hazard ratio of 2.28 can be interpreted in a similar manner as the odds ratio: The risk of mortality at any time in the group on the regorafenib only protocol is approximately twice the risk in the group on the combination treatment. Using the hazard ratio assumes that the hazard or risk of death is the same throughout the time of the study; we will discuss the concept of hazard again in the next chapter.

The Mantel–Haenszel Chi-Square Statistic

Another method for comparing survival distributions is an estimate of the odds ratio developed by Mantel and Haenszel that follows (approximately) a chi-square distribution with 1 degree of freedom. The **Mantel–Haenszel test** combines a series of 2×2 tables formed at different survival times into an overall test of significance of the survival curves. The Mantel–Haenszel statistic is very useful because it can be used to compare any distributions, not simply survival curves.

We again use data from Lin and colleagues (2018) to illustrate the calculation of the Mantel–Haenszel statistic (Table 9–7). The first step is to select the time intervals for which 2×2 tables will be formed; we use the 5-month intervals as displayed in the life table

2. In columns 5 through 7, the number of patients in each group who died during that interval and the total number are listed. This calculation continues through all periods.

3. The last three columns contain the *expected* number of deaths for each group and the total at each period. The expected number of deaths for a given group is found by multiplying the total number of deaths in a given period by the proportion of patients in that group. For example, at 9 months, 21 patients remain in group C and 11 in group R, for a total of 32. One death is recorded; so $1 \times (21/32)$ is the number of deaths expected to occur in group C, and $1 \times (11/32)$ is the number of deaths expected in group R. This calculation is done for all periods.

4. The totals are calculated for each column.

The following expression can be used to test the null hypothesis that the survival distributions are the same in the two groups:

$$\chi^2 = \frac{(O_1 - E_1)^2}{E_1} + \frac{(O_2 - E_2)^2}{E_2}$$

where O_1 is the total number of observed deaths in group C, E_1 is the total number of expected deaths in group C, and so forth. The statistic χ^2 follows an approximate chi-square distribution with 1 degree of freedom. In our example, the calculation is

Table 9-7. Illustration of Mantel–Haenszel using entire sample.

Time Period	Status	Group C	Group R	Total	Odds Ratio ad/n	Odds Ratio bc/n	Observed	Expected	Variance
0–5	Alive	28	19	47	3.672131	1.868852	28	26.19672	2.705563
	Dead	6	8	14					
	Total	34	27	61					
6–10	Alive	22	12	34	1.65	0.9	22	21.25	1.225962
	Dead	3	3	6					
	Total	25	15	40					
11–15	Alive	13	2	15	0.684211	0.315789	13	12.63158	0.443213
	Dead	3	1	4					
	Total	16	3	19					
				Sums	6.006342	3.084642	63	60.0783	4.374738
				Mantel–Haenszel	1.951278				

example. For each interval, the number of patients who remained alive and the number who die are the rows, and the number of patients in each group are the columns of the 2×2 tables.

As with the logrank test, the Mantel–Haenszel test is onerous to compute. The first step estimates a pooled odds ratio, which is useful for descriptive purposes but is not needed for the statistical test itself. The pooled odds ratio is

$$OR = \frac{\sum(a \times d / n)}{\sum(b \times c / n)}$$

where a, b, c, d, and n are defined as they were in the 2×2 table in Table 6–9. The numerator and denominator are calculated in the columns under the heading "Odds Ratio." For the first time period, the ad/n is $(28 \times 8)/61$ or 3.67. The sum of the terms in the numerator is 6.00 and in the denominator is 3.08. The estimate of the odds ratio using the Mantel–Haenszel approach is, therefore, $6.00/3.08=1.95$. The hypothesis to be tested is whether 1.95 is significantly different from 1.

The remaining calculations focus on cell (1, 1) of the table; we first find its expected value and its variance for each 2×2 table. For example, at 6 to 10 months, among the 25 patients on the combination therapy who are alive and who were in the study at least 6 months, 22 remained alive and 3 died during that period. Among the 15 on the regorafenib only therapy, 12 remained alive and 3 died. The expected values are found in the same manner as in the chi-square

test discussed in Chapters 5 and 6. For example, the expected value of cell (1, 1) in this period is the row total times the column total divided by the grand total:

$$E(a_i) = \frac{\text{Row total} \times \text{Column total}}{\text{Grand total}}$$

$$= \frac{34 \times 25}{40} = 21.25$$

In addition, the variance of cell (1, 1) is calculated. Using the notation from Table 6–9, the estimated variance is

$$V(a_i) = \left[\frac{(a + c)(b + d)(a + b)(c + d)}{(n)(n)(n - 1)} \right]$$

For this period, the variance, with rounding, is

$$V(a_i) = \frac{25 \times 34 \times 15 \times 6}{40 \times 40 \times 39} = 1.23$$

After the expected value and the variance are found for each 2×2 table, the values are added, along with the number of observed patients in cell (1, 1) in each table. The three sums are 63, 60.08, and 4.37, as you can see in Table 9–7. The Mantel–Haenszel test is the squared difference between the sum of the observed number minus the sum of the expected number, all divided by the sum of the variances:

$$\text{Mantel} - \text{Haenszel} = \frac{[|\sum a_i - \sum E(a_i)|]}{\sum V(a_i)}$$

$$= \frac{(63 - 60.08)^2}{4.37}$$

$$= 1.95$$

This value is smaller than the value we found for the logrank test, and it is no longer significant. Recall that the critical value for the chi square statistic with one degree of freedom is 3.851 at the 0.05 level. Which statistic should we use? It is not a straightforward choice. The value of the logrank statistic in R is 5.9, significant at $p = 0.02$. We give some general guidelines in the next section.

Summary of Procedures to Compare Survival Distributions

The logrank statistics are used with a great deal of frequency in the medical literature. Several logrank methods are seen in the literature, such as that developed by Peto and Peto (1972). The logrank procedure gives all calculations the same weight, regardless of the time at which an event occurs. In contrast, the Peto logrank test weighs the terms (observed minus expected) by the number of patients at risk at that time, thereby giving more weight to early events when the number of patients at risk is large. Some biostatisticians choose this method because they believe that calculations based on larger sample sizes should receive more weight than calculations based on smaller sample sizes that occur later in time. If the pattern of deaths is similar over time, the Peto logrank statistic and the logrank statistic we illustrated earlier generally lead to the same conclusion. If, however, a higher proportion of deaths occurs during one interval, such as sometimes occurs early in the survival curve, the Peto logrank test and the logrank test may differ.

In truth, the information available to guide investigators in deciding which procedure is appropriate in any given application is quite complex, and, in some situations, readers of journal articles cannot determine which procedure actually was used. It is unfortunate that many of the statistical procedures used to compare survival distributions are called by a variety of names. Part of the confusion has occurred because the same biostatisticians (e.g., Mantel, Gehan, Cox, Peto and Peto, Haenszel) are or have been leading researchers who developed a number of statistical tests. Another source of confusion is that research on biostatistical methods for analyzing survival data is still underway; as a result, the Mantel procedure and the Peto logrank procedure were only recently shown to be equivalent.

The Mantel–Haenszel chi-square test is sometimes referred to as the logrank test in some texts, and although it is technically different, on many occasions it leads to the same conclusion. This statistic actually may be considered an extension of the logrank test because it can be used in more general situations.

For example, the Mantel–Haenszel chi-square test can be used to combine two or more 2×2 tables in other situations, such as a 2×2 table for men and a 2×2 table for women. This procedure is similar to other methods to control for confounding factors, topics discussed in Chapter 10.

To summarize, all logrank tests, regardless of what they are called, and the Mantel–Haenszel chi-square test may be considered similar procedures. The Gehan and Wilcoxon tests, however, are conceptually different. The **Gehan,** or **generalized Wilcoxon test**, is an extension of the Wilcoxon rank sum test illustrated in Chapter 6 modified so that it can be used with censored observations (Gehan, 1965). This test is also referred to in the literature as the Breslow test or the generalized Kruskal–Wallis test for comparison of more than two samples (Kalbfleisch and Prentice, 2002). As with the Peto logrank test, the generalized Wilcoxon test uses the number of patients at risk as weights and, therefore, counts losses that occur early in the survival distribution more heavily than losses that occur late.

Another difference between these two families of tests is that the logrank statistic assumes that the ratio of hazard rates in the two groups stays the same throughout the period of interest. When a constant hazard ratio cannot be assumed, the generalized Wilcoxon procedure is preferred. In the special situation in which the hazard rates are proportional, a method called **Cox's proportional hazard model** can be used; it is increasingly used in the literature because it permits investigators to control for confounding variables (see Chapter 10).

As you can see, the issue is complex and illustrates the advisability of consulting a statistician if performing a survival analysis. Back to our question in the previous section when comparing patients on the two treatment protocols for metastatic colon cancer, should we accept the result from the logrank test, which was significant, or the Mantel–Haenszel test, which was not? Looking at the distribution of mortality across time periods in Table 9–6, a constant hazard appears to be a reasonable assumption. Therefore, we would opt for the logrank statistic and conclude the treatments are different at $p < 0.02$, as did Lin and colleagues (2018). Readers who want more information are referred to the Lee and Wang (2003) text, possibly the most comprehensive text available. An introductory text devoted to survival analysis is that by Kleinbaum (1996). Other texts that discuss survival methods include books by Collett (2003), Fisher and van Belle (1996), Fleiss

(1981, 1999), Hosmer and Lemeshow (1999), and Schlesselman (1982).

Many of the statistical computer programs provide several test statistics for survival, but they generally provide at least one from the Gehan/Wilcoxon family and one from the logrank group. R presents the logrank test and R packages are available to calculate all of the statistics listed above. SPSS provides the logrank test and two others. JMP gives two tests: the Wilcoxon test and the logrank test.

THE HAZARD FUNCTION IN SURVIVAL ANALYSIS

In the introduction to this chapter, we stated that calculating mean survival is generally not useful, and we subsequently illustrated how its value depends on the time when the data are analyzed. Estimates of mean survival that are reasonable can be obtained, however, when the sample size is fairly large. This procedure depends on the **hazard function,** which is the probability that a person dies in the time interval i to $i + 1$, given that the person has survived until time i. The hazard function is also called the conditional failure rate; in epidemiology, the term *force of mortality* is used.

Although the **exponential probability distribution** was not discussed in Chapter 4 when we introduced other probability distributions (i.e., the normal, binomial, and Poisson), many survival curves follow an exponential distribution. It is a continuous distribution that involves the natural logarithm, *ln*, and it depends on a constant rate (which determines the shape of the curve) and on time. It provides a model for describing processes such as radioactive decay.

If an exponential distribution is a reasonable assumption for the shape of a survival curve, then the following formula can be used to estimate the hazard rate, symbolized by the letter *H,* when censored observations occur:

$$H = \frac{d}{\Sigma f + \Sigma c}$$

where d is the number of deaths, Σf is the sum of failure times, and Σc is the sum of censored times. Calculating the hazard rate requires us to add all of the failure times and censored times.

One reason the hazard rate is of interest is that its reciprocal is an estimate of mean survival time. The formulas are complex, and, fortunately, the R computer program calculates the hazard function and its 95% confidence interval as part of the Kaplan–Meier analysis. Details on using the hazard function are given in the comprehensive text on survival analysis by Lee and Wang (2003).

THE INTENTION-TO-TREAT PRINCIPLE

In the methods section of journal articles that report clinical trial results, investigators often state that they analyzed the data on an **intention-to-treat** basis. For instance, in a study of the effectiveness of a 16-week diabetes prevention program (DPP), Ciemins et al (2018) used an intent to treat approach. The primary outcomes variables in this study were body weight loss, meeting physical activity goals, and meeting the daily fat gram goal.

In the method section, the researchers state: "The primary objective of this ITT analysis was to determine whether an intervention delivered simultaneously to multiple communities via telehealth resulted in clinical outcomes comparable to an intervention delivered face-to-face. As an ITT analysis, all patients enrolled in the study were included in the analysis, regardless of attendance …" This statement means that the results for each patient who entered the trial were included in the analysis of the group to which the patient was randomized, regardless of any subsequent events. In Ciemens and coworkers' study (2018), the randomization was based on the rural or urban location of the subjects.

Analyzing data on an intention-to-treat basis is appropriate for several reasons. First is the issue of dropouts, as in the study by Ciemens and coworkers (2018). The ITT approach is appropriate for this study since it is natural for participants in DPPs to drop out at some point in time and therefore the ITT evaluates the impact of the dropouts also. Is it possible that the patients who dropped out of the treatment group had some characteristics that, independent of the treatment, could affect the outcome? Suppose, for instance, that the subjects who dropped out of the study had a higher BMI than those that stayed in the study. Subjects with a higher starting BMI may have more potential weight to lose during the program. If these patients are omitted from the analysis, the results may appear to be better for the rural or urban group than they should; that is, the results are biased. Although there is no indication that this occurred in this study, it is easy to see how such events could affect the conclusions, and these investigators were correct to analyze the data on the intention-to-treat basis.

The intention-to-treat principle is also important in studies in which patients cross over from one treatment group to another. For example, the classic Coronary Artery Surgery Study (CASS, 1983) was a randomized trial of coronary bypass surgery. Patients were assigned to medical treatment or surgical intervention to evaluate the effect of treatment on outcomes for patients with coronary artery disease. As in many studies that compare a conservative treatment with a more aggressive intervention, some patients in the CASS study who were randomized to medical treatment subsequently underwent surgery. And, some patients randomized to surgery were treated medically instead.

The problem with studies in which patients cross over from one treatment to another is that we do not know why the crossover occurred. Did some of the patients originally assigned to medical treatment improve so that they became candidates for surgery? If so, this could cause results in the surgery group to appear better than they really were (because "healthier" patients were removed from the medical group and transferred to the surgery group). On the other hand, perhaps the condition of the patients originally assigned to medical treatment worsened to such a degree that the patient or family insisted on having surgery. If so, this could cause the surgery group results to appear worse than they really were (because "sicker" patients were transferred from the medical to the surgical group). The point is, we do not know why the patients crossed over, and neither do the investigators.

In the past, some investigators presented studies with such a situation analyzed the patients by the group they were in at the end of the study. Other researchers omitted from the analysis any patients who crossed over. It should be easy to see why both of these approaches are potentially biased. The best approach, one recommended by biostatisticians and advocates of **evidence-based medicine,** is to perform all analyses on the original groups to which the patients were randomized. The CASS study occurred several years ago, and no consensus existed at that time on the best way to analyze the findings. Therefore, the CASS investigators performed the analyses in several ways: by the original group (intention-to-treat), by the final groups of the study, and by eliminating all crossovers from the analysis. All of these methods gave the same result, namely that no difference in survival occurred, although later studies showed differences in quality-of-life indicators.

The intention-to-treat principle applies to studies other than those with survival as the outcome. We included the topic here, however, because it is so pertinent to survival studies. Gillings and Koch (1991) provide a comprehensive and very readable discussion.

SUMMARY

Special methods are needed to analyze data from studies of survival time because censored observations occur when patients enter at different times and remain in a study for different periods. Otherwise, investigators would have to wait until all subjects were in the study for a given period before analyzing the data. In medicine, survival curves are commonly drawn by the Kaplan–Meier product limit method and, less frequently, the actuarial (life table) method. The quality of survival studies published in the medical literature was reviewed by Altman and associates (1995). They found that almost half of the papers did not summarize the length of follow-up or clearly define all endpoints. They suggested some guidelines for presenting survival analyses in medical journals.

In the study by Lin and colleagues (2018), there was a statistical difference in the overall survival curve ($p = 0.015$) for patients on regorafenib alone versus a combination treatment. This difference along with the Kaplan–Meier curves were reported in the article.

We illustrated the Kaplan–Meier and actuarial methods for the length of survival time. The Kaplan–Meier method calculates survival each time a patient dies and provides exact estimates. Although generally more time-intensive to calculate, the widespread use of computers has made Kaplan–Meier curves the procedure of choice.

We concluded the chapter with a discussion of the important principle of intention-to-treat, whereby patients are analyzed in the group to which they were originally assigned. We described some of the problems in interpreting the results when this principle is not adhered to, and we pointed out the applicability of the intention-to-treat principle to any study, regardless of whether the outcome is survival or another variable.

 EXERCISES

1. A renal transplant surgeon compared two groups of patients who received kidney transplants.[*] One group underwent transplantation and received azathioprine to retard rejection of the transplanted organ. The other group was treated with cyclosporine, an immunomodulatory substance. Data are given on these two groups in Tables 9–8 and 9–9.

   a. Perform the calculations for Kaplan–Meier survival curves.

   b. Draw the survival curves. Do you think the survival curves are significantly different?

   c. Perform the logrank test, and interpret the results.

Table 9–8. Survival of kidney in patients having a transplant and receiving azathioprine.

Patient	Date of Transplant	Months in Study	Failed (0 = Censored
1	1-11-1978	2	1
2	1-18-1978	23	0
3	1-29-1978	23	0
4	4-4-1978	1	1
5	4-19-1978	20	0
6	5-10-1978	19	0
7	5-14-1978	3	1
8	5-21-1978	5	1
9	6-6-1978	17	1
10	6-17-1978	18	0
11	6-21-1978	18	0
12	7-22-1978	3	1
13	9-27-1978	15	0
14	10-5-1978	3	1
15	10-22-1978	14	0
16	11-15-1978	13	0
17	12-6-1978	12	0
18	12-12-1978	12	0
19	2-1-1979	10	0
20	2-16-1979	10	0
21	4-8-1979	8	0
22	4-11-1979	8	0
23	4-18-1979	8	0
24	6-26-1979	1	1
25	7-3-1979	5	0
26	7-12-1979	5	0
27	7-18-1979	1	1
28	8-23-1979	4	0
29	10-16-1979	2	0
30	12-12-1979	1	0
31	12-24-1979	1	0

Data from Dr. A. Birtch.

Table 9–9. Survival of kidney in patients having a transplant and receiving cyclosporine.

Patient	Date of Transplant	Months in Study	Failed (0 = Censored
1	2-8-1984	22	0
2	2-22-1984	22	0
3	2-25-1984	22	0
4	2-29-1984	8	1
5	3-12-1984	21	0
6	3-22-1984	1	1
7	4-26-1984	20	0
8	5-2-1984	19	0
9	5-9-1984	19	0
10	6-6-1984	18	0
11	7-11-1984	17	0
12	7-20-1984	17	0
13	8-18-1984	16	0
14	9-5-1984	15	0
15	9-15-1984	15	0
16	10-3-1984	14	0
17	11-9-1984	13	0
18	11-27-1984	6	1
19	12-5-1984	12	0
20	12-6-1984	12	0
21	12-19-1984	12	0

Data from Dr. A. Birtch.

a. Which serum MMP-14 level resulted in longer survival times? Was the longer survival sustained over a long period?

b. What is the value of the logrank statistic? What do you conclude from this value?

c. What are the potential biases in drawing conclusions about treatment method in this study?

3. Refer to Figure 9–5, illustrating the survival curves for the patients categorized by treatment (Lin et al, 2018) Is it possible to find the median survival for the two groups? If so, what is the median survival?

4. Kasurinen and colleagues (2018) also classified patients according to the Laurén classification (1 = intestinal, 2 = diffuse). Use the same n = 240 patients with MMP-14 values used in Exercise 2.

a. Use the previously downloaded data on the Kaplan–Meier curves for the number of years of survival for patients with intestinal and diffuse cancer.

b. Based on the graph, what would you conclude about the risk classification used in the study?

2. Kasurinen and colleagues (2018) wanted to determine if the level of serum MMP-14 impacted the survival of patients with gastric cancer.

Use the data to compare survival for patients with serum MMP-14 greater than 0.0729 (deemed high by the authors) to those with a lower MMP-14 level. The data file may be downloaded here: https://ndownloader.figshare.com/files/10158633. To complete the analysis, use only the subject with cancer and values for MMP-14 variable (n = 240).

(Hints: Refer to the article by Fox and Carvalho (2012) to guide your analysis in R. Note that the survival function in R should be coded 1 if died and 0 if censored).

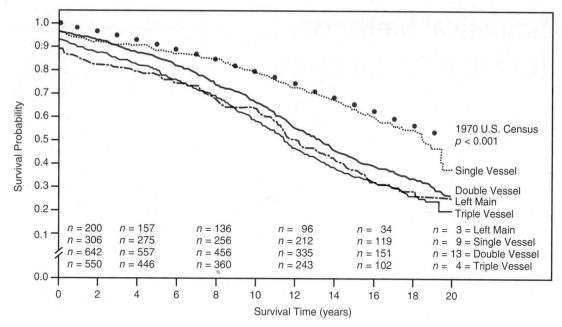

Figure 9–6. Survival probabilities for 1698 patients according to the extent of coronary artery disease before operation. (Reproduced with permission from Lawrie GM, Morris GC Jr, Earle N: Long-term results of coronary bypass surgery. Analysis of 1698 patients followed 15 to 20 years, *Ann Surg*. 1991 May;213(5):377-385.)

5. Refer to the MRFIT study discussed in Chapter 8 and used as a group exercise in that chapter. Refer to Figure 9–2 in the study: cumulative coronary heart disease and total mortality rates for the two groups. What statistical method is optimal for determining whether the two groups differed in either of these outcomes?

6. Outcomes in a cohort of patients who had had coronary artery bypass surgery 20 years earlier were described by Lawrie and coworkers (1991). Follow-up activities included physician visits, questionnaires, and telephone interviews at regular intervals. Data were available on 92% of the patients 20 years after surgery. The investigators examined survival for a number of subgroups and used the expected survival for age- and sex-adjusted population from the U.S. census to provide a baseline. The curves were calculated using the Kaplan–Meier method; groups defined by the vessel involved are given in Figure 9–6 It is important to recognize that coronary artery bypass surgery procedures have changed greatly since the time of this study, and today's patients enjoy more favorable long-term results.

a. Which group had the best survival?

b. Which group had the highest mortality rate?

c. What was the approximate median survival in each group?

Statistical Methods for Multiple Variables

10

KEY CONCEPTS

 The choice of statistical methods depends on the research question, the scales on which the variables are measured, and the number of variables to be analyzed.

 Many of the advanced statistical procedures can be interpreted as an extension or modification of multiple regression analysis.

 Many of the statistical methods used for questions with one independent variable have direct analogies with methods for multiple independent variables.

 The term "multivariate" is used when more than one independent variable is analyzed.

 Multiple regression is a simple and ideal method to control for confounding variables.

 Multiple regression coefficients indicate whether the relationship between the independent and dependent variables is positive or negative.

 Dummy, or indicator, coding is used when nominal variables are used in multiple regression.

 Regression coefficients indicate the amount the change in the dependent variable for each one-unit change in the X variable, holding other independent variables constant.

 Multiple regression measures a linear relationship only.

 The Multiple R statistic is the best indicator of how well the model fits the data—how much variance is accounted for by the model.

 Several methods can be used to select variables in a multivariate regression.

 Polynomial regression can be used when the relationship is curvilinear.

 Cross-validation tell us how applicable the model will be if we used it in another sample of subjects.

 A good rule of thumb is to have ten times as many subjects as variables.

 Analysis of covariance controls for confounding variables; it can be used as part of analysis of variance or in multiple regression.

 Logistic regression predicts a nominal outcome; it is the most widely used regression method in medicine.

 The regression coefficients in logistic regression can be transformed to give odds ratios.

 The Cox model is the multivariate analogue of the Kaplan–Meier curve; it predicts time-dependent outcomes when there are censored observations.

 The Cox model is also called the proportional hazard model; it is one of the most important statistical methods in medicine.

 Meta-analysis provides a way to combine the results from several studies in a quantitative way and is especially useful when studies have come to opposite conclusions or are based on small samples.

 An effect size is a measure of the magnitude of differences between two groups; it is a useful concept in estimating sample sizes.

The Cochrane Collection is a set of very well-designed meta-analyses and is available at libraries and online.

 Several methods are available when the goal is to classify subjects into groups.

 Multivariate analysis of variance, or MANOVA, is analogous to using ANOVA when there are several dependent variables.

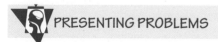 PRESENTING PROBLEMS

Presenting Problem 1

In Chapter 8, we examined the study by Neidert and colleagues (2016), studying the relationship between body composition measurements: plasma DPP-IV activity, gynoid fat, BMI, and lean mass.

The full article may be found here:
Neidert LE, Wainright KS, Zheng C, Babu JR, Kluess HA: Plasma dipeptidyl peptidase IV activity and measures of body composition in apparently healthy people. Heliyon 2016;2:e00097.

https://doi.org/10.1016/j.heliyon.2016.e00097

The data file may be downloaded from this link:
Neidert LE, Wainright KS, Zheng C, Babu JR, Kluess HA: Plasma dipeptidyl peptidase IV activity and measures of body composition in apparently healthy people. Dryad Digital Repository 2016.

https://doi.org/10.5061/dryad.2680t

Presenting Problem 2

Shah and colleagues (2018) studied patients with pulmonary hypertension (PHTN) to determine if their self-reported functional status could be used to predict postoperative outcomes. They used logistic regression to identify patients that may experience an extended length of stay in the hospital (>7 days) based on clinical indications. Shah and his coinvestigators (2018) wanted to develop a model to help hospital staff predict which patients with pulmonary hypertension may experience long postoperative stays in the hospital.

The article may be accessed here:
Shah AC, Ma K, Faraoni D, Oh DCS, Rooke GA, Van Norman GA: Self-reported functional status predicts post-operative outcomes in non-cardiac surgery patients with pulmonary hypertension. PLOS ONE 2018;13(8):e0201914.

https://doi.org/10.1371/journal.pone.0201914

The dataset used for the study may be accessed here:
Shah AC, Ma K, Faraoni D, Oh DCS, Rooke GA, Van Norman GA: Self-reported functional status predicts post-operative outcomes in non-cardiac surgery patients with pulmonary hypertension. Dryad Digital Repository 2018.

https://doi.org/10.5061/dryad.9236ng5

Presenting Problem 3

In the previous chapter, we used data from a study by Lin and colleagues (2018) to illustrate the Kaplan–Meier survival analysis method. The investigators studied two treatments for metastatic colon cancer. Please refer to Chapter 9 for more details.

The full article may be accessed here:
Lin C-Y, Lin T-H, Chen C-C, Chen M-C, Chen C-P: Combination chemotherapy with Regorafenib in metastatic colorectal cancer treatment: A single center, retrospective study. PLoS ONE 2018;13(1):e0190497.

https://doi.org/10.1371/journal.pone.0190497

The accompanying data file may be accessed here:

https://ndownloader.figshare.com/files/10158633

PURPOSE OF THE CHAPTER

The purpose of this chapter is to present a conceptual framework that applies to almost all the statistical procedures discussed so far in this text. We also describe some of the more advanced techniques used in medicine.

A Conceptual Framework

The previous chapters illustrated statistical techniques that are appropriate when the number of observations on each subject in a study is limited. For example, a *t* test is used when two groups of subjects are studied and the measure of interest is a single numerical variable—such as in Presenting Problem 1 in Chapter 6, which discussed differences in self-management activation in subjects with and without chronic disease (Bos-Touwen et al, 2015). When the outcome of interest is nominal, the chi-square test can be used—such as the Anderson et al (2018) study of flu vaccines (Chapter 6, Presenting Problem 3). Regression analysis is used to predict one numerical measure from another, such as in the study predicting percentage body fat (Neidert et al, 2016; Chapter 8, Presenting Problem 1).

Alternatively, each of these examples can be viewed conceptually as involving a set of subjects with two observations on each subject: (1) for the *t* test, one numerical variable, activation score, and one nominal (or group membership) variable, type II diabetes; (2) for the chi-square test, two nominal variables, flu vaccine and flu diagnosis after presenting with symptoms; (3) for regression, two numerical variables, percent body fat and body mass index. It is advantageous to look at research questions from this perspective because ideas are analogous to situations in which many variables are included in a study.

To practice viewing research questions from a conceptual perspective, let us reconsider Presenting Problem 1 in Chapter 7 by Dysangco et al (2017). The objective was to determine whether differences exist in HCL-C in patients who were HIV−, HIV+ with ART, and HIV+ without ART. The research question in this study may be viewed as involving a set of subjects with two observations per subject: one numerical variable, HDL-C, and one nominal (or group membership) variable, HIV status, with three categories. If only two categories were included for HIV status, the *t* test would be used. With more than two groups, however, one-way analysis of variance (ANOVA) is appropriate.

Many problems in medicine have more than two observations per subject because of the complexity involved in studying disease in humans. In fact, many of the presenting problems used in this text have multiple observations, although we chose to simplify the problems by examining only selected variables. One method involving more than two observations per subject has already been discussed: two-way ANOVA. Recall that in Presenting Problem 2 in Chapter 7, activities of daily living (ADL) was examined in various levels of cognitive impairment and gender (Cornelis et al, 2017). For this analysis, the investigators

Table 10–1. Summary of conceptual framework[a] for questions involving two variables.

Independent Variable	Dependent Variable	Method
Nominal	Nominal	Chi-square
Nominal (binary)	Numerical	*t* test[a]
Nominal (more than two values)	Numerical	One-way ANOVA[a]
Nominal	Numerical (censored)	Actuarial methods
Numerical	Numerical	Regression[b]

ANOVA, analysis of variance.
[a]Assuming the necessary assumptions (e.g., normality, independence, etc.) are met.
[b]Correlation is appropriate when neither variable is designated as independent or dependent.

classified subjects according to two nominal variables of cognitive impairment—Alzheimer's disease (AD) versus mild cognitive impairment (MCI) and gender—and one numerical variable, ADL functionality (i-ADL-CDI). If the term **independent variable** is used to designate the group membership variables (e.g., AD or MCI), or the *X* variable (e.g., blood pressure measured by a finger device), and the term **dependent** is used to designate the variables whose means are compared (e.g., i-ADL-CDI), or the *Y* variable (e.g., blood pressure measured by the cuff device), the observations can be summarized as in Table 10–1. (For the sake of simplicity, this summary omits ordinal variables; variables measured on an ordinal scale are often treated as if they are nominal.)

Introduction to Methods for Multiple Variables

Statistical techniques involving multiple variables are used increasingly in medical research, and several of them are illustrated in this chapter. The multiple-regression model, in which several independent variables are used to explain or predict the values of a single numerical response, is presented first, partly because it is a natural extension of the regression model for one independent variable illustrated in Chapter 8. More importantly, however, all the other advanced methods except meta-analysis can be viewed as modifications or extensions of the multiple-regression model. All except meta-analysis involve more than two independent variable observations per subject and are concerned with explanation or prediction.

Table 10–2. Summary of conceptual framework[a] for questions involving two or more independent (explanatory) variables.

Independent Variables	Dependent Variable	Method(s)
Nominal	Nominal	Log-linear
Nominal and numerical	Nominal (binary)	Logistic regression
Nominal and numerical	Nominal (2 or more categories)	Logistic regression Discriminant analysis[a] Cluster analysis Propensity scores CART
Nominal	Numerical	ANOVA[a] MANOVA[a]
Numerical	Numerical	Multiple regression[a]
Nominal and numerical	Numerical (censored)	Cox proportional hazard model
Confounding factors	Numerical	ANCOVA[a] MANOVA[a] GEE[a]
Confounding factors	Nominal	Mantel–Haenszel
Numerical only		Factor analysis

CART, classification and regression tree; ANOVA, analysis of variance; ANCOVA, analysis of covariance; MANOVA, multivariate analysis of variance; GEE, generalized estimating equations.
[a]Certain assumptions (e.g., multivariate normality, independence, etc.) are needed to use these methods.

The goal in this chapter is to present the logic of the different methods listed in Table 10–2 and to illustrate how they are used and interpreted in medical research. These methods are generally not mentioned in traditional introductory texts, and most people who take statistics courses do not learn about them until their third or fourth course. These methods are being used more frequently in medicine, however, partly because of the increased involvement of statisticians in medical research and partly because of the availability of complex statistical computer programs. In truth, few of these methods would be used very much in any field were it not for computers because of the time-consuming and complicated computations involved. To read the literature with confidence, especially studies designed to identify prognostic or risk factors, a reasonable acquaintance with the methods described in this chapter is required. Few of the available elementary books discuss multivariate methods. One that is directed toward statisticians is nevertheless quite readable (Chatfield, 1995); Katz (1999) is intended for readers of the medical literature and contains explanations of many of topics we discuss in this chapter (Dawson, 2000), as does Norman and Streiner (1996).

Before we examine the advanced methods, however, a comment on terminology is necessary. Some statisticians reserve the term "multivariate" to refer to situations that involve more than one dependent (or response) variable. By this strict definition, multiple regression and most of the other methods discussed in this chapter would not be classified as multivariate techniques. Other statisticians, ourselves included, use the term to also refer to methods that examine the simultaneous effect of multiple independent variables. By this definition, all the techniques discussed in this chapter (with the possible exception of some meta-analyses) are classified as multivariate.

MULTIPLE REGRESSION

Review of Regression

Simple linear regression (Chapter 8) is the method of choice when the research question is to predict the value of a response (dependent) variable, denoted Y, from an explanatory (independent) variable X. The regression model is

$$Y = a + bX$$

For simplicity of notation in this chapter we use Y to denote the dependent variable, even though Y', the predicted value, is actually given by this equation. We also use *a* and *b,* the sample estimates, instead of the population parameters, β_0 and β_1, where *a* is the intercept and *b* the **regression coefficient.** Please refer to Chapter 8 if you'd like to review simple linear regression.

Multiple Regression

⑤ The extension of simple regression to two or more independent variables is straightforward. For example, if four independent variables are being studied, the **multiple regression** model is

$$Y = a + b_1X_1 + b_2X_2 + b_3X_3 + b_4X_4$$

where X_1 is the first independent variable and b_1 is the regression coefficient associated with it, X_2 is the second independent variable and b_2 is the regression coefficient associated with it, and so on. This arithmetic equation is called a **linear combination;** thus, the response variable *Y* can be expressed as a (linear) combination of the explanatory variables. Note that a linear combination is really just a weighted average that gives a single number (or index) after the *X*'s are multiplied by their associated *b*'s and the *bX* products are added. The formulas for *a* and *b* were given in Chapter 8, but we do not give the formulas in multiple regression because they become more complex as the number of independent variables increases; and no one calculates them by hand, in any case.

The dependent variable *Y* must be a numerical measure. The traditional multiple-regression model calls for the independent variables to be numerical measures as well; however, nominal independent variables may be used, as discussed in the next section. To summarize, the appropriate technique for numerical independent variables and a single numerical dependent variable is the multiple regression model, as indicated in Table 10–2.

Multiple regression can be difficult to interpret, and the results may not be replicable if the independent variables are highly correlated with each other. In the extreme situation, two variables that are perfectly correlated are said to be collinear. When multicollinearity occurs, the variances of the regression coefficients are large so the observed value may be far from the true value. Ridge regression is a technique for analyzing multiple regression data that suffer from multicollinearity by reducing the size of standard errors. It is hoped that the net effect will be to give more reliable estimates. Another regression technique, principal components regression, is also available, but ridge regression is the more popular of the two methods.

Interpreting the Multiple Regression Equation

In the study by Neidert and colleagues (2016) (Presenting Problem 1 in Chapter 8), the goal of the study was to

Table 10–3. Means and standard deviations broken down by gender.

	Report			
Sex		**Age (yrs)**	**BMI (kg/m²)**	**% Fat**
F	Mean	24.63	23.39	32.28
	N	71	71	71
	Std. Deviation	8.82	3.80	6.54
M	Mean	27.20	24.54	21.36
	N	40	40	40
	Std. Deviation	10.85	3.69	7.84
Total	Mean	25.56	23.80	28.34
	N	111	111	111
	Std. Deviation	9.63	3.79	8.76

Data from Neidert LE, Wainright KS, Zheng C, et al: Plasma dipeptidyl peptidase IV activity and measures of body composition in apparently healthy people, *Heliyon.* 2016 Apr 18;2(4):e00097.

compile statistics regarding BMI, body fat percentage, and Plasma dipeptidyl peptidase IV for healthy people. We provide some basic information on these variables in Table 10–3 and see that the study included 71 females and 40 men.

Table 10–4 shows the regression equation to predict
⑥ percent body fat. Focusing initially on the *Coefficient Section,* we see that all the variables but age are statistically significantly related to percent body fat.

The first variable is a numerical variable, age, with regression coefficient, *b,* of 0.063, is not statistically significant ($p = 0.282$). The second variable, BMI, is also numerical; the regression coefficient of 1.142 indicates that patients with higher BMI also have higher percent body fat, which certainly makes sense.

The third variable, sex, is a binary variable having
⑦ two values. For regression models it is convenient to code binary variables as 0 and 1; in this example, females have a 0 code for sex, and males have a 1. This procedure, called **dummy** or **indicator coding,** allows investigators to include nominal variables in a regression equation in a straightforward manner. The dummy variables are interpreted as follows: A subject who is *male* has the code for males, 1, multiplied by the regression coefficient for sex, -12.389, resulting in 12.389 points being subtracted from his percent body fat. The decision of which value is assigned 1 and which is assigned 0 is an arbitrary decision made by the researcher but can be chosen to facilitate interpretations of interest to the researcher.

The regression coefficients can be used to predict percent body fat by multiplying a given patient's value

Table 10–4. Multiple regression predicting percent body fat.

⇒ Regression

Variables Entered/Removed[a]

Model	Variables Entered	Variables Removed	Method
1	Male, Age (yrs), BMI (kg/m2)[b]	.	Enter

a. Dependent Variable: % Fat

b. All requested variables entered.

Model Summary

Model	R	R Square	Adjusted R Square	Std. Error of the Estimate
1	.794[a]	.630	.620	5.402703898

a. Predictors: (Constant), Male, Age (yrs), BMI (kg/m2)

ANOVA[a]

Model		Sum of Squares	df	Mean Square	F	Sig.
1	Regression	5317.227	3	1772.409	60.721	.000[b]
	Residual	3123.245	107	29.189		
	Total	8440.472	110			

a. Dependent Variable: % Fat

b. Predictors: (Constant), Male, Age (yrs), BMI (kg/m2)

Coefficients[a]

Model		Unstandardized Coefficients		Standardized Coefficients	t	Sig.
		B	Std. Error	Beta		
1	(Constant)	4.008	3.283		1.221	.225
	Age (yrs)	.063	.058	.069	1.082	.282
	BMI (kg/m2)	1.142	.148	.494	7.705	.000
	Male	-12.389	1.083	-.682	-11.439	.000

a. Dependent Variable: % Fat

Data from Neidert LE, Wainright KS, Zheng C, et al: Plasma dipeptidyl peptidase IV activity and measures of body composition in apparently healthy people, *Heliyon.* 2016 Apr 18;2(4):e00097.

for each independent variable X by the corresponding regression coefficient b and then summing to obtain the predicted percent body fat.

Regression coefficients are interpreted differently in multiple regression than in simple regression. In simple regression, the regression coefficient b indicates the amount the predicted value of Y changes each time X increases by 1 unit. In multiple regression, a given regression coefficient indicates how much the predicted value of Y changes each

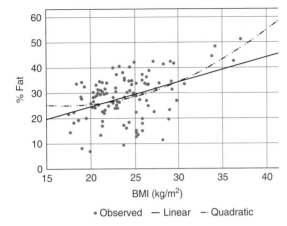

Figure 10–1. Plot illustrating the nonlinear relationship between BMI and percent body fat. Reproduced with permission from Neidert LE, Wainright KS, Zheng C, et al: Plasma dipeptidyl peptidase IV activity and measures of body composition in apparently healthy people, *Heliyon*. 2016 Apr 18;2(4):e00097.

time *X* increases by 1 unit, *holding the values of all other variables in the regression equation constant*—as though all subjects had the same value on the other variables. For example, predicted percent body fat is increased by 1.142 for increase of 1 unit in BMI, assuming all other variables are held constant. This feature of multiple regression makes it an ideal method to control for baseline differences and confounding variables, as we discuss in the section titled "Controlling for Confounding."

It bears repeating that multiple regression measures only the linear relationship between the independent variables and the dependent variable, just as in simple regression. The scatterplot between BMI and percent body fat is displayed in Figure 10–1. The figure indicates a curvilinear relationship, and it may be appropriate to transform BMI by taking its natural logarithm.

Standardized Regression Coefficients

Most authors present regression coefficients that can be used with individual subjects to obtain predicted *Y* values. But the size of the regression coefficients cannot be used to decide which independent variables are the most important, because their size is also related to the scale on which the variables are measured, just as in simple regression. For example, in Neidert and colleagues' study, we coded the sex variable 1 if male and 0 if female, and the variable age was coded as the number of years of age at the time of the first data collection.

Then, if sex and age are equally important in predicting percent body fat, the regression coefficient for sex would be much larger than the regression coefficient for age so that the same amount would be added to the prediction of percent body weight. These regression coefficients are sometimes called *unstandardized*; they cannot be used to draw conclusions about the importance of the variable. The coefficients may only be used to determine if the relationship with the dependent variable is positive or negative.* One way to eliminate the effect of scale is to *standardize* the regression coefficients. Standardization can be done by subtracting the mean value of *X* and dividing by the standard deviation before analysis, so that all variables have a mean of 0 and a standard deviation of 1. After this transformation, it is possible to compare the magnitudes of the regression coefficients and draw conclusions about which explanatory variables play an important role. It is also possible to calculate the standardized regression coefficients after the regression model has been developed.† The larger the standardized coefficient, the larger the value of the *t* statistic. **Standardized regression coefficients** are often referred to as beta (β) coefficients. The major disadvantage of standardized regression coefficients is that they cannot readily be used to predict outcome values. The "Coefficients" section of Table 10–4 also contains the standardized regression coefficients for the variables used to predict percent body fat in Neidert and colleagues' study. Using the standardized coefficients in Table 10–4, can you determine which variable, BMI or sex, has more influence in predicting percent body fat? If you chose sex, you are correct, because the absolute value of its standardized coefficient is larger, 0.682, compared with 0.494 for BMI.

Multiple *R*

Multiple *R* is the multiple-regression analogue of the Pearson product moment correlation coefficient *r*. It is also called the coefficient of multiple determination, but most authors use the shorter term. As an example, suppose percent body fat is calculated for each person in the study by Niedert and colleagues; then, the correlation between predicted percent body fat and the actual percent body fat is calculated. This correlation is the multiple *R*. If the multiple *R* is squared (R^2), it measures how much of the variation in

---

*Technically, it is possible for the regression coefficient and the correlation to have different signs. If so, the variable is called a moderator variable; it affects the relationship between the dependent variable and another independent variable.
†The standardized coefficient = the unstandardized coefficient multiplied by the standard deviation of the *X* variable and divided by the standard deviation of the *Y* variable: $\beta_j = b_j \ (SD_X/SD_Y)$.

the actual depression score is accounted for by knowing the information included in the regression equation. The term R^2 is interpreted in exactly the same way as r^2 in simple correlation and regression, with 0 indicating no variance accounted for and 1.00 indicating 100% of the variance accounted for. Recall that in simple regression, the correlation between the actual value Y of the dependent variable and the predicted value, denoted Y', is the same as the correlation between the dependent variable and the independent variable; that is, $r_{Y'Y} = r_{XY}$. Thus, R and R^2 in multiple regression play the same role as r and r^2 in simple regression. The statistical test for R and R^2, however, uses the F distribution instead of the t distribution.

The computations are time-consuming, and fortunately, computers do them for us. After BMI, age, and race are entered into the regression equation, $R^2 = 0.63$ indicates that more than 63% of the variability in percent body fat is accounted for by knowing patients' BMI, age, and race. Because R^2 is less than 1, we know that factors other than those included in the study also play a role in determining a person's percent body fat.

Selecting Variables for Regression Models

The primary purpose of Neidert and colleagues in their study of DPP-IV activity, BMI and percent body fat was explanation; they used multiple regression analysis to learn how specific characteristics confounded the relationship between DPP-IV activity, BMI and percent body fat. They also wanted to know how the characteristics interacted with one another, such as gender and type of fat. Some research questions, however, focus on the prediction of the outcome, such as using the regression equation to predict of percent body fat in future subjects.

Deciding on the variables that provide the best prediction is a process sometimes referred to as **model building.** Selecting the variables for regression models can be accomplished in several ways. In one approach, all variables are introduced into the regression equation, called the "enter" method in SPSS and used in the linear model procedure in R. Then, especially if the purpose is prediction, the variables that do not have significant regression coefficients are eliminated from the equation. The regression equation may be recalculated using only the variables retained because the regression coefficients have different values when some variables are removed from the analysis.

Computer programs also contain routines to select an optimal set of explanatory variables. One such procedure is called **forward selection.** Forward selection begins with one variable in the regression equation; then, additional variables are added one at a time until all statistically significant variables are included in the equation. The first variable in the regression equation is the X variable that has the highest correlation with the response variable Y. The next X variable considered for the regression equation is the one that increases R^2 by the largest amount. If the increment in R^2 is statistically significant by the F test, it is included in the regression equation. This step-by-step procedure continues until no X variables remain that produce a significant increase in R^2. The values for the regression coefficients are calculated, and the regression equation resulting from this forward selection procedure can be used to predict outcomes for future subjects.

A similar **backward elimination** procedure can also be used; in it, all variables are initially included in the regression equation. The X variable that would reduce R^2 by the smallest increment is removed from the equation. If the resulting decrease is not statistically significant, that variable is permanently removed from the equation. Next, the remaining X variables are examined to see which produces the next smallest decrease in R^2. This procedure continues until the removal of an X variable from the regression equation causes a significant reduction in R^2. That X variable is retained in the equation, and the regression coefficients are calculated.

When features of both the forward selection and the backward elimination procedures are used together, the method is called **stepwise regression** (stepwise selection). Stepwise selection is commonly used in the medical literature; it begins in the same manner as forward selection. After each addition of a new X variable to the equation, however, all previously entered X variables are checked to see whether they maintain their level of significance. Previously entered X variables are retained in the regression equation only if their removal would cause a significant reduction in R^2. The forward versus backward versus stepwise procedures have subtle advantages related to the correlations among the independent variables that cannot be covered in this text. They do not generally produce identical regression equations, but conceptually, all approaches determine a "parsimonious" equation using a subset of explanatory variables.

Some statistical programs examine all possible combinations of predictor values and determine the one that produces the overall highest R^2. We do not recommend this procedure, however, and suggest that a more appealing approach is to build a model in a logical way. Variables are sometimes grouped according to their function, such as all demographic characteristics, and added to the regression equation as a group or block; this process is often called **hierarchical regression;** see Exercise 7 for an example. The advantage of a logical approach to building a regression model is that, in general, the results tend to be more stable and reliable and are more likely to be replicated in similar studies.

Polynomial Regression

Polynomial regression is a special case of multiple regression in which each term in the equation is a power of X. Polynomial regression provides a way to fit a regression model to curvilinear relationships and is an alternative to transforming the data to a linear scale. For example, the following equation can be used to predict a quadratic relationship:

$$Y = b_0 + b_1 X + b_2 X^2$$

If a linear and cubic term do not provide an adequate fit, a cubic term, a fourth-power term, and so on, can also be included until an adequate fit is obtained.

Neidert and colleagues (2016) did not use polynomial regression to fit curves for DPP-IV, but we can evaluate the potential fit for polynomial regression. Two approaches to polynomial regression can be used. The first method calculates squared terms, cubic terms, and so on; these terms are then entered one at a time using multiple regression. Another approach is to use a program that permits curve fitting, such as the regression curve estimation procedure in SPSS.

Missing Observations

When studies involve several variables, some observations on some subjects may be missing. Controlling the problem of missing data is easier in studies in which information is collected prospectively; it is much more difficult when information is obtained from already existing records, such as patient charts. Two important factors are the percentage of observations that is missing and whether missing observations are randomly missing or missing because of some causal factor.

For example, suppose a researcher designs a case–control study to examine the effect of leg length inequality on the incidence of loosening of the femoral component after total hip replacement. Cases are patients who developed loosening of the femoral component, and controls are patients who did not. In reviewing the records of routine follow-up, the researcher found that leg length inequality was measured in some patients by using weight-bearing anterior–posterior (AP) hip and lower extremity films, whereas other patients had measurements taken using non-weight-bearing films. The type of film ordered during follow-up may well be related to whether the patient complained of hip pain; patients with symptoms were more likely to have received the weight-bearing films, and patients without symptoms were more likely to have had the routine non-weight-bearing films. A researcher investigating this question must not base the leg length inequality measures on weight-bearing films only, because controls are less likely than cases to have weight-bearing film measures in their records. In this situation, the missing leg length information occurred because of symptoms and not randomly.

The potential for missing observations increases in studies involving multiple variables. Depending on the cause of the missing observations, solutions include dropping subjects who have missing observations from the study, deleting variables that have missing values from the study, or substituting some value for the missing data, such as the mean or a predicted value, called imputing. SPSS has an option to estimate missing data with the mean for that variable calculated with the subjects who had the data. R provides the option removing records with missing values or substituting either the mean or a predicted score. Investigators in this situation should seek advice from a statistician on the best way to handle the problem.

Cross Validation

The statistical procedures for all regression models are based on correlations among the variables, which, in turn, are related to the amount of variation in the variables included in the study. Some of the observed variation in any variable, however, occurs simply by chance; and the same degree of variation does not occur if another sample is selected and the study is replicated. The mathematical procedures for determining the regression equation cannot distinguish between real and chance variation. If the equation is to be used to predict outcomes for future subjects, it should, therefore, be validated on a second sample, a process called **cross validation.** The regression equation is used to predict the outcome in the second sample, and the predicted outcomes are compared with the actual outcomes; the correlation between the predicted and actual values indicates how well the model fits. Cross-validating the regression equation gives a realistic evaluation of the usefulness of the prediction it provides.

In medical research we rarely have the luxury of cross-validating the findings on another sample of the same size. Several alternative methods exist. First, researchers can hold out a proportion of the subjects for cross validation, perhaps 20% or 25%. The holdout sample should be randomly selected from the entire sample prior to the original analysis. The predicted outcomes in the holdout sample are compared with the actual outcomes, often using R^2 to judge how well the findings cross-validate.

Another method is the **jackknife** in which one observation is left out of the sample, call it x_1; regression is performed using the $n − 1$ observations, and the results are applied to x_1. Then this observation is returned to the sample, and another, x_2, is held out.

This process continues until there is a predicted outcome for each observation in the sample; the predicted and actual outcomes are then compared.

The **bootstrap** method works in a similar manner, although the goal is different. The bootstrap can be used with small samples to estimate the standard error and confidence intervals. A small hold-out sample is randomly selected and the statistic of interest calculated. Then the hold-out sample is returned to the original sample, and another hold-out sample is selected. After a fairly large number of samples is analyzed, generally a minimum of 200, standard errors and confidence intervals can be estimated. In essence, the bootstrap method uses the data itself to determine the sampling distribution rather than the central limit theorem discussed in Chapter 4.

Both the jackknife and bootstrap are called resampling methods; they are very computer-intensive and require special software.

It is possible to estimate the magnitude of R or R^2 in another sample without actually performing the cross validation. This R^2 is smaller than the R^2 for the original sample, because the mathematical formula used to obtain the estimate removes the chance variation. For this reason, the formula is called a formula for *shrinkage*. Many computer programs, including R, SPSS, and SAS, provide both R^2 for the sample used in the analysis as well as R^2 adjusted for shrinkage, often referred to as the adjusted R^2. Refer to Table 10–4 where SPSS gives the "Adjusted R Square" in the Model Summary section of the analysis.

Sample Size Requirements

The only easy way to determine how large a sample is needed in multiple regression or any multivariate technique is to use a computer program. Some rules of thumb, however, may be used for guidance. A common recommendation by statisticians calls for ten times as many subjects as the number of independent variables. For example, this rule of thumb prescribes a minimum of 60 subjects for a study predicting the outcome from six independent variables. Having a large ratio of subjects to variables decreases problems that may arise because assumptions are not met.

Assumptions about normality in multiple regression are complicated, depending on whether the independent variables are viewed as fixed or random (as in fixed-effects model or random-effects model in ANOVA), and they are beyond the scope of this text. To ensure that estimates of regression coefficients and multiple R and R^2 are accurate representatives of actual population values, we suggest that investigators never perform regression without at least five times as many subjects as variables.

A more accurate estimate is found by using a computer power program. We used the G*power program to find the power of a study using five predictor variables. We posed the question: How many subjects are needed to test whether a given variable increases R^2 by 0.05, given that four variables are already in the regression equation and they collectively provide an R^2 of 0.50? The output from the program is shown in Box 10–1. The power analysis indicates that a sample of 85 gives power of 0.80, assuming an α or p value of 0.05. The accompanying graph shows the power curve for different sample sizes and different values of α.

CONTROLLING FOR CONFOUNDING

Analysis of Covariance

Analysis of covariance (ANCOVA) is the statistical technique used to control for the influence of a confounding variable. **Confounding variables** occur most often when subjects cannot be assigned at random to different groups, that is, when the groups of interest already exist. Guo and colleagues (2018) (Chapters 7 and 8) predicted overall fitness as measured by VO2_max based on the Ruffier Index (RI); they wanted to control for age of the subjects and did so by adding age to the regression equation. When RI alone is used to predict fitness (VO2max mlO2/min/kg), the regression equation is

$$VO2max = 44.237 - 0.793 \times RI$$

where VO2max is the fitness level. Using this equation, a fitness level is predicted to decrease by 0.793 for each increase of 1 in RI. For instance, a woman with a RI of 10 has a predicted VO2max of 36.3. What would happen, however, if age were also related to VO2max? A way to control for the possible confounding effect of age is to include that variable in the regression equation. The equation with age included is

$$VO2max = 59.650 - 0.952 \times RI - 0.446 \times AGE$$

Using this equation, fitness level is predicted to decrease by 0.952 for each increase of 1 in RI, *holding age constant* or *independent of age*. A 30-year-old with a RI of 10 has a predicted VO2max of 36.75, whereas a 20-year-old with the same RI of 10 has a predicted VO2max of 41.21.

A more traditional use of ANCOVA is illustrated by a study of the negative influence of smoking on the cardiovascular system. Investigators wanted to know whether smokers have more ventricular wall motion abnormalities than nonsmokers (Hartz et al, 1984). They might use a t test to determine whether the mean number of wall motion abnormalities differ in these two groups. The investigators know, however,

BOX 10-1. ESTIMATION OF SAMPLE SIZE FOR MULTIPLE REGRESSION USING G*POWER.

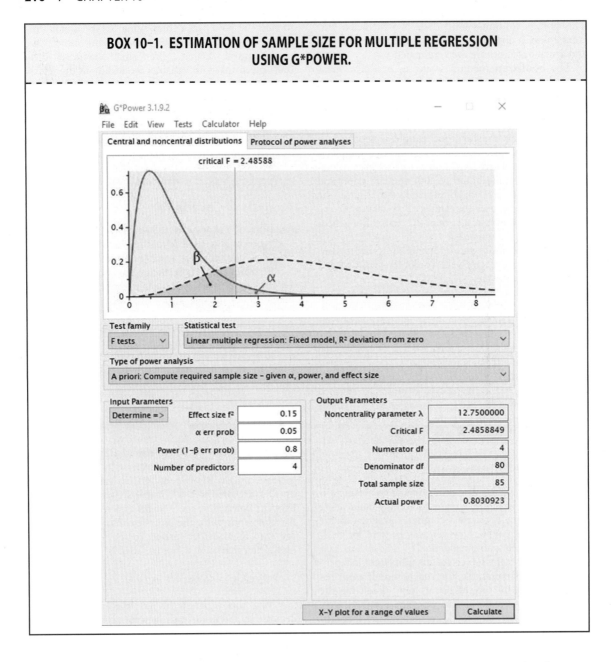

that wall motion abnormalities are also related to the degree of coronary stenosis, and smokers generally have a greater degree of coronary stenosis. Thus, any difference observed in the mean number of wall abnormalities between smokers and nonsmokers may really be a difference in the amount of coronary stenosis between these two groups of patients.

This situation is illustrated in the graph of hypothetical data in Figure 10–2; in the figure, the relationship between occlusion scores and wall motion abnormalities appears to be the same for smokers and nonsmokers. Nonsmokers, however, have both lower occlusion scores and lower numbers of wall motion abnormalities; smokers have higher occlusion scores and higher numbers of wall motion abnormalities. The question is whether the difference in wall motion abnormalities is due to smoking, to occlusion, or to both.

In this study, the investigators must control for the degree of coronary stenosis so that it does not confound (or confuse) the relationship between smoking and wall motion abnormalities. Useful methods to control for confounding variables are analysis of covariance (ANCOVA) and the Mantel–Haenszel chi-square procedure. Table 10–2 specifies ANCOVA when the dependent variable is numerical (e.g., wall motion) and the independent measures are grouping variables on a nominal scale (e.g., smoking vs. nonsmoking), and confounding variables occur (e.g., degree of coronary occlusion). If the dependent measure is also nominal, such as whether a patient has survived to a given time, the Mantel–Haenszel chi-square discussed in Chapter 9 can be used to control for the effect of a confounding (nuisance) variable. ANCOVA can be performed by using the methods of ANOVA; however, most medical studies use one of the regression methods discussed in this chapter.

If ANCOVA is used in this example, the occlusion score is called the **covariate,** and the mean number of wall motion abnormalities in smokers and nonsmokers is said to be *adjusted for* the occlusion score (or degree of coronary stenosis). Put another way, ANCOVA simulates the Y outcome observed if the value of X is held constant, that is, if all the patients had the same degree of coronary stenosis. This adjustment is achieved by calculating a regression equation to predict mean number of wall motion abnormalities from the covariate, degree of coronary stenosis, and from a dummy variable coded 1 if the subject is a member of the group (i.e., a smoker) and 0 otherwise. For example, the regression equation determined for the hypothetical observations in Figure 10–2 is

$$Y = -0.19 + 0.01 \times \text{Occlusion score} + 1.28 \text{ if a smoker}$$

The equation illustrates that smokers have a larger number of predicted wall motion abnormalities, because 1.28 is added to the equation if the subject is a smoker. The equation can be used to obtain the mean number of wall motion abnormalities in each group, adjusted for degree of coronary stenosis.

If the relationship between coronary stenosis and ventricular motion is ignored, the mean number of wall motion abnormalities, calculated from the observations in Figure 10–2, is 3.33 for smokers and 1.00 for nonsmokers. If, however, ANCOVA is used to control for degree of coronary stenosis, the adjusted mean wall motion is 2.81 for smokers and 1.53 for nonsmokers, a difference of 1.28, represented by the regression coefficient for the dummy variable for smoking. In ANCOVA, the adjusted Y mean for a given group is obtained by (1) finding the difference between the

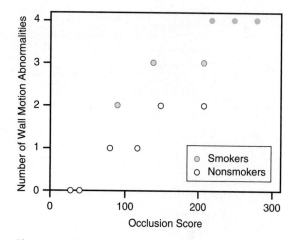

Figure 10–2. Relationship between degree of coronary stenosis and ventricular wall motion abnormalities in smokers and nonsmokers (hypothetical data).

group's mean on the covariate variable X, denoted, and the grand mean; (2) multiplying the difference by the regression coefficient; and (3) subtracting this product from the unadjusted mean. Thus, for group j, the adjusted mean is (See Exercise 1.)

$$\text{Adjusted } \overline{Y}_j = \text{Unadjusted } \overline{Y}_j - b(\overline{X}_j - \overline{\overline{X}})$$

This result is consistent with our knowledge that coronary stenosis alone has some effect on abnormality of wall motion; the unadjusted means contain this effect as well as any effect from smoking. Therefore, controlling for the effect of coronary stenosis results in a smaller difference in number of wall motion abnormalities, a difference related only to smoking.

Using hypothetical data, Figure 10–3 illustrates schematically the way ANCOVA adjusts the mean of the dependent variable if the covariate is important. Using unadjusted means is analogous to using a separate regression line for each group. For example, the mean value of Y for group 1 is found by using the regression line drawn through the group 1 observations to project the mean value $\overline{X}_1$ onto the Y-axis, denoted $\overline{Y}_1$ in Figure 10–3. Similarly, the mean of group 2 is found at $\overline{Y}_2$ by using the regression line to project the mean $\overline{X}_2$ in that group. The Y means in each group *adjusted for the covariate* (stenosis) are analogous to the projections based on the overall mean value of the covariate; that is, as though the two groups had the same mean value for the covariate. The adjusted means for groups 1 and 2, Adj. $\overline{Y}_1$ and Adj. $\overline{Y}_2$, are illustrated

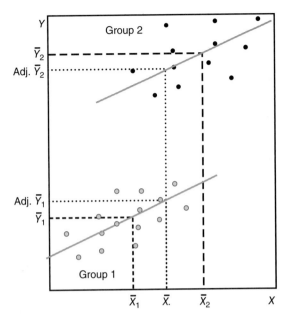

Figure 10–3. Illustration of means adjusted using analysis of covariance.

by the dotted line projections of $\overline{X}$ from each separate regression line in Figure 10–3.

ANCOVA assumes that the relationship between the covariate (X variable) and the dependent variable (Y) is the same in both groups, that is, that any relationship between coronary stenosis and wall motion abnormality is the same for smokers and nonsmokers. This assumption is equivalent to requiring that the regression slopes be the same in both groups; geometrically, ANCOVA asks whether a difference exists between the intercepts, assuming the slopes are equal.

ANCOVA is an appropriate statistical method in many situations that occur in medical research. For example, age is a variable that affects almost everything studied in medicine; if preexisting groups in a study have different age distributions, investigators must adjust for age before comparing the groups on other variables, just as Gonzalo and colleagues (1996) recognized. The methods illustrated in Chapter 3 to adjust mortality rates for characteristics such as age and birth weight are used when information is available on groups of individuals; when information is available on individuals themselves, ANCOVA is used.

Before leaving this section, we point out some important aspects of ANCOVA. First, although only two groups were included in the example, ANCOVA can be used to adjust for the effect of a confounding variable in more than two groups. In addition, it is possible to adjust for more than one confounding variable in the same study, and the confounding variables may be either nominal or numerical. Thus, it is easy to see why the multiple regression model for analysis of covariance provides an ideal method to incorporate confounding variables.

Finally, ANCOVA can be considered as a special case of the more general question of comparing two regression lines (discussed in Chapter 8). In ANCOVA, we assume that the slopes are equal, and attention is focused on the intercept. We can also perform the more global test of both slope and intercept, however, by using multiple regression. In Presenting Problem 1 in Chapter 8 on percent body fat (Neidert et al, 2016), interest focused on comparing the regression lines predicting percent body fat from body mass index (BMI) in men and women. ANCOVA can be used for this comparison using dummy coding. If we let X be BMI, Y be percent body fat, and Z be a dummy variable, where $Z = 1$ for men and $Z = 0$ for women, then the multiple-regression model for testing whether the two regression lines are the same (coincident) is

$$Y = a + b_1 X + b_2 Z + b_3 XZ$$

The regression lines have equal slopes and are parallel when b_3 is 0, that is, no interaction between the independent variable X and the group membership variable Z. The regression lines have equal intercepts and equal slopes (are coincident) if both b_2 and b_3 are 0; thus, the model becomes the simple regression equation $Y = a + bX$. The statistical test for b_2 and b_3 is the t test discussed in the section titled, "Statistical Tests for the Regression Coefficient."

Generalized Estimating Equations (GEE)

Many research designs, including both observational studies and clinical trials, concern observations that are clustered or hierarchical. A group of methods has been developed for these special situations. To illustrate, a study to examine the effect of different factors on complication rates following total knee arthroplasty was undertaken in a province of Canada (Kreder et al, 2003). Outcomes included length of hospital stay, inpatient complications, and mortality. Can the researchers examine the outcomes for patients and conclude that any differences are due to the risk factors? The statistical methods we have examined thus far assume that one observation is independent from another. The problem with this study design, however, is that the outcome for patients operated on by the same surgeon may be related to factors other than the surgical method, such as the skill level of the surgeon. In this situation, patients are said to be nested within physicians.

Many other examples come to mind. Comparing the efficacy of medical education curricula is difficult because students are nested within medical schools. Comparing health outcomes for children within a community is complicated by the fact that children are nested within families. Many clinical trials create nested situations, such as when trials are carried out in several medical centers. The issue arises of how to define the unit of analysis—should it be the students or the school? The children or the families? The patients or the medical center?

The group of methods that accommodates these types of research questions include generalized estimating equations (GEE), multilevel modeling, and the analysis of hierarchically structured data. Most of these methods have been developed within the last decade and statistical software is just now becoming widely available. In addition to some specialized statistical packages R, SAS, Stata, and SPSS contain procedures to accommodate hierarchical data. Using these models is more complex than some of the other methods we have discussed, and it is relatively easy to develop a model that is meaningless or misleading. Investigators who have research designs that involve nested subjects should consult a biostatistician for assistance.

PREDICTING NOMINAL OR CATEGORICAL OUTCOMES

In the regression model discussed in the previous section, the outcome or dependent Y variable is measured on a numerical scale. When the outcome is measured on a nominal scale, other approaches must be used. Table 10–2 indicates that several methods can be used to analyze problems with several independent variables when the dependent variable is nominal. First we discuss logistic regression, a method that is frequently used in the health field. One reason for the popularity of logistic regression is that many outcomes in health are nominal, actually binary, variables—they either occur or do not occur. The second reason is that the regression coefficients obtained in logistic regression can be transformed into odds ratios. So, in essence, logistic regression provides a way to obtain an odds ratio for a given risk factor that controls for, or is adjusted for, confounding variables; in other words, we can do analysis of covariance with logistic regression as well as with multiple linear regression.

Other methods are log-linear analysis and several methods that attempt to classify subjects into

groups. These methods appear occasionally in the medical literature, and we provide a brief illustration, primarily so that readers can have an intuitive understanding of their purpose. The classification methods are discussed in the section titled "Methods for Classification."

Logistic Regression

Logistic regression is commonly used when the independent variables include both numerical and nominal measures and the outcome variable is binary (dichotomous). Logistic regression can also be used when the outcome has more than two values (Hosmer and Lemeshow, 2000), but its most frequent use is as in Presenting Problem 2, which illustrates the use of logistic regression to identify patients that may experience an extended length of stay in the hospital (>7 days) based on clinical indications. Shah and his coinvestigators (2018) wanted to develop a model to help hospital staff predict which patients with pulmonary hypertension may experience long postoperative stays in the hospital. The logistic model gives the probability that the outcome, such as length of stay longer than 7 days, occurs as an exponential function of the independent variables. For example, with three independent variables, the model is

$$P_X = \frac{1}{1 + \exp[-(b_0 + b_1 X_1 + b_2 X_2 + b_3 X_3)]}$$

where b_0 is the intercept, b_1, b_2, and b_3 are the regression coefficients, and exp indicates that the base of the natural logarithm (2.718) is taken to the power shown in parentheses (i.e., the antilog). The equation can be derived by specifying the variables to be included in the equation or by using a variable selection method similar to the ones for multiple regression. A chi-square test (instead of the t or F test) is used to determine whether a variable adds significantly to the prediction.

In the study described in Presenting Problem 2, the variables used by the investigators to predict long hospital stays included the variables listed in Table 10–5. The investigators coded the values of the independent variables as 0 and 1, a method useful both for dummy variables in multiple regression and for variables in logistic regression. This practice makes it easy to interpret the odds ratio. In addition, if a goal is to develop a score, as is the case in the study by Shah and coinvestigators, the coefficient associated with a given variable needs to be included in the score only if the patient has a 1 on that variable. For instance, if patients are more likely to

Table 10–5. Variables, codes, and frequencies for variables.[a]

	Value	Frequency
ASA		
<= 3	0	420
>3	1	130
Poor Functional Status		
No	0	277
Yes	1	273
Severe Hypertension		
Yes	0	365
No	1	185
Open Surgical Approach		
No	0	258
Yes	1	292
Procedure Length		
<= 2 hours	0	350
>2 hours	1	197
Severe PHTN		
No	0	477
Yes	1	50

[a]Not all totals are the same because of missing data on some variables.
Data from Shah AC , Ma K, Faraoni D, et al: Self-reported functional status predicts post-operative outcomes in non-cardiac surgery patients with pulmonary hypertension, *PLoS One.* 2018 Aug 16;13(8):e0201914.

have a LOS >7 for a procedure less than 2 hours, the score associated with length of procedure would not be included, since the value of the procedure length variable would be 0. The results of the analysis are given in Table 10–6.

We need to know which value is coded 1 and which 0 in order to interpret the results. Interpreting the equation for the variables indicates that patients with ASA >3, poor function status, no severe HTN (sHTN) with an open surgical procedure of duration longer than 2 hours are at the most risk for a length of stay longer than 7 days. The column in Table 10–6 labeled "Exp(B)" is the relative risk for the value of 1 versus 0 for each risk factor. Any coefficients with an Exp(B) of greater than 1 increases the risk of a length of stay longer than 7; those with an Exp(B) of less than 1 are protective.

The logistic equation can be used to find the probability for any given individual. For instance, let us find the probability that a patient with an ASA of 1, poor functional status, no sHTN, and a 1-hour open surgical procedure has a length of stay longer than 7 days. The regression coefficients from Table 10–6 are:

$$-3.246$$
$$+0.887 \times [ASA > 3]$$
$$+0.754 \times [\text{poor functional status}]$$
$$+0.632 \times [\text{No sHTN}]$$
$$+1.084 \times [\text{open approach}]$$
$$+0.838 \times [\text{longer than 2 hours}]$$

and we evaluate it as follows:

$$-3.246 +$$
$$0.887 \times [0]$$
$$+0.754 \times [1]$$
$$+0.632 \times [1]$$
$$+1.084 \times [1]$$
$$+0.838 \times [0]$$
$$= -0.776$$

Substituting -0.776 in the equation for the probability:

$$p_x = \frac{1}{1 + \exp[-(b_0 + b_1 X_1 + b_2 X_2 + b_3 X_3)]}$$
$$= \frac{1}{1 + \exp[-(-0.776)]} = \frac{1}{1 + 2.173} = 0.315$$

Therefore, the chance that this patient has a long LOS is 31.5%. See Exercise 3 to determine the likelihood of a patient with an ASA = 1, poor functional status, and severe hypertension, undergoing an open surgical procedure of 1.5 hours, stays longer than 7 days.

One advantage of logistic regression is that it requires no assumptions about the distribution of the independent variables. Another is that the regression coefficient can be interpreted in terms of relative risks in cohort studies or odds ratios in case–control studies. In other words, the relative risk of a LOS >7 after a surgical procedure over 2 hours is exp (0.838) = 2.31. The relative risk for a short procedure is the reciprocal, 1/2.31 = 0.433; therefore, patients undergoing a procedure over 2 hours in duration are more than two times more likely to have a long length of stay as those having shorter duration procedures.

How can readers easily tell which relative risks are statistically significant? Recall from Chapter 8 that if the 95% confidence interval does not include 1, we can

Table 10–6. Logistic regression model for LOS greater than 7

		B	S.E.	Wald	df	Sig.	Exp(B)	95% C.I.for EXP(B)	
Variables in the Equation									
								Lower	Upper
Step 1[a]	ASA<=3;>3(1)	.887	.240	13.717	1	.000	2.428	1.518	3.883
	POOR Functional Status(1)	.754	.234	10.378	1	.001	2.126	1.344	3.364
	NO sHTN(1)	.632	.236	7.153	1	.007	1.882	1.184	2.990
	OPEN Surgical Approach (1)	1.084	.249	18.968	1	.000	2.957	1.815	4.817
	Proc Length <=2/>2(1)	.838	.230	13.271	1	.000	2.311	1.473	3.628
	Constant	−3.246	.305	113.039	1	.000	.039		

Classification Table[b]

			Predicted		
			CORRECT LOS >7		Percentage Correct
	Observed		0	1	
Step 1	CORRECT LOS > 7	0	409	22	94.9
		1	90	26	22.4
	Overall Percentage				79.5

[a]Variable(s) entered on step 1: ASA<=3/>3, POOR Functional Status, NO sHTN, OPEN Surgical Approach , Proc Length <=2/>2.
[b]The cut value is .500.
Data from Shah AC , Ma K, Faraoni D, et al: Self-reported functional status predicts post-operative outcomes in non-cardiac surgery patients with pulmonary hypertension, *PLoS One.* 2018 Aug 16;13(8):e0201914.

be 95% sure that the factor associated with the odds ratio either is a significant risk or provides a significant level of protection. Do any of the independent variables in Table 10–6 have a 95% confidence interval for the odds ratio that contains 1?

The overall results from a logistic regression may be tested with **Hosmer and Lemeshow's goodness of fit test.** The test is based on the chi-square distribution. A p value ≥ 0.05 means that the model's estimates fit the data at an acceptable level.

There is no straightforward statistic to judge the overall logistic model as R^2 is used in multiple regression. Some statistical programs give R^2, but it cannot be interpreted as in multiple regression because the predicted and observed outcomes are nominal. Several other statistics are available as well, including Cox and Snell's R^2 and a modification called Nagelkerke's R^2, which is generally larger than Cox and Snell's R^2.

Before leaving the topic of logistic regression, it is worthwhile to inspect the classification table in Table 10–6. This table gives the actual and the predicted number of patients with LOS greater than 7 versus 7 or less. The logistic equation tends to under predict those with long LOS: 46 are predicted versus the 116 who actually had LOS >7. Overall, the

prediction using the logistic equation correctly classified 79.5% of these patients. Although this sounds rather impressive, it is important to compare this percentage with the baseline: 78.8% of the time we would be correct if we simply predicted each patient to have a LOS of 7 or less. Can you recall an appropriate way to compensate for or take the baseline into consideration? Although computer programs typically do not provide the kappa statistic, discussed in Chapter 5, it provides a way to evaluate the percentage correctly classified (see Exercise 4). Other measures of association are used so rarely in medicine that we did not discuss them in Chapter 8. SPSS provides two nonparametric correlations, the lambda correlation and the tau correlation, that can be interpreted as measures of strength of the relationship between observed and predicted outcomes.

Log-Linear Analysis

Psoriasis, a chronic, inflammatory skin disorder characterized by scaling erythematous patches and plaques of skin, has a strong genetic influence—about one-third of patients have a positive family history. Stuart and colleagues (2002) conducted a study to determine differences in clinical manifestation between patients with

Table 10–7. Frequency of joint complaints by familial status, stratified by age at examination.

Age at Examination (years)	Joint Complaints (%)		Relative risk	Pearson X^2	p value
	Sporadic	Familial			
0–20	0.0	0.0	—	—	—
21–30	14.6	19.4	1.41	0.32	0.57
31–40	26.6	40.9	1.91	3.33	0.068
41–50	20.5	26.8	1.42	0.43	0.51
51–60	47.1	47.3	1.01	0.00024	0.99
>60	28.6	45.3	2.07	0.72	0.40
Total	312	34.0	2.09	13.32	0.00026

Reproduced with permission from Stuart P, Malick F, Nair RP, et al: Analysis of phenotypic variation in psoriasis as a function of age at onset and family history, *Arch Dermatol Res*. 2002 Jul;294(5):207-213.

positive and negative family histories of psoriasis and with early-onset versus late-onset disease. This study was used in Exercise 5 in Chapter 7.

The hypothesis was that the variables age at onset (in 10-year categories), onset (early or late), and familial status (sporadic or familial) had no effect on the occurrence of joint complaints. Results from the analysis of age, familial status, and frequency of joint complaints are given in Table 10–7.

Each independent variable in this research problem is measured on a categorical or nominal scale (age, onset, and familial status), as is the outcome variable (occurrence of joint complaints). If only two variables are being analyzed, the chi-square method introduced in Chapter 6 can be used to determine whether a relationship exists between them; with three or more nominal or categorical variables, a statistical method called log-linear analysis is appropriate. **Log-linear analysis** is analogous to a regression model in which all the variables, both independent and dependent, are measured on a nominal scale. The technique is called log-linear because it involves using the logarithm of the observed frequencies in the contingency table.

Stuart and colleagues (2002) concluded that joint complaints and familial psoriasis were conditionally independent given age at examination, but that age at examination was not independent of either joint complaints or a family history.

Log-linear analysis may also be used to analyze multidimensional contingency tables in situations in which no distinction exists between independent and dependent variables, that is, when investigators simply want to examine the relationship among a set of nominal measures. The fact that log-linear analysis does not require a distinction between independent and dependent variables points to a major difference between it and other regression models—namely, that the regression coefficients are not interpreted in log-linear analysis.

PREDICTING A CENSORED OUTCOME: COX PROPORTIONAL HAZARD MODEL

In Chapter 9, we found that special methods must be used when an outcome has not yet been observed for all subjects in the study sample. Studies of time-limited outcomes in which there are censored observations, such as survival, naturally fall into this category; investigators usually cannot wait until all patients in the study experience the event before presenting information.

Many times in clinical trials or cohort studies, investigators wish to look at the simultaneous effect of several variables on length of survival. For example, Martínez and her colleagues (2017) wanted to evaluate the relationship of marital status on breast cancer survival. They analyzed data from the California Cancer Registry (CCR). The data included HER2 status, tumor stage, ICD-O site codes as well as address, source of payment and treatment modalities. Since the CCR data is self-reported by hospitals, it is censored at the time of the abstraction and analysis.

Table 10–2 indicates that the regression technique developed by Cox (1972) is appropriate when time-dependent censored observations are included. This technique is called the **Cox regression,** or **proportional hazard, model.** In essence this model allows the covariates (independent variables) in the regression equation to vary with time. The dependent variable is the survival time of the *j*th patient, denoted Y_j. Both numerical and nominal independent variables may be used in the model.

The Cox regression coefficients can be used to determine the relative risk or odds ratio (introduced in Chapter 3) associated with each independent variable and the outcome variable, adjusted for the effect of all other variables in the equation. Thus, instead of giving adjusted means, as ANCOVA does in regression, the Cox model gives adjusted relative risks. We can also use a variety of methods to select the independent variables that add significantly to the prediction of the outcome, as in multiple regression; however, a chi-square test (instead of the F test) is used to test for significance.

The Cox proportional hazard model involves a complicated exponential equation (Cox, 1972). Although we will not go into detail about the mathematics involved in this model, its use is so common in medicine that an understanding of the process is needed by readers of the literature. Our primary focus is on the application and interpretation of the Cox model.

Understanding the Cox Model

Recall from Chapter 9 that the survival function gives the probability that a person will survive the next interval of time, given that they have survived up until that time. The hazard function, also defined in Chapter 9, is in some ways the opposite: it is the probability that a person will die (or that there will be a failure) in the next interval of time, given that they have survived until the beginning of the interval. The hazard function plays a key role in the Cox model.

The Cox model examines two pieces of information: the amount of time since the event first happened to a person and the person's observations on the independent variables. Using the Martinez example, the amount of time might be 3 years, and the observations would be the patient's age, race, first course of treatment, and marital status. In the Cox model, the length of time is evaluated using the hazard function, and the linear combination of the independent values (like the linear combination we obtain when we use multiple regression) is the exponent of the natural logarithm, e. For example, for the Martinez study, the model is written as

$$h(t, X_1 X_2 \ldots X_5) = h_0(t)e^{b_1 X_1 + b_2 X_1 + \ldots + b_5 X_5}$$

In words, the model is saying that the probability of dying in the next time interval, given that the patient has lived until this time and has the given values for age, race, first course of treatment, marital status, and so on, can be found by multiplying the baseline hazard (h_0) by the natural log raised to the power of the linear combination of the independent variables. In other words, a given person's probability of dying is influenced by how commonly patients die and the given person's individual characteristics. If we take the antilog of the linear combination, we

multiply rather than add the values of the covariates. In this model, the covariates have a multiplicative, or proportional, effect on the probability of dying—thus, the term "proportional hazard" model.

An Example of the Cox Model

In the Martínez et al study (2017), researchers used the Cox proportional hazard model to examine the relationship between marital status and survival. The investigators wanted to control for possible confounding variables, including the age at diagnosis (continuous), race/ethnicity, subtype (for analysis of all patients), lymph node involvement, tumor size, grade, histological subtypes, first course of treatment, insurance status; AJCC stage I–IV. The outcome is a censored variable, the amount of time before the patient's death, so the Cox proportional hazard model is the appropriate statistical method. We use the results of analysis from Table 3 in the manuscript, reproduced in Table 10–8, to point out some salient features of the method.

As in logistic regression, the regression coefficients in the Cox model can be interpreted in terms of relative risks or odds ratios (by finding the antilog) if they are based on independent binary variables, such as triple negative. For this reason, many researchers divide independent variables into two categories, even though this practice can be risky if the correct cutpoint is not selected. The neighborhood SES was recoded into five dummy variables to facilitate interpretation in terms of odds ratios for each stage. The MRR are mortality rate ratios and can be interpreted in the same way as risk ratios. Note that since the 95% confidence interval for the MRR does not contain 1, the odds ratio is statistically significant (consistent with the p value).

Importance of the Cox Model

The Cox model is very useful in medicine, and it is easy to see why it is being used with increasing frequency. It provides the only valid method of predicting a time-dependent outcome, and many health-related outcomes are related to time. If the independent variables are divided into two categories (dichotomized), the exponential of the regression coefficient, exp (b), is the odds ratio, a useful way to interpret the risk associated with any specific factor. In addition, the Cox model provides a method for producing survival curves that are adjusted for confounding variables. The Cox model can be extended to the case of multiple events for a subject, but that topic is beyond our scope. Investigators who have repeated measures in a time-to-survival study are encouraged to consult a statistician.

Table 10–8. Results from Cox proportional hazard model using both pretreatment and posttreatment variables.

	Total mortality		
	No. of deaths Unmarried	No. of deaths Married	MRR[a] (95%CI) Unmarried vs. Married
By Race/ethnicity			
Non-Hispanic white	8761	5858	1.31 (1.26–1.36)
Black	1599	614	1.17 (1.05–1.30)
Hispanic	1943	1750	1.15 (1.07–1.24)
Asian/Pacific Islander	894	1006	1.29 (1.16–1.43)
Other/unknown	109	76	1.06 (0.74–1.53)
P-heterogeneity[b]			<0.001
Among APIs by ethnic group			
Chinese	167	227	1.21 (0.95–1.54)
Japanese	125	92	1.33 (0.96–1.83)
Filipino	305	321	1.24 (1.03–1.50)
Other Asian	138	135	1.35 (1.02–1.79)
Korean	52	68	1.38 (0.89–2.15)
South Asian	47	84	0.84 (0.53–1.33)
Vietnamese	60	79	1.03 (0.68–1.56)
P-heterogeneity[b]			0.6183
Among Hispanics by nativity			
US-born	948	727	1.23(1.10–1.37)
Foreign-born	995	1023	1.07 (0.97–1.18)
P-heterogeneity[b]			0.010
Among APIs by nativity			
US-born	168	128	1.62 (1.25–2.11)
Foreign-born	722	876	1.25 (1.12–1.41)
P-heterogeneity[b]			0.425
By Neighborhood SES			
1st (lowest)	2526	1357	1.22 (1.13–1.32)
2nd	2918	1804	1.26 (1.18–1.35)
3rd	2857	2009	1.33 (1.24–1.42)
4th	2751	2068	1.22 (1.14–1.30)
5th (highest)	2254	2066	1.32 (1.24–1.42)
P-heterogeneity[b]			0.009
By Tumor Subtype			
HR+/HER2−	5939	4102	1.32 (1.26–1.37)
HR+/HER2+	1157	899	1.18 (1.07–1.30)
HR−/HER2+	779	705	1.21(1.07–1.35)
Triple negative	1961	1803	1.16 (1.08–1.25)
Unclassified	3470	1795	1.35(1.25–1.46)
P-heterogeneity[b]			<0.0001

[a]Estimated from Cox proportional hazard models, stratified by stage (AJCC stage I-IV or unknown) and adjusted for: age (continuous): race/ethnicity (NHW, non-Hispanic white, black, Hispanic, Asian/Pacific Islander, other/unknown); tumor subtype HR+/HER2−, HR+/HER2+, HR−/HER2, triple negative, and unclassified); first course of treatment (Y/N for surgery, radiation, hormone therapy); lymph node involvement (negative, positive, unknown); tumor size (continuous); grade (I, II, II/IV, unknown); histology (ductal, lobular, other); insurance status (no insurance, private insurance only, Medicare only/Medicare + private insurance, any public/Medical/military insurance, unknown); and neighborhood socioeconomic status (quintiles).
[b]Likelihood ratio test for interaction computed based on cross-product terms.
Reproduced with permission from Martínez ME, Unkart JT, Tao L, et al: Prognostic significance of marital status in breast cancer survival: A population-based study, *PLoS One.* 2017 May 5;12(5):e0175515.

META-ANALYSIS

Meta-analysis is a way to combine results of several independent studies on a specific topic. Meta-analysis is different from the methods discussed in the preceding sections because its purpose is not to identify risk factors or to predict outcomes for individual patients; rather, this technique is applicable to any research question. We briefly introduced meta-analysis in Chapter 2. Because we could not talk about it in detail until the basics of statistical tests (confidence limits, *p* values, etc.) were explained, we include it in this chapter. It is an important technique increasingly used for studies in health and it can be looked on as an extension of multivariate analysis.

The idea of summarizing a set of studies in the medical literature is not new; review articles have long had an important role in helping practicing physicians keep up to date and make sense of the many studies on any given topic. Meta-analysis takes the review article a step further by using statistical procedures to combine the results from different studies. Glass (1977) developed the technique because many research projects are designed to answer similar questions, but they do not always come to similar conclusions. The problem for the practitioner is to determine which study to believe, a problem unfortunately too familiar to readers of medical research reports.

Sacks and colleagues (1987) reviewed meta-analyses of clinical trials and concluded that meta-analysis has four purposes: (1) to increase statistical power by increasing the sample size, (2) to resolve uncertainty when reports do not agree, (3) to improve estimates of effect size, and (4) to answer questions not posed at the beginning of the study. Purpose 3 requires some expansion because the concept of effect size is central to meta-analysis. Cohen (1988) developed this concept and defined **effect size** as the *degree* to which the phenomenon is present in the population. An effect size may be thought of as an index of how much difference exists between two groups—generally, a treatment group and a control group. The effect size is based on means if the outcome is numerical, on proportions or odds ratios if the outcome is nominal, or on correlations if the outcome is an association. The effect sizes themselves are statistically combined in meta-analysis.

Bellou and colleagues (2018) used meta-analysis to evaluate the risk factors for type 2 diabetes mellitus. They examined the literature by searching PubMed from inception to 2/10/2016 for publications containing the words *diabetes and (systematic review or meta-analysis)* and found 7,303 studies. Of these, 86 met the inclusion criteria. They performed an additional PubMed search to find Mendelian randomization

(MR) studies. They excluded studies that focused on impaired glucose tolerance or insulin resistance as the outcome.

Two authors independently read and evaluated each article. They reviewed the risk factors and the number of studies considered. They also extracted study specific risk estimates such as odds ratio and risk ratios.

The authors of the meta-analysis article calculated the odds ratios and 95% confidence intervals for each study and used a statistical method to determine summary odds ratios over all the studies. These risk factors and associated effect sizes are displayed in Figure 10–5. This figure illustrates the typical way findings from meta-analysis studies are presented. Generally the results from each study are shown, and the summary or combined results are given at the bottom of the figure. When the summary statistic is the odds ratio, a line representing the value of 1 is drawn to make it easy to see which of the studies have a significant outcome.

A meta-analysis does not simply add the means or proportions across studies to determine an "average" mean or proportion. Although several different methods can be used to combine results, they all use the same principle of determining an effect size in each study and then combining the effect sizes in some manner. The methods for combining the effect sizes include the *z* approximation for comparing two proportions (Chapter 6); the *t* test for comparing two means (Chapter 6); the *p* values for the comparisons; and the odds ratio as shown in Bellou and colleagues' study (2018). The values corresponding to the effect size in each study are the numbers combined in the meta-analysis to provide a pooled (overall) *p* value or confidence interval for the combined studies. The most commonly used method for reporting meta-analyses in the medical literature is the odds ratio with confidence intervals.

In addition to being potentially useful when published studies reach conflicting conclusions, meta-analysis can help raise issues to be addressed in future clinical trials. The procedure is not, however, without its critics, and readers should be aware of some of the potential problems in its use. To evaluate meta-analysis, LeLorier and associates (1997) compared the results of a series of large randomized, controlled trials with relevant previously published meta-analyses. Their results were mixed: They found that meta-analysis accurately predicted the outcome in only 65% of the studies; however, the difference between the trial results and the meta-analysis results was statistically significant in only 12% of the comparisons. Ioannidis and colleagues (1998) determined that the discrepancies in the conclusions were attributable to different disease risks, different study protocols, varying quality of the studies,

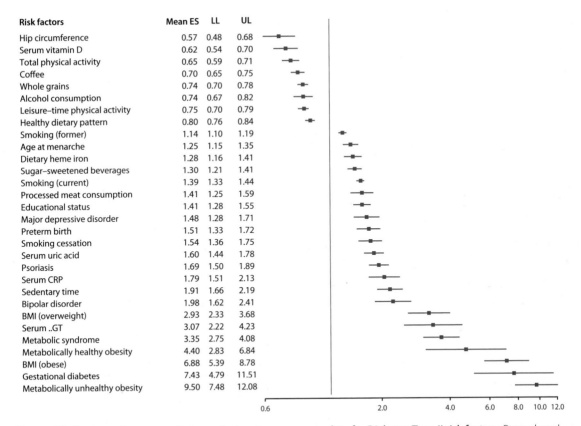

Risk factors	Mean ES	LL	UL
Hip circumference	0.57	0.48	0.68
Serum vitamin D	0.62	0.54	0.70
Total physical activity	0.65	0.59	0.71
Coffee	0.70	0.65	0.75
Whole grains	0.74	0.70	0.78
Alcohol consumption	0.74	0.67	0.82
Leisure–time physical activity	0.75	0.70	0.79
Healthy dietary pattern	0.80	0.76	0.84
Smoking (former)	1.14	1.10	1.19
Age at menarche	1.25	1.15	1.35
Dietary heme iron	1.28	1.16	1.41
Sugar–sweetened beverages	1.30	1.21	1.41
Smoking (current)	1.39	1.33	1.44
Processed meat consumption	1.41	1.25	1.59
Educational status	1.41	1.28	1.55
Major depressive disorder	1.48	1.28	1.71
Preterm birth	1.51	1.33	1.72
Smoking cessation	1.54	1.36	1.75
Serum uric acid	1.60	1.44	1.78
Psoriasis	1.69	1.50	1.89
Serum CRP	1.79	1.51	2.13
Sedentary time	1.91	1.66	2.19
Bipolar disorder	1.98	1.62	2.41
BMI (overweight)	2.93	2.33	3.68
Serum ..GT	3.07	2.22	4.23
Metabolic syndrome	3.35	2.75	4.08
Metabolically healthy obesity	4.40	2.83	6.84
BMI (obese)	6.88	5.39	8.78
Gestational diabetes	7.43	4.79	11.51
Metabolically unhealthy obesity	9.50	7.48	12.08

Figure 10–5. Example meta-analysis graph showing aggregate data for Diabetes Type II risk factors. Reproduced with permission from Bellou V, Belbasis L, Tzoulaki I, et al: Risk factors for type 2 diabetes mellitus: An exposure-wide umbrella review of meta-analyses, *PLoS One*. 2018 Mar 20;13(3):e0194127.

and possible publication bias (discussed in a following section). These reports serve as a useful reminder that well-designed clinical trials remain a critical source of information.

Studies designed in dissimilar manners should not be combined. In performing a meta-analysis, investigators should use clear and well-accepted criteria for deciding whether studies should be included in the analysis, and these criteria should be stated in the published meta-analysis.

Most meta-analyses are based on the published literature, and some people believe it is easier to publish studies with results than studies that show no difference. This potential problem is called publication bias. Researchers can take at least three important steps to reduce publication bias. First, they can search for unpublished data, typically done by contacting the authors of published articles. Second, researchers can perform an analysis to see how sensitive the conclusions

are to certain characteristics of the studies. For instance, Bellou and colleagues assessed sources of heterogeneity or variation among the studies and reported that excluding these studies had no substantive effect on the conclusions. Third, investigators can estimate how many studies showing no difference would have to be done but not published to raise the pooled p value above the 0.05 level or produce a confidence interval that includes 1 so that the combined results would no longer be significant. The reader can have more confidence in the conclusions from a meta-analysis that finds a significant effect if a large number of unpublished negative studies would be required to repudiate the overall significance. The increasing use of computerized patient databases may lessen the effect of publication bias in future meta-analyses.

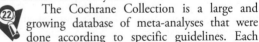 The Cochrane Collection is a large and growing database of meta-analyses that were done according to specific guidelines. Each

meta-analysis contains a description and an assessment of the methods used in the articles that constitute the meta-analysis. Graphs such as Figure 10–5 are produced, and, if appropriate, graphs for subanalyses are presented. For instance, if both cohort studies and clinical trials have been done on a given topic, the Cochrane Collection presents a separate figure for each. The Cochrane Collection is available on CD-ROM or via the Internet for an annual fee. The Cochrane Web site states that: "Cochrane reviews (the principal output of the Collaboration) are published electronically in successive issues of The Cochrane Database of Systematic Reviews. Preparation and maintenance of Cochrane reviews is the responsibility of international collaborative review groups."

No one has argued that meta-analyses should replace clinical trials. Bellou and his colleagues (2018) conclude that a large trial may be warranted to confirm their findings. Despite their shortcomings, meta-analyses can provide guidance to clinicians when the literature contains several studies with conflicting results, especially when the studies have relatively small sample sizes. Furthermore, based on the increasingly large number of published meta-analyses, it appears that this method is here to stay. As with all types of studies, however, the methods used in a meta-analysis need to be carefully assessed before the results are accepted.

METHODS FOR CLASSIFICATION

Several multivariate methods can be used when the research question is related to classification. When the goal is to classify subjects into groups, discriminant analysis, cluster analysis, and propensity score analysis are appropriate. These methods all involve multiple measurements on each subject, but they have different purposes and are used to answer different research questions.

Discriminant Analysis

Logistic regression is used extensively in the biologic sciences. A related technique, **discriminant analysis,** although used with less frequency in medicine, is a common technique in the social sciences. It is similar to logistic regression in that it is used to predict a nominal or categorical outcome. It differs from logistic regression, however, in that it assumes that the independent variables follow a multivariate normal distribution, so it must be used with caution if some X variables are nominal.

The procedure involves determining several discriminant functions, which are simply linear combinations of the independent variables that separate or discriminate among the groups defined by the outcome measure as much as possible. The number of discriminant functions needed is determined by a multivariate test statistic called Wilks' lambda. The discriminant functions' coefficients can be standardized and then interpreted in the same manner as in multiple regression to draw conclusions about which variables are important in discriminating among the groups.

Howcroft and coworkers (2017) wanted to identify characteristics that differentiate among elderly subjects who were of high risk for falling. Range in anterior-posterior and medial-lateral pressure were measures using a Wii Balance Board. Discriminant analysis is useful when investigators want to evaluate several explanatory variables and the goal is to classify subjects into two or more categories or groups, such as that defined by the fall risk categories.

Although discriminant analysis is most often employed to explain or describe factors that distinguish among groups of interest, the procedure can also be used to classify future subjects. Howcroft et al (2017) used discriminant analysis for this purpose. Classification involves determining a separate prediction equation corresponding to each group that gives the probability of belonging to that group, based on the explanatory variables. For classification of a future subject, a prediction is calculated for each group, and the individual is classified as belonging to the group they most closely resemble. They were able to create a discriminant function based on four variables that classified subjects into fallers and non-fallers. The function further identified those subjects most likely to be multi-fallers.

Factor Analysis

Andrewes and colleagues (2003) wanted to know how scores on the Emotional and Social Dysfunction Questionnaire (ESDQ) can be used to help decide the level of support needed following brain surgery. Similarly, the Medical Outcomes Study Short Form 36 (MOSSF36) is a questionnaire commonly used to measure patient outcomes (Stewart et al, 1988). In examples such as these, tests with a large number of items are developed, patients or other subjects take the test, and scores on various items are combined to produce scores on the relevant factors.

The MOS-SF36 is probably used more frequently than any other questionnaire to measure functional outcomes and quality of life; it has been used all over the world and in patients with a variety of medical conditions. The questionnaire contains 36 items that are combined to produce a patient profile on eight concepts: physical functioning, role-physical, bodily pain, general health, vitality, social functioning, role-emotional, and mental health. The first four concepts are combined to give a measure of physical health, and the last four concepts are combined to give a measure of mental health. The developers used **factor analysis** to decide how to combine the questions to develop these concepts.

In a research problem in which factor analysis is appropriate, all variables are considered to be independent; in other words, there is no desire to predict one on the basis of others. Conceptually, factor analysis works as follows: First, a large number of people are measured on a set of items; a rule of thumb calls for at least ten times as many subjects as items. The second step involves calculating correlations. To illustrate, suppose 500 patients answered the 36 questions on the MOS-SF36. Factor analysis answers the question of whether some of the items group together in a logical way, such as items that measure the same underlying component of physical activity. If two items measure the same component, they can be expected to have higher correlations with each other than with other items.

In the third step, factor analysis manipulates the correlations among the items to produce linear combinations, similar to a regression equation without the dependent variable. The difference is that each linear combination, called a **factor,** is determined so that the first one accounts for the most variation among the items, the second factor accounts for the most residual variation after the first factor is taken into consideration, and so forth. Typically, a small number of factors account for enough of the variation among subjects that it is possible to draw inferences about a patient's score on a given factor. For example, it is much more convenient to refer to scores for physical functioning, role-physical, bodily pain, and so on, than to refer to scores on the original 36 items. Thus, the fourth step involves determining how many factors are needed and how they should be interpreted.

Andrewes and colleagues (2003) analyzed the ESDQ, a questionnaire designed for brain-damaged populations. They performed a factor analysis of the ratings by the partner or caretaker of 211 patients. They found that the relationships among the questions could be summarized by eight factors, including anger, helplessness, emotional dyscontrol, indifference, inappropriateness, fatigue, maladaptive behavior, and insight. The researchers subsequently used the scores on the factors for a discriminant analysis to differentiate between the brain-damaged patients and a control group with no cerebral dysfunction and found significant discrimination.

Investigators who use factor analysis usually have an idea of what the important factors are, and they design

the items accordingly. Many other issues are of concern in factor analysis, such as how to derive the linear combinations, how many factors to retain for interpretation, and how to interpret the factors. Using factor analysis, as well as the other multivariate techniques, requires considerable statistical skill.

Cluster Analysis

A statistical technique similar conceptually to factor analysis is **cluster analysis.** The difference is that cluster analysis attempts to find similarities among the subjects that were measured instead of among the measures that were made. The object in cluster analysis is to determine a classification or taxonomic scheme that accounts for variance among the subjects. Cluster analysis can also be thought of as similar to discriminant analysis, except that the investigator does not know to which group the subjects belong. As in factor analysis, all variables are considered to be independent variables.

Cluster analysis is frequently used in archeology and paleontology to determine if the existence of similarities in objects implies that they belong to the same taxon. Biologists use this technique to help determine classification keys, such as using leaves or flowers to determine appropriate species. A study by Penzel and colleagues (2003) used cluster analysis to examine the relationships among chromosomal imbalances in thymic epithelial tumors. Journalists and marketing analysts also use cluster analysis, referred to in these fields as Q-type factor analysis, as a way to classify readers and consumers into groups with common characteristics.

Propensity Scores

The propensity score method is an alternative to multiple regression and analysis of covariance. It provides a creative method to control for an entire group of confounding variables. Conceptually, a propensity score is found by using the confounding variables as predictors of the group to which a subject belongs; this step is generally accomplished by using logistic regression. For example, many cohort studies are handicapped by the problem of many confounding variables, such as age, gender, race, comorbidities, and so forth. Once the outcome is known for the subjects in the cohort, the confounding variables are used to develop a logistic regression equation to predict whether a patient has the outcome or not. This prediction, based on a combination of the confounding variables, is calculated for all subjects and then used as the confounding variable in subsequent analyses. Developers of the technique maintain it does a better job of controlling for confounding variables (Rubin, 1997). See Katzan and colleagues (2003) for an example of the application of propensity score analysis in a clinical study to determine the effect of pneumonia on mortality in patients with acute stroke.

Classification and Regression Tree (CART) Analysis

Classification and regression tree (CART) analysis is an approach to analyzing large databases to find significant patterns and relationships among variables. The patterns are then used to develop predictive models for classifying future subjects. As an example, CART was used in a study of 105 patients with stage IV colon or rectal cancer (Dixon et al, 2003). CART identified optimal cut points for carcinoembryonic antigen (CEA) and albumen (ALB) to form four groups of patients: low CEA with high ALB, low CEA with low ALB, high CEA with high ALB, and high CEA with low ALB. A survival analysis (Kaplan–Meier) was then used to compare survival times in these four groups. The method requires special software and extensive computing power.

MULTIPLE DEPENDENT VARIABLES

Multivariate analysis of variance and canonical correlation are similar to each other in that they both involve *multiple dependent* variables as well as multiple independent variables.

Multivariate Analysis of Variance

Multivariate analysis of variance (MANOVA) conceptually (although not computationally) is a simple extension of the ANOVA designs discussed in Chapter 7 to situations in which two or more dependent variables are included. As with ANOVA, MANOVA is appropriate when the independent variables are nominal or categorical and the outcomes are numerical. If the results from the MANOVA are statistically significant, using the multivariate statistic called Wilks' lambda, follow-up ANOVAs may be done to investigate the individual outcomes.

Weiner and Rudy (2002) wanted to identify nursing home resident and staff attitudes that are barriers to effective pain management. They collected information from nurses, nursing assistants, and residents in seven long-term care facilities. They designed questionnaires to collect beliefs about 12 components of chronic pain management and administered them to these three groups. They wanted to know if there were attitudinal differences among the three groups on the 12

components. If analysis of variance is used in this study, they would need to do 12 different ANOVAs, and the probability of any one component being significant by chance is increased. With these multiple dependent variables, they correctly chose to use MANOVA. Results indicated that residents believed that chronic pain does not change, and they were fearful of addiction. The nursing staff believed that many complaints were unheard by busy staff. Note that this study used a nested design (patients and staff within nursing homes) and would be a candidate for GEE or multilevel model analysis.

The motivation for doing MANOVA prior to univariate ANOVA is similar to the reason for performing univariate ANOVA prior to *t* tests: to eliminate doing many significance tests and increasing the likelihood that a chance difference is declared significant. In addition, MANOVA permits the statistician to look at complex relationships among the dependent variables. The results from MANOVA are often difficult to interpret, however, and it is used sparingly in the medical literature.

Canonical Correlation Analysis

Canonical correlation analysis also involves both multiple independent and multiple dependent variables. This method is appropriate when *both* the independent variables and the outcomes are numerical, and the research question focuses on the relationship between the set of independent variables and the set of dependent variables. For example, suppose researchers wish to examine the overall relationship between indicators of health outcome (physical functioning, mental health, health perceptions, age, gender, etc.) measured at the beginning of a study and the set of outcomes (physical functioning, mental health, social contacts, serious symptoms, etc.) measured at the end of the study. Canonical correlation analysis forms a linear combination of the independent variables to predict not just a single outcome measure, but a linear combination of outcome measures. The two linear combinations of independent variables and dependent variables, each resulting in a single number (or index), are determined so the correlation between them is as large as possible. The correlation between the pair of linear combinations (or numbers or indices) is called the **canonical correlation.** Then, as in factor analysis, a second pair of linear combinations is derived from the residual variation after the effect of the first pair is removed, and the third pair from those remaining, and so on. The canonical coefficients in the linear combinations are interpreted in the same manner as regression coefficients in a multiple regression equation, and the canonical correlations as multiple *R*. Generally, the first two or three pairs of linear combinations account for sufficient variation, and they can be interpreted to gain insights about related factors or dimensions.

The relationship between personality and symptoms of depression was studied in a community-based sample of 804 individuals. Grucza and colleagues (2003) used the Temperament and Character Inventory (TCI) to assess personality and the Center for Epidemiologic Studies Depression scale (CES-D) to measure symptoms of depression. Both of these questionnaires contain multiple scales or factors, and the authors used canonical correlation analysis to learn how the factors on the TCI are related to the factors on the CES-D. They discovered several relationships and concluded that depression symptom severity and patterns are partially explained by personality traits.

SUMMARY OF ADVANCED METHODS

The advanced methods presented in this chapter are used in approximately 10% to 15% of the articles in medical and surgical journals. Unfortunately for readers of the medical literature, these methods are complex and not easy to understand, and they are not always described adequately. As with other complex statistical techniques, investigators should consult with a statistician if an advanced statistical method is planned. Table 10–2 gives a guide to the selection of the appropriate method(s), depending on the number independent variables and the scale on which they are measured.

EXERCISES

1. Using the following formula, verify the adjusted mean number of ventricular wall motion abnormalities in smokers and nonsmokers from the hypothetical data in the section titled, "Controlling for Confounding." That is,

$$\text{Adjusted } \overline{Y}_j = \text{Unadjusted } \overline{Y}_j - b(\overline{X}_j - \overline{\overline{X}})$$

2. Refer to the study by Shah and coinvestigators (2018). Find the probability that a patient with an ASA = 1, poor functional status, severe hypertension undergoing an open surgical procedure of 1.5 hours stays longer than 7 days.

3. Refer to the study by Shah and coinvestigators (2018). From Table 10–6, find the value of the kappa statistic for the agreement between the predicted and actual number of patients with lengths of stay longer than 7 days.

4. Bale and associates (1986) performed a study to consider the physique and anthropometric variables of athletes in relation to their type and amount of training and to examine these variables as potential predictors of distance running performance. Sixty runners were divided into three groups: (1) elite runners with 10-km runs in less than 30 min; (2) good runners with 10-km times between 30 and 35 min, and (3) average runners with 10-km times between 35 and 45 min. Anthropometric data included body density, percentage fat, percentage absolute fat, lean body mass, ponderal index, biceps and calf circumferences, humerus and femur widths, and various skinfold measures. The authors wanted to determine whether the anthropometric variables were able to differentiate between the groups of runners. What is the best method to use for this research question?

5. Ware and collaborators (1987) reported a study of the effects on health for patients in health maintenance organizations (HMO) and for patients in fee-for-service (FFS) plans. Within the FFS group, some patients were randomly assigned to receive free medical care and others shared in the costs. The health status of the adults was evaluated at the beginning and again at the end of the study. In addition, the number of days spent in bed because of poor health was determined periodically throughout the study. These measures, recorded at the beginning of the study—along with information on the participant's age, gender, income, and the system of health care to which he or she was assigned (HMO, free FFS, or pay FFS)—were the independent variables used in the study. The dependent variables were the values of these same 13 measures at the end of the study. The results from a multiple-regression analysis to predict number of bed days are given in Table 10–9. Use the regression equation to predict the number of bed-days during

Table 10–9. Regression coefficients and t test values for predicting bed-days in RAND study.

Explanatory Variables and Other Measures (X)	Dependent-Variable Equation	
	Coefficient (b)	t Test
Intercept	0.613	22.36
FFS freeplan	−0.017	−2.17
FFS payplan	−0.014	−2.18
Personal functioning	−0.0002	−1.35
Mental health	−0.00006	0.25
Health perceptions	−0.002	−5.17
Age	−0.0001	−0.54
Male	−0.026	−4.58
Income	−0.021	−1.65
Three-year term	0.002	0.44
Took physical	−0.003	−0.56
Bed-day	0.105	6.15
Sample size	1568	
R^2	0.12	
Residual standard error	0.01	

FFS, fee for service.
Data from Ware JE, Brook RH, Rogers WH, et al: Health Outcomes for Adults in Prepaid and Fee-for-Service Systems of Care. Santa Monica, CA: The RAND Corporation; 1987.

Table 10–10. Values for prediction equation.

Variable	Value
Personal functioning	80
Mental health	80
Health perceptions	75
Age	70
Income	10 (from a formula used in the RAND study)
Three-year term[a]	Yes
Took physical[a]	Yes
Bed-day	14

[a]Indicates a dummy variable with 1 = yes and 0 = no.

a 30-day period for a 70-year-old woman in the FFS pay plan who has the values on the independent variables shown in Table 10–10 (asterisks [[a]] designate dummy variables given a value of 1 if yes and 0 if no).

6. Symptoms of depression in the elderly may be more subtle than in younger patients, but recognizing depression in the elderly is important because it can be treated. In Australia, Henderson and colleagues (1997) studied a group of more than 1,000 elderly, all aged 70 years or older. They examined the outcome of depressive states 3–4 years after initial diagnosis to identify factors associated with persistence of depressive symptoms and to test the hypothesis that depressive symptoms in the elderly are a risk factor for dementia or cognitive decline. They used the Canberra Interview for the Elderly (CIE), which measures depressive symptoms and cognitive performance, and referred to the initial measurement as "wave 1" and the follow-up as "wave 2." The regression equation predicting depression at wave 2 for 595 people who completed the interview on both occasions is given in Table 10–11. The variables have been entered into the regression equation in blocks, an example of hierarchical regression.

   a. Based on the regression equation in Table 10–11, what is the relationship between depression score initially and at follow-up?

   b. The regression coefficient for age is –0.014. Is it significant? How would you interpret it?

   c. Once a person's depression score at wave 1 is known, which group of variables accounts for more of the variation in depression at wave 2?

7. Hindmarsh and Brook (1996) examined the final height of 16 short children who were treated with growth hormone. They studied several variables they thought might predict height in these children, such as the mother's height, the father's height, the child's chronologic and bone age, dose of the growth hormone during the first year, age at the start of therapy, and the peak response to an insulin-induced hypoglycemia test. All anthropometric indices were expressed as standard deviation scores; these scores express height in terms of standard deviations from the mean in a norm group. For example, a height score of –2.00 indicates the child is 2 standard deviations below the mean height for their age group.

Table 10–11. Regression results for predicting depression at wave 2.

Predictor Variable[a]	b	Beta[b]	P	R^2	R^2 Change
Depression Score					
Wave 1	0.267	0.231	0.000	0.182	0.182
Sociodemographic					
Age	−0.014	−0.024	0.538	0.187	0.005
Sex	0.165	0.034	0.370		
Psychologic Health					
Neuroticism, wave 1	0.067	0.077	0.056	0.0237	0.050
Past history of depression	0.320	0.136	0.000		
Physical Health					
ADL, wave 1	−0.154	−0.103	0.033	0.411	0.174
ADL, wave 2	0.275	0.283	0.012		
ADL squared, wave 2	−0.013	−0.150	0.076		
Number of current symptoms, wave 2	0.115	0.117	0.009		
Number of medical conditions, wave 2	0.309	0.226	0.000		
BP, systolic, wave 2	−0.010	−0.092	0.010		
Global health rating change	0.284	0.079	0.028		
Sensory impairment change	−0.045	−0.064	0.073		
Social support/inactivity					
Social support—friends, wave 2	−1.650	−0.095	0.015	0.442	0.031
Social support—visits, wave 2	−1.229	−0.087	0.032		
Activity level, wave 2	0.061	0.095	0.025		
Services (community residents only), wave 2	0.207[c]	0.135[c]	0.001[c]	0.438[c]	0.015[c]

ADL, adult daily living; BP, blood pressure.

[a]Only those variables are shown that were included in the final model.

[b]Standardized beta value, controlling for all other variables in the regression, except service use. Based on community and institutional residents.

[c]Regression limited to community sample only; coefficients for other variables vary only very slightly from those obtained with regression on the full sample.

Modified with permission from Henderson AS, Korten AE, Jacomb PA, et al: The course of depression in the elderly: a longitudinal community-based study in Australia, *Psychol Med*. 1997 Jan;27(1):119-129.

Data are given in Table 10–12.

a. Use the data to perform a stepwise regression and interpret the results. We reproduced a portion of the output in Table 10–13.

b. What variable entered the equation on the first iteration (model 1)? Why do you think it entered first?

c. What variables are in the equation at the final model? Which of these variables makes the greatest contribution to the prediction of final height?

d. Why do you think the variable that entered the equation first is not in the final model?

e. Using the regression equation, what is the predicted height of the first child? How close is this to the child's actual final height (in SDS scores)?

Table 10–12. Case summaries.[a]

	Final Height SDS	Age	Dose	Father's Height	Mother's Height	Height SDS Chronologic Age	Height SDS Bone Age
1	−2.18	6.652	20.00	−2.14	−2.20	−3.07	−1.75
2	−2.15	10.383	16.00	−2.78	−0.15	−2.20	−2.43
3	−1.65	10.565	16.00	−1.91	−1.87	−2.62	−0.90
4	−1.18	10.104	15.00	0.84	−1.63	−2.43	−2.06
5	−1.31	11.145	14.00	−1.80	−0.70	−1.92	−1.49
6	−1.35	9.682	14.00	0.09	0.38	−1.38	−0.54
7	−1.18	9.863	16.00	−0.26	−1.70	−2.08	−1.32
8	−2.51	9.463	15.00	−3.62	−0.75	−2.36	−0.45
9	−1.61	7.704	19.00	−2.11	−1.25	−1.98	1.23
10	−2.15	5.858	25.00	1.31	0.23	−2.43	−1.95
11	0.80	5.153	22.00	−0.14	−1.83	−2.36	−0.39
12	−0.20	6.986	21.00	−0.14	−1.83	−2.09	−0.98
13	0.20	8.967	17.00	−0.14	−1.83	−1.38	−0.19
14	−0.71	6.970	21.00	0.50	1.63	−1.09	0.49
15	−1.71	6.515	13.00	0.84	−0.10	−1.98	−0.18
16	−2.32	7.548	21.00	−2.89	−0.20	−3.30	−2.25
Total N	16	16	16	16	16	16	16

SDS, standard deviation score.
[a]Limited to first 100 cases.
Data from Hindmarsh PC, Brook CG: Final height of short normal children treated with growth hormone, *Lancet*. 1996 Jul 6; 348(9019):13-16.

Table 10–13. Results from stepwise multiple regression to predict final height in standard deviation scores.[a]

		Unstandardized Coefficients		Standardized Coefficients		
Model		B	SE	β	t	Significance
1	(Constant)	−1.055	0.248		−4.261	0.001
	Father's height	0.302	0.142	0.494	2.126	0.052
2	(Constant)	−1.335	0.284		−4.705	0.000
	Father's height	0.337	0.135	0.552	2.503	0.026
	Mother's height	−0.343	0.200	−0.378	−1.715	0.110
3	(Constant)	0.205	0.734		0.280	0.785
	Father's height	0.211	0.131	0.345	1.612	0.133
	Mother's height	−0.478	0.185	−0.527	−2.581	0.024
	Height SDS chronologic age	0.820	0.368	0.505	2.230	0.046
4	(Constant)	−1.110	0.927		−1.198	0.256
	Father's height	0.128	0.124	0.210	1.035	0.323
	Mother's height	−0.559	0.170	−0.617	−3.284	0.007
	Height SDS chronologic age	1.132	0.363	0.697	3.116	0.010
	Dose	0.104	0.052	0.385	2.009	0.070
5	(Constant)	−1.138	0.929		−1.225	0.244
	Mother's height	−0.575	0.170	−0.634	−3.381	0.005
	Height SDS chronologic age	1.325	0.313	0.816	4.229	0.001
	Dose	0.121	0.049	0.451	2.487	0.029

SE, standard error; SDS, standard deviation scores.
[a]Dependent variable: final height SDS.
Note: Because the sample size is small, we set probability for variables to enter the regression equation at 0.15 and for variables to be removed at 0.20.
Data from Hindmarsh PC, Brook CG: Final height of short normal children treated with growth hormone, *Lancet*. 1996 Jul 6; 348(9019):13-16.

Survey Research

11

KEY CONCEPTS

 Survey research is one of the most common forms of research.

 Survey research generally involves asking people about a topic, although some surveys may be based on existing data sources.

 A clear research question and specific objectives help guide the design of a survey and questionnaire.

 Survey topics may need to be investigated with focus groups in order to know the specific issues that are important to study.

 Survey methods are determined by the research question. They include interviews and self-administered questionnaires using the mail or telephone. They may be web-based, or given in person.

 The most appropriate types of questions and response scales should be selected, and questions should be free from bias.

 Questions that have a predetermined list of possible responses are easier to analyze than open-ended questions.

 The choice of scale (nominal, ordinal, numerical) has ramifications for ways in which the results can be analyzed.

 Answers need to be balanced with equal numbers of positive and negative response options.

 In general, responses should be specific and avoid vague adjectives.

 Response categories need to be homogeneous and mutually exclusive.

 Potentially objectionable questions can sometimes be softened so they are more acceptable to the subject.

 Questions permitting subjects to select as many options as they choose can present challenges at the time of analysis.

 People often find ranking scales difficult if more than three choices are to be ranked.

 Likert scales are popular and easy for respondents to understand.

 Reliability indicates whether the results from a test or questionnaire are reproducible.

 Validity indicates whether a test or questionnaire is measuring what it is intended to measure.

 Pilot testing is essential and need not use a large sample.

 A high response rate provides more confidence in the findings.

 Effective follow-up is the most important way to increase response rates.

 A well-crafted cover letter should accompany all questionnaires.

Incentives, both monetary and nonmonetary, appear to have a large effect on response rates.

 Ethical considerations and institutional review boards require that respondents be assured that their responses will be kept confidential.

 Appropriate sampling methods lead to more valid studies so long as the type of respondent is pertinent to the research question.

 Determining the required number of subjects is part of the survey design process.

 Survey results are analyzed using the methods previously discussed in this book.

 PRESENTING PROBLEMS

Presenting Problem 1

The Patient Dignity Inventory (PDI) measures the dignity-related stress experienced by a cancer patient. Li and colleagues (2018) studied the validity and reliability of translation of the PDI into Mandarin 9PDI-MV). Each time a survey instrument is translated into a new language, the reliability and validity should be retested in that language to ensure that the survey is still fulfilling its purpose in the new language.

The full paper may be accessed here:

Li Y-C, Wang H-H, Ho C-H: Validity and reliability of the Mandarin version of Patient Dignity Inventory (PDI-MV) in cancer patients. PLoS ONE 2018;13(9):e0203111.

https://doi.org/10.1371/journal.pone.0203111

Presenting Problem 2

With the number of surveys sent to physicians increasing each day, the challenge of optimizing the response rate is a difficult one to overcome. Brtnikova et al (2018) studied a number of different sampling and reminder methods including email, hard copy mail, and post cards. They found that response rates varied from 66% to 83% and discovered different levels of response among specialties.

The article may be accessed here:

Brtnikova M, Crane LA, Allison MA, Hurley LP, Beaty BL, Kempe A: A method for achieving high response rates in national surveys of U.S. primary care physicians. PLoS ONE 2018;13(8):e0202755.

https://doi.org/10.1371/journal.pone.0202755

The data may be accessed at this link:

https://ndownloader.figshare.com/files/12852026

Presenting Problem 3

Urinary tract infections (UTIs) are among the most common bacterial infections, accounting for 7 million outpatient visits and 1 million hospital admissions in the United States each year. They are usually caused by Escherichia coli and are often treated empirically with trimethoprim–sulfamethoxazole. Recent guidelines from the Infectious Disease Society of America recommend this drug as standard therapy with specific fluoroquinolones as second-line choices. Two important factors in the selection of treatment are the health care costs of drug therapy and emergence of resistance to trimethoprim–sulfamethoxazole among E. coli strains causing UTIs. Huang and Stafford (2002) used survey data from the National Ambulatory Medical Care Survey (NAMCS) to assess the demographics and clinical characteristics of women who visit primary care physicians and specialists for UTIs.

THE RESEARCH QUESTIONS

With a little common sense and the information from this chapter, you can develop questionnaires to evaluate courses, learn student preferences for use in an educational program, and other undertakings in which you want to gather information locally. For more extensive projects, especially those related to a research project, you may wish to consult a biostatistician, epidemiologist, or other professional with survey expertise.

Everyone knows about surveys. In fact, the average person's opinion of statistics is greatly based on the results of polls and marketing surveys. Many people associate surveys with the U.S. census, which occurs every 10 years, but a census is not really a survey. A census queries everyone in the population, whereas a survey queries only a sample from the population. Survey research became more prominent

Table 11–1. Advantages and disadvantages of different survey methods.

	Self-Administered Mail/Email	Self-Administered in Person	Interview by Phone	Interview in Person
Cost	++	+	–	–
Time	++	+	–	–
Standardization	+	+	+/–	+/–
Depth/detail	–	–	+	++
Response rate	–	++	+	++
Missing responses	–	++	++	++

+, Advantage; –, Disadvantage; +/–, Neutral.

after World War II as manufacturers began to market products to the public and hired marketing experts to learn what would make the product sell. At the same time, political pollsters began to have an increasing presence garnering public opinion about specific issues and learning which candidate was leading during an election campaign. Today, surveys seem omnipresent, and, as a result, many people think that survey research is easy—just design some questions and get some people to answer them. The purpose of this chapter is to acquaint you with some of the issues in designing, administering, and interpreting surveys.

The term *poll* is generally associated with political polls, but it simply means asking questions in order to learn information or opinions. The Gallup Organization and the Roper Center are two of the largest polling organizations in the United States. They both use proper methods to design surveys and to select random samples of respondents.

A large number of excellent resources exist for those who want to design a survey. We have selected some salient issues to discuss in this chapter, and we have used a number of resources that you may wish to consult if you desire further information: Dillman (2014), Fink and Kosecoff (1998), Korn and Graubard (1999), Litwin and Fink (1995), and Rea and Parker (1997).

Determining the Research Question

The need to know the answer to a question generally motivates survey research, such as those in the Presenting Problems. As with any other research question, a crucial first step is to review the literature to learn what is known on the topic and what other methods have been used previously.

It may be difficult to specify the precise issues that should be addressed in a survey. For instance, suppose a researcher wants to know how health care workers view the elderly, and after performing a MEDLINE search can find little information on the subject. In this situation, **focus groups** may help refine the issues. Focus groups are interviews of a small number of people, generally 6 to 10, rather than individual interviews, and are done in person or over the telephone. One can get a great deal of information during a focus group session by obtaining in-depth responses to a few general questions. Of course, asking an expert, if one is available, is always advisable—in developing a research question as well as in reviewing a draft questionnaire.

Decide on the Survey Method

Most surveys use self-administered questionnaires —either in person or via mail or email, or interviews —again in person or over the telephone. Advantages and disadvantages exist for each method, some of which are illustrated in Table 11–1.

When interviews are used for survey research, they are often called structured interviews, in which the same questions are administered to each subject in the same order, and no coaching is permitted. In other words, the researcher tries to make the questions and the manner in which they are asked identical for all persons being interviewed. In other situations, less-structured interviews that permit the investigator to probe areas can yield rich results, although the data do not lend themselves to the quantitative methods we have used in this book. A famous example was the pioneering work in human sexuality by Alfred Kinsey in the 1940s in which he interviewed many people to learn about their sexual habits. Book 4 in the *Survey Kit* by Litwin and Fink (1995) is devoted to how to conduct interviews in person and by telephone.

The majority of the studies in the medical literature use self-administered questionnaires, these may be self-administered and mail surveys like the patient satisfaction surveys distributed by many health care providers. Researchers are also turning to national databases to answer survey questions, such as the study by Robbins et al (2018).

Surveys are generally thought of as cross-sectional and measuring the current situation, and certainly most surveys fit this category. However, questionnaires

Table 11–2. Open versus closed questions.

	Use Open	Use Closed
Purpose	Actual words or quotes	Most common answers
Respondents	Capable of providing answers in their words	Willing to answer only if easy and quick; may write illegibly
Asking the question	Choices are unknown	Choices can be anticipated
Analyzing results	Content analysis; time-consuming	Counting or scoring
Reporting results	Individual or grouped responses	Statistical data

---

BOX 11–1. OPEN VERSUS CLOSED QUESTIONS.

Open Question

What is the importance of reputation in choosing a fellowship?

Please describe: _____

Closed question

What is the importance of reputation in choosing a fellowship?
- ❑ Definitely important
- ❑ Probably important
- ❑ Probably unimportant
- ❑ Definitely unimportant

---

are used in cohort and case–control studies as well. The Nurses' Health study is a good example; this study began in the late 1970s with follow-up questionnaires mailed to over 280,000 nurses every 2 years (Colditz et al, 1997).

Developing the Questions

Many ways to ask questions exist, and survey designers want to state questions so that they are clear and obtain the desired information. We discuss a number of examples, some of which are modeled on the text by Dillman and colleagues (2014) and subsequently modified to reflect medical content by Dr. Laura Q. Rogers.

Decide Format of Questions—Open-Ended Versus Closed: Open-ended questions are ones that permit the subject to respond in his or her own words. They are sometimes appropriate, as shown in Table 11–2, such as when the topic has not been studied before, and it is important to obtain answers that have not been cued by any listed responses. Many researchers analyze the content of the answers and try to classify them into categories. A primary advantage of open-ended questions is the capability to report some of the prototypic answers using a subject's own words. Closed-response questions are more difficult to write, but their payoff is the ease with which the answers can be analyzed and reported. Many of the statistical methods discussed in this text can be used to analyze survey responses. A compromise approach can be taken by using a set of responses gleaned from the literature or focus groups, but also adding an opportunity for subjects to write in a brief answer if none from the responses fits. These questions generally have an "Other—please explain" at the end of the response set.

An example of a question with open versus closed questions is given in Box 11–1. Does the closed response set have an answer with which you would be comfortable?

Decide on the Scale for the Answer: If closed questions are used, the researcher needs to decide the level of detail required in the answers. The scale helps determine which methods can be used to analyze the results. Sometimes knowing only whether a subject agrees with the question is sufficient (nominal), such as whether a large city location is important in the choice of a training program (Box 11–2). An ordinal scale may be used if knowing gradations of importance is desired. Alternatively, an ordinal scale giving a choice of city sizes provides more specific information. At the other end of the spectrum is an open-ended question in which the subject provides a number (numerical). Depending on the question, we generally recommend that researchers collect data in as much detail as is reasonable; for instance, it is always possible to form categories of age for tables or graphs later (see Chapter 3). On the other hand, too much detail is not necessary and leads to unreliable data. For the question about city size, we would opt for one of the two ordinal response sets.

Balancing Positive and Negative Categories: Questions using an ordinal response should provide as many positive as negative options. Box 11–3 shows two sets of options regarding students' satisfaction with the Introduction to Clinical Medicine course. The first set places the neutral answer in the fourth position and provides only one answer in which students can express dissatisfaction. The second set is more likely to provide valid responses, with the neutral answer in the middle position and the same number of positive and negative options.

BOX 11-2. CHOOSING THE SCALE FOR THE QUESTION.

Nominal

Is a large city environment important in choosing a fellowship?
- ❑ Yes
- ❑ No

Ordinal

How important is a large city environment in choosing a fellowship?
- ❑ Definitely important
- ❑ Somewhat important
- ❑ Doesn't matter
- ❑ Somewhat unimportant
- ❑ Definitely unimportant

How large a city is important in choosing a fellowship?
- ❑ 25,000 or less
- ❑ 25,001 to 50,000
- ❑ 50,001 to 100,000
- ❑ 100,001 to 500,000
- ❑ Larger than 500,000

Numerical

How large a city is important in choosing a fellowship?

BOX 11-3. BALANCED RESPONSES.

Problem:

How satisfied were you with the Introduction to Clinical Medicine Course?
- ❑ Completely satisfied
- ❑ Mostly satisfied
- ❑ Somewhat satisfied
- ❑ Neither satisfied or dissatisfied
- ❑ Dissatisfied

Revision to balance responses:

How satisfied were you with the Introduction to Clinical Medicine Course?
- ❑ Completely satisfied
- ❑ Mostly satisfied
- ❑ Neither satisfied or dissatisfied
- ❑ Mostly dissatisfied
- ❑ Completely dissatisfied

BOX 11-4. AVOIDING VAGUE QUALIFIERS.

Problem:

How many alcoholic beverages did you drink during the past week?
- ❑ None
- ❑ A few
- ❑ Several
- ❑ Many

Revision to be less vague:

How many alcoholic beverages did you drink during the past week?
- ❑ Zero
- ❑ 1–5
- ❑ 6–10
- ❑ 20
- ❑ >20

Avoid Vague Qualifiers: What are the potential problems in using terms like *sometimes, often, rarely,* and so on? Box 11–4 illustrates two questions that ask the amount of alcohol consumed weekly. The choices specifying actual numbers of drinks is much less ambiguous and will be easier to interpret.

Use Mutually Exclusive Categories: In filling out a questionnaire, how many times have you encountered a question in which you don't understand the issue being addressed? This may result because the options are not mutually exclusive. For example, the question in Box 11–5 is confusing because it is mixing educational activities and sources of information. The easiest solution is to form two questions, each of which has mutually exclusive answers.

Potentially Objectionable Questions: Some questions are viewed as very personal, and people hesitate to divulge the information. Examples include income, sexual activity, and personal habits; see Box 11–6. These questions can be dealt with in two ways. First is to soften the manner in which the question is asked, perhaps by asking for less detail; it is generally better to obtain an approximate answer than none at all. Second is placement in the questionnaire itself; some survey experts recommend placement near the end of the questionnaire, after people have become comfortable with answering questions.

13 **Check All-That-Apply Items:** Items in which subjects can choose as many options as they wish are often used when survey questions ask about qualities of a product or why consumers selected

a specific model, school, or service. They do not force the subject to single out one best feature. They can, however, be tricky to analyze. The best approach is to treat each option as a yes/no variable and calculate the percentage of time each was selected. Box 11–7 shows that how they used the responses of ask/don't ask for each question.

Using "Don't Know": No consensus exists in the use of a "Don't Know" or "Undecided" category. Some researchers do not like to provide an opportunity for a subject not to commit to an answer. Others point out that not providing this type of option forces respondents to indicate opinions they do not really hold. If these categories are used, placement at the end of the

---

BOX 11-5. NONHOMOGENEOUS AND MUTUALLY EXCLUSIVE CATEGORIES.

Problem:

Which of the following sources provided you with the most information concerning smoking cessation?
- ❏ Medical school training
- ❏ Residency training
- ❏ Attending physician
- ❏ Colleague
- ❏ Printed medical journal
- ❏ Web site or other web-related resource
- ❏ Published book/pamphlet
- ❏ Drug salesperson

Revision to be mutually exclusive:

Which educational experience provided you with the most information concerning smoking cessation?
- ❏ Medical school training
- ❏ Residency training
- ❏ Continuing education

Which source provided you with the most information concerning smoking cessation?
- ❏ Colleague
- ❏ Printed medical journal
- ❏ Web site or other web-related resource
- ❏ Published book/pamphlet
- ❏ Drug salesperson

BOX 11-6. SOFTENING POTENTIALLY OBJECTIONAL QUESTIONS.

Problem:

What was your total income from all sources in 2019?

$_____Total income for 2019

Softening objectional questions:

Which of the following broad categories best describes your total income from all sources in 2019?
- ❏ $10,000 or less
- ❏ $10,001 to $20,000
- ❏ $20,001 to $35,000
- ❏ $35,001 to $50,000
- ❏ $50,001 to $100,000
- ❏ More than $100,000

BOX 11-7. ILLUSTRATION OF YES/NO SCALES INSTEAD OF CHECK-ALL-THAT-APPLY.

For your patients who you believe do **NOT** exercise adequately, about which of the following aspects do you ask routinely?

	Ask	Don't Ask
10. Why they do not exercise	1	0
11. What previous types of exercise they have done	1	0
12. What their attitude is toward exercise	1	0
13. What their beliefs are about exercise	1	0
14. What type of exercise their friends or family get	1	0
15. What they know about how to exercise to improve health	1	0

Modified with permission from Rogers LQ, Bailey JE, Gutin B, et al: Teaching resident physicians to provide exercise counseling: a needs assessment, *Acad Med.* 2002 Aug;77(8):841-844.

question rather than in the middle of the question has been shown to increase the completion rate of questions by 9%.

⑭ Ranking Versus Rating: In general, subjects confuse ranking scales in which they are asked to rank a number of choices from 1 to whatever. We believe that ranking options is fine when the researcher wants to know which choice is viewed as the "best" by most subjects. Selecting the top 3 choices also works well; however, beyond that, many people begin to have difficulty. For instance, some people omit one number and/or rank two options with the same number. Furthermore, although most people can discriminate among a limited number of choices, they have trouble when the list becomes long. Rating scales have difficulties as well, including the tendency for responses often to cluster at one end of the scale.

Summary of Suggestions for Writing Questions: Responses will be more valid and response rates will be higher if user-friendly questions are used on a survey. User-friendly questions have clear instructions with short, specific questions and are stated in a neutral manner. They avoid jargon and abbreviations that may be confusing, check-all-that-apply questions, and questions with too much detail (e.g., *how many minutes do you spend …*).

⑮ Issues Regarding Scales

If questions with ordinal scales are used, the researcher must decide among different options. Likert scales are commonly used on many surveys. They allow answers that range from "strongly disagree" to "strongly agree," from "most important" to "least important," and so on. We used Likert scales in the questions in Boxes 11–2 and 11–3 and listed the options vertically. When several questions use the same scale, the options may be listed in a row. Box 11–8 shows an excerpt from the survey by Caiola and Litaker (2000) in which several questions are asked about the quality of a fellowship. Note that the researchers provide an opportunity for respondents to add another quality if they wish.

No consensus exists in the survey literature about the number of categories to use. An even number of categories, such as the first question in Box 11–9, forces a respondent to choose some level of importance or unimportance, even if they are totally neutral. Our personal preference is for an odd number of categories with either five or seven categories, as illustrated in the second and third questions in Box 11–9. The choice of the number of categories can have a major effect on conclusions.

QUESTIONNAIRE LAYOUT

No hard and fast rules dictate the way a questionnaire is formatted, but some general, common sense guidelines apply. The first issue is length; although shorter surveys are generally preferable to longer surveys, Dillman and colleagues (2014) cite several studies that show that questionnaires up to four pages in length have similar response rates.

Well-designed questions place instructions where needed, even when it means repeating the instructions at the top of a continuation page. Avoid skipping or branching questions if possible; if not, use directional arrows and other visual guides to assist the subject.

BOX 11–8. ILLUSTRATION OF LIKERT SCALE.

Perceived Quality of a Fellowship Program:

Q–3. How important were the following factors as you **decided** on your fellowship program?
(Please circle **ONE** number, with **1** being **Not Very Important** and **5** being **Very Important**)

	Not Very Important				Very Important
1. National reputation of excellence	1	2	3	4	5
2. Academic placement of graduates	1	2	3	4	5
3. Renowned in research in your area of interest	1	2	3	4	5
4. Government sponsorship (e.g., GIM Faculty Development Program from HRSA)	1	2	3	4	5
5. Robert Wood Johnson Sponsorship	1	2	3	4	5
6. Other (*specify*)_____	1	2	3	4	5

Data from Caiola E, Litaker D: Factors influencing the selection of general internal medicine fellowship programs: a national survey, *J Gen Intern Med*. 2000 Sep;15(9):656-658.

Most researchers opt to place easier questions first and to list questions in logical order so that questions about the same topic are grouped together. When scales are used, subjects are less confused when the scale direction is listed in a consistent manner, such as from very important to very unimportant. Although no consensus exists on whether to place demographic items at the beginning or end of the questionnaire, we opt for the latter.

BOX 11–9. NUMBER OF RESPONSE OPTIONS.

Even number

How important is a large city environment in choosing a fellowship?
- ❏ Definitely important
- ❏ Somewhat important
- ❏ Somewhat unimportant
- ❏ Definitely unimportant

Odd number

How important is a large city environment in choosing a fellowship?
- ❏ Definitely important
- ❏ Somewhat important
- ❏ Doesn't matter
- ❏ Somewhat unimportant
- ❏ Definitely unimportant

Odd number with more than 5 options

How important is a large city environment in choosing a fellowship?
- ❏ Very important
- ❏ Moderately important
- ❏ Somewhat important
- ❏ Doesn't matter
- ❏ Somewhat unimportant
- ❏ Moderately unimportant
- ❏ Very unimportant

RELIABILITY AND VALIDITY OF SURVEY INSTRUMENTS

We advise researchers to use existing questionnaires or instruments if possible. Not only does this save time and effort in developing the questionnaire, it also avoids the need to establish the reliability and validity of the instrument. Furthermore, it is possible to make more direct comparisons between different studies if they use the same instrument. If an existing instruments meets 80% or more of the needs of a researcher, we recommend using it; additional questions that are deemed to be crucial can be included on a separate page.

Ways to Measure Reliability

We briefly discussed intra- and interrater reliability in Chapter 5 when we introduced the kappa statistic as a measure of agreement between observers. Questionnaires need to be reliable as well. The basic question answered by **reliability** is how reproducible the findings would be if the same measurement were repeatedly made on the same subject.

Five different types of reliability are listed in Table 11–3, along with methods to measure each type. An instrument's capacity to provide the same measurement on different occasions is called the **test–retest** reliability. Because it is difficult to administer the same instrument to the same people on more than one occasion, questionnaire developers and testing agencies often use internal consistency reliability as an estimate of test–retest reliability. Reliability as measured in these ways can be thought of as the correlation between two scores; it ranges from 0 to 1.00; an acceptable level of reliability is 0.80 or higher.

The **internal consistency** reliability of the items on the instrument or questionnaire indicates how strongly the items are related to one another; that is, whether they are measuring a single characteristic. Testing agencies that create examinations, such as the SAT or National Board USMLE Examinations, sometimes refer to the internal consistency reliability as Cronbach's alpha. (Note that this is not the same alpha as we use to measure a type I error in hypothesis testing.) Li and

Table 11–3. Types of reliability.

Type	Characteristics	How Measured
Test–retest	Responses are stable over time	Administer twice (generally estimated)
Internal consistency	Agreement among items (measuring the same thing)	Cronbach's alpha ("average" correlation)
Alternative form	Different items measure same topic	Correlation between item scores
Intraobserver	Observer is consistent	Intraclass correlation or McNemar statistic
Interobserver	Different observers agree	Intraclass correlation or kappa

Table 11–4. Types of validity.

Type	Characteristics	How Measured
Content	Appropriateness of content by experts	Subjective
Face	It looks on target by nonexperts	Subjective
Criterion-concurrent	Is associated with similar skills at present time	Correlation between scores on instruments
Criterion-predictive	Predicts similar skills in future	Correlation between scores on instruments
Construct (convergent & divergent)	Theoretical measure	Correlation with other measures

colleagues (2018) set out to test the reliability and validity of the Patient Dignity Inventory (PDI-MV) after a translation to Mandarin. The PDI was tested for reliability and validity in the English language version (Chochinov et al, 2008), but survey instruments must be retested when translated to other languages. They found an overall Chronbach's alpha of 0.95.

Our discussion of intra- and interrater reliability in Chapter 5 referred to nominal measurement, such as positive versus negative. If the measurement is numerical, such as the score on a test or a section of a questionnaire, intra- and interobserver agreement is measured by the intraclass correlation coefficient. The ordinary correlation coefficient is sensitive only to random error, also called noise, in a measurement. The intraclass correlation, however, is sensitive to both random error and systematic error, also called statistical bias. Statistical bias occurs when one observer always scores candidates higher by the same amount than another observer. More details about psychological measurement can be found in classic texts on measurement, such as the one by Anastasi and Urbina (1997).

Validity of Measurements

Validity is a term for how well an instrument (or measurement procedure) measures what it purports to measure. The issue of validity motivates many questions about measuring specific characteristics in medicine, such as how accurate the arthritis functional status scale is for indicating a patient's level of activity; how accurate the National Board Examination is in measuring students' knowledge of medicine; or, in the case of questionnaires, how well the Medical Outcomes Study Short Form 36 (MOS SF-36) measures quality of life.

Commonly used measures of validity are content, face, criterion, and construct validity. For a test or questionnaire, **content validity** indicates the degree to which the items on the instrument are representative of the knowledge being tested or the characteristic being investigated. **Face validity** refers to the degree to which

a questionnaire or test appears to be measuring what it is supposed to measure. In other words, a questionnaire about domestic violence training should have questions related to that issue.

Criterion validity refers to the instrument's capacity to predict a characteristic that is associated with the characteristic. For example, the criterion validity of the MOS SF-36 could be measured by comparing its quality-of-life score with subject interviews and physical examinations. The criterion may indicate either a concurrent or a future state. Ideally, criterion validity is established by comparing the measurement to a gold standard, if one exists. The final type of validity, **construct validity,** is more abstract and difficult to define. It consists of demonstrating that the instrument is related to other instruments that assess the same characteristic and not related to instruments that assess other characteristics. It is generally established by using several instruments or tests on the same group of individuals and investigating the pattern of relationships among the measurements (Table 11–4).

ADMINISTRATION OF SURVEYS

Several issues related to the design and administration of questionnaires, along with recommendations from the survey research literature, are listed in Table 11–5.

Pilot Testing

Almost everyone who has consulted with the author on questionnaire design has lamented, once the results are in, that they wish they had included another question, or asked a question in a different way, or provided other response options, and so on. It is almost impossible to carry out a perfect survey, but many problems can be caught by pilot testing the instrument. A pilot test is carried out after the questionnaire is designed but before it is printed or prepared for administration. Pilot testing may reveal that the reading level is not appropriate for the intended subjects, that some questions are unclear or are objectionable and need to be modified, or that instructions are unclear.

Table 11–5. Summary of issues related to administration of questionnaires.

Issue	Effect on Success of Survey
Response rates	Should be between 50% and 85%
Follow-up	Four to five every 2 weeks increases response rates significantly
Pilot testing	Critical to success of any survey
Cover letter	Provides purpose of survey and why response is important
Prenotification	Increases response rates by 7–8%
Return stamped envelope	Increases response rates by 6–9%
Providing incentives with survey	
Monetary	Increases response rates by 16–30%
Nonmonetary	Increases response rates by 8%
First-class postage, stamps	Small increase
Color of questionnaire	No known effect
Confidentiality	Must be guaranteed; required by IRBs

A large sample is not required to pilot test an instrument; it is more important to choose people who will provide feedback after completing the questionnaire. In most cases, the best subjects will not be your friends or colleagues, unless, of course, they are representative of the group who will receive the survey. If a large number of changes are required, it may be necessary to repeat the pilot test with another group of subjects.

Response Rates

Brtnikova and colleagues (2018) studied the response rates for questionnaires mailed to physicians and assessed the effectiveness of various methods used to increase response. They found that the overall response rate varied from 66% to 83% across 13 surveys regarding vaccine practices sent over Internet and mail from 2008 to 2013. For the mailed questionnaires, Brtnikova and colleagues followed Dillman's Tailored Design Method: a pre-letter explaining the importance of the survey, questionnaire and pre-stamped envelope 5 days later, and finally a reminder postcard after 5 more days.

A high response rate increases our confidence in the validity of the results and the likelihood that the results will be used. If demographic information on the sampled group is available, researchers can compare characteristics, such as sex, age, and other important variables, to learn if the distribution of these characteristics is the same in the subjects who returned the questionnaire. Brtnikova was able to assess the nonresponse bias for each survey.

Many suggestions on ways to go about follow-up have been made. The consensus indicates that the best response occurs with three to four follow-ups at approximately 2-week intervals. Each subsequent follow-up has a smaller yield, so it may be wise to stop with fewer follow-ups. Brtnikova and colleagues (2018) received an additional 15% and 11% response, respectively, with their second and third mailings. Chances are a fourth mailing would have little yield. For the Internet survey, the initial response was 18%; reminders every 3 days resulted in an additional 11% and 7%. Reminders after the third email yielded less than 5% additional responses. An extra handwritten letter to the Internet group did yield an additional 11% response.

Colleagues and students often ask what constitutes a good response rate. Far too many surveys report response rates less than 40%. With effort, it should be possible to obtain responses of 50% or more. If people are very interested in the topic, response rates often approach 70%, but it is possible to obtain as much as 85% or more in a highly selected sample or a "captive population." For this reason, some teachers require students to complete a questionnaire before receiving a grade; in continuing-education courses, someone often stands at the door to collect the course evaluations as attendees leave. The documentation for the National Ambulatory Medical Care Survey database used by Robbins and colleagues (2018) had annual response rates ranging from 54% to 73%.

Advance Notification

Many survey specialists recommend notifying the people who are to receive the survey in advance of its administration. Prenotification may by be done by letter, telephone, or, increasingly, by email. The prenotification should include information on who is doing the survey, what its purpose is, why the subject has been selected to receive the survey, how the results will be used, whether responses will be anonymous, and when the questionnaire will be mailed (or emailed) or the interview scheduled. Prenotification has been reported to increase response rate by 7% to 8%.

Cover Letters and Return Envelopes

If a questionnaire is administered directly, such as to a group of physicians in a continuing-education course, it is not necessary to include a cover letter. Otherwise, one is essential. Cover letters should be short, relevant, on letterhead, and signed. Information on the letter includes the purpose of the survey, why the recipient's response is important, and how the data will be used. Some researchers offer to share the results. To maintain anonymity, a separate postcard can be included for the recipient to return indicating a desire for a copy of the results. More questionnaires are returned when a stamped envelope is included; this practice is reported to increase response rates by 6% to 9%.

Incentives

Providing incentives to complete a questionnaire is controversial, but research has shown that it may increase response rates more than any other single action, except repeated follow-ups. Monetary incentives, even modest ones of a few dollars, are reported to increase responses by 16% to 30% and nonmonetary incentives by up to 8%. Response rates are similar, regardless of whether the incentive is sent with the questionnaire or as a reward after it is returned. Material incentives also increase response rates, but by only about half as much, and lotteries or chances to win tickets or prizes have relatively little effect. Dillman (2014) provides an extensive discussion of these and other issues related to improving response rates.

Anonymity and Confidentiality

The cover letter should contain information on anonymity or confidentiality. Depending on the purpose and sensitivity of the questionnaire, it may be advisable to make the returns completely anonymous. The researcher can still keep track of who returns the questionnaire by asking the responder to mail a separate postcard at the time he or she returns the questionnaire. Only the postcard and not the questionnaire itself contains any information that can be used to identify the respondent. This practice permits the researcher to remove the responder's name from the follow-up list, thereby saving administrative costs and potentially annoying the responder.

Confidentiality of responses is a different issue. If questionnaires can be identified with a number or code, it is easier to know who has returned the questionnaire and streamlines the follow-up process. Regardless, subjects always need to be assured that their responses will be kept confidential. No individual's response can be identified in any information reported or otherwise communicated. With the increasing protection for human subjects, confidentiality is almost always required by institutional review boards (IRBs) as a prerequisite to approving the survey.

SELECTING THE SAMPLE & DETERMINING N

Properly done survey research is based on the principle that a randomly selected sample can represent the responses of all people. Randomly selected samples are, in fact, more accurate than questioning everyone. For instance, the U.S. census is well known to have a problem with undercounting certain populations, and the American Statistical Association has recommended the use of sampling to deal with this shortcoming. The U.S. census continues to use a census rather than random samples, largely for political rather than statistical reasons; the results are used to reallocate seats in the House of Representatives and form the foundation for allocation of federal funds to states. Research has shown that properly selected samples provide more accurate estimates of underrepresented populations than the census, and random samples are generally used to correct the census undercount.

Review of Sampling Methods

We discussed random sampling methods in Chapter 4 and very briefly review them here. A simple random sample is one in which every subject has an equal chance of being selected.

Random samples are typically selected using computer-generated random numbers or a table of random numbers, as we illustrated in Chapter 4. A systematic random sample is one in which every kth item is selected, where k is determined by dividing the number of items in the sampling frame by the desired sample size. Systematic sampling is simple to use and effective as long as no cyclic repetition is inherent in the sampling frame.

A stratified random sample is one in which the population is first divided into strata or subgroups, and a random sample is then selected from each stratum. This method, if properly used, requires the smallest sample size, and it is the method used for most sponsored surveys and by most professional polling organizations. The database used by Robbins (2018) was a random sample of U.S. physicians stratified by geographic region and specialty. Stratified sampling requires great care in analyzing the data, because a response from one physician may represent 10 other physicians, whereas the response from a second physician may represent 25 other physicians. A cluster random sample occurs when the population is divided into clusters and a subset of the clusters is randomly selected. Cluster sampling requires a larger sample size than other methods and presents even greater challenges for analysis. Recall that nonprobability sampling to obtain quota or convenience samples does not fulfill the requirements of randomness needed to estimate sampling errors and use statistical methods.

Finding the Sample Size for a Survey

Many national survey organizations, such as Gallup, use approximately 1,000 people in a given poll, and, as previously noted, large sponsored surveys typically use complicated sampling designs. However, many of the studies published in the medical literature use samples selected by the investigators.

When determining a sample size, we first ask, "What are study outcomes?" Is it the percentage of people who respond a given way? The "average" response (based on a scale of some sort)? The difference between two or more types of respondents (either percentages or averages)? or, The relationship among questions, such as: Do people who exercise regularly also eat a proper diet? By this point in this book, you probably recognize each of these situations as those we covered in Chapter 5 (for a proportion or mean), Chapters 6 and 7 (comparing two or more proportions or means), or Chapter 8 (correlations among variables). In each of these chapters we illustrated methods for finding a sample size, so we review these very briefly here and refer you back to the previous chapters for more detail. Recall that power is the sample size needed to have a reasonable chance of finding an effect if there is one.

Dyrbye and colleagues (2018) wanted to estimate the percentage of residents that reported symptoms of burn out. They might have expected that approximately 50% would view research as an important factor. Using the G*Power program, we see from Box 11–10 that a sample of 199 is sufficient for a 95% confidence interval if the proportion is around 50 and we wish to detect a 10% shift from the 50%. Dyrbye and colleagues had responses from 3,588 of the 4,732 eligible residents, so they can be assured that their finding of 45.2% is within ± 3.5% of the true proportion.

None of our presenting problems involved estimating means, but, for the sake of illustration, we'll assume that a researcher wanted to estimate the mean score for the sum of the six questions dealing with the ability of exercise to prevent disease or improve health: decreases overall mortality, decreases coronary heart disease mortality, decreases COPD mortality, improves blood sugar control, improves lipoprotein profile, prevents hip fractures. Suppose they want to form a 95% confidence interval about the mean score for these six items. Box 11–11 shows the output from G*Power when the standard deviation of the sum is estimated to be 3, and the desired confidence interval is within ± 0.5. A sample size of 285 is sufficient.

ANALYSIS OF SURVEY RESULTS

Almost all of the statistical procedures we discussed in Chapters 3 to 10 are used to analyze survey data. Confidence limits for proportions, means, the difference between proportions or means, and correlations are all relevant, in addition to chi-square and other nonparametric tests; t tests; analysis of variance; and regression, including logistic regression. Procedures that are rarely used include those that analyze time-dependent outcomes, such as Kaplan–Meier curves and the Cox model, because surveys rarely ask subjects the length of time until an event occurs.

Analyzing Dyrbye and Colleagues

Dyrbye and colleagues reported the relative risk of burnout for female residents as well as other factors.

Analyzing Brtnikova and Colleagues

Brtnikova et al used chi-square tests and descriptive statistics to describe the impact of various survey models on response rate. Table 11–6 is reproduced from the study and lists a number of responder characteristics and the rates of response. The p values are the results of chi-square tests for association of the sample characteristic and the level of response.

Analyzing Robbins and Colleagues

A situation we have not discussed before is the use of weights in analyzing data. As we mentioned with stratified samples, not all subjects represent the same number of nonsampled subjects. For instance, suppose a researcher wants to survey 500 physicians in each of the states of Illinois, New York, and California. The estimated 2010 census for these states was 12.8, 19.3, and 37.2 million, respectively. Assuming that the number of physicians is similarly distributed, a randomly sampled physician in California would "represent" almost twice as many other physicians as in New York and almost three times as many as in Illinois. Thus, a single response would have these approximate weights: 1 if from Illinois, 1.5 if from New York, and 2.9 if from California. These weights are used in any analysis that involves responses from more than one state.

Robbins et al (2018) had to include weights to reflect a complicated sampling plan. Their data was from the National Ambulatory Medical Care Survey (NAMCS) from 2005 through 2012. Each year NAMCS uses master lists from the American Medical Association and American Osteopathic Association to select a random sample of physicians, stratified by geographic area and specialty. For each participating physician, patient visits during a randomly selected

BOX 11-10. G*POWER SAMPLE SIZE CALCULATION TO ESTIMATE PERCENTAGE OF RESIDENTS WITH SYMPTOMS OF BURN OUT.

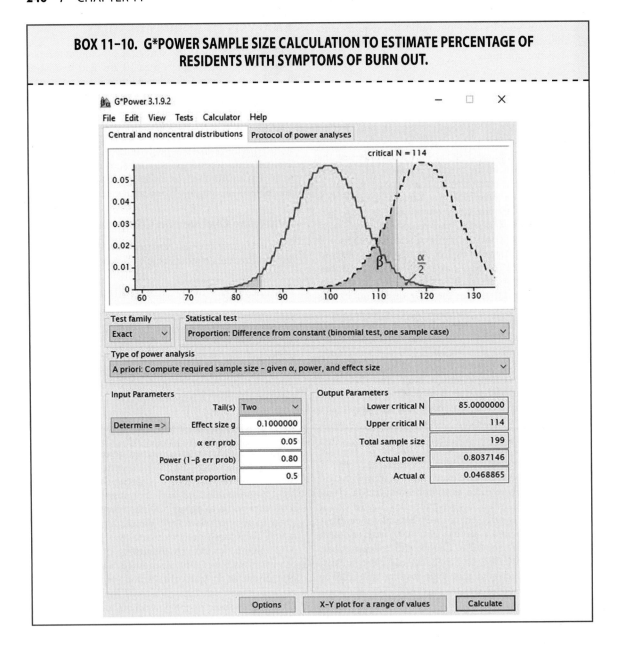

week are systematically sampled. Robbins et al selected hypertension patient visits where sleep apnea diagnosis or complaint was recorded. They subsequently excluded any women who had codes for urologic procedures, pregnancy, diabetes mellitus, cancer, and several other comorbid conditions. The result was a sample of 2,612 unweighted patient visits or 3 million weighted visits. Because of the complex sampling system, Robbins had to include different weights for each individual subject according to the analysis they were doing.

SUMMARY

We discussed three survey articles in this chapter. Brtnikova and colleagues (2018) studied factors that impact the response rate for surveys of physicians. They studied both email and mailed surveys. The impact of a number of reminder strategies were evaluated in addition to the impact of multiple surveys on response rates.

Dyrbye and colleagues (2018) studied the factors that may lead to physician burnout. They found that

BOX 11-11. EXAMPLE USE OF G*POWER TO CALCULATE SAMPLE SIZE REQUIRED TO ESTIMATE MEAN FROM SURVEY.

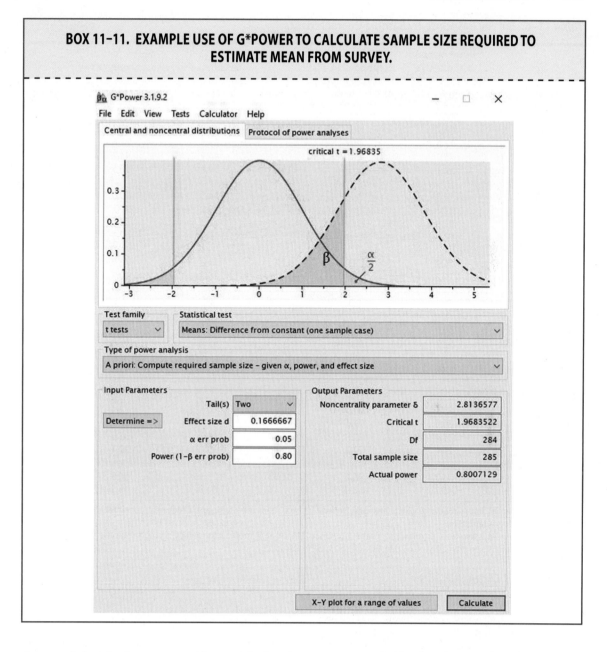

the rate of physician burnout varied by specialty based on a survey of over 3,500 second-year residents. They reported the relative risk of burnout for a number of characteristics including gender, specialty, and level of anxiety in medical school.

Robbins and colleagues (2018) evaluated patterns in physician management of sleep apnea for patients with hypertension. They found that there were differences in the pattern in ordering of a behavioral treatment for patients; patients with obesity were more likely to

receive an order for this treatment (OR 4.96 [2.93 to 8.38]) while smokers were less likely to receive behavioral treatment (OR 0.54 [0.32 to 0.93]). Medication was offered less often to patients of non-Hispanic Black race/ethnicity (OR 0.19 [0.06 to 0.65]).

We reviewed some of the important factors when designing and administering a survey. We provided only a general overview of survey research, but provided a number of references for those readers who want to learn more. We recommend that researchers

Table 11–6. Survey Response by Sample Characteristics.

Characteristic	Did not respond to all surveys (n = 2111, 55%) Column %	Responded to all surveys (n = 1740, 45%) Column %	p value	Responded to none (n = 497, 13%) Column %	Responded at least to one survey (n = 3354, 87%) Column %	p value
Specialty						
FM	36.7	28.7	<.0001	31.8	33.3	0.80
GIM	18.4	28.0		23.3	22.6	
Peds	45.0	43.3		44.9	44.1	
Male, %	52.1	51.2	0.57	59.6	50.5	0.0002
Provider Age						
Less than 40	19.3	17.3	0.01	14.3	19.0	0.002
40–49	32.0	28.7		35.9	29.7	
50–59	31.8	36.1		30.1	34.2	
Over 60	17.0	17.9		19.8	17.1	
Practice setting, %						
Private practice	76.9	77.5	0.12	79.3	76.9	0.49
Community/ hospital based	19.2	17.5		16.9	18.7	
HMO or MCO	3.8	5.0		3.8	4.4	
Practice location, %						
Urban, Inner city	30.6	39.5	<.0001	33.8	34.7	0.04
Urban, non-inner/ Suburban	52.7	43.3		52.7	47.8	
Rural	16.8	17.2		13.5	17.5	
Region of the Country, %						
Midwest	23.6	23.5	0.10	24.6	23.4	0.005
Northeast	20.6	22.4		23.5	21.1	
South	35.4	32.0		36.8	33.5	
West	20.4	22.2		15.1	22.1	
Providers in practice						
1–5	53.3	48.4	0.003	55.5	50.5	0.06
6 or more	46.7	51.6		44.5	49.5	

Peds, pediatricians; FM, family medicine physicians; GIM, general internal medicine physicians; HMO, health maintenance organization; MCO, managed care organization.
Reproduced with permission from Brtnikova M, Crane LA, Allison MA, et al: A method for achieving high response rates in national surveys of U.S. primary care physicians, *PLoS One*. 2018 Aug 23;13(8):e0202755.

consider using a standard questionnaire if at all possible; it is much faster because the work of writing questions and pilot testing has already been done. If standard questionnaires are used, researchers can compare their results with other studies, and the reliability and validity of the instrument has generally been established.

We expect that the surveys using email and the Internet will become increasingly popular. Already, some researchers are using them and others use fax machines for responses to short questionnaires. Dillman et al (2014) is an excellent source for information on email and Internet surveys. Several first-rate software packages are available for those interested in designing questionnaires and using the Internet including SurveyMonkey and Qualtrics.

A number of excellent resources are available on the Internet. They include:

American Statistical Association Section on Survey Research http://www.amstat.org/sections/srms/

StatPack Survey Software http://www.statpac.com/surveys/

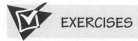

EXERCISES

1. What are the difficulties, if any, with the following surveys:

   a. Questionnaires handed out on an airplane to measure customer satisfaction

   b. A poll in which people sign onto the Internet and vote on an issue

   c. Satisfaction questionnaires mailed to all patients by hospitals and clinics

   d. Requiring students to hand in a course evaluation before receiving their final grade

2. If you wanted to analyze the information in Table 11–6 using statistical methods, what procedure(s) would you use?

3. A pediatrician is planning to survey the parents of a random sample of patients and wants to know how many hours their child watches TV each month. How would you ask this question?

4. A clinic manager wants to survey a random sample of patients to learn how they view some recent changes made in the clinic operation. The manager has drafted a questionnaire and wants you to review it. One of the questions asks, "Do you agree that the new clinic hours are an improvement over the old ones?" What advice will you give the manager about the wording of this question?

5. Suppose you would like to know how far physicians are willing to travel to attend continuing-education course, assuming that some number of hours is required each year. In addition, you want to learn topics they would like to have included in future programs. You plan to publish the results of your study. How would you select the sample of physicians to include in your survey?

   a. All physicians who attended last year's programs

   b. All physicians who attend the two upcoming programs

   c. A random sample of physicians who attended last year's programs

   d. A random sample of physicians obtained from a list maintained by the state medical society

   e. A random sample of physicians in each county obtained from a list maintained by the county medical societies

Methods of Evidence-Based Medicine and Decision Analysis

12

KEY CONCEPTS

 Selecting the appropriate diagnostic procedure depends, in part, on the clinician's index of suspicion.

 The threshold model for testing contains two decision points: when the index of suspicion is high enough to order a diagnostic procedure, and when the index of suspicion is so high that results from a procedure will not influence subsequent actions.

 Two components of evaluating diagnostic procedures are sensitivity and specificity.

 Sensitivity is a procedure's ability to detect a disease if one is present.

 Specificity is a procedure's ability to give a negative result if no disease is present.

 Two errors are possible: false-positive results occur when the procedure is positive but no disease is present; false-negative results occur when the procedure is negative but a disease is present.

 Sensitivity and specificity must be combined with the clinician's index of suspicion to properly interpret a procedure.

 The 2 × 2 table method provides a simple way to use sensitivity and specificity to determine how to interpret the diagnostic procedure after it is done.

 After sensitivity and specificity are applied to the clinician's index of suspicion, the probability of a disease based on a positive test and the probability of no disease with a negative test can be found. They are the predictive values of a positive and negative test, respectively.

 A likelihood ratio is the ratio of true-positives to false-positives; it is used with the prior odds of a disease (instead of the prior probability) to determine the odds after the test is done.

 A decision tree may be used to find predictive values.

 Bayes' theorem gives the probability of one outcome, given that another outcome has occurred. It is another way to calculate predictive values.

 A sensitive test is best to rule out a disease; a specific test is used to rule in a disease.

 ROC (receiver operating characteristic) curves are used for diagnostic procedures that give a numerical result, rather than simply being positive and negative.

 Decision analysis, often using decision trees, is an optimal way to model approaches to diagnosis or management.

 Outcomes for the decision analysis may be costs, quality-of-life adjusted survival, or subjective utilities measuring how the patient values different outcomes.

 The optimal decision from a decision tree may be analyzed to learn how sensitive the decision is to various assumptions regarding probabilities, costs, and so on.

Decision analysis can be used to compare two or more alternative approaches to diagnosis or management (or both).

 Decision analysis can be used to compare the timing for diagnostic testing.

 Journal articles should not publish predictive values without reminding readers that these values depend on the prevalence or index of suspicion.

 PRESENTING PROBLEMS

Presenting Problem 1

A 57-year-old man presents with a history of low back pain. The pain is aching in quality, persists at rest, and is made worse by bending and lifting. The pain has been getting progressively worse, and in the past 6 weeks has been awakening him at night. Within the past 10 days, he has noticed numbness in the right buttock and thigh and weakness in the right lower extremity. He denies fever, but has had a slight loss of appetite and a 10-lb weight loss over a period of 4 months. He has no prior history of low back pain and his general health has been good. The physical examination reveals a temperature of 99.6°F, tenderness in the lower lumbar spine, a decrease in sensation over the dorsal and lateral aspect of the right foot, and weakness of right ankle eversion. Deep tendon reflexes were normal.

*Based on your review of the literature, the patient's history, and physical examination, you suspect the man has a 20% to 30% chance of a spinal malignancy. You must decide whether to order an erythrocyte sedimentation rate (ESR) or directly order imaging studies, such as a lumbar MRI. Joines and colleagues (2001) compared several strategies for diagnosing cancer in patients with low back pain. These results were later reevaluated and confirmed by Deyo et al (2014). They reported the **sensitivity** and **specificity** for different diagnostic procedures, including an ESR ≥20 mm/h and several imaging studies. They reported a sensitivity of 78% and specificity of 67% for an ESR ≥20 mm/h and sensitivity and specificity of 95% for lumbar MRI. They developed several diagnostic strategies, or **decision trees,** for investigating the possibility of cancer in primary care outpatients with low back pain and determined the cost for each diagnostic strategy using data from the year 2000 Medicare reimbursements. Strategies were arranged in order of cost per patient and compared with the number of cases of cancer found per 1,000 patients. We use information from their study to illustrate sensitivity and specificity of a diagnostic procedure and again to illustrate the use of decision trees to compare strategies.*

Presenting Problem 2

Abraham et al (2017) studied various neurological examinations to determine which might be more effective in detecting polyneuropathy. They evaluated 312 patients to determine the sensitivity and specificity of the tests. Data summarizing some of their findings are given in the section titled, "Measuring the Accuracy of Diagnostic Procedures." We use some of these findings to illustrate sensitivity and specificity.

The full article and relevant data may be accessed here:

Abraham A, Alabdali M, Alsulaiman A, et al: The sensitivity and specificity of the neurological examination in polyneuropathy patients with clinical and electrophysiological correlations. PLoS ONE 2017;12(3):e0171597.

https://doi.org/10.1371/journal.pone.0171597

Presenting Problem 3

Dabi and colleagues (2017) validated a model that may be used to predict preterm delivery. They further analyzed the model to determine an optimal cutoff for the scores derived from the model. They used ROC curves and nomograms to evaluate the model.

The full article may be accessed at this link:

Dabi Y, Nedellec S, Bonneau C, Trouchard B, Rouzier R, Benachi A: Clinical validation of a model predicting the risk of preterm delivery. PLoS ONE 2017;12(2):e0171801.

https://doi.org/10.1371/journal.pone.0171801

The relevant data is included in the link above also.

Presenting Problem 4

As the cost of health care continues to grow, cost effectiveness analysis is becoming an important component in clinical decision-making. Gurusamy et al (2017) studied the cost-effectiveness of laparoscopic versus open distal pancreatectomy for the treatment of prostate cancer. They used cost-utility analysis as well as quality-adjusted life years (QALYs) to make their conclusions.

The manuscript may be accessed at this link:
Gurusamy KS, Riviere D, van Laarhoven CJH, et al: Cost-effectiveness of laparoscopic versus open distal pancreatectomy for pancreatic cancer. PLoS ONE 2017;12(12):e0189631.

https://doi.org/10.1371/journal.pone.0189631

The relevant data is reported along with the paper.

Presenting Problem 5

Nguyen and Adang (2018) evaluated the cost and benefits of implementing mammography for breast cancer screening for women in Vietnam. They report that the breast cancer incidence is increasing in Vietnam and that the survival rate is much lower than other countries. They use decision analysis including incremental cost-effectiveness ratios (ICERs) as well as incremental net monetary benefits (INMBs) to evaluate screening for various age groups.

The full article may be accessed here:
Nguyen CP, Adang EMM: Cost-effectiveness of breast cancer screening using mammography in Vietnamese women. PLoS ONE 2018;13(3):e0194996.

https://doi.org/10.1371/journal.pone.0194996

The data is reported in the paper and in the files in the paper supporting information.

INTRODUCTION

"Decision-making" is a term that applies to the actions people take many times each day. Many decisions—such as what time to get up in the morning, where and what to eat for lunch, and where to park the car—are often made with little thought or planning. Others—such as how to prepare for a major examination, whether or not to purchase a new car and, if so, what make and model—require some planning and may even include a conscious outlining of the steps involved. This chapter addresses the second type of decision-making as applied to problems within the context of medicine. These problems include evaluating the accuracy of diagnostic procedures, interpreting the results of a positive or negative procedure in a specific patient, **modeling** complex patient problems, and selecting the most appropriate approach to the problem. These topics are very important in using and applying **evidence-based medicine**; they are broadly defined as methods in **medical decision-making** or **analysis.** They are applications of probabilistic and statistical principles to *individual patients*, although they are not usually covered in introductory biostatistics textbooks.

Medical decision-making has become an increasingly important area of research in medicine for evaluating patient outcomes and informing health policy. More and more quality-assurance articles deal with topics such as evaluating new diagnostic procedures, determining the most cost-effective approach for dealing with certain diseases or conditions, and evaluating options available for treatment of a specific patient. These methods also form the basis for cost–benefit analysis.

Correct application of the principles of evidence-based medicine helps clinicians and other health care providers make better diagnostic and management decisions. Ioannidis (2017) discusses the abuse of statistics in evidence-based medicine.

Those who read the medical literature and wish to evaluate new procedures and recommended therapies for patient care need to understand the basic principles discussed in this chapter.

We begin the presentation with a discussion of the threshold model of decision-making, which provides a unified way of deciding whether to perform a diagnostic procedure. Next, the concepts of sensitivity and specificity are defined and illustrated. Four different methods that lead to equivalent results are presented. Then, an extension of the diagnostic testing problem in which the test results are numbers, not simply positive or negative, is given using the ROC curves. Finally, more complex methods that use decision trees and algorithms are introduced.

EVALUATING DIAGNOSTIC PROCEDURES WITH THE THRESHOLD MODEL

Consider the patient described in Presenting Problem 1, the 57-year-old man who is concerned about increasing low back pain. Before deciding how to proceed with diagnostic testing, the physician must consider the probability that the man has a spinal malignancy. This probability may simply be the **prevalence** of a particular disease if a screening test is being considered. If a history and a physical examination have been performed, the prevalence is adjusted, upward or downward, according to the patient's characteristics (e.g., age, gender, and race), symptoms, and signs.

Physicians use the term "index of suspicion" for the probability of a given disease prior to performing a diagnostic procedure; it is also called the **prior probability.** It may also be considered in the context of a threshold model (Pauker and Kassirer, 1980).

The **threshold model** allows a physician to balance the likelihood that patient has a disease with the decision of whether or not to perform a diagnostic test. The physician's estimate that the patient has the disease, from information available without using the diagnostic test, is called the probability of disease. It helps to think of the probability of disease as a line that extends from 0 to 1. According to this model, the **testing threshold,** T_t, is the point on the probability line at which no difference exists between the value of not treating the patient and performing the test. Similarly, the **treatment threshold,** T_{rx}, is the point on the probability line at which no difference exists between the value of performing the test and treating the patient without doing a test. The points at which the thresholds occur depend on several factors: the risk of the diagnostic test, the benefit of the treatment to patients who have the disease, the risk of the treatment to patients with and without the disease, and the accuracy of the test.

Consider the situation in which the test is quite accurate and has very little risk to the patient. In this situation, the physician is likely to test at a lower probability of disease as well as at a high probability of disease. In the opposite situation, in which the test has low accuracy or is risky to the patient, the test is less likely to be performed.

MEASURING THE ACCURACY OF DIAGNOSTIC PROCEDURES

The accuracy of a diagnostic test or procedure has two aspects. The first is the test's ability to detect the condition it is testing for, thus being positive in patients who actually have the condition; this is called the **sensitivity** of the test. If a test has high sensitivity, it has a low **false-negative** rate; that is, the test does not falsely give a negative result in many patients who have the disease.

Sensitivity can be defined in many equivalent ways: the probability of a positive test result in patients who have the condition; the proportion of patients with the condition who test positive; the **true-positive** rate. Some people use aids such as *positivity in disease* or *sensitive to disease* to help them remember the definition of sensitivity.

The second aspect of accuracy is the test's ability to identify those patients who do *not* have the condition, called the **specificity** of the test. If the specificity of a test is high, the test has a low **false-positive** rate; that is, the test does not falsely give a positive result in many patients without the disease. Specificity can also be defined in many equivalent ways: the probability of a negative test result in patients who do not have the condition; the proportion of patients without the condition who test negative; 1 minus the false-positive rate. The phrases for remembering the definition of specificity are *negative in health* or *specific to health.*

Sensitivity and specificity of a diagnostic procedure are commonly determined by administering the test to two groups: a group of patients known to have the disease (or condition) and another group known not to have the disease (or condition). The sensitivity is then calculated as the proportion (or percentage) of patients known to have the disease who test positive; specificity is the proportion of patients known to be free of the disease who test negative. Of course, we do not always have a **gold standard** immediately available or one totally free from error. Sometimes, we must wait for autopsy results for definitive classification of the patient's condition, as with Alzheimer's disease.

In Presenting Problem 2, Abraham and colleagues (2017) wanted to evaluate the accuracy of components of a neurological examination and electrophysiological to identify patients with polyneuropathy. They identified 312 diagnosed with polyneuropathy and 47 controls. The investigators reviewed the neurological exam findings and noted the features present; information is given in Table 12–1.

Let us use the information associated with impaired reflexes in the knee to develop a 2 × 2 table from which we can calculate sensitivity and specificity of this finding. Table 12–2 illustrates the basic setup for the 2 × 2 table method. Traditionally, the columns represent the disease (or condition), using D^+ and D^- to denote the presence and absence of disease (polyneuropathy, in this example). The rows represent the tests, using T^+ and T^- for positive and negative test results, respectively (impaired reflexes of knee or not).

True-positive (TP) results go in the upper left cell, the T^+D^+ cell. False-positives (FP) occur when the test is positive but no ST segment elevation is present, the upper right T^+D^- cell. Similarly, **true-negatives** (TN) occur when the test is negative in patient presentations that do not have an MI, the T^-D^- cell in the lower right; and false-negatives (FN) are in the lower left T^-D^+ cell corresponding to a negative test in patient presentations with an MI.

In Abraham and colleagues' study, 312 patient presentations were positive for polyneuropathy; therefore, 312 goes at the bottom of the first column, headed by D^+. Forty-seven patient presentations were without polyneuropathy, and this is the total of the second (D^-) column. Because 52% among the 312

Table 12–1. Comparison of abnormal neurological examination findings between patients and controls

	Total Cohort (n = 312)	Controls (n = 47)	Specificity	PPV	NPV
Impaired reflexes					
Knee	52%	4%	96%	99%	24%
Ankle	74%	38%	62%	92%	27%
Sensory deficits					
Vibration	73%	23%	77%	95%	31%
Pinprick	72%	9%	91%	98%	34%
Temperature	60%	11%	89%	97%	27%
Light touch	45%	4%	96%	98%	23%
Proprioception	36%	2%	98%	99%	20%

PPV-Positive Predictive Value; NPV-Negative Predictive Value. $p < 0.0001$ for each comparison between groups.
Reproduced with permission from Abraham A, Alabdali M, Alsulaiman A, et al: The sensitivity and specificity of the neurological examination in polyneuropathy patients with clinical and electrophysiological correlations, *PLoS ONE.* 2017 Mar 1;12(3):e0171597.

Table 12–2. Basic setup for 2 × 2 table.

Test	Disease	
	Positive D$^+$	Negative D$^-$
Positive T$^+$	TP (true-positive)	FP (false-positive)
Negative T$^-$	FN (false-negative)	TN (true-negative)

Table 12–3. 2 × 2 table for evaluating sensitivity and specificity of test for impaired reflexes of the knee.

Exam Finding	Polyneuropathy		Total
	Present	Absent	
Impaired reflexes - Knee	162 (TP)	2 (FP)	164
No Impaired reflexes - Knee	150 (FN)	45 (TN)	195
Total	312	47	359

TP, true-positive; FP, false-positive; FN, false-negative; TN, true-negative.
Data from Abraham A, Alabdali M, Alsulaiman A, et al: The sensitivity and specificity of the neurological examination in polyneuropathy patients with clinical and electrophysiological correlations, *PLoS ONE.* 2017 Mar 1;12(3):e0171597.

presentations with polyneuropathy, 162 goes in the T^+D^+ (true-positive) cell of the table, leaving 150 of the 312 samples as false-negatives. Among the 47 presentations without polyneuropathy, 45 did not have impaired reflexes of the knee, so 45 is placed in the true-negative cell (T^-D^-). The remaining 2 presentations are called false-positives and are placed in the T^+D^- cell of the table. Table 12–3 shows the completed table.

Using Table 12–3, we can calculate sensitivity and specificity of the knee reflex criterion for the development of polyneuropathy. Try it before reading further. (The sensitivity of impair knee reflexes is the proportion of presentations with polyneuropathy that exhibit this criterion, 162 of 312, or 52%. The specificity is the proportion of presentations without polyneuropathy that do not have impaired knee reflexes, 45 of 47, or 96%.)

USING SENSITIVITY & SPECIFICITY TO REVISE PROBABILITIES

The values of sensitivity and specificity cannot be used alone to determine the value of a diagnostic test in a specific patient; they are combined with a clinician's index of suspicion (or the prior probability) that the patient has the disease to determine the probability of disease (or nondisease) given knowledge of the test result. An index of suspicion is not always based on probabilities determined by experiments or observations; sometimes, it must simply be a best guess, which is simply an estimate lying somewhere between the prevalence of the disease being investigated in this particular patient population and certainty. A physician's best guess generally begins with baseline prevalence and then is revised upward (or downward) based on clinical signs and symptoms. Some vagueness is acceptable in the initial estimate of the index of suspicion; in the section titled, "Decision Analysis," we discuss a technique called *sensitivity analysis* for evaluating the effect of the initial estimate on the final decision.

We present four different methods because some people prefer one method to another. We personally find the first method, using a 2 × 2 table, to be the easiest in terms of probabilities. The likelihood ratio method is superior if you can think in terms of odds, and it is important for clinicians to understand because it is used in evidence-based medicine. You can use the method that makes the most sense to you or is the easiest to remember and apply.

The 2 × 2 Table Method

In Presenting Problem 1, a decision must be reached on whether to order an ESR or proceed directly with imaging studies (lumbar MRI). This decision depends on three pieces of information: (1) the probability of spinal malignancy (index of suspicion) prior to performing any tests; (2) the accuracy of ESR in detecting malignancies among patients who are subsequently shown to have spinal malignancy (sensitivity); and (3) the frequency of a negative result for the procedure in patients who subsequently do not have spinal malignancy (specificity).

What is your index of suspicion for spinal malignancy in this patient before the ESR? Considering the age and history of symptoms in this patient, a reasonable prior probability is 20% to 30%; let us use 20% for this example.

How will this probability change with the positive ESR? With a negative ESR? To answer these questions, we must know how sensitive and specific the ESR is for spinal malignancy and use this information to revise the probability. These new probabilities are called the **predictive value of a positive test** and the **predictive value of a negative test,** also called *posterior probabilities.* If positive, we order a lumbar MRI and if negative, a radiograph, according to the decision rules used by Joines and colleagues (2001) and later reevaluated and confirmed by Deyo et al (2014). Then we must repeat the process by determining the predictive values of the lumbar MRI or radiograph to revise the probability after interpreting the ESR.

The first step in the 2 × 2 table method for determining predictive values of a diagnostic test incorporates the index of suspicion (or prior probability) of disease. We find it easier to work with whole numbers rather than percentages when evaluating diagnostic procedures. Another way of saying that the patient has a 20% chance of having a spinal malignancy is to say that 200 out of 1,000 patients like this one would have spinal malignancy. In Table 12–4, this number (200) is written at the bottom of the D^+

Table 12–4. Step one: Adding the prior probabilities to the 2 × 2 table.

Test	Disease	
	D^+	D^-
T^+	(TP)	(FP)
T^-	(FN)	(TN)
	200	800

TP, true-positive; FP, false-positive; FN, false-negative; TN, true-negative.

Table 12–5. Step 2: Using sensitivity and specificity to determine number of true-positives, false-negatives, true-negatives, and false-positives in 2 × 2 table.

Test	Disease	
	D^+	D^-
T^+	(TP)	(FP)
	156	264
T^-	(FN)	(TN)
	44	536
	200	800

TP, true-positive; FP, false-positive; FN, false-negative; TN, true-negative.

column. Similarly, 800 patients out of 1,000 would not have a spinal malignancy, and this number is written at the bottom of the D^- column.

The second step is to fill in the cells of the table by using the information on the test's sensitivity and specificity. Table 12–4 shows that the true-positive rate, or sensitivity, corresponds to the T^+D^+ cell (labeled TP). Deyo and colleagues (2014) reported 78% sensitivity and 67% specificity for the ESR ($\geq$20 mm/h) in detecting spinal malignancy. Based on their data, 78% of the 200 patients with spinal malignancy, or 156 patients are true-positives, and 200 − 156 = 44, are false-negatives (Table 12–5). Using the same reasoning, we find that a test that is 67% specific results in 536 true-negatives in the 800 patients without spinal malignancy, and 800 − 536 = 264 false-positives.

The third step is to add across the rows. From row 1, we see that 156 + 264 = 420 people like this patient would have a positive ESR (Table 12–6). Similarly, 580 patients would have a negative ESR.

The fourth step involves the calculations for predictive values. Of the 420 people with a positive test, 156 actually have spinal malignancy, giving 156/420 = 37%. Similarly, 536 of the

Table 12–6. Step 3: Completed 2 × 2 table for calculating predictive values.

Test	A. Completed Table		
	Disease		
	D$^+$	D$^-$	
	(TP)	(FP)	
T$^+$	156	264	420
	(FN)	(TN)	
T$^-$	44	536	580
	200	800	1000

B. Step 4	
Predictive value of a positive test	PV$^+$ = TP/(TP + FP) = 156/420 = 0.371
Predictive value of a negative test	PV$^-$ = TN/(TN + FN) = 536/580 = 0.924

TP, true-positive; FP, false-positive; FN, false-negative; TN, true-negative.

Table 12–7. Completed 2 × 2 table for ultrasound examination from Presenting Problem 1.

Test	A. Completed Table		
	Disease		
	D$^+$	D$^-$	
	(TP)	(FP)	
T$^+$	351.5	31.5	383
	(FN)	(TN)	
T$^-$	18.5	598.5	617
	370	630	1000

B. Step 4	
Predictive value of a positive test	PV$^+$ = TP/(TP + FP) = 351.5/383 = 0.918
Predictive value of a negative test	PV$^-$ = TN/(TN + FN) = 598.5/617 = 0.970

TP, true-positive; FP, false-positive; FN, false-negative; TN, true-negative.

580 patients with a negative test, or 92%, do not have spinal malignancy. The percentage 37% is called the **predictive value of a positive test,** abbreviated PV$^+$, and gives the percentage of patients with a positive test result who actually have the condition (or the probability of spinal malignancy, given a positive ESR). The percentage 92% is the **predictive value of a negative test,** abbreviated PV$^-$, and gives the probability that the patient does not have the condition when the test is negative. Two other probabilities can be estimated from this table as well, although they do not have specific names: 264/420 = 0.63 is the probability that the patient does not have the condition, even though the test is positive; and 44/580 = 0.08 is the probability that the patient does have the condition, even though the test is negative.

To summarize so far, the ESR is moderately sensitive and specific for detecting spinal malignancy when used with a low index of suspicion. It provides only a fair amount of information; it increases the probability of spinal malignancy from 20% to 37% when positive, and it increases the probability of no spinal malignancy from 67% to 92% when negative. Thus, in general, tests that have high sensitivity are useful for ruling out a disease in patients when the test is negative; for that reason, most screening tests have high sensitivity.

Now we repeat the previous reasoning for the subsequent procedure, assuming that the man's ESR was positive; from Table 12–6, we know that the probability of spinal malignancy with a positive ESR is 37%. When a second diagnostic test is performed, the results from the first test determine the prior probability. Based on a positive ESR, 37%, or 370 out of 1,000 patients, are likely to have spinal malignancy, and 630 are not. These numbers are the column totals in Table 12–7. Lumbar MRI was shown by Joines and colleagues to be 95% sensitive and 95% specific for spinal malignancy; applying these statistics gives (0.95)(370), or 351.5, true-positives and (0.95)(630), or 598.5, true-negatives. Subtraction gives 18.5 false-negatives and 31.5 false-positives. After adding the rows, the predictive value of a positive lumbar MRI is 351.5/383, or 91.8%, and the predictive value of a negative lumbar MRI is 97% (see Table 12–7).

Joines and colleagues (2001) and Deyo and colleagues (2014) concluded that the ESR with a cutoff of ≥20 mm/h is of minimal utility. We will refer to these studies again in the section titled, "Using Decision Analysis to Compare Strategies."

The Likelihood Ratio

An alternative method for incorporating information provided by the sensitivity and specificity of a test is the likelihood ratio; it uses **odds** rather than probabilities. The likelihood ratio is being used with increasing frequency in the medical literature, especially within the context of evidence-based medicine. Even if you decide not to use this particular approach to revising probabilities, you need to know how to interpret the likelihood ratio. Because it makes calculating predictive values very simple, many people prefer it after becoming familiar with it.

The **likelihood ratio** expresses the odds that the test result occurs in patients with the disease versus the odds that the test result occurs in patients without the disease. Thus, a positive test has one likelihood ratio and a negative test another. For a positive test, the likelihood ratio is the sensitivity divided by the false-positive rate. The likelihood ratio is multiplied by the prior, or **pretest odds,** to obtain the **posttest odds** of a positive test. Thus,

$$\text{Pretest odds} \times \text{ikelihood ratio} = \text{Posttest odds}$$

In Presenting Problem 1, the sensitivity of the ESR for spinal malignancy is 78%; and the specificity is 67%, giving a false-positive rate of 100% − 67% = 33%. The likelihood ratio (*LR*) for a positive test is therefore

$$LR = \frac{0.78}{0.33} = 2.36$$

To use the likelihood ratio, we must convert the prior probability into prior odds. The prior probability of spinal malignancy is 0.20, and the odds are found by dividing the probability by 1 minus the probability, giving

$$\text{Pretest odds} = \frac{\text{Prior probability}}{1 - \text{Prior probability}}$$
$$= \frac{0.20}{1 - 0.20}$$
$$= \frac{0.20}{0.80} = 0.25$$

It helps to keep in mind that the probability is a proportion: It is the number of times a given outcome occurs divided by all the occurrences. If we take a sample of blood from a patient five times, and the sample is positive one time, we can think of the probability as being 1 in 5, or 0.20. The odds, on the other hand, is a ratio: It is the number of times a given outcome occurs divided by the number of times that specific outcome does not occur. With the blood sample example, the odds of a positive sample is 1 to 4, or 1/(5 − 1). This interpretation is consistent with the relative risk and odds ratio, which indicate the risk in a population with a risk factor divided by the risk in a population without the risk factor.

Continuing with the ESR example, we multiply the pretest odds by the likelihood ratio to obtain the posttest odds:

$$\text{Posttest odds} = 0.25 \times 2.36 = 0.59$$

Because the posttest odds are really 0.59 to 1, although the "to 1" part does not appear in the preceding formula, these odds can be used by clinicians simply as they are. Because the odds are less than 1, or less than 50–50, we know the probability will be less than 0.5. Alternatively, the odds can be converted back to a probability by dividing the odds by 1 plus the odds. That is,

$$\text{Posterior probability} = \frac{\text{Posttest odds}}{1 + \text{Posttest odds}}$$
$$= \frac{0.59}{1 + 0.59} = 0.37$$

The posterior probability is, of course, the predictive value of a positive test and is the same result we found earlier.

Many journal articles that present likelihood ratios use the LR as just defined, which is actually the likelihood ratio for a positive test. The evidence-based medicine literature sometimes uses the notation of ⁺LR to distinguish it from the LR for a negative test, generally denoted by ⁻LR. The negative likelihood ratio can be used to find the odds of disease, even if the test is negative. It is the ratio of false-negatives to true-negatives (FN/TN).

To illustrate the use of the negative likelihood ratio, let us find the probability of spinal malignancy if the ESR is negative. The ⁻LR in this example is 0.22 (1 minus sensitivity) divided by 0.67 (true-negatives), or 0.328. Multiplying the ⁻LR by the prior odds of the disease gives 0.328 × 0.25 = 0.082, the posttest odds of disease with a negative test. We can again convert the odds to a probability by dividing 0.082 by 1 + 0.082 to obtain 0.076, or 7.6%. This value tells us that a person such as our patient, about whom our index of suspicion is 20%, has a posttest probability of spinal malignancy, even with a negative test, of approximately 7.6%. This result is consistent with the predictive value of a negative test of 92.4% (see the section titled, "The 2 × 2 Table Method."). So, another way to interpret the ⁻LR is that it is analogous to 1 minus PV⁻.

Absolutely nothing is wrong with thinking in terms of odds instead of probabilities. If you are comfortable using odds instead of probabilities, the calculations are really quite streamlined. One way to facilitate conversion between probability and odds is to recognize the simple pattern that results. We list some common probabilities in Table 12–8, along with the odds and the action to take with the likelihood ratio to find the posttest odds.

To use the information in Table 12–8, note that the odds in column 2 are <1 when the probability is <0.50, are equal to 1 when the probability is 0.50, and are >1 when the probability is >0.50. The last column shows that we divide the likelihood ratio to obtain the posttest odds when the prior probability is <0.50 and multiply when it is >0.50. To illustrate, suppose your index of suspicion, prior to ordering a diagnostic procedure, is about 25%. A probability of 0.25 gives 1 to 3 odds, so the likelihood ratio is divided by 3. If your index of suspicion is 75%, the odds are 3 to 1, and the likelihood ratio is multiplied by 3. Once the posttest odds are found, columns 2 and 1 can be used to convert back to probabilities.

A major advantage of the likelihood ratio method is the need to remember only one number, the ratio, instead of two numbers, sensitivity and specificity. Sackett and colleagues (1991) indicate that likelihood ratios are much more stable (or robust) for indicating changes in prevalence than are sensitivity and specificity; these authors also give the likelihood

ratios for some common symptoms, signs, and diagnostic tests.

The Decision Tree Method

Using Presenting Problem 1 again, we illustrate the **decision tree** method for revising the initial probability, a 20% chance of spinal malignancy in this example. Trees are useful for diagramming a series of events, and they can easily be extended to more complex examples as we will see in Presenting Problem 4. Figure 12–1 illustrates that prior to ordering a test, the patient can be in one of two conditions: with the disease (or condition) or without the disease (or condition). These alternatives are represented by the branches, with one labeled D^+, indicating a disease present and the other labeled D^- representing no disease.

The prior probabilities are included on each branch, 20% on the D^+ branch and 100% – 20% or 80% on the D^- branch. The test can be either positive or negative, regardless of the patient's true condition. These situations are denoted by T^+ for a positive test and T^- for a negative test and are illustrated in the decision tree by the two branches connected to both the D^+ and D^- branches.

In the next step, information on sensitivity and specificity of the test is added to the tree. Concentrating on the D^+ branch, an ESR is positive in approximately 78% of these patients. Figure 12–2 shows the 78% sensitivity of the test written on the T^+ line. In 22% of the cases (100% – 78%), the test is negative, written on the T^- line. This information is then combined to obtain the numbers at the end of the lines: The result for 78% of the 20% of the men with spinal malignancy, or (20%)(78%) = 15.6%, is written at the end of the D^+T^+ branch; the result (20%)(22%) = 4.4% for men with spinal malignancy who have a negative test is written at the end of the D^+T^- branch.

Similar calculations are done for the 80% of men who do not have spinal malignancy. Note that the percentages at the ends of the four branches add to 100%. At this point, the decision tree is complete.

Table 12–8. Conversion table for changing probabilities to odds and action to take with likelihood ratio to obtain posttest odds.

Prior Probability	Prior Odds	Posttest Odds = Likelihood Ratio
0.10	1 to 9	÷ by 9
0.20	1 to 4	÷ by 4
0.25	1 to 3	÷ by 3
0.33	1 to 2	÷ by 2
0.50	1 to 1	× by 1
0.66	2 to 1	× by 2
0.75	3 to 1	× by 3
0.80	4 to 1	× by 4
0.90	9 to 1	× by 9

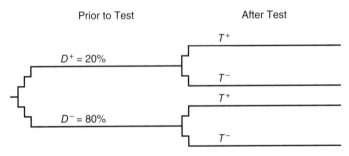

Figure 12–1. Decision tree with test result branches.

However, the tree can also be used to find predictive values by "reversing" the tree. Figure 12–2 is replicated in Figure 12–3, showing that the first two lines are the results of the tests, T^+ and T^-, and the disease state of D^+ and D^- is associated with each. The values at the end of each line are simply transferred; that is, 16.6% corresponding to D^+T^+ is placed on the T^+D^+ line, etc. The two outcomes related to a positive test are added to obtain 42%. The predictive values can now be determined. If this man has a positive ESR, the revised probability is found by dividing 15.6% by 42%, giving a 37.1% chance, the same as the conclusions reached by using the 2 × 2 table method. Other predictive values are equally easy to find.

Bayes' Theorem

Another method for calculating the predictive value of a positive test involves the use of a mathematical formula. Bayes' theorem is not new; it was developed in the eighteenth century by an English clergyman and mathematician, Thomas Bayes, but was not published until after his death. It had little influence at the time, but two centuries later it became the basis for a different way to approach statistical inference, called Bayesian statistics. Although it was used in the early clinical epidemiology literature, the 2 × 2 table and likelihood ratio are seen today with much greater frequency and are, therefore, worth knowing.

The formula for Bayes' theorem gives the predictive value of a positive test, or the chance that a patient with a positive test has the disease. The symbol P stands for the probability that an event will happen (see Chapter 4), and $P(D^+|T^+)$ is the probability that the disease is present, given that the test is positive. As we discussed in Chapter 4, this probability is a **conditional probability** in which the event of the disease being present is dependent, or conditional, on having a positive test result. The formula, known as **Bayes' theorem,** can be rewritten from the form we used in Chapter 4, as follows:

$$P(D^+\mid T^+) = \frac{P(T^+\mid D^+)P(D^+)}{P(T^+\mid D^+)P(D^+) + P(T^+\mid D^-)P(D^-)}$$

This formula specifies the probability of disease, given the occurrence of a positive test. The two probabilities in the numerator are (1) the probability that a test is positive, given that the disease is present (or the sensitivity of the test) and (2) the best guess (or prior probability) that the patient has the disease to begin

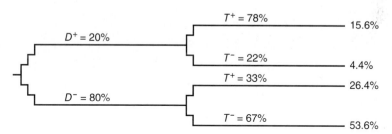

Figure 12–2. Decision tree with test result information.

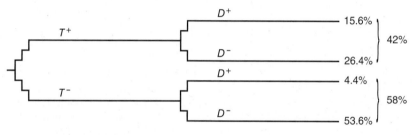

Figure 12–3. Reversing tree to correspond with situation facing physicians.

with. The denominator is simply the probability that a positive test occurs at all, $P(T^+)$, which can occur in one of two ways: a positive test when the disease is present, and a positive test when the disease is not present, each weighted by the prior probability of that outcome. The first quantity in this term is simply the false-positive rate, and the second can be thought of as 1 minus the probability that the disease is present.

Rewriting Bayes' theorem in terms of sensitivity and specificity, we obtain

$$\frac{\text{Sensitivity} \times \text{Prior probability}}{\{\text{Sensitivity} \times \text{Prior probability} + [(\text{False} - \text{positive rate} \times (1 - \text{Prior probability}))]\}}$$

We again use Presenting Problem 1 to illustrate the use of Bayes' formula. Recall that the prior probability of spinal malignancy is 0.20, and sensitivity and specificity of the ESR for spinal malignancy are 78% and 67%, respectively. In the numerator, the sensitivity times the probability of disease is (0.78)(0.20). In the denominator, that quantity is repeated and added to the false-positive rate, 0.33, times 1 minus the probability of malformation, 0.80. Thus, we have

$$P(D^+ \mid T^+) = \frac{0.78 \times 0.20}{(0.78 \times 0.20) + (0.33 \times 0.80)}$$

$$= \frac{0.156}{0.156 + 0.264} = 0.37$$

This result, of course, is exactly the same as the result obtained with the 2×2 table and the decision tree methods.

A similar formula may be derived for the predictive value of a negative test:

$$P(D^- \mid T^-) = \frac{P(T^- \mid D^-)P(D^-)}{P(T^- \mid D^-)P(D^-) + P(T^- \mid D^+)P(D^+)}$$

Calculation of the predictive value using Bayes' theorem for a negative test in the ESR example is left as an exercise.

Using Sensitivity and Specificity in Clinical Medicine

Fairly typical in medicine is the situation in which a very sensitive test (95–99%) is used to detect the presence of a disease with low prevalence (or prior probability); that is, the test is used in a screening capacity. By itself, these tests have little diagnostic meaning.

When used indiscriminately to screen for diseases that have low prevalence (e.g., 1 in 1,000), the rate of false positivity is high. Tests with these statistical characteristics become more helpful in making a diagnosis when used in conjunction with clinical findings that suggest the possibility of the suspected disease. To summarize, when the prior probability is very low, even a very sensitive and specific test increases the posttest probability only to a moderate level. For this reason, a positive result based on a very sensitive test is often followed by a very specific test, such as following a positive antinuclear antibody test (ANA) for systemic lupus erythematosus with the anti-DNA antibody procedure.

Another example of a test with high sensitivity is the serum calcium level. It is a good screening test because it is almost always elevated in patients with primary hyperparathyroidism—meaning, it rarely "misses" a person with primary hyperparathyroidism. However, serum calcium level is not specific for this disease, because other conditions, such as malignancy, sarcoidosis, multiple myeloma, or vitamin D intoxication, may also be associated with elevated serum calcium. A more specific test, such as radioimmunoassay for parathyroid hormone, may therefore be ordered after finding an elevated level of serum calcium. The posterior probability calculated by using the serum calcium test becomes the new index of suspicion (prior probability) for analyzing the effect of the radioimmunoassay.

The diagnosis of HIV in low-risk populations provides an example of the important role played by prior probability. Some states in the United States require premarital testing for the HIV antibody in couples applying for a marriage license. The enzyme-linked immunosorbent assay (ELISA) test is highly sensitive and specific; some estimates range as high as 99% for each. The prevalence of HIV antibody in a low-risk population, such as people getting married in a Midwestern community, however, is very low; estimates range from 1 in 1,000 to 1 in 10,000. How useful is a positive test in such situations? For the higher estimate of 1 in 1,000 for the prevalence and 99% sensitivity and specificity, 99% of the people with the antibody test positive (99% × 1 = 0.99 person), as do 1% of the 999 people without the antibody (9.99 people). Therefore, among those with a positive ELISA test (0.99 + 9.99 = 10.98 people), less than 1 person is truly positive (the positive predictive value is actually about 9% for these numbers).

The previous examples illustrate three important points:

1. To *rule out* a disease, we want to be sure that a negative result is really negative; therefore, not very many false-negatives should occur. A sensitive test is the best choice to obtain as few false-negatives as possible if factors such as cost and risk are similar; that is, high

sensitivity helps rule out if the test is negative. As a handy acronym, if we abbreviate sensitivity by **SN,** and use a sensitive test to rule **OUT,** we have **SNOUT.**

2. To find evidence of a disease, we want a positive result to indicate a high probability that the patient has the disease—that is, a positive test result should really indicate disease. Therefore, we want few false-positives. The best method for achieving this is a highly specific test—that is, high specificity helps rule in if the test is positive. Again, if we abbreviate specificity by **SP,** and use a specific test to rule **IN,** we have **SPIN.**

3. To make accurate diagnoses, we must understand the role of prior probability of disease. If the prior probability of disease is extremely small, a positive result does not mean very much and should be followed by a test that is highly specific. The usefulness of a negative result depends on the sensitivity of the test.

Assumptions

The methods for revising probabilities are equivalent, and you should feel free to use the one you find easiest to understand and remember. All the methods are based on two assumptions: (1) The diseases or diagnoses being considered are mutually exclusive and include the actual diagnosis; and (2) the results of each diagnostic test are independent from the results of all other tests.

The first assumption is easy to meet if the diagnostic hypotheses are stated in terms of the probability of disease, $P(D^+)$, versus the probability of no disease, $P(D^-)$, as long as D^+ refers to a specific disease.

The second assumption of mutually independent diagnostic tests is more difficult to meet. Two tests, T_1 and T_2, for a given disease are independent if the result of T_1 does not influence the chances associated with the result of T_2. When applied to individual patients, independence means that if T_1 is positive in patient A, T_2 is no more likely to be positive in patient A than in any other patient in the population that patient A represents. Even though the second assumption is sometimes violated in medical applications of decision analysis, the methods described in this chapter appear to be fairly robust.

Finally, it is important to recognize that the values for the sensitivity and specificity of diagnostic procedures assume the procedures are interpreted without error. For example, variation is inherent in determining the value of many laboratory tests. As mentioned in Chapter 3, the coefficient of variation is used as a measure of the replicability of assay measurements. In Chapter 5 we discussed the concepts of intrarater and interrater reliability, including the statistic kappa to measure interjudge agreement. Variability in test determination or in test interpretation is ignored in calculating for sensitivity, specificity, and the predictive values of tests.

ROC CURVES

The preceding methods for revising the prior (pretest) probability of a disease or condition on the basis of information from a diagnostic test are applicable if the outcome of the test is simply positive or negative. Many tests, however, have values measured on a **numerical scale.** When test values are measured on a continuum, sensitivity and specificity levels depend on where the cutoff is set between positive and negative. This situation can be illustrated by two normal (Gaussian) distributions of laboratory test values: one distribution for people who have the disease and one for people who do not have the disease. Figure 12–4 presents two hypothetical distributions corresponding to this situation in which the mean value for people with the disease is 75 and that for those without the disease is 45. If the cutoff point is placed at 60, about 10% of the people without the disease are incorrectly classified as abnormal (false-positive) because their test value is greater than 60, and about 10% of the people with the disease are incorrectly classified as normal (false-negative) because their test value is less than 60. In other words, this test has a sensitivity of 90% and a specificity of 90%.

Suppose a physician wants a test with greater sensitivity, meaning that the physician prefers to have more

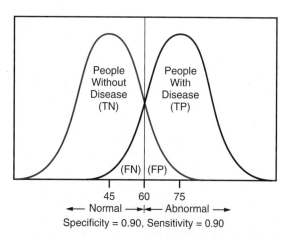

Figure 12–4. Two hypothetical distributions with cutoff at 60. (TN, true-negative; TP, true-positive; FN, false-negative; FP, false-positive).

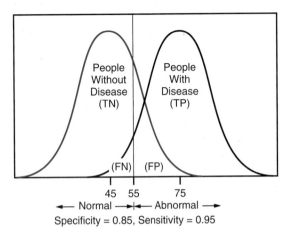

Figure 12–5. Two hypothetical distributions with cutoff at 55. (TN, true-negative; TP, true-positive; FN, false-negative; FP, false-positive).

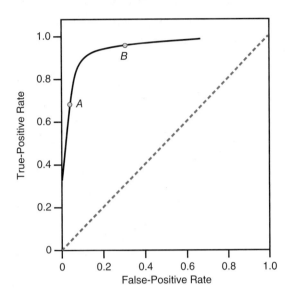

Figure 12–6. Receiver operating characteristic curve.

false-positives than to miss people who really have the disease. Figure 12–5 illustrates what happens if the sensitivity is increased by lowering the cutoff point to 55 for a normal test. The sensitivity is increased, but at the cost of a lower specificity.

A more efficient way to display the relationship between sensitivity and specificity for tests that have continuous outcomes is with **receiver operating characteristic,** or **ROC, curves.** ROC curves were developed in the communications field as a way to display signal-to-noise ratios. If we think of true-positives as being the correct signal from a diagnostic test and false-positives as being noise, we can see how this concept applies. The ROC curve is a plot of the sensitivity (or true-positive rate) to the false-positive rate. The dotted diagonal line in Figure 12–6 corresponds to a test that is positive or negative just by chance. The closer an ROC curve is to the upper left-hand corner of the graph, the more accurate it is, because the true-positive rate is 1 and the false-positive rate is 0. As the criterion for a positive test becomes more stringent, the point on the curve corresponding to sensitivity and specificity (point *A*) moves down and to the left (lower sensitivity, higher specificity); if less evidence is required for a positive test, the point on the curve corresponding to sensitivity and specificity (point *B*) moves up and to the right (higher sensitivity, lower specificity).

ROC curves are useful graphic methods for comparing two or more diagnostic tests or for selecting cutoff levels for a test. For example, in Presenting

Problem 3, Dabi and colleagues (2017) performed a retrospective study to validate the use of a nomogram (http://www.perinatology.com/calculators/TRANSFER.htm) to estimate two probabilities: delivery within 48 hours and delivery before 32 weeks. They had to decide where to put the cutoff level for the probabilities. These investigators' ROC curve for delivery within 48 hours is reproduced in (Box 12–1). The ROC curve illustrates that lowering the probability is considered a positive finding results in higher sensitivity but increasing false-positives (or decreasing sensitivity).

A statistical test can be performed to evaluate an ROC curve or to determine whether two ROC curves are significantly different. A commonly used procedure involves determining the area under each ROC curve and uses a modification of the Wilcoxon rank sum procedure to compare them. Box 12–1 shows that the area under the curve for the nomogram is 0.88 with a 95% confidence interval from 0.86 to 0.90. Is the curve significant? The answer is yes, because it does not contain 0.5.

DECISION ANALYSIS

Decision analysis can be applied to any problem in which a choice is possible among different alternative actions. Any decision has two major components: specifying the alternative actions and determining the possible outcomes from each alternative action. Figure 12–7 illustrates the components for

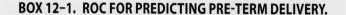

BOX 12-1. ROC FOR PREDICTING PRE-TERM DELIVERY.

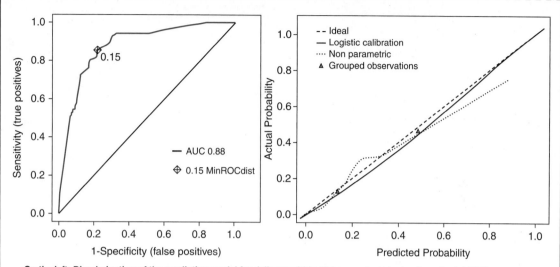

On the left: Discrimination of the prediction model for delivery within 48 hours of admission for cohort 1.ROC curve of the nomogram for the prediction of premature birth wihtin 48 hours. Concordance index: 0.88 (95% CI: 0.86–0.90). **On the right: Calibration of the prediction model for delivery within 48 hours of admission for cohort 1.**The x-axis represents the probability of delivery within 48 hours after transfer calculated using the nomogram, and the y-axis represents the actual rate of delivery within 48 hours. The dashed line represents the performance of an ideal nomogram. The predicted and observed rates of delivery within 48 hours are plotted as the grouped observations and logistic calibration.

Reproduced with permission from Dabi Y, Nedellec S, Bonneau C, et al: Clinical validation of a model predicting the risk of preterm delivery, *PLoS One.* 2017 Feb 9;12(2):e0171801.

the study of laparoscopic versus open distal pancreatectomy for pancreatic cancer (Gurusamy et al, 2017). The alternative actions to use a laparoscopic or open approach. If the open approach is used, there is a possibility of complications or no complications. If the laparoscopic approach is used, then there a possibility of conversion to an open approach as well as the complication/no complication outcomes. The point at which a branch occurs is called a *node*; in Figure 12–7, nodes are identified by either a square or a circle. The square denotes a decision node—a point at which the decision is under the control of the decision maker, whether or not to enforce the strict policy in this example. The circle denotes a chance node, or point at which the results occur by chance; thus, whether lead poisoning recurs is a chance outcome of a decision to or not to enforce the policy.

Determining Probabilities

The next step in developing a decision tree is to assign a probability to each branch leading from each chance node.

To determine the probabilities for the decision tree, the investigators may survey the medical literature and incorporate the results from previous studies. Gurusamy and colleagues took this approach. These probabilities are written in the boxes above the branches in Figure 12–8. Note that the combined probabilities for any set of outcomes, such as for complications and no complications, equal 1.

Deciding the Value of the Outcomes

The final step in defining a decision problem requires *assigning a value*, or *utility*, to each outcome. With some decision problems, the outcome is cost, and dollar amounts can be used as the utility of each outcome.

Objective versus subjective outcomes: Outcomes based on objective probabilities, such as costs, numbers of years of life, quality-adjusted years of life (QALYs), or other variables that have an inherent numeric value, can be used as the utilities for a decision. When outcomes are based on **subjective probabilities**, investigators must find a way to give them a value. This process

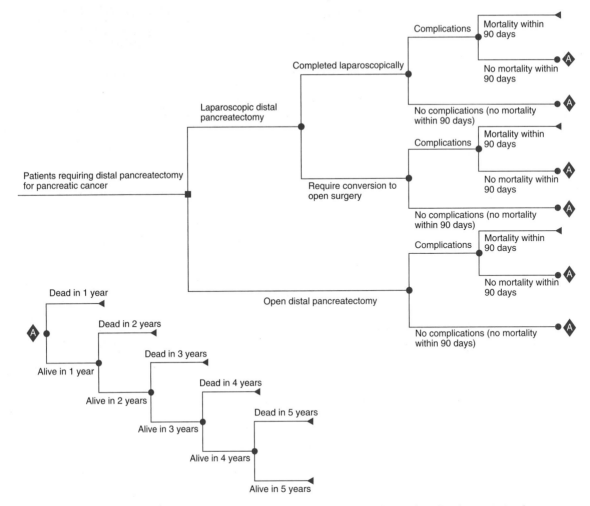

Figure 12–7. Decision tree for open versus laparoscopic pancreatectomy. (Reproduced with permission from Gurusamy KS, Riviere D, van Laarhoven CJH, et al: Cost-effectiveness of laparoscopic versus open distal pancreatectomy for pancreatic cancer, *PLoS ONE.* 2017 Dec 22;12(12):e0189631.)

is known as assigning a utility to each outcome. The scale used for utilities is arbitrary, although a scale from 0 for least desirable outcome, such as death, to 1 or 100 for most desirable outcome, such as perfect health, is frequently used.

An example of determining subjective utilities: Subjective utilities can be obtained informally or by a more rigorous process called a lottery technique. This technique involves a process called **game theory.** To illustrate, suppose we ask you to play a game in which you can choose a prize of $50 or you can play the game with a 50–50 chance of winning $100 (and nothing if you lose). Here, the **expected value** of playing the game is 0.50 × $100 = $50,

the same as the prize. Do you take the sure $50 or play the game? If you choose not to gamble and take $50 instead, then we ask whether you will play the game if the chance of winning increases from 50% to 60%, resulting in an expected value of $60, $10 more than the prize. If you still take $50, then we increase the chance to 70%, and so on, until it reaches a point at which you cannot decide whether to play the game or take the prize, called the point of indifference. This is the value you attach to playing this game. We say you are risk-averse when you refuse to gamble even when the odds are in your favor, that is, when the expected value of the game is more than the prize.

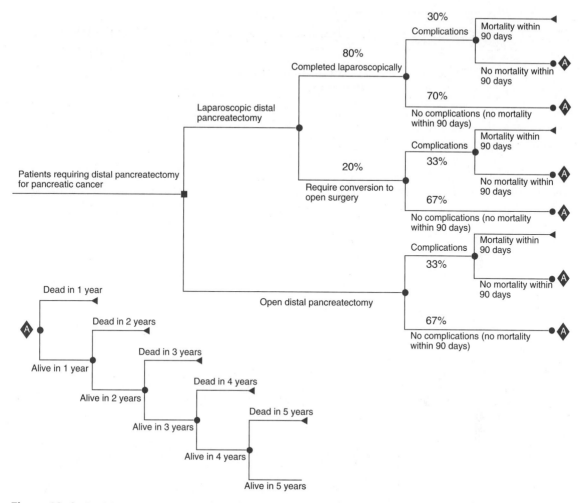

Figure 12–8. Decision tree open versus laparoscopic pancreatectomy with probabilities. (Adapted with permission from Gurusamy KS, Riviere D, van Laarhoven CJH, et al: Cost-effectiveness of laparoscopic versus open distal pancreatectomy for pancreatic cancer, *PLoS ONE.* 2017 Dec 22;12(12):e0189631.)

Suppose now that a colleague plays the game and chooses the $50 prize when the chance of winning $100 is 50–50. Then, we ask whether the colleague will still play if the chance of winning $100 is only 40%, and so on, until the point of indifference is reached. We describe your colleague as risk-seeking when they are willing to gamble even when the odds are unfavorable and the expected value of the game is less than the prize.

Completing the Decision Tree

The analysis of the decision tree involves combining the probabilities of each action with the utility of each so that the optimal decision can be made at the decision nodes. To decide whether to perform an open or laparoscopic procedure, the Gurusamy study in Presenting

Problem 4 defined the decision alternatives and possible outcomes, along with estimated probabilities and costs.

The decision tree is analyzed by a process known as *calculating the expected utilities*. The results of that calculation are displayed in Figure 12–9, which is a copy of Table 2 from the original manuscript. Notice that the raw cost of the open distal pancreatectomy is more than the laparoscopic approach, but when the costs and probabilities of the various end points are taken, difference in both cost and QALYs favor the laparoscopic approach.

Conclusions from the Decision Analysis

The investigator concluded that "This shows that laparoscopic distal pancreatectomy results in decreased costs and increased QALYs compared to open distal pancreatectomy, with a higher net monetary benefit. Therefore,

Treatment	Costs	QALYs	Net monetary benefit*	
			£20,000	£30,000
Laparoscopic distal pancreatectomy	£7,676	1.6472	£25,267.54	£41,739.31
Open distal pancreatectomy	£8,539	1.4974	£21,409.10	£36,383.12
Incremental	-£863	0.1498	£3,858.45	£5,356.20

* Calculated at willingness to pay thresholds of £20,000 and £30,000 per QALY gained.

Figure 12–9. Results of decision analysis. (QALY, quality adjusted life year.) (Reproduced with permission from Gurusamy KS, Riviere D, van Laarhoven CJH, et al: Cost-effectiveness of laparoscopic versus open distal pancreatectomy for pancreatic cancer, *PLoS ONE*. 2017 Dec 22;12(12):e0189631.)

laparoscopic distal pancreatectomy dominates open distal pancreatectomy, and the incremental NMB is positive."

The optimal decision is the one with the lowest cost or largest expected value, and the decision maker's choice is relatively easy. When the expected costs or utilities of two decisions are very close, the situation is called a toss-up, and considerations such as the estimates used in the analysis become more important.

Evaluating the Decision: Sensitivity Analysis

Accurate probabilities for each branch in a decision tree are frequently difficult to obtain from the literature. Investigators often have to use estimates made for related situations. For example, in Presenting Problem 4, the authors provide a sensitivity analysis showing the impact of various values of incremental cost and QALY. The procedure for evaluating the way the decision changes as a function of changing probabilities and utilities is called **sensitivity analysis.** It is possible to perform an analysis to determine the sensitivity of the final decision to two or more assumptions simultaneously. Most statisticians and researchers in decision analysis recommend that all published reports of a decision analysis include a sensitivity analysis to help readers know the range of applications is which the results are applicable.

USING DECISION ANALYSIS TO COMPARE STRATEGIES

No consensus exists about which diagnostic approach is the best for follow-up in a patient with low back pain and suspected spinal malignancy. Among the available diagnostic procedures are erythrocyte sedimentation rate (ESR), lumbosacral radiograph, bone scan, lumbar MRI, and biopsy under fluoroscopic guidance. An ideal diagnostic protocol would combine these tests so that all cancers could be found without undue costs, risks, or discomfort to the patient. The ideal does not exist, however, because none of the tests is perfect; and as more tests are done, the costs and risks increase accordingly.

Several protocols have been recommended in the literature, and the range of procedures used in actual practice varies widely. Joines and colleagues (2001) designed a decision analysis to determine the most effective protocol. They examined several protocols; these are outlined in Figure 12–10A and 12–10B. We discuss several of the protocols and illustrate the way in which Joines and colleagues evaluated their effectiveness.

Protocols Evaluated

The strategies evaluated are lettered A through F. Figure 12–10A shows strategy **A** as a rather complex algorithm. If a patient has a history of cancer and the ESR is <20, a radiograph is done, which, if positive, leads to imaging studies. With a history of cancer and an ESR ≥20, the patient goes directly to imaging studies. On the other hand, if there is no history of cancer, the approach is based on the number of risk factors the patient has (age ≥50 years, weight loss, or failure to improve). Several other strategies are illustrated in Figure 12–10B and require either a history of cancer or one of the previously mentioned three risk factors. A summary of several strategies follows.

B. ESR, if <20, is followed by radiograph. If radiograph is positive, it is followed by imaging studies. If ESR ≥20, imaging studies are done.

B2. If a history of cancer, or ESR ≥20, or positive radiograph, perform imaging studies.

C. Imaging studies are done on all patients.

D. ESR, if ≥20, is followed by imaging studies.

E. Radiograph, if positive, is followed by imaging studies.

E2. If a history of cancer or positive radiograph, perform imaging studies.

F. ESR, if ≥20, is followed by radiograph. If radiograph is positive, it is followed by imaging studies.

Assumptions Made in the Analysis

A decision problem of this scope required the investigators to estimate the sensitivity and specificity of a number of patient characteristics and diagnostic tests for spinal malignancy. The values of the patient characteristics and costs for the diagnostic tests are given in Table 12–9.

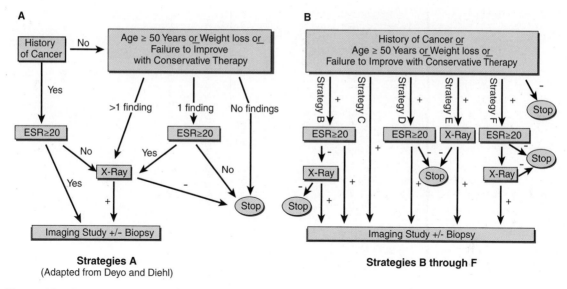

Strategies A
(Adapted from Deyo and Diehl)

Strategies B through F

Figure 12–10. Screening strategies for spinal malignancy. (Reproduced with permission from Joines JD, McNutt RA, Carey TS, et al: Finding cancer in primary care outpatients with low back pain: a comparison of diagnostic strategies, *J Gen Intern Med*. 2001 Jan;16(1):14–23.)

Table 12–9. Clinical findings and diagnostic tests used in the decision model.

	Sensitivity (range)	Specificity (range)	Cost (range)[d]
Clinical findings			
History of cancer[a]	0.31 (0.10–0.61)	0.98 (0.97–0.99)	
Age >50 years[a]	0.77 (0.46–0.94)	0.71 (0.69–0.73)	
Failure to improve with conservative therapy[a]	0.31 (0.10–0.61)	0.90 (0.89–0.91)	
Weight loss[a]	0.15 (0.03–0.46)	0.94 (0.93–0.95)	
Any one or more of above[b]	0.91 (0.58–0.99)	0.59 (0.55–0.63)	
Diagnostic test			
ESR ≥20[a]	0.78	0.67	$5 (5–50)
ESR ≥50[a]	0.56	0.97	$5 (5–50)
Lumbosacral x-ray[a]	0.70	0.95	$38 (10–100)
Bone scan[c]	0.95	0.70	$211
Lumbar MRI	0.95 (0.85–1.00)	0.95	$562 (100–1200)
Biopsy under fluoroscopic guidance	0.85	1.00	$297 (100–1200)

ESR, erythrocyte sedimentation rate; MRI, magnetic resonance imaging.
[a]Sensitivity and specificity from Deyo and Diehl (1988).
[b]Calculated assuming conditional independence of tests.
[c]Sensitivity and specificity from Mazanec (1999).
[d]Cost is shown rounded to the nearest dollar.
Reproduced with permission from Joines JD, McNutt RA, Carey TS, et al: Finding cancer in primary care outpatients with low back pain: a comparison of diagnostic strategies, *J Gen Intern Med*. 2001 Jan;16(1):14–23.

Results of the Decision Analysis

The investigators developed a decision tree for each of the protocols evaluated in their study. Using a computer program, they evaluated each tree to determine the effectiveness of the protocol. The results for the five dominant strategies are given in Table 12–10. In general, the relationship between the sensitivity of a strategy and its cost is positive, but the relationship is not linear. The procedure that detects the most cancers is strategy C, imaging all patients; however, it has the lowest specificity (resulting in more false-positives), and

Table 12-10. Comparison of the five dominant strategies in the baseline analysis.[a]

Strategy	Description	Strategy Sensitivity	Strategy Specificity[b]	Cases Found Per 1,000 Patients	Cases Missed Per 1,000 Patients	Patients Biopsied Without Cancer Per 1,000 Patients	Total Number of Biopsies Per 1,000 Patients	Cost Per Patient	Cost Per Case Found	Incremental Cost Per Additional Case Found
F	Image if ESR+ and x-ray+	0.400	0.9997	2.6	4.0	0.3	3.4	$14	$5,283	
A	Selective testing	0.525	0.9992	3.5	3.1	0.8	4.8	$21	$6,026	$8,397
E2	Image if HxCa+ or x-ray+	0.588	0.9980	3.9	2.7	2.0	6.5	$42	$10,706	$50,020
B2	Image if HxCa+ or ESR+ or x-ray+	0.701	0.9919	4.6	2.0	8.1	13.5	$110	$23,703	$91,428
C	Image everyone	0.732	0.9794	4.8	1.8	20.4	26.1	$241	$49,814	$624,781

ESR, erythrocyte sedimentation rate; HxCa, history of cancer; MRI, magnetic resonance imaging.
[a]Assuming MRI as imaging test. ESR cutoff point of 20, prevalence of cancer 0.66%, baseline estimates of sensitivities and specificities, baseline estimates of costs, and a single biopsy. Strategies are arranged in order of increasing cost.
[b]Defined as proportion of patients without spinal malignancy who were spared a biopsy.

Reproduced with permission from Joines JD, McNutt RA, Carey TS, et al: Finding cancer in primary care outpatients with low back pain: a comparison of diagnostic strategies, *J Gen Intern Med.* 2001 Jan;16(1):14–23.

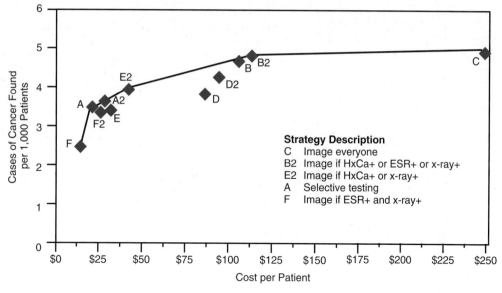

Figure 12–11. Receiver operating curve for testing for spinal malignancy. (Reproduced with permission from Joines JD, McNutt RA, Carey TS, et al: Finding cancer in primary care outpatients with low back pain: a comparison of diagnostic strategies, *J Gen Intern Med*. 2001 Jan;16(1):14–23.)

it is the most costly ($241 per patient). Protocol B2 is almost as sensitive, is more specific, and costs only $110 per patient. A number of other interesting criteria with which to judge the strategies are given in Table 12–10.

The authors prepared a graph comparing the numbers of cases of cancers found per 1,000 patients and the cost per patient. The graph is reproduced in Figure 12–11 and clearly illustrates the conclusions we just described.

Conclusions from the Decision Analysis

From the results of the decision analysis of the different strategies, the investigators recommended strategy B2: imaging patients with a clinical finding (history of cancer, age ≥50 years, weight loss, or failure to improve) if there is an elevated ESR (≥50 mm/h) or a positive radiograph, or directly imaging patients with a history of cancer.

USING DECISION ANALYSIS TO EVALUATE TIMING & METHODS

In Presenting Problem 5, Nguyen and Adang (2018) evaluated the cost-effectiveness (CE) of breast cancer screening via mammography for women in Vietnam. Although mammography for breast cancer screening is well-supported in the United States, it is not the standard in Vietnam. This study aims to calculate the CE of implementing the practice.

The investigators compared the cost and outcomes of screening with three scenarios:

1. No screening
2. 5% private screening and 95% no screening
3. 10% private screening and 90% no screening

The investigators used a theoretical cohort of women and assumed that screening starts at four different age groups: 45 to 49, 50 to 54, 55 to 59 and 60 to 64.

The result of the CE analysis for 100,000 Vietnamese women is reproduced in Figure 12–12. They measured both ICER and incremental net monetary benefits (INMB)

Figure 12–13 presents the INMBs for the age to start screening and the proportion of women screened. In reviewing the figures in Figure 12–13, you can see that the INMB is highest for all of the screening scenarios for the 50- to 54-year age group.

QALY was not used in this study. Recall that the concept behind a QALY is that 1 year of life with perfect health is worth 1, and 1 year of life with less than perfect health is worth less than 1. To illustrate, suppose a patient will live 1 year without treatment, but that treatment will extend the patient's life to 3 years but at

Strategy	Cost (USS)	Life year gained	ICER (USS) Per patient	INMB (USS)
Women aged 45–49 years				
No screening	115,603	100,520		
Mammography screening	1,169,942	100,640	8,782.70	–294.117
Women aged 50–54 years				
No screening	104,134	100,096		
Mammography screening	1,157,487	100,385	3,647.06	775,674
Women aged 55–59 years				
No screening	99,351	99,689		
Mammography screening	1,148,683	99,928	4,405.44	459,055
Women aged 60–64 years				
No screening	79,603	98,897		
Mammography screening	1,110,692	99,060	6,335.84	–512

Figure 12–12. Cost-effectiveness of scenarios for mammography in Vietnamese women. (Reproduced with permission from Nguyen CP, Adang EMM: Cost-effectiveness of breast cancer screening using mammography in Vietnamese women, *PLoS ONE.* 2018 Mar 26;13(3):e0194996.)

Group	INMB (USS) of base case	INMB (USS) of Screening vs.		INMB (USS) of 23.6% screening vs. no screening
		95% no screening+ 5% individual screening	90% no screening+ 10% individual screening	
45–49 years	–294,117	–279,465	–264,815	–69,412
50–54 years	775,674	736,811	697,948	183,059
55–59 years	459,055	436,289	413,244	108,337
60–64 years	–512	–486	–460	–121

Figure 12–13. Comparison of INMB for age groups and uptake percentages for mammography in Vietnamese women. (Reproduced with permission from Nguyen CP, Adang EMM: Cost-effectiveness of breast cancer screening using mammography in Vietnamese women, *PLoS ONE.* 2018 Mar 26;13(3):e0194996).

a lower quality of life, say 0.75. Then the number of QALYs gained if the treatment is used is: 3 years of life with a utility of 0.75 is 2.25; subtracting 1 year of life at reduced quality (1 – 0.75 = 0.25) gives 2 QALYs. Nguyen and Adang opted to measure "life year gained" with a measure that is not quality adjusted.

COMPUTER PROGRAMS FOR DECISION ANALYSIS

Several computer programs have been written for researchers who wish to model clinical decision-making problems. These programs are generally single-purpose programs and are not included in the general statistical analysis programs illustrated in earlier chapters in this book.

Decision Analysis by TreeAge (DATA) software is a decision analysis program that lets the researcher build decision trees interactively on the computer screen. Once the tree is developed, TreeAge performs the calculations for the expected utilities to determine the optimal pathway for the decision. It also performs sensitivity analysis. The researcher who uses computers to model decision problems is able to model complex problems, update or alter them as needed, and perform a variety of sensitivity analyses with relative ease.

SUMMARY

Topics in this chapter are departures from the topics considered in traditional introductory biostatistics textbooks. The increase in medical studies using methods in decision-making and the growing emphasis on evidence-based medicine, however, indicate that practitioners should be familiar with the concepts. Equally important, the methods discussed in this chapter for calculating the probability of disease are ones that every clinician must be able to use in everyday patient care. These methods allow clinicians to integrate the results of published studies into their own practice of medicine.

We presented four equivalent methods for determining how likely a disease (or condition) is in a given patient based on the results of a diagnostic procedure. Three pieces of information are needed: (1) the probability of the disease or condition prior to any procedure, that is, the base rate (or prevalence); (2) the accuracy of the procedure in identifying the condition when it is present (sensitivity); and (3) the accuracy of the procedure in identifying the absence of the condition when it is indeed absent (specificity). We can draw an analogy with hypothesis testing: A false-positive is similar to a type I error, falsely declaring a significant difference; and sensitivity is like power, correctly detecting a difference when it is present.

The logic discussed in this chapter is applicable in many situations other than diagnostic testing. For example, the answer to each history question or the finding from each action of the physical examination may be interpreted in a similar manner. When the outcome from a procedure or inquiry is expressed as a numerical value, rather than as the positive or negative evaluation, ROC curves can be used to evaluate the ramifications of decisions, such as selecting a given cutoff value or comparing the efficacy of two or more diagnostic methods.

Articles in the literature sometimes report predictive values using the same subjects that were used to determine sensitivity and specificity, ignoring the fact that predictive values change as the prior probability or prevalence changes. As readers, we can only assume these investigators do not recognize the crucial role that prior probability (or prevalence) plays in interpreting the results of both positive and negative procedures.

We extended these simple applications to more complex situations. A diagnostic procedure is often part of a complex decision, and the methods in this chapter can be used to determine probabilities for branches of the decision tree. These methods allow research findings to be integrated into the decisions physicians must make in diagnosing and managing diseases and conditions. A procedure called sensitivity analysis can be performed to determine which assumptions are important and how changes in the probabilities used in the decision analysis will change the decision.

Decision analysis can also be used to determine the most efficient approach for dealing with a problem. Because increasing attention is being focused on the cost of medical care, increasing numbers of articles dealing with decision analysis now appear in the literature. Decision analysis can help decision makers who must choose between committing resources to one program or another.

We also reviewed a novel but effective application of decision analysis to evaluating protocols recommended by experts but not subjected to clinical trial. The protocols outlined the steps to take in doing workups for patients with low back pain who may be at risk of spinal malignancy.

Finally, we described a study that seeks to assess the cost-effectiveness of extending mammography for screening for breast cancer in Vietnamese women.

Not many introductory texts discuss topics in medical decision-making, partly because it is not viewed as mainstream biostatistics. A survey of the biostatistics curriculum in medical schools (Dawson-Saunders et al, 1987), however, found that these topics were taught at 87% of the medical schools. In summary, we note that published articles (Davidoff, 1999; Greenhalgh, 1997a; Pauker and Kassirer, 1987; Raiffa, 1997) and texts (Eddy, 1996; Ingelfinger et al, 1994; Locket, 1997; Sackett et al, 1991 Weinstein and Fineberg, 1998) discuss the role of decision analysis in medicine, and you may wish to consult these resources for a broader discussion of the issues. One advantage of performing a well-defined analysis of a medical decision problem is that the process itself forces explicit consideration of all factors that affect the decision.

EXERCISES

1. Suppose a 70-year-old woman comes to your office because of fatigue, pain in her hands and knees, and intermittent, sharp pains in her chest. Physical examination reveals an otherwise healthy female—the cardiopulmonary examination is normal, and no swelling is present in her joints. A possible diagnosis in this case is systemic lupus erythematosus (SLE). The question is whether to order an ANA (antinuclear antibody) test and, if so, how to interpret the results. Tan and coworkers (1982) reported that the ANA test is very sensitive to SLE, being positive 95% of the time when the disease is present. It is, however, only about 50% specific: Positive results are also obtained with connective tissue diseases other than SLE, and the occurrence of a positive ANA in the normal healthy population also increases with age.

   a. Assuming this patient has a baseline 2% chance of SLE, how will the results of an ANA test that is 95% sensitive and 50% specific for SLE change the probabilities of lupus if the test is positive? Negative?

   b. Suppose the woman has swelling of the joints in addition to her other symptoms of fatigue, joint pain, and intermittent, sharp chest pain. In this case, the probability of lupus is higher, perhaps 20%. Recalculate the probability of lupus if the test is positive and if it is negative.

2. Use Bayes' theorem and the likelihood ratio method to calculate the probability of no lupus when the ANA test is negative, using a pretest probability of lupus of 2%.

3. Joines and colleagues (2001) examined two cut-off values for ESR.

   a. What is the effect on the sensitivity of ESR for spinal malignancy if the threshold for positive is increased from ESR ≥ 20 mm/h to ESR ≥ 0 mm/h?

   b. What is the effect on the number of false-positives?

4. A 43-year-old white male comes to your office for an insurance physical examination. Routine urinalysis reveals glucosuria. You recently learned of a newly developed test that produced positive results in 138 of 150 known diabetics and in 24 of 150 persons known not to have diabetes.

   a. What is the sensitivity of the new test?

   b. What is the specificity of the new test?

   c. What is the false-positive rate of the new test?

   d. Suppose a fasting blood sugar is obtained with known sensitivity and specificity of 0.80 and 0.96, respectively. If this test is applied to the same group that the new test used (150 persons with diabetes and 150 persons without diabetes), what is the predictive validity of a positive test?

   e. For the current patient, after the positive urinalysis, you think the chance that he has diabetes is about 90%. If the fasting blood sugar test is positive, what is the revised probability of disease?

5. Consider a 22-year-old woman who comes to your office with palpitations. Physical examination shows a healthy female with no detectable heart murmurs. In this situation, your guess is that this patient has a 25–30% chance of having mitral valve prolapse, from prevalence of the disease and physical findings for this particular patient. Echocardiograms are fairly sensitive for detecting mitral valve prolapse in patients who have it—approximately 90% sensitive. Echocardiograms are also quite specific, showing only about 5% false-positives; in other words, a negative result is correctly obtained in 95% of people who do not have mitral valve prolapse.

   a. How does a positive echocardiogram for this woman change your opinion of the 30% chance of mitral valve prolapse? That is, what is your best guess on mitral valve prolapse with a positive test?

   b. If the echocardiogram is negative, how sure can you be that this patient does not have mitral valve prolapse?

6. No consensus exists regarding the management of incidental intracranial saccular aneurysms. Some experts advocate surgery; others point out that the prognosis is relatively benign even without surgery, especially for aneurysms smaller than 10 mm. The decision is complicated because rupture of an incidental aneurysm is a long-term risk, spread out over many years, whereas surgery represents an immediate risk. Some patients may prefer to avoid surgery, even at the cost of later excess risk; others may not.

   Van Crevel and colleagues (1986) approached this problem by considering a fictitious 45-year-old woman with migraine (but otherwise healthy) who had been having attacks for the past 2 years. Her attacks were right-sided and did not respond to medication. She had no family history of migraine. The neurologist suspected an arteriovenous malformation and ordered four-vessel angiography, which showed an aneurysm of 7 mm on the left middle cerebral artery. Should the neurologist advise the patient to have preventive surgery? The decision is diagrammed in Figure 12–14.

   The investigators developed a scale for the utility of each outcome, ranging from 0 for death to 100 for perfect health. They decided that disability following surgery should be valued at 75.

   If no surgery is performed, the possibility of a rupture is considered. A utility of 100 is still used for no rupture and for recovery following a rupture. Disability following a rupture at some time in the future is considered more positive, however, than disability following immediate surgery and is given a utility of 90.1. Similarly, death following a future rupture is preferred to death immediately following surgery and is given a utility of 60.2. These utilities are given in Figure 12–14.

   a. What is the expected utility of the three outcomes if there is a rupture?

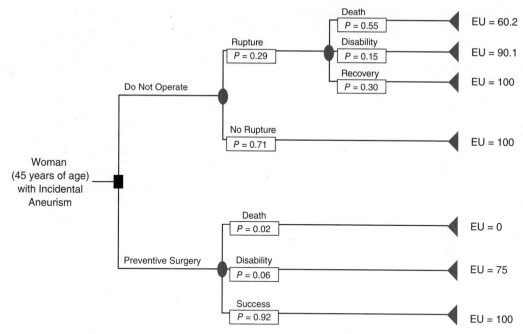

Figure 12–14. Decision tree for aneurysms with probabilities and utilities included. (EU, expected utility.) (Adapted with permission from van Crevel H, Habbema JD, Braakman R: Decision analysis of the management of incidental intracranial saccular aneurysms, *Neurology.* 1986 Oct;36(10):1335–1339.)

b. What is the expected utility of the decision not to operate?

c. What is the expected utility of the decision to operate?

d. Which approach has the highest utility?

8. A decision analysis for managing ulcerative colitis points out that patients with this condition are at high risk of developing colon cancer (Gage, 1986). The analysis compares the decisions of colectomy versus colonoscopy versus no test or therapy. The decision tree developed for this problem is shown in Figure 12–15. The author used information from the literature for the data listed on the tree. The utilities are 5-year survival probabilities (multiplied by 100).

a. What is the probability of colon cancer used in the analysis?

b. The author gave a range of published values for sensitivity and specificity of colonoscopy with biopsy but did not state the precise values used in the analysis. Can you tell what sensitivity and specificity were used in the analysis?

c. The expected utility of the colonoscopy arm is calculated as 94.6. Calculate the expected utility of the no-test-or-therapy arm and the colectomy arm. What is the procedure with the highest expected utility, that is, what is the recommended decision?

9. Group Exercise. Select a diagnostic problem of interest and perform a literature search to find published articles on the sensitivity and specificity of diagnostic procedures used with the problem.

a. What terminology is used for sensitivity and specificity? Are these terms used, or are results discussed in terms of false-positives and false-negatives?

b. Are actual numbers given or simply the values for sensitivity and specificity?

c. Does a well-accepted gold standard exist for the diagnosis? If not, did investigators provide information on the validity of the assessment used for the gold standard?

| Choices | Probabilities | Outcomes | Utilities |

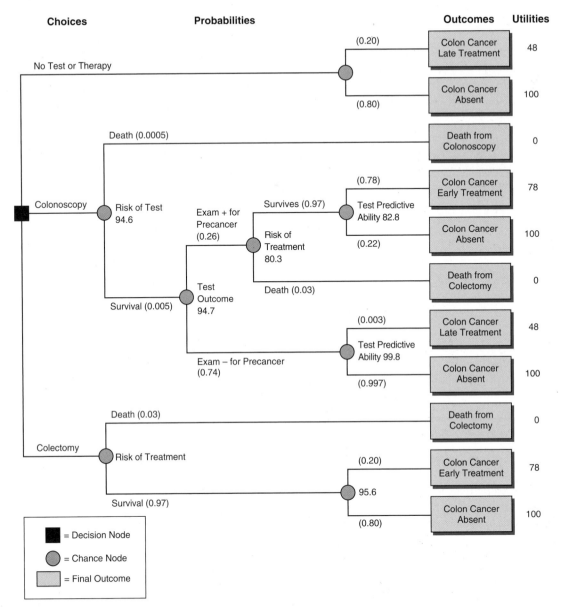

Figure 12–15. Decision tree for ulcerative colitis. (Adapted with permission from Gage TP: Managing the cancer risk in chronic ulcerative colitis. A decision-analytic approach, *J Clin Gastroenterol*. 1986 Feb;8(1):50–57.)

d. *Did investigators discuss the reasons for false-positives? Were the selection criteria used for selecting persons with and without the disease appropriate?*

e. *Did authors cite predictive values for positive and negative tests? If so, why is this inappropriate?*

10. **Group Exercise.** *The CAGE questionnaire was designed as a screening device for alcoholism (Bush et al, 1987). The questionnaire consists of four questions:*

a. *Have you ever felt you should Cut down on your drinking?*

b. Have people Annoyed you by criticizing your drinking?

c. Have you ever felt bad or Guilty about your drinking?

d. Have you ever had a drink first thing in the morning to steady your nerves or get rid of a hangover (Eye-opener)?

The questionnaire is scored by counting the number of questions to which the patient says yes. Buchsbaum and coworkers (1991) studied the predictive validity of CAGE scores. Obtain a copy of the article and calculate the predictive validity for 0, 1, 2, 3, and 4 positive answers. Draw an ROC curve for the questionnaire. Do you think this questionnaire is a good screening tool?

e. Discuss the pros and cons of using this questionnaire with women with node-negative breast cancer and of using similar instruments for patients with other diseases. What are some possible advantages? Disadvantages? Would you use this instrument or a similar one with your patients?

Reading the Medical Literature

PURPOSE OF THE CHAPTER

This final chapter has several purposes. Most importantly, it ties together concepts and skills presented in previous chapters and applies these concepts very specifically to reading medical journal articles. Throughout the text, we have attempted to illustrate the strengths and weaknesses of some of the studies discussed, but this chapter focuses specifically on those attributes of a study that indicate whether we, as readers of the medical literature, can use the results with confidence. The chapter begins with a brief summary of major types of medical studies. Next, we examine the anatomy of a typical journal article in detail, and we discuss the contents of each component—abstract or summary, introduction, methods, results, discussion, and conclusions. In this examination, we also point out common shortcomings, sources of bias, and threats to the validity of studies.

Clinicians read the literature for many different reasons. Some articles are of interest because you want only to be aware of advances in a field. In these instances, you may decide to skim the article with little interest in how the study was designed and carried out. In such cases, it may be possible to depend on experts in the field who write review articles to provide a relatively superficial level of information. On other occasions, however, you want to know whether the conclusions of the study are valid, perhaps so that they can be used to determine patient care or to plan a research project. In these situations, you need to read and evaluate the article with a critical eye in order to detect poorly done studies that arrive at unwarranted conclusions.

To assist readers in their critical reviews, we present a checklist for evaluating the validity of a journal article. The checklist notes some of the characteristics of a well-designed and well-written article. The checklist is based on experiences of previous edition authors with medical students, house staff, journal clubs, and interactions with physician colleagues. It also reflects the opinions expressed in an article describing how journal editors and statisticians can interact to improve the quality of published medical research (Marks et al, 1988).

A number of authors have found that only a minority of published studies meet the criteria for scientific adequacy. The checklist should assist you in using your time most effectively by allowing you to differentiate valid articles from poorly done studies so that you can concentrate on the more productive ones.

Two guidelines recently published increase our optimism that the quality of the published literature will continue to improve. The International Conference on Harmonization (ICH) E9 guideline "Statistical Principles for Clinical Trials" (1999) addresses issues of statistical methodology in the design, conduct, analysis, and evaluation of clinical trials. Application of the principles is intended to facilitate the general acceptance of analyses and conclusions drawn from clinical trials.

The International Committee of Medical Journal Editors published the "Uniform Requirements of Manuscripts Submitted to Biomedical Journals" in 1997. Under Statistics, the document states:

> Describe statistical methods with enough detail to enable a knowledgeable reader with access to the original data to verify the reported results.... When data are summarized in the results section, specify the statistical methods used to analyze them.

The requirements also recommend the use of confidence intervals and to avoid depending solely on p values.

REVIEW OF MAJOR STUDY DESIGNS

Chapter 2 introduced the major types of study designs used in medical research, broadly divided into **experimental studies** (including **clinical trials**); **observational studies** (cohort, case–control, cross-sectional/surveys, case–series); and meta-analyses. Each design has certain advantages over the others as well as some specific disadvantages; they are briefly summarized in the following paragraphs. (A more detailed discussion is presented in Chapter 2.)

Clinical trials provide the strongest evidence for causation because they are experiments and, as such, are subject to the least number of problems or biases. Trials with randomized controls are the study type of choice when the objective is to evaluate the effectiveness of a treatment or a procedure. Drawbacks to using clinical trials include their expense and the generally long time needed to complete them.

Cohort studies are the best observational study design for investigating the causes of a condition, the course of a disease, or **risk factors.** Causation cannot be proved with cohort studies, because they do not involve interventions and are not randomized. Because they are **longitudinal studies,** they incorporate the correct time sequence to provide strong evidence for possible causes and effects. In addition, in cohort studies that are **prospective,** as opposed to **historical,** investigators can control many sources of bias. Cohort studies have disadvantages, of course. If they take a long time to complete, they are frequently weakened by patient attrition. They are also expensive to carry out if the disease or outcome is rare (so that a large number of subjects needs to be followed) or requires a long time to develop.

Case–control studies are an efficient way to study rare diseases, examine conditions that take a long time to develop, or investigate a preliminary hypothesis. They are the quickest and generally the least expensive studies to design and carry out. Case–control studies also are the most vulnerable to possible biases, however, and they depend entirely on high-quality existing records. A major issue in case–control studies is the selection of an appropriate control group. Some statisticians have recommended the use of two control groups: one similar in some ways to the cases (such as having been hospitalized or treated during the same period) and another made up of healthy subjects.

Cross-sectional studies and **surveys** are best for determining the status of a disease or condition at a particular point in time; they are similar to case–control studies in being relatively quick and inexpensive to complete. Because cross-sectional studies provide only a snapshot in time, they may lead to misleading conclusions if interest focuses on a disease or other time-dependent process.

Case–series studies are the weakest kinds of observational studies and represent a description of typically unplanned observations; in fact, many would not call them studies at all. Their primary use is to provide insights for research questions to be addressed by subsequent, planned studies.

Studies that focus on **outcomes** can be experimental or observational. Clinical outcomes remain the major focus, but emphasis is increasingly placed on functional status and quality-of-life measures. It is important to use properly designed and evaluated methods to collect outcome data. **Evidence-based medicine** makes great use of outcome studies.

Meta-analysis may likewise focus on clinical trials or observational studies. Meta-analyses differ from the traditional review articles in that they attempt to evaluate the quality of the research and quantify the summary data. They are helpful when the available evidence is based on studies with small sample sizes or when studies come to conflicting conclusions. Meta-analyses do not, however, take the place of well-designed clinical trials.

THE ABSTRACT & INTRODUCTION SECTIONS OF A RESEARCH REPORT

Journal articles almost always include an abstract or summary of the article prior to the body of the article itself. Most of us are guilty of reading *only* the abstract on occasion, perhaps because we are in a great hurry or have only a cursory interest in the topic. This practice is unwise when it is important to know whether the conclusions stated in the article are justified and can be used to make decisions. This section discusses the abstract and introduction portions of a research report and outlines the information they should contain.

The Abstract

The major purposes of the abstract are (1) to tell readers enough about the article so they can decide whether to read it in its entirely and (2) to identify the focus of the study. The International Committee of Medical Journal Editors (2018) recommended that the abstract "state the purposes of the study or investigation, basic procedures (selection of study subjects or experimented animals; observational and analytic methods), main findings (specific data and their statistical significance, if possible) and the principal conclusions."

We suggest asking two questions to decide whether to read the article: (1) If the study has been properly designed and analyzed, would the results be important and worth knowing? (2) If the results are statistically significant, does the magnitude of the change or effect also have clinical significance; if the results are not statistically significant, was the sample size sufficiently large to detect a meaningful difference or effect? If the answers to these questions are yes, then it is worthwhile to continue to read the report. Structured abstracts are a boon to the busy reader and frequently contain enough information to answer these two questions.

The Introduction or Abstract

At one time, the following topics were discussed (or should have been discussed) in the introduction section; however, with the advent of the structured abstract, many of these topics are now addressed directly in that section. The important issue is that the information be available and easy to identify.

Reason for the Study: The introduction section of a research report is usually fairly short. Generally, the authors briefly mention previous research that indicates the need for the present study. In some situations, the study is a natural outgrowth or the next logical step of previous studies. In other circumstances, previous studies have been inadequate in one way or another. The overall purpose of this information is twofold: to provide the necessary background information to place the present study in its proper context and to provide reasons for doing the present study. In some journals, the main justification for the study is given in the discussion section of the article instead of in the introduction.

Purpose of the Study: Regardless of the placement of background information on the study, the introduction section is where the investigators communicate the purpose of their study. The purpose of the study is frequently presented in the last paragraph or last sentences at the end of the introduction. The purpose should be stated clearly and succinctly, in a manner analogous to a 15-second summary of a patient case. For example, in the study described in Chapter 10, Shah and colleagues (2018) do this very well; they stated their objective as follows:

> *We analyzed whether self-reported exercise tolerance predicts outcomes (hospital length of-stay [LOS], mortality and morbidity) in PHTN patients (WHO Class I±V) undergoing anesthesia and surgery.*

This statement concisely communicates the population of interest (PHTN patients), the focus of the study or independent variable (self-reported exercise tolerance), and the outcome (LOS, mortality and morbidity). As readers, we should be able to determine whether the purpose for the study was conceived prior to data collection or if it evolved after the authors viewed their data; the latter situation is much more likely to capitalize on chance findings. The lack of a clearly stated research question is the most common reason medical manuscripts are rejected by journal editors (Springer, 2019).

Population Included in the Study: In addition to stating the purpose of the study, the structured abstract or introduction section may include information on the study's location, length of time, and subjects. Alternatively, this information may be contained in the methods sections. This information helps readers decide whether the location of the study and the type of subjects included in the study are applicable in the readers' own practice environment.

The time covered by a study gives important clues regarding the **validity** of the results. If the study on a particular therapy covers too long a period, patients entering at the beginning of the study may differ in important ways from those entering at the end. For example, major changes may have occurred in the way the disease in question is diagnosed, and patients entering near the end of the study may have had their disease diagnosed at an earlier stage than did patients who entered the study early (see detection **bias,** in the section of that title). If the purpose of the study is to examine sequelae of a condition or procedure, the period covered by the study must be sufficiently long to detect consequences.

THE METHOD SECTION OF A RESEARCH REPORT

The method section contains information about how the study was done. Simply knowing the study design provides a great deal of information, and this information is often given in a structured abstract. In addition, the method section contains information regarding subjects who participated in the study or, in animal or inanimate studies, information on the animals or materials. The procedures used should be described in sufficient detail that the reader knows how measurements were made. If methods are novel or require interpretation, information should be given on the reliability of the assessments. The study outcomes should be specified along with the criteria used to assess them. The method section also should include information on the sample size for the study and on the statistical methods used to analyze the data; this information is often placed at the end of the method section. Each of these topics is discussed in detail in this section.

How well the study has been designed is of utmost importance. The most critical statistical errors, according to a statistical consultant to the *New England Journal of Medicine,* involve improper research design: "Whereas one can correct incorrect analytical techniques with a simple reanalysis of the data, an error in research design is almost always fatal to the study—one cannot correct for it subsequent to data collection" (Marks et al, 1988, p. 1004). Many statistical advances have occurred in recent years, especially in the methods used to design, conduct, and analyze clinical trials, and investigators should offer evidence that they have obtained expert advice.

Subjects in the Study

Of foremost importance is how the patients were selected for the study and, if the study is a clinical trial, how treatment assignments were made.

Randomized selection or assignment greatly enhances the generalizability of the results and avoids biases that otherwise may occur in patient selection (see the section titled, "Bias Related to Subject Selection."). Some authors believe it is sufficient merely to state that subjects were randomly selected or treatments were randomly assigned, but most statisticians recommend that the type of randomization process be specified as well. Authors who report the randomization methods provide some assurance that randomization actually occurred, because some investigators have a faulty view of what constitutes randomization. For example, an investigator may believe that assigning patients to the treatment and the control on alternate days makes the assignment random. As we emphasized in Chapter 4, however, randomization involves one of the precise methods that ensure that each subject (or treatment) has a known probability of being selected.

Eligibility Criteria: The authors should present information to illustrate that major selection biases (discussed in the section titled, "Bias Related to Subject Selection.") have been avoided, an aspect especially important in **nonrandomized trials.** The issue of which patients serve as controls was discussed in Chapter 2 in the context of case–control studies. In addition, the eligibility criteria for both inclusion and exclusion of subjects in the study must be specified in detail. We should be able to state, given any hypothetical subject, whether this person would be included in or excluded from the study. Cai and coworkers (2014) gave the following information on patients included in their study:

Exclusion criteria included hip hemiarthroplasty, uni-compartmental knee arthroplasty, TJA for fracture treatment, conversion TJA, and revision TJA.

Patient Follow-up: For similar reasons, sufficient information must be given regarding the procedures the investigators used to follow up patients, and they should state the numbers lost to follow-up. Some articles include this information under the results section instead of in the methods section.

The description of follow-up and dropouts should be sufficiently detailed to permit the reader to draw a diagram of the information. Occasionally, an article presents such a diagram, as was done by Bos-Touwen and colleagues (2015) in their study of patient activation, reproduced in Figure 13–1. Such a diagram makes very clear the number of patients who were eligible, those who were not eligible because of specific reasons, the dropouts, and so on.

Bias Related to Subject Selection

Bias in studies should not happen; it is an error related to selecting subjects or procedures or to measuring a characteristic. Biases are sometimes called **measurement errors** or **systematic errors** to distinguish them from **random error** (**random variation**), which occurs any time a sample is selected from a population. This section discusses selection bias, a type of bias common in medical research.

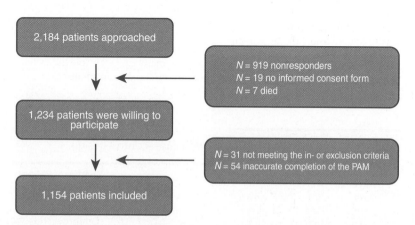

Figure 13–1. Flow of the subjects through the study. (Data from Bos-Touwen I, Schuurmans M, Monninkhof EM, et al: Patient and disease characteristics associated with activation for self-management in patients with diabetes, chronic obstructive pulmonary disease, chronic heart failure and chronic renal disease: a cross-sectional survey study, *PLoS One.* 2015 May 7;10(5):e0126400.)

Selection biases can occur in any study, but they are easier to control in clinical trials and cohort designs. It is important to be aware of selection biases, even though it is not always possible to predict exactly how their presence affects the conclusions. Sackett (1979) enumerated 35 different biases. We discuss some of the major ones that seem especially important to the clinician. If you are interested in a more detailed discussion, consult the article by Sackett and the text by Feinstein (1985), which devotes several chapters to the discussion of bias (especially Chapter 4, in the section titled "The Meaning of the Term Probability," and Chapters 15–17).

Prevalence or Incidence Bias: Prevalence bias occurs when a condition is characterized by early fatalities (some subjects die before they are diagnosed) or silent cases (cases in which the evidence of exposure disappears when the disease begins). Prevalence bias can result whenever a time gap occurs between exposure and selection of study subjects and the worst cases have died. A cohort study begun prior to the onset of disease is able to detect occurrences properly, but a case–control study that begins at a later date consists only of the people who did not die. This bias can be prevented in cohort studies and avoided in case–control studies by limiting eligibility for the study to newly diagnosed or incident cases. The practice of limiting eligibility is common in population-based case–control studies in cancer epidemiology.

To illustrate prevalence or incidence bias, let us suppose that two groups of people are being studied: those with a risk factor for a given disease (e.g., hypertension as a risk factor for stroke) and those without the risk factor. Suppose 1,000 people with hypertension and 1,000 people without hypertension have been followed for 10 years. At this point, we might have the situation shown in Table 13–1.

A cohort study begun 10 years ago would conclude correctly that patients with hypertension are more likely to develop cerebrovascular disease than patients without hypertension (300–100) and far more likely to die from it (250–20).

Suppose, however, a case–control study is undertaken at the end of the 10-year period without limiting eligibility to newly diagnosed cases of cerebrovascular disease. Then the situation illustrated in Table 13–2 occurs.

The **odds ratio** is calculated as $(50 \times 900)/(80 \times 700) = 0.80$, making it appear that hypertension is actually a protective factor for the disease! The bias introduced in an improperly designed case–control study of a disease that kills off one group faster than the other can lead to a conclusion exactly the opposite of the correct conclusion that would be obtained from a well-designed case–control study or a cohort study.

Admission Rate Bias: Admission rate bias (Berkson's fallacy) occurs when the study admission rates differ, which causes major distortions in risk ratios. As an example, admission rate bias can occur in studies of hospitalized patients when patients (cases) who have the risk factor are admitted to the hospital more frequently than either the cases without the risk factor or the controls with the risk factor.

This fallacy was first pointed out by Berkson (1946) in evaluating an earlier study that had concluded that tuberculosis might have a protective effect on cancer. This conclusion was reached after a case–control study found a negative association between tuberculosis and cancer: The frequency of tuberculosis among hospitalized cancer patients was less than the frequency of tuberculosis among the hospitalized control patients who did not have cancer. These counterintuitive results occurred because a smaller proportion of patients who had both cancer and tuberculosis were hospitalized and thus available for selection as cases in the study; chances are that patients with both diseases were more likely to die than patients with cancer or tuberculosis alone.

It is important to be aware of admission rate bias because many case–control studies reported in the medical literature use hospitalized patients as sources for

Table 13–1. Illustration of prevalence bias: Actual situation.

Patients	Number of Patients in 10-Year Cohort Study		
	Alive with Cerebrovascular Disease	Dead from Stroke	Alive with No Cerebrovascular Disease
With hypertension	50	250	700
Without hypertension	80	20	900

Table 13–2. Illustration of prevalence bias: Result with case–control design.

Patients	Number of Patients in Case–Control Study at End of 10 Years	
	With Cerebrovascular Disease	Without Cerebrovascular Disease
With hypertension	50	700
Without hypertension	80	900

both cases and controls. The only way to control for this bias is to include an unbiased control group, best accomplished by choosing controls from a wide variety of disease categories or from a population of healthy subjects. Some statisticians suggest using two control groups in studies in which admission bias is a potential problem.

Nonresponse Bias and the Volunteer Effect: Several steps discussed in Chapter 11 can be taken to reduce potential bias when subjects fail to respond to a survey. Bias that occurs when patients either volunteer or refuse to participate in studies is similar to nonresponse bias. This effect was studied in the nationwide Salk polio vaccine trials in 1954 by using two different study designs to evaluate the effectiveness of the vaccine (Meier, 1989). In some communities, children were randomly assigned to receive either the vaccine or a placebo injection. Some communities, however, refused to participate in a randomized trial; they agreed, instead, that second graders could be offered the vaccination and first and third graders could constitute the controls. In analysis of the data, researchers found that families who volunteered their children for participation in the nonrandomized study tended to be better educated and to have a higher income than families who refused to participate. They also tended to be absent from school with a higher frequency than nonparticipants.

Although in this example we might guess how absence from school could bias results, it is not always easy to determine how selection bias affects the outcome of the study; it may cause the experimental treatment to appear either better or worse than it should. Investigators should therefore reduce the potential for nonresponse bias as much as possible by using all possible means to increase the response rate and obtain the participation of most eligible patients. Using databases reduces response bias, but sometimes other sources of bias are present, that is, reasons that a specific group or selected information is underrepresented in the database.

Membership Bias: Membership bias is essentially a problem of preexisting groups. It also arises because one or more of the same characteristics that cause people to belong to the groups are related to the outcome of interest. For example, investigators have not been able to perform a clinical trial to examine the effects of smoking; some researchers have claimed it is not smoking itself that causes cancer but some other factor that simply happens to be more common in smokers. As readers of the medical literature, we need to be aware of membership bias because it cannot be prevented, and it makes the study of the effect of potential risk factors related to lifestyle very difficult.

A problem similar to membership bias is called the healthy worker effect; it was recognized in epidemiology when workers in a hazardous environment were unexpectedly found to have a higher survival rate than the general public. After further investigation, the cause of this incongruous finding was determined: Good health is a prerequisite in persons who are hired for work, but being healthy enough to work is not a requirement for persons in the general public.

Procedure Selection Bias: Procedure selection bias occurs when treatment assignments are made on the basis of certain characteristics of the patients, with the result that the treatment groups are not really similar. This bias frequently occurs in studies that are not randomized and is especially a problem in studies using historical controls. A good example is the comparison of a surgical versus a medical approach to a problem such as coronary artery disease. In early studies comparing surgical and medical treatment, patients were not randomized, and the evidence pointed to the conclusion that patients who received surgery were healthier than those treated medically; that is, only healthier patients were subjected to the risks associated with surgery. The Coronary Artery Surgery Study (CASS, 1983) was undertaken in part to resolve these questions. It is important to be aware of procedure selection bias because many published studies describe a series of patients, some treated one way and some another way, and then proceed to make comparisons and draw inappropriate conclusions as a result.

Procedures Used in the Study and Common Procedural Biases

Terms and Measurements: The procedures used in the study are also described in the method section. Here, authors provide definitions of measures used in the study, especially any operational definitions developed by the investigators. If unusual instruments or methods are used, the authors should provide a reference and a brief description. For example, the study of screening for domestic violence in emergency department patients by Bos-Touwen and colleagues (2015) carefully defined their primary outcome variable:

> *The primary outcome was activation for self-management, which was assessed with the 13-item Patient Activation Measure (PAM-13). The PAM was considered the best generic measure, since it assesses self-reported knowledge, skills and confidence for self-management irrespective of the underlying chronic condition.*

The journal *Stroke* has the practice of presenting the abbreviations and acronyms used in the article in a box.

This makes the abbreviations clear and also easy to refer to in reading other sections of the article. For example, in reporting their study of sleep-disordered breathing and stroke, Good and colleagues (1996) presented a list of abbreviations at the top of the column that describe the subjects and methods in the study.

Several biases may occur in the measurement of various patient characteristics and in the procedures used or evaluated in the study. Some of the more common biases are described in the following subsections.

Procedure Bias: Procedure bias, discussed by Feinstein (1985), occurs when groups of subjects are not treated in the same manner. For example, the procedures used in an investigation may lead to detection of other problems in patients in the treatment group and make these problems appear to be more prevalent in this group. As another example, the patients in the treatment group may receive more attention and be followed up more vigorously than those in another group, thus stimulating greater compliance with the treatment regimen. The way to avoid this bias is by carrying out all maneuvers except the experimental factor in the same way in all groups and examining all outcomes using similar procedures and criteria.

Recall Bias: Recall bias may occur when patients are asked to recall certain events, and subjects in one group are more likely to remember the event than those in the other group. For example, people take aspirin commonly and for many reasons, but patients diagnosed as having peptic ulcer disease may recall the ingestion of aspirin with greater accuracy than those without gastrointestinal problems.

Insensitive-Measure Bias: Measuring instruments may not be able to detect the characteristic of interest or may not be properly calibrated. For example, routine x-ray films are an insensitive method for detecting osteoporosis because bone loss of approximately 30% must occur before a roentgenogram can detect it. Newer densitometry techniques are more sensitive and thus avoid insensitive-measure bias.

Detection Bias: Detection bias can occur because a new diagnostic technique is introduced that is capable of detecting the condition of interest at an earlier stage. Survival for patients diagnosed with the new procedure inappropriately appears to be longer, merely because the condition was diagnosed earlier.

A spin-off of detection bias, called the Will Rogers phenomenon (because of his attention to human phenomena), was described by Feinstein and colleagues (1985). They found that a cohort of subjects with lung cancer first treated in 1953 to 1954 had lower 6-month survival rates for patients with each of the three main stages (localized, nodal involvement, and metastases) as well as for the total group than did a 1977 cohort treated at the same institutions. Newer imaging procedures were used with the later-stage group; however, according to the old diagnostic classification, this group had a prognostically favorable zero-time shift in that their disease was diagnosed at an earlier stage. In addition, by detecting metastases in the 1977 group that were missed in the earlier group, the new technologic approaches resulted in stage migration; that is, members of the 1977 cohort were diagnosed as having a more advanced stage of the disease, whereas they would have been diagnosed as having earlier-stage disease in 1953 to 1954. The individuals who migrated from the earlier-stage group to the later-stage group tended to have the poorest survival in the earlier-stage group; so removing them resulted in an increase in survival rates in the earlier group. At the same time, these individuals, now assigned to the later-stage group, were better off than most other patients in this group, and their addition to the group resulted in an increased survival in the later-stage group as well. The authors stated that the 1953 to 1954 and 1977 cohorts actually had similar survival rates when patients in the 1977 group were classified according to the criteria that would have been in effect had there been no advances in diagnostic techniques.

Compliance Bias: Compliance bias occurs when patients find it easier or more pleasant to comply with one treatment than with another. For example, in the treatment of hypertension, a comparison of α-methyldopa versus hydrochlorothiazide may demonstrate inaccurate results because some patients do not take α-methyldopa owing to its unpleasant side effects, such as drowsiness, fatigue, or impotence in male patients.

Assessing Study Outcomes

Variation in Data: In many clinics, a nurse collects certain information about a patient (e.g., height, weight, date of birth, blood pressure, pulse) and records it on the medical record before the patient is seen by a physician. Suppose a patient's blood pressure is recorded as 140/88 on the chart; the physician, taking the patient's blood pressure again as part of the physical examination, observes a reading of 148/96. Which blood pressure reading is correct? What factors might be responsible for the differences in the observation? We use blood pressure and other clinical information to examine sources of variation in data and ways to measure the reliability of observations. Two classic articles in the *Canadian Medical Association Journal* (McMaster University Health Sciences Centre, Department of

Clinical Epidemiology and Biostatistics, 1980a; 1980b) discuss sources of clinical disagreement and ways disagreement can be minimized.

Factors that Contribute to Variation in Clinical Observations: Variation, or variability in measurements on the same subject, in clinical observations and measurements can be classified into three categories: (1) variation in the characteristic being measured, (2) variation introduced by the examiner, and (3) variation owing to the instrument or method used. It is especially important to control variation due to the second two factors as much as possible so that the reported results will generalize as intended.

Substantial variability may occur in the measurement of biologic characteristics. For example, a person's blood pressure is not the same from one time to another, and thus blood pressure values vary. A patient's description of symptoms to two different physicians may vary because the patient may forget something. Medications and illness can also affect the way a patient behaves and what information they remember to tell a nurse or physician.

Even when no change occurs in the subject, different observers may report different measurements. When examination of a characteristic requires visual acuity, such as the reading on a sphygmomanometer or the features on an x-ray film, differences may result from the varying visual abilities of the observers. Such differences can also play a role when hearing (detecting heart sounds) or feeling (palpating internal organs) is required. Some individuals are simply more skilled than others in history taking or performing certain examinations.

Variability also occurs when the characteristic being measured is a behavioral attribute. Two examples are measurements of functional status and measurements of pain; here the additional component of patient or observer interpretation can increase apparent variability. In addition, observers may tend to observe and record what they expect based on other information about the patient. These factors point out the need for a standardized protocol for data collection.

The instrument used in the examination can be another source of variation. For instance, mercury column sphygmomanometers are less inherently variable than aneroid models. In addition, the environment in which the examination takes place, including lighting and noise level, presence of other individuals, and room temperature, can produce apparent differences. Methods for measuring behavior-related characteristics such as functional status or pain usually consist of a set of questions answered by patients and hence are not as precise as instruments that measure physical characteristics.

Several steps can be taken to reduce variability. Taking a history when the patient is calm and not heavily medicated and checking with family members when the patient is incapacitated are both useful in minimizing errors that result from a patient's illness or the effects of medication. Collecting information and making observations in a proper environment is also a good strategy. Recognizing one's own strengths and weaknesses helps one evaluate the need for other opinions. **Blind** assessment, especially of subjective characteristics, guards against errors resulting from preconceptions. Repeating questionable aspects of the examination or asking a colleague to perform a key aspect (blindly, of course) reduces the possibility of error. Having well-defined operational guidelines for using classification scales helps people use them in a consistent manner. Ensuring that instruments are properly calibrated and correctly used eliminates many errors and thus reduces variation.

Ways to Measure Reliability and Validity: A common strategy to ensure the **reliability** or reproducibility of measurements, especially for research purposes, is to replicate the measurements and evaluate the degree of agreement. We discussed **intra-** and **interrater reliability** in Chapter 5 and discussed reliability and validity in detail in Chapter 11.

One approach to establishing the reliability of a measure is to repeat the measurements at a different time or by a different person and compare the results. When the outcome is nominal, the kappa statistic is used; when the scale of measurement is numerical, the statistic used to examine the relationship is the correlation coefficient (Chapter 8) or the intraclass correlation (Chapter 11).

Blinding: Another aspect of assessing the outcome is related to ways of increasing the objectivity and decreasing the subjectivity of the assessment. In studies involving the comparison of two treatments or procedures, the most effective method for achieving objective assessment is to have both patient and investigator be unaware of which method was used. If only the patient is unaware, the study is called **blind;** if both patient and investigator are unaware, it is called **double-blind.**

Blinding helps to reduce a priori biases on the part of both patient and physician. Patients who are aware of their treatment assignment may imagine certain side effects or expect specific benefits, and their expectations may influence the outcome. Similarly, investigators who know which treatment has been assigned to a given patient may be more watchful for certain side effects or benefits. Although we might suspect an investigator who is not blinded to be more favorable to the new treatment or procedure, just the opposite may happen; that is, the investigator may bend over backward to keep from being prejudiced by their knowledge and, therefore, may err in favor of the control.

Knowledge of treatment assignment may be somewhat less influential when the outcome is straightforward, as is true for mortality. With mortality, it is difficult to see how outcome assessment can be biased. Many examples exist in which the outcome appears to be objective, however, even though its evaluation contains subjective components. Many clinical studies attempt to ascribe reasons for mortality or morbidity, and judgment begins to play a role in these cases. For example, mortality is often an outcome of interest in studies involving organ transplantation, and investigators wish to differentiate between deaths from failure of the organ and deaths from an unrelated cause. If the patient dies in an automobile accident, for example, investigators can easily decide that the death is not due to organ rejection; but in most situations, the decision is not so easy.

The issue of blinding becomes more important as the outcome becomes less amenable to objective determination. Research that focuses on quality-of-life outcomes, such as chest pain status, activity limitation, or recreational status, require subjective measures. Although patients cannot be blinded in many studies, the subjective outcomes can be assessed by a person, such as another physician, a psychologist, or a physical therapist, who is blind to the treatment the patient received.

Data Quality and Monitoring: The method section is also the place where steps taken to ensure the accuracy of the data should be described. Increased variation and possibly incorrect conclusions can occur if the correct observation is made but is incorrectly recorded or coded. Dual or duplicate entry decreases the likelihood of errors because it is unusual for the same entry error to occur twice.

Multicenter studies provide additional data quality challenges. It is important that an accurate and complete protocol be developed to ensure that data are handled the same way in all centers.

Determining an Appropriate Sample Size

Specifying the sample size needed to detect a difference or an effect of a given magnitude is one of the most crucial pieces of information in the report of a medical study. Recall that missing a significant difference is called a **type II error,** and this error can happen when the sample size is too small. We provide many illustrations in the chapters that discuss specific statistical methods, especially Chapters 5 to 8 and 10 to 11.

Determination of sample size is referred to as power analysis or as determining the **power** of a study. An assessment of power is essential in negative studies, studies that fail to find an expected difference or relationship; we feel so strongly about this point that we recommend that readers disregard negative studies that do not provide information on power.

Lin et al (2018) studied the use of regorafenib versus a combination chemotherapy alternative. They stated:

The study was designed to confirm our hypothesis that combination therapy would extend median PFS and OS. The PFS in the study group was expected to be 3.5 months compared with 1.7 month based on the results of a previous study. A two-sided log rank test with an overall sample size of 68 subjects (34 in the control group and 34 in the treatment group) achieves 80.4% power at a 0.050% significance level to detect a hazard ratio of 0.4857.

We repeatedly emphasize the need to perform a power analysis prior to beginning a study and have illustrated how to estimate power using statistical programs for that purpose. Investigators planning complicated studies or studies involving a number of variables are especially advised to contact a statistician for assistance.

Observational studies sometimes suffer from a phenomenon called overpowering. Studies with very large sample sizes may detect differences that are not clinically meaningful. In these cases, the researcher should determine if the statistically significant differences detected also meet the criteria for **minimum clinical significance**.

Evaluating the Statistical Methods

Statistical methods are the primary focus of this text, and only a brief summary and some common problems are listed here. At the risk of oversimplification, the use of statistics in medicine can be summarized as follows: (1) to answer questions concerning differences; (2) to answer questions concerning associations; and (3) to control for confounding issues or to make predictions. If you can determine the type of question investigators are asking (from the stated purpose of the study) and the types and numbers of measures used in the study (**numerical, ordinal, nominal**), then the appropriate statistical procedure should be relatively easy to specify. Tables 10–1 and 10–2 in Chapter 10 and the flowcharts in Appendix C were developed to assist with this process. Some common biases in evaluating data are discussed in the next sections.

Fishing Expedition: A fishing expedition is the name given to studies in which the investigators do not have clear-cut research questions guiding the research. Instead, data are collected, and a search is carried out for results that are *significant.* The problem with this approach is that it capitalizes on chance occurrences and leads to conclusions that may not hold up if the study is replicated. Unfortunately, such studies are rarely repeated, and incorrect conclusions can remain a part of accepted wisdom.

Multiple Significance Tests: Multiple tests in statistics, just as in clinical medicine, result in increased chances of making a type I, or false-positive, error when the results from one test are interpreted as being independent of the results from another. For example, a **factorial design** for analysis of variance in a study involving four groups measured on three independent variables has the possibility of 18 comparisons (6 comparisons among the four groups on each of three variables), ignoring interactions. If each comparison is made for $p \leq 0.05$, the probability of finding one or more comparisons significant by chance is considerably greater than 0.05. The best way to guard against this bias is by performing the appropriate global test with analysis of variance prior to making individual group comparisons (Chapter 7) or using an appropriate method to analyze multiple variables (Chapter 10).

A similar problem can occur in a clinical trial if too many interim analyses are done. Sometimes, it is important to analyze the data at certain stages during a trial to learn if one treatment is clearly superior or inferior. Many trials are stopped early when an interim analysis determines that one therapy is markedly superior to another. For instance, the Women's Health Initiative trial on estrogen plus progestin (Rossouw et al, 2002) and the study of finasteride and the development of prostate cancer (Thompson et al, 2003) were both stopped early. In the estrogen study, the conclusion was that overall health risks outweighed the benefits, whereas finasteride was found to prevent or delay prostate cancer in a significant number of men. In these situations, it is unethical to deny patients the superior treatment or to continue to subject them to a risky treatment. Interim analyses should be planned as part of the design of the study, and the overall probability of a type I error (the α level) should be adjusted to compensate for the multiple comparisons.

Migration Bias: Migration bias occurs when patients who drop out of the study are also dropped from the analysis. The tendency to drop out of a study may be associated with the treatment (e.g., its side effects), and dropping these subjects from the analysis can make a treatment appear more or less effective than it really is. Migration bias can also occur when patients cross over from the treatment arm to which they were assigned to another treatment. For example, in **crossover studies** comparing surgical and medical treatment for coronary artery disease, patients assigned to the medical arm of the study sometimes require subsequent surgical treatment for their condition. In such situations, the appropriate method is to analyze the patient according to their original group; this is referred to as analysis based on the **intention-to-treat** principle.

Entry Time Bias: Entry time bias may occur when time-related variables, such as survival or time to remission, are counted differently for different arms of the study. For example, consider a study comparing survival for patients randomized to a surgical versus a medical treatment in a clinical trial. Patients randomized to the medical treatment who die at any time after randomization are counted as treatment failures; the same rule must be followed with patients randomized to surgery, even if they die prior to the time surgery is performed. Otherwise, a bias exists in favor of the surgical treatment.

THE RESULTS SECTION OF A RESEARCH REPORT

The results section of a medical report contains just that: results of (or findings from) the research directed at questions posed in the introduction. Typically, authors present tables or graphs (or both) of quantitative data and also report the findings in the text. Findings generally consist of both **descriptive statistics** (means, standard deviations, risk ratios, etc.) and results of **statistical tests** that were performed. Results of statistical tests are typically given as either **p values** or **confidence limits;** authors seldom give the value of the statistical test itself but, rather, give the p value associated with the statistical test. The two major aspects for readers evaluating the results section are the adequacy of information and the sufficiency of the evidence to withstand possible threats to the validity of the conclusions.

Assessing the Data Presented

Authors should provide adequate information about measurements made in the study. At a minimum, this information should include sample sizes and either means and standard deviations for numerical measures or proportions for nominal measures. For example, in describing the effect of sex, race, and age on estimating percentage body fat from body mass index, Kluess and colleagues (2016) specified the independent variables in the method section along with how they were coded for the regression analysis. They also gave the equation of the standard error of the estimate that they used to evaluate the fit of the regression models. In the results section, they included a table of means and standard deviations of the variables broken down by sex and race.

In addition to presenting adequate information on the observations in the study, good medical reports use tables and graphs appropriately. As we outlined in Chapter 3, tables and graphs should be clearly labeled so that they can be interpreted without referring to the text of the article. Furthermore, they should be properly constructed, using the methods illustrated in Chapter 3.

Assuring the Validity of the Data

A good results section should have the following three characteristics. First, authors of medical reports should provide information about the baseline measures of the group (or groups) involved in the study as did Kluess and colleagues (2016) in Table 1 of their article. Tables like this one typically give information on the gender, age, and any important risk factors for subjects in the different groups and are especially important in observational studies. Even with randomized studies, it is always a good idea to show that, in fact, the randomization worked and the groups were similar. Investigators often perform statistical tests to demonstrate the lack of significant difference on the baseline measures. If it turns out that the groups are not equivalent, it may be possible to make adjustments for any important differences by one of the covariance adjusting methods discussed in Chapter 10.

Second, readers should be alert for the problem of multiple comparisons in studies in which many statistical tests are performed. **Multiple comparisons** can occur because a group of subjects is measured at several points in time, for which repeated-measures analysis of variance should be used. They also occur when many study outcomes are of interest; investigators should use multivariate procedures in these situations. In addition, multiple comparisons result when investigators perform many subgroup comparisons, such as between men and women, among different age groups, or between groups defined by the absence or presence of a risk factor. Again, either multivariate methods or clearly stated a priori hypotheses are needed. If investigators find unexpected differences that were not part of the original hypotheses, these should be advanced as tentative conclusions only and should be the basis for further research.

Third, it is important to watch for inconsistencies between information presented in tables or graphs and information discussed in the text. Such inconsistencies may be the result of typographic errors, but sometimes they are signs that the authors have reanalyzed and rewritten the results or that the researchers were not very careful in their procedures. In any case, more than one inconsistency should alert us to watch for other problems in the study.

THE DISCUSSION & CONCLUSION SECTIONS OF A RESEARCH REPORT

The discussion and conclusion section(s) of a medical report may be one of the easier sections for clinicians to assess. The first and most important point to watch for is consistency among comments in the discussion, questions posed in the introduction, and data presented in the results. In addition, authors should address the consistency or lack of same between their findings and those of other published results. Careful readers will find that a surprisingly large number of published studies do not address the questions posed in their introduction. A good habit is to refer to the introduction and briefly review the purpose of the study just prior to reading the discussion and conclusion.

The second point to consider is whether the authors extrapolated beyond the data analyzed in the study. For example, are there recommendations concerning dosage levels not included in the study? Have conclusions been drawn that require a longer period of follow-up than that covered by the study? Have the results been generalized to groups of patients not represented by those included in the study?

Finally, note whether the investigators point out any shortcomings of the study, especially those that affect the conclusions drawn, and discuss research questions that have arisen from the study or that still remain unanswered. No one is in a better position to discuss these issues than the researchers who are intimately involved with the design and analysis of the study they have reported.

A CHECKLIST FOR READING THE LITERATURE

It is a rare article that meets all the criteria we have included in the following lists. Many articles do not even provide enough information to make a decision about some of the items in the checklist. Nevertheless, practitioners do not have time to read all the articles published, so they must make some choices about which ones are most important and best presented. Bordage and Dawson (2003) developed a set of guidelines for preparing a study and writing a research grant that contains many topics that are relevant to reading an article as well. Greenhalgh (1997b) presents a collection of articles on various topics published in the *British Medical Journal,* and the *Journal of the American Medical Association* has published a series of excellent articles under the general title of "Users' Guides to the Medical Literature."

The following checklist is fairly exhaustive, and some readers may not want to use it unless they are reviewing an article for their own purposes or for a report.

The items on the checklist are included in part as a reminder to the reader to look for these characteristics. Its primary purpose is to help clinicians decide whether a journal article is worth reading and, if so, what issues are important when deciding if the results are useful. The items in *italics* can often be found in a structured abstract. An asterisk (*) designates items that we believe are the most critical; these items are the ones readers should use when a less comprehensive checklist is desired.

Reading the Structured Abstract

*A. Is the topic of the study important and worth knowing about?

*B. What is the purpose of the study? Is the focus on a difference or a relationship? The purpose should be clearly stated; one should not have to guess.

C. What is the main outcome from the study? Does the outcome describe something measured on a numerical scale or something counted on a categorical scale? The outcome should be clearly stated.

D. Is the population of patients relevant to your practice—can you use these results in the care of your patients? The population in the study affects whether or not the results can be generalized.

*E. If statistically significant, do the results have clinical significance as well?

Reading the Introduction

If the article does not contain a structured abstract, the introduction section should include all of the preceding information plus the following information.

*A. What research has already been done on this topic and what outcomes were reported? The study should add new information.

Reading the Methods

*A. *Is the appropriate study design used (clinical trial, cohort, case–control, cross-sectional, meta-analysis)?*

B. Does the study cover an adequate period of time? Is the follow-up period long enough?

*C. *Are the criteria for inclusion and exclusion of subjects clear? How do these criteria limit the applicability of the conclusions? The criteria also affect whether or not the results can be generalized.*

*D. *Were subjects randomly sampled (or randomly assigned)? Was the sampling method adequately described?*

E. Are standard measures used? Is a reference to any unusual measurement/procedure given if needed? Are the measures reliable/replicable?

F. What other outcomes (or dependent variables) and risk factors (or independent variables) are in the study? Are they clearly defined?

*G. Are statistical methods outlined? Are they appropriate? (The first question is easy to check; the second may be more difficult to answer.)

*H. Is there a statement about power—the number of patients that are needed to find the desired outcome? A statement about sample size is essential in a negative study.

I. In a clinical trial:

  1. How are subjects recruited?

  *2. *Are subjects randomly assigned to the study groups? If not:*

   a. How are patients selected for the study to avoid selection biases?

   b. If historical controls are used, are methods and criteria the same for the experimental group; are cases and controls compared on prognostic factors?

  *3. *Is there a control group? If so, is it a good one?*

  4. Are appropriate therapies included?

  5. *Is the study blind? Double-blind? If not, should it be?*

  6. How is compliance ensured/evaluated?

  *7. If some cases are censored, is a survival method such as Kaplan–Meier or the Cox model used?

J. In a cohort study:

  *1. How are subjects recruited?

  2. *Are subjects randomly selected from an eligible pool?*

  *3. *How rigorously are subjects followed? How many dropouts does the study have and who are they?*

  *4. If some cases are censored, is a survival method such as Kaplan–Meier curves used?

K. In a case–control study:

  *1. *Are subjects randomly selected from an eligible pool?*

  2. *Is the control group a good one (bias-free)?*

  3. Are records reviewed independently by more than one person (thereby increasing the reliability of data)?

L. In a cross-sectional (survey, epidemiologic) study:

  1. Are the questions unbiased?

  *2. *Are subjects randomly selected from an eligible pool?*

  *3. *What is the response rate?*

M. In a meta-analysis:

  *1. *How is the literature search conducted?*

  2. Are the criteria for inclusion and exclusion of studies clearly stated?

  *3. Is an effort made to reduce publication bias (because negative studies are less likely to be published)?

  *4. Is there information on how many studies are needed to change the conclusion?

Reading the Results

*A. *Do the reported findings answer the research questions?*

*B. Are actual values reported—means, standard deviations, proportions—so that the magnitude of differences can be judged by the reader?

C. Are many *p* values reported, thus increasing the chance that some findings are bogus?

*D. Are groups similar on baseline measures? If not, how did investigators deal with these differences (confounding factors)?

E. Are the graphs and tables, and their legends, easy to read and understand?

*F. If the topic is a diagnostic procedure, is information on both sensitivity and specificity (false-positive rate) given? If predictive values are given, is the dependence on prevalence emphasized?

Reading the Conclusion and Discussion

*A. Are the research questions adequately discussed?

*B. Are the conclusions justified? Do the authors extrapolate more than they should, for example, beyond the length of time subjects were studied or to populations not included in the study?

C. Are the conclusions of the study discussed in the context of other relevant research?

D. Are shortcomings and limitations of the research addressed?

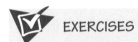

EXERCISES

For Questions 1–56, choose the single best answer.

1. Table 2 from Hodgson and Cutler (1997) is reproduced in Table 13–3. Which variable is most closely associated with anticipatory dementia?

   a. CES-D

   b. Psych symptoms

   c. Life satisfaction

   d. Health status

Questions 2–3

2. Henderson and colleagues (1997) studied a community sample of elderly subjects for a period of 3–4 years. One of their goals was to predict the level of depression, as measured by a depression score, at the end of the study period. Table 13–4 gives the list of measures used in their analysis. What type of statistical method was used to produce this information?

Table 13–3. Association between anticipatory dementia and well-being by sample group.

	Anticipatory Dementia	
	Adult Children (*n* = 25)	Control (*n* = 25)
CES-D		
r	0.352	0.266
p	0.085	0.200
Psych symptoms		
r	0.341	0.433
p	0.095	0.031
Life satisfaction		
r	−0.419	−0.283
p	0.037	0.171
Health status		
r	−0.173	−0.446
p	0.409	0.026

CES-D, Center for Epidemiological Studies Depression Scale
Reproduced with permission from Hodgson LG, Cutler SJ: Anticipatory dementia and well-being, *Am J Alzheimer's Dis* 1997 March 1; 12(2):62–66.

   a. Multiple regression

   b. Logistic regression

   c. Cox proportional hazard model

   d. Paired t tests

   e. Wilcoxon signed rank test

3. Which set of variables increased the prediction of depression score by the largest amount?

   a. Sociodemographic variables

   b. Age

   c. Psychological health variables

   d. Physical health variables

   e. ADL at wave 2

4. In study of mortality from selected diseases in England and Wales by Barker (1989), the author stated that the trend in deaths from thyrotoxicosis rose to a peak in the 1930s and declined thereafter. A graph from this investigation is given in Figure 13–2. Based on this figure, which of the following statements is true?

   a. Iodine deficiency during childhood was not a problem among people born in Britain in the 1800s.

   b. Age-specific rates of thyrotoxicosis rose progressively beginning in 1836 and reached a peak in 1880.

Table 13–4. Predictors of depression score at wave 2.

Predictor Variable[a]	Beta[b]	p	R^2	R^2 change
Depression score, wave 1	0.231	0.000	0.182	0.182
Sociodemographic variables				
Age	–0.024	0.528	0.187	0.005
Sex	0.034	0.370		
Psychologic health variables				
Neuroticism, wave 1	0.077	0.056	0.237	0.050
Past history of depression or nervous breakdown, wave 2	0.136	0.000		
Physical health variables				
ADL, wave 1	–0.103	0.033	0.411	0.174
ADL, wave 2	0.283	0.012		
ADL squared, wave 2	–0.150	0.076		
Number current symptoms, wave 2	0.117	0.009		
Number medical conditions, wave 2	0.226	0.000		
Blood pressure: systolic, wave 2	–0.092	0.010		
Global health rating change between waves	0.079	0.028		
Sensory impairment change between waves	–0.064	0.073		
Social support/inactivity				
Social support—friends, wave 2	–0.095	0.015	0.442	0.031
Social support—social visits, wave 2	–0.087	0.032		
Activity level, wave 2	0.095	0.025		
Services (community residents only)				
Total services used, wave 2	0.135[c]	0.001[c]	0.438[c]	0.015[c]

[a]Only the variables shown were included in the final model.
[b]Standardized beta value, controlling for all other variables in the regression, except service use. Based on community and institutional residents.
[c]Regression limited to community sample only; coefficients for other variables vary only very slightly from those obtained with regression on the full sample.
Reproduced with permission from Henderson AS, Korten AE, Jacomb PA, et al: The course of depression in the elderly: a longitudinal community-based study in Australia, *Psychol Med.* 1997 Jan;27(1):119–129.

    c. People who are iodine-deficient in youth are more able to adapt to increased iodine intake in later life.

    d. People exposed to increased levels of iodine during their adult years are more likely to develop thyrotoxicosis.

Questions 5–6

In a sample of 49 individuals, the mean total leukocyte count is found to be 7,600 cells/mm3, with a standard deviation of 1,400 cells/mm3.

    5. *If it is reasonable to assume that total leukocyte counts follow a normal distribution, then approximately 50% of the individuals will have a value*

        a. Between 6,200 and 9,000

        b. Between 7,400 and 7,800

        c. Below 6,200 or above 9,000

        d. Below 7,600

        e. Above 9,000

    6. *Again assuming a normal distribution of total leukocyte counts, a randomly selected individual has a total leukocyte count lower than 4,800 cells/mm³*

        a. 1% of the time

        b. 2.5% of the time

        c. 5% of the time

        d. 10% of the time

        e. 16.5% of the time

    7. *If the correlation between two measures of functional status is 0.80, we can conclude that*

        a. The value of one measure increases by 0.80 when the other measure increases by 1.

        b. 64% of the observations fall on the regression line.

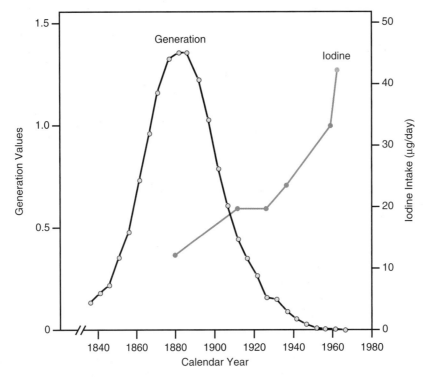

Figure 13–2. Relative mortality from thyrotoxicosis in successive generations of women in England and Wales according to year of birth, together with estimated per capita daily iodine intake from milk, meat, and fish. (Reproduced with permission from Barker DJ: Rise and fall of Western diseases, *Nature.* 1989 Mar 30;338(6214):371–372.)

c. 80% of the observations fall on the regression line.

d. 80% of the variation in one measure is accounted for by the other.

e. 64% of the variation in one measure is accounted for by the other.

Questions 8–10

An evaluation of an antibiotic in the treatment of possible occult bacteremia was undertaken. Five hundred children with fever but no focal infection were randomly assigned to the antibiotic or to a placebo. A blood sample for culture was obtained prior to beginning therapy, and all patients were reevaluated after 48 hours.

8. The design used in this study is best described as a

  a. Randomized clinical trial

  b. Placebo-controlled trial

  c. Controlled clinical trial

  d. Cohort study

  e. Crossover study

9. The authors reported the proportion of children with major infectious morbidity among those with bacteremia was 13% in the placebo group and 10% in the antibiotic group. The 95% confidence interval for the difference in proportions was −2.6% to +8.6%. Thus, the most important conclusion is that

  a. The difference in major infectious morbidity between placebo and antibiotic is statistically significant.

  b. The proportion of children with major infectious morbidity is the same with placebo and antibiotic.

  c. No statistically significant difference exists in the proportions that received placebo and antibiotic.

  d. The study has low power to detect a difference owing to the small sample size, and no conclusions should be drawn until a larger study is done.

  e. Using a chi-square test to determine significance is preferable to determining a confidence interval for the difference.

10. What is the approximate number needed to treat to prevent one patient from developing occult bacteremia?

   a. 15

   b. 6.7 or 7

   c. 65

   d. 3

   e. 33.3 or 33

11. The statistical method most appropriate to analyze the means of the four groups is

   a. Analysis of variance

   b. Correlation

   c. Independent groups t test

   d. Simple linear regression

   e. Trend analysis

12. Table 1 from the study of glucose tolerance and insulin sensitivity in normal and overweight hyperthyroid women is reproduced below in Table 13–5 (Gonzalo et al, 1996). Which statistical procedure is best if the authors wanted to compare the baseline glucose (mmol/L) in the women to see if weight or thyroid level have an effect?

   a. Correlation

   b. Independent-groups t test

   c. Paired t test

   d. One-way ANOVA

   e. Two-way ANOVA

13. If the relationship between two measures is linear and the coefficient of determination has a value near 1, a scatterplot of the observations

   a. Is a horizontal straight line

   b. Is a vertical straight line

   c. Is a straight line that is neither horizontal nor vertical

   d. Is a random scatter of points about the regression line

   e. Has a positive slope

Questions 14–17

A study was undertaken to evaluate the use of computed tomography (CT) in the diagnosis of lumbar disk herniation. Eighty patients with lumbar disk herniation confirmed by surgery were evaluated with CT, as were 50 patients without herniation. The CT results were positive in 56 of the patients with herniation and in 10 of the patients without herniation.

14. The sensitivity of CT for lumbar disk herniation in this study is

   a. 10/50, or 20%

   b. 24/80, or 30%

   c. 56/80, or 70%

   d. 40/50, or 80%

   e. 56/66, or 85%

15. The false-positive rate in this study is

   a. 10/50, or 20%

   b. 24/80, or 30%

   c. 56/80, or 70%

   d. 40/50, or 80%

   e. 56/66, or 85%

16. Computed tomography is used in a patient who has a 50–50 chance of having a herniated lumbar disk, according to the patient's history and physical examination. What are the chances of herniation if the CT is positive?

   a. 35/100, or 35%

   b. 50/100, or 50%

   c. 35/50, or 70%

Table 13–5. Clinical and metabolic details.[a,b]

Subjects	Age (years)	BMI (kg/m^2)	Basal Glucose (mmol/L)	Basal Insulin (pmol/L)	KG (%/min)
NW-HT (n = 8)	39.4 ± 5.0 (20–62)	23.5 ± 0.6 (21.4 –25)	4.99 ± 0.26	84.8 ± 13.6	2.45 ± 0.41
OW-HT (n = 6)	42.7 ± 5.7 (23–60)	28.0 ± 0.7 (26–31.4)	5.05 ± 0.11	134 ± 23.6	1.84 ± 0.20
Total-HT (n = 14)	40.8 ± 3.7 (20–62)	25.4 ± 0.8 (21.4 –31.4)	5.02 ± 0.15	105.9 ± 13.9	2.19 ± 0.26
NW-C (n = 11)	42.8 ± 5.0 (22–66)	21.3 ± 0.9 (18–24)	4.81 ± 0.11	79.6 ± 7.0	2.35 ± 0.13
OW-C (n = 8)	45.0 ± 4.7 (26–62)	29.0 ± 0.8 (25.5–31.6)	5.0 ± 0.22	112.5 ± 20.5	2.65 ± 0.35
Total-C (n = 19)	43.7 ± 3.4 (22–66)	24.5 ± 1.0 (18–31.6)	4.89 ± 0.11	15.5 ± 1.6	2.47 ± 0.16

BMI, body mass index; NW, normal weight; OW, overweight; HT, hyperthyroid patients; C, control subjects.
[a]Numbers in parentheses are range values.
[b]Data presented as mean plus or minus the standard error of the mean.
Reproduced with permission from Gonzalo MA, Grant C, Moreno I, et al: Glucose tolerance, insulin secretion, insulin sensitivity and glucose effectiveness in normal and overweight hyperthyroid women, *Clin Endocrinol (Oxf)*. 1996 Dec;45(6):689–697.

d. 40/55, or 73%

e. 35/45, or 78%

17. The likelihood ratio is

 a. 0.28

 b. 0.875

 c. 1.0

 d. 3.5

 e. 7.0

18. In a placebo-controlled trial of the use of oral aspirin–dipyridamole to prevent arterial restenosis after coronary angioplasty, 38% of patients receiving the drug had restenosis, and 39% of patients receiving placebo had restenosis. In reporting this finding, the authors stated that $p > 0.05$, which means that

 a. Chances are greater than 1 in 20 that a difference would again be found if the study were repeated.

 b. The probability is less than 1 in 20 that a difference this large could occur by chance alone.

 c. The probability is greater than 1 in 20 that a difference this large could occur by chance alone.

 d. Treated patients were 5% less likely to have restenosis.

 e. The chance is 95% that the study is correct.

19. A study of the relationship between the concentration of lead in the blood and hemoglobin resulted in the following prediction equation: $Y = 15 - 0.1(X)$, where Y is the predicted hemoglobin and X is the concentration of lead in the blood. From the equation, the predicted hemoglobin for a person with blood lead concentration of 20 mg/dL is

 a. 13

 b. 14.8

 c. 14.9

 d. 15

 e. 20

Questions 20–21

20. D'Angio and colleagues (1995) studied a group of extremely premature infants to learn whether they have immunologic responses to tetanus toxoid and polio vaccines that are similar to the response of full-term infants. Figure 1 from their study contains the plots of the antitetanus titers before and after the vaccine was given (reproduced in Figure 13–3). The authors calculated the geometric means. Which statistical test is best to learn if the titer level increases in

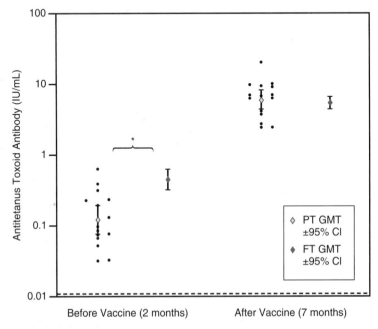

Figure 13–3. Antitetanus toxoid antibody levels. (PT, preterm; FT, full term; GMT, geometric mean titer; *, $p < 0.001$.) (Reproduced with permission from D'Angio CT, Maniscalco WM, Pichichero ME, et al: Immunologic response of extremely premature infants to tetanus, *Haemophilus influenzae*, and polio immunizations, *Pediatrics*. 1995 Jul;96(1 Pt 1):18–22.)

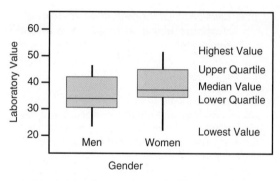

Figure 13–4. Gender-specific distributions of values on a laboratory test.

the preterm group after they were given the vaccine?

a. One-group t test

b. Paired t test

c. Wilcoxon signed rank test

d. Two independent-groups t test

e. Wilcoxon rank sum test

21. Based on Figure 13–3, which is the appropriate conclusion?

a. No difference exists between preterm and full-term infants before and after the vaccine.

b. No difference exists between preterm and full-term infants before the vaccine, but a difference does occur after the vaccine.

c. A difference exists between preterm and full-term infants before and after the vaccine.

d. A difference exists between preterm and full-term infants before the vaccine but not after.

Questions 22–23

Figure 13–4 summarizes the gender-specific distribution of values on a laboratory test.

22. From Figure 13–4, we can conclude that

a. Values on the laboratory test are lower in men than in women.

b. The distribution of laboratory values in women is bimodal.

c. Laboratory values were reported more often for women than for men in this study.

d. Half of the men have laboratory values between 30 and 43.

e. The standard deviation of laboratory values is equal in men and women.

23. The most appropriate statistical test to compare the distribution of laboratory values in men with that in women is

a. Chi-square test

b. Paired t test

c. Independent-groups t test

d. Correlation

e. Regression

24. A study was undertaken to evaluate any increased risk of breast cancer among women who use birth control pills. The relative risk was calculated. A type I error in this study consists of concluding

a. A significant increase in the relative risk when the relative risk is actually 1

b. A significant increase in the relative risk when the relative risk is actually greater than 1

c. A significant increase in the relative risk when the relative risk is actually less than 1

d. No significant increase in the relative risk when the relative risk is actually 1

e. No significant increase in the relative risk when the relative risk is actually greater than 1

Questions 25–26

25. A graph of the lowest oxyhemoglobin percentage in the patients studied overnight in the study by Good and colleagues (1996) is given in Figure 1 from their article (see Figure 13–5). What is the best way to describe the distribution of these values?

a. Normal distribution

b. Chi-square distribution

c. Binomial distribution

d. Negatively skewed distribution

e. Positively skewed distribution

26. If the investigators wanted to compare oxyhemoglobin levels in patients who died within 12 months with the levels of oxyhemoglobin percentage in patients who survived, what method should they use?

a. t test for two independent groups

b. Wilcoxon rank sum test

c. Analysis of variance

d. Chi-square test

e. Kaplan–Meier curves

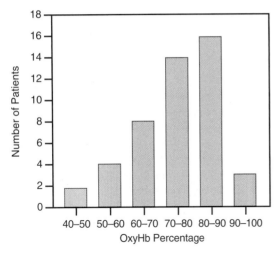

Figure 13–5. Distribution of lowest oxyhemoglobin (OxyHb) values for each patient during overnight oximetry. (Reproduced with permission from Good DC, Henkle JQ, Gelber D, et al: Sleep-disordered breathing and poor functional outcome after stroke, *Stroke.* 1996 Feb;27(2):252–259.)

27. The scale used in measuring cholesterol is
    a. Nominal
    b. Ordinal
    c. Interval
    d. Discrete
    e. Qualitative

28. The scale used in measuring presence or absence of a risk factor is
    a. Binary
    b. Ordinal
    c. Interval
    d. Continuous
    e. Quantitative

29. Which of the following sources is most likely to provide an accurate estimate of the prevalence of multiple sclerosis (MS) in a community?
    a. A survey of practicing physicians asking how many MS patients they are currently treating
    b. Information from hospital discharge summaries
    c. Data from autopsy reports
    d. A telephone survey of a sample of randomly selected homes in the community asking how many people living in the home have the disease

    e. Examination of the medical records of a representative sample of people living in the community

Questions 30–31

In an epidemiologic study of carbon-black workers, 500 workers with respiratory disease and 200 workers without respiratory disease were selected for study. The investigators obtained a history of exposure to carbon-black dust in both groups of workers. Among workers with respiratory disease, 250 gave a history of exposure to carbon-black dust; among the 200 workers without respiratory disease, 50 gave a history of exposure.

30. The odds ratio is
    a. 1.0
    b. 1.5
    c. 2.0
    d. 3.0
    e. Cannot be determined from the preceding information

31. This study is best described as a
    a. Case–control study
    b. Cohort study
    c. Cross-sectional study
    d. Controlled experiment
    e. Randomized clinical trial

32. A physician wishes to study whether a particular risk factor is associated with some disease. If, in reality, the presence of the risk factor leads to a relative risk of disease of 4.0, the physician wants to have a 95% chance of detecting an effect this large in the planned study. This statement is an illustration of specifying
    a. A null hypothesis
    b. A type I, or alpha, error
    c. A type II, or beta, error
    d. Statistical power
    e. An odds ratio

33. The most likely explanation for a lower crude annual mortality rate in a developing country than in a developed country is that the developing country has
    a. An incomplete record of deaths
    b. A younger age distribution
    c. An inaccurate census of the population
    d. A less stressful lifestyle
    e. Lower exposure to environmental hazards

Questions 34–35

34. The distribution of variation in heart rate to deep breathing and the Valsalva ratio from the study by Gelber and colleagues (1997) is given in Figure 1 in their article and is reproduced below in Figure 13–6. What is the best way to describe the distribution of these values?
    a. Normal distribution
    b. Chi-square distribution
    c. Binomial distribution
    d. Negatively skewed distribution
    e. Positively skewed distribution

35. What is the best method to find the normal range of values for the Valsalva ratio?
    a. The values determined by the mean $\pm$ 2 standard deviations
    b. The values determined by the mean $\pm$ 2 standard errors
    c. The values determined by the upper and lower 5% of the distribution
    d. The values determined by the upper and lower 2.5% of the distribution
    e. The highest and lowest values defined by the whiskers on a box plot

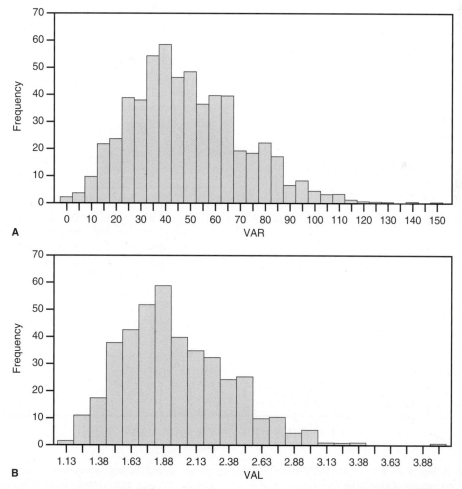

Figure 13–6. **A:** Distribution of normative values for heart rate variation to deep breathing (VAR) and **B:** Valsalva ratio (VAL) for the entire study population. (Reproduced with permission from Gelber DA, Pfeifer M, Dawson B, et al: Cardiovascular autonomic nervous system tests: determination of normative values and effect of confounding variables, *J Auton Nerv Syst.* 1997 Jan 12;62(1-2):40–44.)

36. A study of the exercise tolerance test for detecting coronary heart disease had the characteristics shown in Table 13–6. The authors concluded the exercise stress test has positive predictive value in excess of 75%. The error in this conclusion is that
   a. Not enough patients are included in the study for precise estimates.
   b. The sample sizes should be equal in these kinds of studies.
   c. The positive predictive value is really 80%.
   d. The prevalence of coronary heart disease (CHD) is assumed to be 33%.
   e. No gold standard exists for D.

Table 13–6. Results of test.

	CHD Present	CHD Absent
Positive test	80	50
Negative test	20	150

CHD, coronary heart disease.

Questions 37–39

37. Hébert and colleagues (1997) studied functional decline in a very elderly population of community-dwelling subjects. They used the Functional Autonomy Measurement System (SMAF) questionnaire to measure several indices of functioning. Figure 2 from their article displays box plots of scores for men and women at baseline and is reproduced in Figure 13–7. Based on the plots, men and women had the most similar scores on which measure?
   a. ADL (adult daily living)
   b. Mobility
   c. Communication
   d. Mental
   e. IADL (instrumental activities of daily living)
   f. Total score
   g. Impossible to tell

38. Among men, which measure has the most symmetric distribution?
   a. ADL (adult daily living)
   b. Mobility

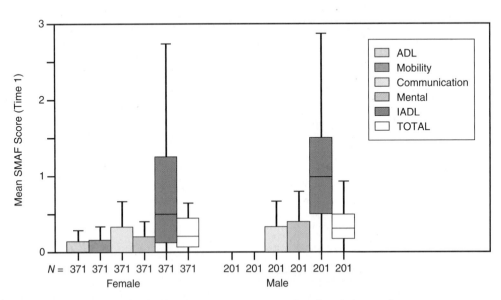

Figure 13–7. Box plots of the mean SMAF score and subscores at baseline (T1) according to sex, among a representative sample of elderly people living at home in Sherbrooke, Canada, 1991–1993. (SMAF, Functional Autonomy Measurement System; ADL, activities of daily living; IADL, instrumental activities of daily living.)
(Reproduced with permission from Hébert R, Brayne C, Spiegelhalter D: Incidence of functional decline and improvement in a community-dwelling very elderly population, *Am J Epidemiol.* 1997 May 15;145(10):935–944.)

c. Communication

d. Mental

e. IADL (instrumental activities of daily living)

f. Total score

g. Impossible to tell

39. What is the median mental score for women?

a. 0

b. 0.15

c. 0.3

d. 0.7

e. Impossible to tell

Questions 40–41

Several studies have shown that men with low blood cholesterol levels as well as those with high levels have an increased risk of early death. A study by Dr Carlos Iribarren and colleagues (1995) at the University of Southern California on a cohort of 8,000 Japanese-American men followed for 23 years. The purpose was to study further the link between low blood cholesterol levels and higher death rate. The men were divided into four groups: healthy men, men with chronic disorders of the stomach or liver, heavy smokers, and heavy drinkers. Within each group, subjects were stratified according to their cholesterol level. Among men with cholesterol levels below 189 mg/dL, death rates were higher in the chronic illness, heavy smoker, and heavy drinker groups but not in the group of healthy men.

40. This study highlights a potential threat that may have occurred in previous studies that suggested that low cholesterol is linked to higher death rates. The most likely threat in the previous studies is

a. Selection bias

b. Length of follow-up

c. A confounding variable

d. Inappropriate sample size

41. Using the guidelines in Table 10–2, select the most appropriate statistical method to analyze the data collected in this study.

a. Mantel–Haenszel chi-square

b. ANOVA

c. Multiple regression

d. Log-linear methods

Questions 42–43

42. Figure 2 in Dennison and colleagues (1997) shows the relationship between the age of children and daily consumption of fruit juice (see Figure 13–8). What is the best method to learn

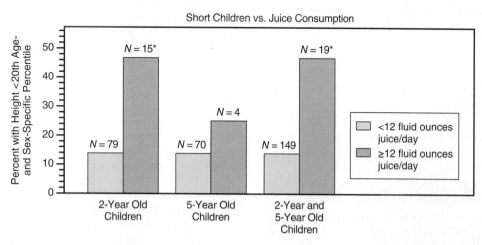

Figure 13–8. The prevalence of children with decreased stature (height less than 20th age- and sex-specific percentile) between children drinking less than 12 fl oz/day of fruit juice and children drinking more than 12 fl oz/day of fruit juice. (* Indicates Fisher's exact test $p < 0.01$.) (Reproduced with permission from Dennison BA, Rockwell HL, Baker SL: Excess fruit juice consumption by preschool-aged children is associated with short stature and obesity, *Pediatrics*. 1997 Jan;99(1):15–22.)

if a difference exists between 2-year-old and 5-year-old children?

a. Chi-square test

b. Fisher's exact test

c. Fisher's z distribution

d. Paired t test

e. Pearson correlation

43. What is the best way to describe the magnitude of the relationship between the age of children and daily consumption of fruit juice?

a. Kappa

b. Odds ratio

c. Pearson correlation

d. Spearman correlation

e. r^2

44. Birth weights of a population of infants at 40 weeks gestational age are approximately normally distributed, with a mean of 3,000 g. Roughly 68% of such infants weigh between 2,500 and 3,500 g at birth. If a sample of 100 infants were studied, the standard error would be

a. 50

b. 100

c. 250

d. 500

e. None of the above

45. A significant positive correlation has been observed between alcohol consumption and the level of systolic blood pressure in men. From this correlation, we may conclude that

a. No association exists between alcohol consumption and systolic pressure.

b. Men who consume less alcohol are at lower risk for increased systolic pressure.

c. Men who consume less alcohol are at higher risk for increased systolic pressure.

d. High alcohol consumption can cause increased systolic pressure.

e. Low alcohol consumption can cause increased systolic pressure.

46. In a randomized trial of patients who received a cadaver renal transplant, 100 were treated with cyclosporin and 50 were treated with conventional immunosuppression therapy. The difference in treatments was not statistically significant at the 5% level. Therefore

a. This study has proven that cyclosporin is not effective.

b. Cyclosporin could be significant at the 1% level.

c. Cyclosporin could be significant at the 10% level.

d. The groups have been shown to be the same.

e. The treatments should not be compared because of the differences in the sample sizes.

47. The statistical method used to develop guidelines for diagnostic-related groups (DRGs) was

a. Survival analysis

b. t tests for independent groups

c. Multiple regression

d. Analysis of covariance

e. Correlation

48. Suppose the confidence limits for the mean of a variable are 8.55 and 8.65. These limits are

a. Less precise but have a higher confidence than 8.20 and 9.00

b. More precise but have a lower confidence than 8.20 and 9.00

c. Less precise but have a lower confidence than 8.20 and 9.00

d. More precise but have a higher confidence than 8.20 and 9.00

e. Indeterminate because the level of confidence is not specified

49. A senior medical student wants to plan her elective schedule. The probability of getting an elective in endocrinology is 0.8, and the probability of getting an elective in sports medicine is 0.5. The probability of getting both electives in the same semester is 0.4. What is the probability of getting into endocrinology or sports medicine or both?

a. 0.4

b. 0.5

c. 0.8

d. 0.9

e. 1.7

50. A manager of a multispecialty clinic wants to determine the proportion of patients who are referred by their primary care physician to another physician within the group versus a physician outside the group. Every 100th patient chart is selected and reviewed for a letter from a physician other than the primary care physician. This procedure is best described as

a. Random sampling

b. Stratified sampling

c. Quota sampling

d. Representative sampling

e. Systematic sampling

51. The probability is 0.6 that a medical student will receive his first choice of residency programs. Four senior medical students want to know the probability that they all will obtain their first choice. The solution to this problem is best found by using

 a. The binomial distribution

 b. The normal distribution

 c. The chi-square distribution

 d. The z test

 e. Correlation

52. The graph in Figure 13–9 gives the 5-year survival rates for patients with cancer at various sites. From this figure, we can conclude

 a. That breast and uterine corpus cancer are increasing at higher rates than other cancers

 b. That lung cancer is the slowest growing cancer

 c. That few patients are diagnosed with distant metastases

 d. That survival rates for patients with regional involvement are similar, regardless of the primary site of disease

 e. None of the above

53. A study was undertaken to compare treatment options in black and white patients who are diagnosed as having breast cancer. The 95% confidence interval for the odds ratio for blacks being more likely to be untreated than whites was 1.1 to 2.5. The statement that most accurately describes the meaning of these limits is that

 a. Ninety-five percent of the odds ratios fall within these limits.

 b. Black women are up to 2.5 times more likely than whites to be untreated.

 c. Ninety-five percent of the time blacks are more likely than whites to be untreated.

 d. Blacks are 95 times more likely than whites to receive no treatment for breast cancer.

 e. No difference exists in the treatment of black and white women.

54. What statistical technique can the investigators use to control for differences in any of the

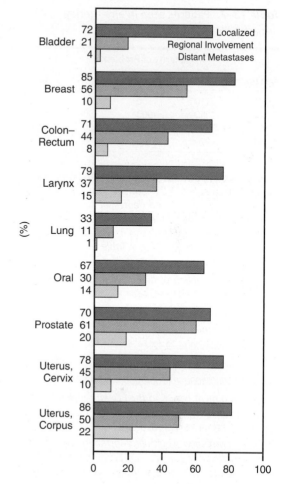

Figure 13–9. Five-year survival rates for patients with cancer. (Data from Rubin P: *Clinical oncology for medical students and physicians: a multidisciplinary approach,* 6th ed. Atlanta, GA: American Cancer Society; 1983.)

sociodemographic characteristics in the two groups that might confound the statistical analysis of mortality?

 a. Paired t test

 b. Analysis of variance

 c. Chi-square test

 d. Regression

 e. Logistic regression

Questions 55–56

Physicians wish to determine whether the emergency department (ED) at the local hospital is being

Table 13–7. Patients seen in emergency department.

| Age (years) | Severity of Problem | | | Total |
	Low	Medium	High	
<5	1100	300	200	1600
5–14	500	900	300	1700
>14	600	500	600	1700
Total	2200	1700	1100	5000

overused by patients with minor health problems. A random sample of 5,000 patients was selected and categorized by age and degree of severity of the problem that brought them to the ED; severity was measured on a scale of 1 to 3, with 3 being most severe; the results are given in Table 13–7.

55. The joint probability that a 3-year-old patient with a problem of high severity is selected for review is

   a. 200/5000 = 0.04
   b. 200/1600 = 0.125
   c. 1600/5000 = 0.32
   d. 1100/5000 = 0.22
   e. 1600/5000 + 1100/5000 = 0.54

56. If a patient comes to the ED with a problem of low severity, how likely is it that the patient is older than 14 years of age?

   a. 1700/5000 2200/5000 = 0.15
   b. 600/2200 = 0.27
   c. 1700/5000 = 0.34
   d. 600/1700 = 0.35
   e. 2200/5000 = 0.44

Questions 57–61

These questions constitute a set of extended matching items. For each of the situations outlined here, select the most appropriate statistical method to use in analyzing the data from the choices a–i that follow. Each choice may be used more than once.

   a. *Independent-groups t test*
   b. *Chi-square test*
   c. *Wilcoxon rank sum test*
   d. *Pearson correlation*
   e. *Analysis of variance*
   f. *Mantel–Haenszel chi-square*
   g. *Multiple regression*
   h. *Paired t test*
   i. *Odds ratio*

57. *Investigating average body weight before and after a supervised exercise program*

58. *Investigating gender of the head of household in families of patients whose medical costs are covered by insurance, Medicaid, or self*

59. *Investigating a possible association between exposure to an environmental pollutant and miscarriage*

60. *Investigating blood cholesterol levels in patients who follow a diet either low or moderate in fat and who take either a drug to lower cholesterol or a placebo*

61. *Investigating physical functioning in patients with diabetes on the basis of demographic characteristics and level of diabetic control*

Appendix A: Tables

Table A–1. Random numbers.

927415	956121	168117	169280	326569	266541
926937	515107	014658	159944	821115	317592
867169	388342	832261	993050	639410	698969
867169	542747	032683	131188	926198	371071
512500	843384	085361	398488	774767	383837
062454	423050	670884	840940	845839	979662
806702	881309	772977	367506	729850	457758
837815	163631	622143	938278	231305	219737
926839	453853	767825	284716	916182	467113
854813	731620	978100	589512	147694	389180
851595	452454	262448	688990	461777	647487
449353	556695	806050	123754	722070	935916
169116	586865	756231	469281	258737	989450
139470	358095	528858	660128	342072	681203
433775	761861	107191	515960	759056	150336
221922	232624	398839	495004	881970	792001
740207	078048	854928	875559	246288	000144
525873	755998	866034	444933	785944	018016
734185	499711	254256	616625	243045	251938
773112	463857	781983	078184	380752	492215
638951	982155	747821	773030	594005	526828
868888	769341	477611	628714	250645	853454
611034	167642	701316	589251	330456	681722
379290	955292	664549	656401	320855	215201
411257	411484	068629	050150	106933	900095
407167	435509	578642	268724	366564	511815
895893	438644	330273	590506	820439	976891
986683	830515	284065	813310	554920	111395
335421	814351	508062	663801	365001	924418
927660	793888	507773	975109	625175	552278
957559	236000	471608	888683	146821	034687
694904	499959	950969	085327	352611	335924
863016	494926	871064	665892	076333	990558
876958	865769	882966	236535	541645	819783
619813	221175	370697	566925	705564	472934

(continued)

Table A–1. Random numbers. (*continued*)

476626	646911	337167	865652	195448	116729
578292	863854	145858	206557	430943	591126
286553	981699	232269	819656	867825	890737
819064	712344	033613	457019	478176	342104
383035	043025	201591	127424	771948	762990
879392	378486	198814	928028	493486	373709
924020	273258	851781	003514	685749	713570
502523	157212	472643	439301	718562	196269
815316	651530	080430	912635	820240	533626
914984	444954	053723	079387	530020	703312
312248	619263	715357	923412	252522	913950
030964	407872	419563	426527	565215	243717
870561	984049	445361	315827	651925	464440
820157	006091	670091	478357	490641	082559
519649	761345	761354	794613	330132	319843

Table A–2. Area under the standard normal curve.

z	Area in One Tail ($<-z$ or $>+z$)	Area in Two Tails ($<-z$ and $>+z$)	Area between $-z$ and $+z$
3.50	0.000	0.000	1.000
3.45	0.000	0.001	0.999
3.40	0.000	0.001	0.999
3.35	0.000	0.001	0.999
3.30	0.000	0.001	0.999
3.25	0.001	0.001	0.999
3.20	0.001	0.001	0.999
3.15	0.001	0.002	0.998
3.10	0.001	0.002	0.998
3.05	0.001	0.002	0.998
3.00	0.001	0.003	0.997
2.95	0.002	0.003	0.997
2.90	0.002	0.004	0.996
2.85	0.002	0.004	0.996
2.80	0.003	0.005	0.995
2.75	0.003	0.006	0.994
2.70	0.003	0.007	0.993
2.65	0.004	0.008	0.992
2.60	0.005	0.009	0.991
2.55	0.005	0.011	0.989
2.50	0.006	0.012	0.988
2.45	0.007	0.014	0.986
2.40	0.008	0.016	0.984
2.35	0.009	0.019	0.981
2.30	0.011	0.021	0.979
2.25	0.012	0.024	0.976
2.20	0.014	0.028	0.972

(*continued*)

Table A–2. Area under the standard normal curve. (*continued*)

z	Area in One Tail ($<-z$ or $>+z$)	Area in Two Tails ($<-z$ and $>+z$)	Area between $-z$ and $+z$
2.15	0.016	0.032	0.968
2.10	0.018	0.036	0.964
2.05	0.020	0.040	0.960
2.00	0.023	0.046	0.954
1.95	0.026	0.051	0.949
1.90	0.029	0.057	0.943
1.85	0.032	0.064	0.936
1.80	0.036	0.072	0.928
1.75	0.040	0.080	0.920
1.70	0.045	0.089	0.911
1.65	0.049	0.099	0.901
1.60	0.055	0.110	0.890
1.55	0.061	0.121	0.879
1.50	0.067	0.134	0.866
1.45	0.074	0.147	0.853
1.40	0.081	0.162	0.838
1.35	0.089	0.177	0.823
1.30	0.097	0.194	0.806
1.25	0.106	0.211	0.789
1.20	0.115	0.230	0.770
1.15	0.125	0.250	0.750
1.10	0.136	0.271	0.729
1.05	0.147	0.294	0.706
1.00	0.159	0.317	0.683
0.95	0.171	0.342	0.658
0.90	0.184	0.368	0.632
0.85	0.198	0.395	0.605
0.80	0.212	0.424	0.576
0.75	0.227	0.453	0.547
0.70	0.242	0.484	0.516
0.65	0.258	0.516	0.484
0.60	0.274	0.549	0.451
0.55	0.291	0.582	0.418
0.50	0.309	0.617	0.383
0.45	0.326	0.653	0.347
0.40	0.345	0.689	0.311
0.35	0.363	0.726	0.274
0.30	0.382	0.764	0.236
0.25	0.401	0.803	0.197
0.20	0.421	0.841	0.159
0.15	0.440	0.881	0.119
0.10	0.460	0.920	0.080
0.05	0.480	0.960	0.040
0.00	0.500	1.000	0.000

Table A–3. Critical values for the t distribution.

Degrees of Freedom	Area in 1 Tail				
	0.05	0.025	0.01	0.005	0.0005
	Area in 2 Tails				
	0.1	0.05	0.02	0.01	0.001
1	6.314	12.706	31.821	63.657	636.619
2	2.920	4.303	6.965	9.925	31.599
3	2.353	3.182	4.541	5.841	12.924
4	2.132	2.776	3.747	4.604	8.610
5	2.015	2.571	3.365	4.032	6.869
6	1.943	2.447	3.143	3.707	5.959
7	1.895	2.365	2.998	3.499	5.408
8	1.860	2.306	2.896	3.355	5.041
9	1.833	2.262	2.821	3.250	4.781
10	1.812	2.228	2.764	3.169	4.587
11	1.796	2.201	2.718	3.106	4.437
12	1.782	2.179	2.681	3.055	4.318
13	1.771	2.160	2.650	3.012	4.221
14	1.761	2.145	2.624	2.977	4.140
15	1.753	2.131	2.602	2.947	4.073
16	1.746	2.120	2.583	2.921	4.015
17	1.740	2.110	2.567	2.898	3.965
18	1.734	2.101	2.552	2.878	3.922
19	1.729	2.093	2.539	2.861	3.883
20	1.725	2.086	2.528	2.845	3.850
21	1.721	2.080	2.518	2.831	3.819
22	1.717	2.074	2.508	2.819	3.792
23	1.714	2.069	2.500	2.807	3.768
24	1.711	2.064	2.492	2.797	3.745
25	1.708	2.060	2.485	2.787	3.725
26	1.706	2.056	2.479	2.779	3.707
27	1.703	2.052	2.473	2.771	3.690
28	1.701	2.048	2.467	2.763	3.674
29	1.699	2.045	2.462	2.756	3.659
30	1.697	2.042	2.457	2.750	3.646
35	1.690	2.030	2.438	2.724	3.591
40	1.684	2.021	2.423	2.704	3.551
45	1.679	2.014	2.412	2.690	3.520
50	1.676	2.009	2.403	2.678	3.496
120	1.658	1.980	2.358	2.617	3.373
Infinite (N(0,1))	1.645	1.960	2.326	2.576	3.291

Table A-4. Critical values for F distribution. Areas represent upper tail of the distribution.

Upper Tail Area = 0.10																	
Denominator Degrees of Freedom	Numerator Degrees of Freedom																
	1	2	3	4	5	6	7	8	9	10	15	20	25	30	40	50	60
1	39.863	49.500	53.593	55.833	57.240	58.204	58.906	59.439	59.858	60.195	61.220	61.740	62.055	62.265	62.529	62.688	62.794
2	8.526	9.000	9.162	9.243	9.293	9.326	9.349	9.367	9.381	9.392	9.425	9.441	9.451	9.458	9.466	9.471	9.475
3	5.538	5.462	5.391	5.343	5.309	5.285	5.266	5.252	5.240	5.230	5.200	5.184	5.175	5.168	5.160	5.155	5.151
4	4.545	4.325	4.191	4.107	4.051	4.010	3.979	3.955	3.936	3.920	3.870	3.844	3.828	3.817	3.804	3.795	3.790
5	4.060	3.780	3.619	3.520	3.453	3.405	3.368	3.339	3.316	3.297	3.238	3.207	3.187	3.174	3.157	3.147	3.140
6	3.776	3.463	3.289	3.181	3.108	3.055	3.014	2.983	2.958	2.937	2.871	2.836	2.815	2.800	2.781	2.770	2.762
7	3.589	3.257	3.074	2.961	2.883	2.827	2.785	2.752	2.725	2.703	2.632	2.595	2.571	2.555	2.535	2.523	2.514
8	3.458	3.113	2.924	2.806	2.726	2.668	2.624	2.589	2.561	2.538	2.464	2.425	2.400	2.383	2.361	2.348	2.339
9	3.360	3.006	2.813	2.693	2.611	2.551	2.505	2.469	2.440	2.416	2.340	2.298	2.272	2.255	2.232	2.218	2.208
10	3.285	2.924	2.728	2.605	2.522	2.461	2.414	2.377	2.347	2.323	2.244	2.201	2.174	2.155	2.132	2.117	2.107
15	3.073	2.695	2.490	2.361	2.273	2.208	2.158	2.119	2.086	2.059	1.972	1.924	1.894	1.873	1.845	1.828	1.817
20	2.975	2.589	2.380	2.249	2.158	2.091	2.040	1.999	1.965	1.937	1.845	1.794	1.761	1.738	1.708	1.690	1.677
25	2.918	2.528	2.317	2.184	2.092	2.024	1.971	1.929	1.895	1.866	1.771	1.718	1.683	1.659	1.627	1.607	1.593
30	2.881	2.489	2.276	2.142	2.049	1.980	1.927	1.884	1.849	1.819	1.722	1.667	1.632	1.606	1.573	1.552	1.538
40	2.835	2.440	2.226	2.091	1.997	1.927	1.873	1.829	1.793	1.763	1.662	1.605	1.568	1.541	1.506	1.483	1.467
50	2.809	2.412	2.197	2.061	1.966	1.895	1.840	1.796	1.760	1.729	1.627	1.568	1.529	1.502	1.465	1.441	1.424
60	2.791	2.393	2.177	2.041	1.946	1.875	1.819	1.775	1.738	1.707	1.603	1.543	1.504	1.476	1.437	1.413	1.395

(continued)

Table A-4. Critical values for F distribution. Areas represent upper tail of the distribution. (*continued*)

Upper Tail Area = 0.05																	
Denominator Degrees of Freedom	Numerator Degrees of Freedom																
	1	2	3	4	5	6	7	8	9	10	15	20	25	30	40	50	60
1	161.448	199.500	215.707	224.583	230.162	233.986	236.768	238.883	240.543	241.882	245.950	248.013	249.260	250.095	251.143	251.774	252.196
2	18.513	19.000	19.164	19.247	19.296	19.330	19.353	19.371	19.385	19.396	19.429	19.446	19.456	19.462	19.471	19.476	19.479
3	10.128	9.552	9.277	9.117	9.013	8.941	8.887	8.845	8.812	8.786	8.703	8.660	8.634	8.617	8.594	8.581	8.572
4	7.709	6.944	6.591	6.388	6.256	6.163	6.094	6.041	5.999	5.964	5.858	5.803	5.769	5.746	5.717	5.699	5.688
5	6.608	5.786	5.409	5.192	5.050	4.950	4.876	4.818	4.772	4.735	4.619	4.558	4.521	4.496	4.464	4.444	4.431
6	5.987	5.143	4.757	4.534	4.387	4.284	4.207	4.147	4.099	4.060	3.938	3.874	3.835	3.808	3.774	3.754	3.740
7	5.591	4.737	4.347	4.120	3.972	3.866	3.787	3.726	3.677	3.637	3.511	3.445	3.404	3.376	3.340	3.319	3.304
8	5.318	4.459	4.066	3.838	3.687	3.581	3.500	3.438	3.388	3.347	3.218	3.150	3.108	3.079	3.043	3.020	3.005
9	5.117	4.256	3.863	3.633	3.482	3.374	3.293	3.230	3.179	3.137	3.006	2.936	2.893	2.864	2.826	2.803	2.787
10	4.965	4.103	3.708	3.478	3.326	3.217	3.135	3.072	3.020	2.978	2.845	2.774	2.730	2.700	2.661	2.637	2.621
15	4.543	3.682	3.287	3.056	2.901	2.790	2.707	2.641	2.588	2.544	2.403	2.328	2.280	2.247	2.204	2.178	2.160
20	4.351	3.493	3.098	2.866	2.711	2.599	2.514	2.447	2.393	2.348	2.203	2.124	2.074	2.039	1.994	1.966	1.946
25	4.242	3.385	2.991	2.759	2.603	2.490	2.405	2.337	2.282	2.236	2.089	2.007	1.955	1.919	1.872	1.842	1.822
30	4.171	3.316	2.922	2.690	2.534	2.421	2.334	2.266	2.211	2.165	2.015	1.932	1.878	1.841	1.792	1.761	1.740
40	4.085	3.232	2.839	2.606	2.449	2.336	2.249	2.180	2.124	2.077	1.924	1.839	1.783	1.744	1.693	1.660	1.637
50	4.034	3.183	2.790	2.557	2.400	2.286	2.199	2.130	2.073	2.026	1.871	1.784	1.727	1.687	1.634	1.599	1.576
60	4.001	3.150	2.758	2.525	2.368	2.254	2.167	2.097	2.040	1.993	1.836	1.748	1.690	1.649	1.594	1.559	1.534

(*continued*)

Denominator Degrees of Freedom	Numerator Degrees of Freedom																
	1	2	3	4	5	6	7	8	9	10	15	20	25	30	40	50	60
1	4,052.181	4,999.500	5,403.352	5,624.583	5,763.650	5,858.986	5,928.356	5,981.070	6,022.473	6,055.847	6,157.285	6,208.730	6,239.825	6,260.649	6,286.782	6,302.517	6,313.030
2	98.503	99.000	99.166	99.249	99.299	99.333	99.356	99.374	99.388	99.399	99.433	99.449	99.459	99.466	99.474	99.479	99.482
3	34.116	30.817	29.457	28.710	28.237	27.911	27.672	27.489	27.345	27.229	26.872	26.690	26.579	26.505	26.411	26.354	26.316
4	21.198	18.000	16.694	15.977	15.522	15.207	14.976	14.799	14.659	14.546	14.198	14.020	13.911	13.838	13.745	13.690	13.652
5	16.258	13.274	12.060	11.392	10.967	10.672	10.456	10.289	10.158	10.051	9.722	9.553	9.449	9.379	9.291	9.238	9.202
6	13.745	10.925	9.780	9.148	8.746	8.466	8.260	8.102	7.976	7.874	7.559	7.396	7.296	7.229	7.143	7.091	7.057
7	12.246	9.547	8.451	7.847	7.460	7.191	6.993	6.840	6.719	6.620	6.314	6.155	6.058	5.992	5.908	5.858	5.824
8	11.259	8.649	7.591	7.006	6.632	6.371	6.178	6.029	5.911	5.814	5.515	5.359	5.263	5.198	5.116	5.065	5.032
9	10.561	8.022	6.992	6.422	6.057	5.802	5.613	5.467	5.351	5.257	4.962	4.808	4.713	4.649	4.567	4.517	4.483
10	10.044	7.559	6.552	5.994	5.636	5.386	5.200	5.057	4.942	4.849	4.558	4.405	4.311	4.247	4.165	4.115	4.082
15	8.683	6.359	5.417	4.893	4.556	4.318	4.142	4.004	3.895	3.805	3.522	3.372	3.278	3.214	3.132	3.081	3.047
20	8.096	5.849	4.938	4.431	4.103	3.871	3.699	3.564	3.457	3.368	3.088	2.938	2.843	2.778	2.695	2.643	2.608
25	7.770	5.568	4.675	4.177	3.855	3.627	3.457	3.324	3.217	3.129	2.850	2.699	2.604	2.538	2.453	2.400	2.364
30	7.562	5.390	4.510	4.018	3.699	3.473	3.304	3.173	3.067	2.979	2.700	2.549	2.453	2.386	2.299	2.245	2.208
40	7.314	5.179	4.313	3.828	3.514	3.291	3.124	2.993	2.888	2.801	2.522	2.369	2.271	2.203	2.114	2.058	2.019
50	7.171	5.057	4.199	3.720	3.408	3.186	3.020	2.890	2.785	2.698	2.419	2.265	2.167	2.098	2.007	1.949	1.909
60	7.077	4.977	4.126	3.649	3.339	3.119	2.953	2.823	2.718	2.632	2.352	2.198	2.098	2.028	1.936	1.877	1.836

Table A-5. Critical values for Chi square distribution.

Degrees of Freedom	Upper Tail Area			
	0.1	0.05	0.01	0.001
1	2.706	3.841	6.635	10.828
2	4.605	5.991	9.210	13.816
3	6.251	7.815	11.345	16.266
4	7.779	9.488	13.277	18.467
5	9.236	11.070	15.086	20.515
6	10.645	12.592	16.812	22.458
7	12.017	14.067	18.475	24.322
8	13.362	15.507	20.090	26.124
9	14.684	16.919	21.666	27.877
10	15.987	18.307	23.209	29.588
11	17.275	19.675	24.725	31.264
12	18.549	21.026	26.217	32.909
13	19.812	22.362	27.688	34.528
14	21.064	23.685	29.141	36.123
15	22.307	24.996	30.578	37.697
16	23.542	26.296	32.000	39.252
17	24.769	27.587	33.409	40.790
18	25.989	28.869	34.805	42.312
19	27.204	30.144	36.191	43.820
20	28.412	31.410	37.566	45.315
25	34.382	37.652	44.314	52.620
30	40.256	43.773	50.892	59.703
35	46.059	49.802	57.342	66.619
40	51.805	55.758	63.691	73.402
45	57.505	61.656	69.957	80.077
50	63.167	67.505	76.154	86.661
60	74.397	79.082	88.379	99.607
70	85.527	90.531	100.425	112.317
80	96.578	101.879	112.329	124.839
90	107.565	113.145	124.116	137.208
100	118.498	124.342	135.807	149.449

Table A–6. z transformation[a] of the correlation coefficient (r).

r	z	r	z
0	–	0.50	0.549
0.01	0.010	0.51	0.563
0.02	0.020	0.52	0.576
0.03	0.030	0.53	0.590
0.04	0.040	0.54	0.604
0.05	0.050	0.55	0.618
0.06	0.060	0.56	0.633
0.07	0.070	0.57	0.648
0.08	0.080	0.58	0.662
0.09	0.090	0.59	0.678
0.10	0.100	0.60	0.693
0.11	0.110	0.61	0.709
0.12	0.121	0.62	0.725
0.13	0.131	0.63	0.741
0.14	0.141	0.64	0.758
0.15	0.151	0.65	0.775
0.16	0.161	0.66	0.793
0.17	0.172	0.67	0.811
0.18	0.182	0.68	0.829
0.19	0.192	0.69	0.848
0.20	0.203	0.70	0.867
0.21	0.213	0.71	0.887
0.22	0.224	0.72	0.908
0.23	0.234	0.73	0.929
0.24	0.245	0.74	0.950
0.25	0.255	0.75	0.973
0.26	0.266	0.76	0.996
0.27	0.277	0.77	1.020
0.28	0.288	0.78	1.045
0.29	0.299	0.79	1.071
0.30	0.310	0.80	1.099
0.31	0.321	0.81	1.127
0.32	0.332	0.82	1.157
0.33	0.343	0.83	1.188
0.34	0.354	0.84	1.221
0.35	0.365	0.85	1.256
0.36	0.377	0.86	1.293
0.37	0.388	0.87	1.333
0.38	0.400	0.88	1.376
0.39	0.412	0.89	1.422
0.40	0.424	0.90	1.472
0.41	0.436	0.91	1.528
0.42	0.448	0.92	1.589
0.43	0.460	0.93	1.658
0.44	0.472	0.94	1.738
0.45	0.485	0.95	1.832
0.46	0.497	0.96	1.946
0.47	0.510	0.97	2.092
0.48	0.523	0.98	2.298
0.49	0.536	0.99	2.647

[a]$z = 1/2 \{\ln[(1 + r)/(1 - r)]\}$.

Appendix B: Answers to Exercises

CHAPTER 2

1. This is a retrospective cohort or case–control study because the study leverages data from an historical data source and includes both case and control groups.

2. This is an observational longitudinal study that is best categorized as a cohort study. The cohort here is newly diagnosed cancer patients.

3. This study design is interesting, and some might be tempted to call it case–control. The purpose was to compare self-reported therapy with actual therapy. Both of these measures (self-reported and actual) occurred at the same time, so the study also has some characteristics of a cross-sectional study. Our opinion is that the study is case–control, but it illustrates the difficulty in classifying studies cleanly into any scheme.

4. The study is observational and is a matched case–control study.

5. The study is a placebo-controlled randomized clinical trial.

6. The group of subjects was identified and initial data collection occurred in 1976; the same subjects were followed up in future years. The study design is, therefore, best described as a cohort or prospective study to identify risk factors.

7. Several study designs are possible, but the most realistic is an observational study. A case–control study provides information faster, but several case–control studies are required; a group of cases for each cause of death and type of cardiovascular morbidity needs to be identified. We suggest you use one of the electronic search programs to see if you can locate a copy of a cohort study, and, if so, read and discuss the pros and cons of how the study was done.

CHAPTER 3

1. The sum of the deviations (22.26, 3.36, 15.46, 6.96, ... −7.84, −17.04, −0.14) is zero.

2. a. Using the Numerical Summary in R Commander or the Descriptives program in SPSS, the mean SF-12 Total Score for the 1,132 subjects was 58.0 with a standard deviation of 24.8.

   b. See Table B–1.

   c. See Figure B–1.

3.

			SF12_total_score			
age_cat	N	Mean	Median	Std. Deviation	Mini-mum	Maxi-mum
≤60	223	61.31	67.08	24.82	5.42	97.92
61–70	366	62.76	67.29	24.25	3.33	100.00
71–80	358	56.09	55.21	24.58	5.00	100.00
>80	182	47.89	42.82	22.95	3.75	94.17
Total	1129	57.96	59.17	24.79	3.33	100.00

Age was available for 1,129 patients. The mean age must be estimated using the weighted means formula. It is found by multiplying the midpoint of each age interval by the count:

$$[(223 \times 55.5) + (366 \times 65.5) + (358 \times 75.5)$$
$$+ (182 \times 85.5)]/1129 = 69.92$$

The mean SF-12 Total Score is estimated by multiplying the count by the mean in each age group:

$$[(223 \times 61.31) + (366 \times 62.76) + (358 \times 56.09)$$
$$+ (182 \times 47.89)]/1129 = 57.96$$

The means calculated from the raw data are 69.4 years and 57.96. The SF-12 total score is a

Table B–1. Frequency distribution of SF-12 Total Score.

SF-12 Group	Count	Cumulative Count	Percent	Cumulative Percent
0–20	78	78	7.2%	7.2%
21–40	251	329	23.2%	30.4%
41–60	229	558	21.1%	51.5%
61–80	249	807	23.0%	74.5%
81–100	276	1083	25.5%	100.0%

Data from Bos-Touwen I, Schuurmans M, Monninkhof EM, et al: Patient and disease characteristics associated with activation for self-management in patients with diabetes, chronic obstructive pulmonary disease, chronic heart failure and chronic renal disease: a cross-sectional survey study, *PLoS One*. 2015 May 7;10(5):e0126400.

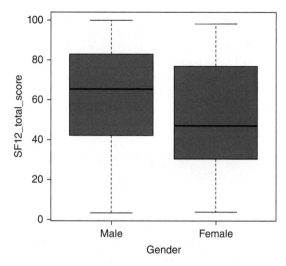

Figure B–1. Box plot of SF-12 total score for male and female subjects.

very good estimate because the means in each age group are used. The age is a good estimate because this table follows the rules for good frequency construction by choosing class limits so that most of the observations in the class are closer to the midpoint of the class than to either end of the class.

4. See Table B–2. The odds ratio is $(55 \times 2,847)/(229 \times 1,438) = 0.476$ and indicates the risk of a confirmed flu diagnosis for patient with symptoms is half as much in the inpatient hospital setting.

5. **a.** Bimodal with one peak in the early 20s and with a smaller peak in the 40s and 50s.

   b. Skewed positively, with many physicians delivering 30–60 babies (family or general practitioners) and fewer delivering 200–250

Table B–2. Contingency table for flu diagnosis and collection site and odds ratio.

Collection Site	Flu Diagnosis		
	Yes	No	Total
Inpatient department	55	229	284
Outpatient department	1438	2847	4285
Total	1493	3076	4569

Data from Anderson KB, Simasathien S, Watanaveeradej V, et al: Clinical and laboratory predictors of influenza infection among individuals with influenza-like illness presenting to an urban Thai hospital over a five-year period, *PLoS One*. 2018 Mar 7;13(3): e0193050.

(obstetricians); the distribution might also be bimodal with one mode at 50 babies and another at 225.

c. Probably bell-shaped, with a few hospitals referring a very small number of patients and a few referring a very large number of patients, but with the majority referring moderate numbers of patients.

6. See Figures B–2 and B–3.

7.
$$SD = \sqrt{\frac{\sum X^2 - \frac{(\sum X)^2}{n}}{n - 1}}$$

$$SD = \sqrt{\frac{52,990.37 - \left(\frac{911,452.09}{18}\right)}{18 - 1}}$$

$$= \sqrt{138.48} = 11.77$$

8. **a.** Salaries probably do not follow a bell-shaped curve; they tend to have a positive skew, with a few physicians making relatively

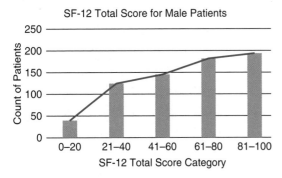

Figure B–2. Distribution of SF-12 total score for male patients.

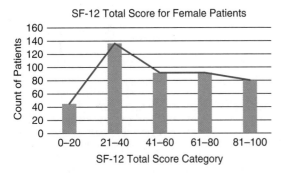

Figure B–3. Distribution of SF-12 total score for female patients.

larger salaries. The median and either the range or the interquartile range are therefore best.

b. Standardized ability and achievement tests administered to large numbers of examinees tend to follow a bell-shaped curve; therefore, the mean and the standard deviation are appropriate.

c. A bell-shaped distribution is a reasonable assumption, so the mean and the standard deviation are used.

d. The number of tender joints probably has a positively skewed distribution, so the median and the range or interquartile range are appropriate.

e. Presence of diarrhea either occurs or does not; therefore, this is a nominal characteristic, and proportions or percentages are correct.

f. This ordinal scale calls for the use of the median and the range; alternatively, proportions or percentages may be used.

g. Somewhat negatively skewed, with the majority of females developing the disease at ages 50–70 years, so the median and range are appropriate.

h. Assuming compliance is fairly good, the distribution has a positive skew, with most patients having a low pill count, and the median and range may be used.

9. A correlation of 0.27 represents a positive correlation—as activation score increases, so does SF-12 total score. The correlation of 0.19 between age and SF-12 total score means that as age increases, SF-12 total score decreases.

10. a. Approximately 25 lb, or 11.5 kg.

b. Approximately 18.9 in., or 48 cm.

c. Approximately 16 lb, or 7 kg.

11. The coefficient of variation for men is 10.84/54.47, or 19.9%; for women it is 10.71/53.58, or 20.0%. Therefore, the variation is nearly identical for men and women in this sample.

12. The odds that a person with a stroke abuses drugs are

$$\frac{(73/214)}{(141/214)} = \frac{73}{141}$$

$$= 0.518$$

The odds that a person without a stroke abuses drugs are

$$\frac{(18/214)}{(196/214)} = \frac{18}{196} = 0.092$$

Therefore, the odds ratio is 0.518/0.092 = 5.64; that is, a person in this study who abuses drugs is more than five times more likely to have a stroke.

13. a. The purpose of the study was to learn about acute effects of acetylsalicylic acid (ASA) on the gastroduodenal mucosa in young and old healthy men.

b. The study design was an experiment because a manipulation was made, and each subject was used as his own control; therefore, it is a self-controlled clinical trial.

c. Two groups were used because part of the purpose was to determine if differences existed between young and old men.

d. Figure B–1 in Moore and colleagues (1991) indicates that a dose-response relationship exists between the total number of lesions observed on endoscopic study: The smallest number was observed under the placebo condition, and the largest number when subjects received 1,300 mg aspirin. The long whiskers and dots representing the extreme values when subjects received 1,300 mg aspirin show that considerable variability exists between subjects in the total number of lesions observed.

e. Figure B–2 in Moore and colleagues (1991) indicates that significantly more variability occurs between subjects at the higher ranges of pH values than at the lower ranges. The figure legend points out that the median or middle value for three of the plots is at the very bottom of the plot; this means that half of the men had pH values under 1.0.

CHAPTER 4

1. **a.** To show that gender and blood type are independent, we must show that

$$P(A)P(B) = P(A \text{ and } B)$$

for each cell in the table:

$$0.42 \times 0.50 = 0.21$$
$$0.43 \times 0.50 = 0.215$$
$$0.11 \times 0.50 = 0.055$$
$$0.04 \times 0.50 = 0.02$$

b. $P(\text{male and type O}) = P(\text{male} \mid \text{type O})$
$$\times P(\text{type O})$$
$$= \frac{0.21}{0.42} \times \frac{0.42}{1.00}$$
$$= (0.50) \times (0.42) = 0.21$$

This demonstrates that $P(\text{male} \mid \text{type O}) = P(\text{male})$ when these are independent.

2. Assuming 47 patients were in the study,

a. $P(\text{chronic}) = \dfrac{7 + 3 + 2}{42}$
$$= 0.29$$

b. $P(\text{acute}) = \dfrac{6 + 2 + 2}{47} = 0.21$

c. $P(\text{acute} \mid \text{seroconvert}) = \dfrac{2}{18} = 0.11$

d. $P(\text{seropositive} \mid \text{died}) = \dfrac{2}{8} = 0.25$

e. $P(\text{seronegative}) = \dfrac{17}{47} = 0.36$

Using the binomial distribution, we get

$$P(4 \text{ out of } 8) = \frac{8!}{4!4!}(0.36)^4(0.64)^4$$
$$= \frac{40,320}{(24)(24)}(0.0168)(0.1678)$$
$$= 0.1973, \text{ or } 0.20$$

3. **a.** $P(\text{flu virus A}) = 34,329/48,291 = 0.71$
   b. $P(\text{flu virus B}\mid 25\text{-}64) = 4,618/16,021 = 0.29$

4. Use the binomial distribution.
   a. $P(\text{infection}) = 0.30$

$$P(1 \text{ infection in } 8 \text{ patients}) = \frac{8!}{1!7!}(0.30)^1(0.70)^7$$
$$= 8(0.30)(0.0824)$$
$$= 0.1977, \text{ or } 0.20$$

   b. $P(\text{survival}) = 0.80$

$$P(7 \text{ survivals in } 8 \text{ patients}) = \frac{8!}{1!7!}(0.80)^7(0.20)^1$$
$$= 8(0.2097)(.020)$$
$$= 0.3355, \text{ or } 0.34$$

5. $\lambda = 1487 / 390 = 3.81$. The probability of exactly five hospitalizations is

$$P(X = 5) = (3.81^5)\frac{e^{-3.81}}{5!}$$
$$= \frac{(802.83)(0.022)}{120} = 0.147$$

6. **a.** The probability that a normal healthy adult has a serum sodium above 147 mEq/L is $P(z > 2) = 0.023$.

   b. $P[z < (130 - 141)/3] = P(z < -3.67) < 0.001$

   c. $P\left[\dfrac{132 - 141}{3} < z < \dfrac{150 - 141}{3}\right]$
   $$= P(-3 < z < +3) = 0.997$$

   d. The top 1% of the standard normal distribution is found at $z = 2.326$; therefore, $2.326 = (X - 141)/3$, or $X = 147.98$. So a serum sodium level of approximately 148 mEq/L puts a patient in the upper 1% of the distribution.

   e. The bottom 10% of the standard normal distribution is found at $z = -1.28$; therefore,

Table B–3. Binomial distributions for different values of the parameter, π.

Probability	$\pi = 0.1$	$\pi = 0.3$	$\pi = 0.5$
$P(X = 0)$	0.531	0.118	0.016
$P(X = 1)$	0.354	0.303	0.094
$P(X = 2)$	0.098	0.324	0.234
$P(X = 3)$	0.015	0.185	0.313
$P(X = 4)$	0.001	0.060	0.234
$P(X = 5)$	<0.001	0.010	0.094
$P(X = 6)$	<0.001	0.001	0.016

$-1.28 = (X - 141)/3$, or $X = 137.16$. So a serum sodium level of approximately 137 mEq/L puts a patient in the lower 10% of the distribution.

7. The distributions are given in Table B–3. Thus,

$$P(X = 4 \text{ when } \pi = 0.3) = \left[\frac{6!}{4! \times 2!}\right](0.3)^4(0.7)^2$$

$$= \left[\frac{720}{(24 \times 2)}\right](0.008)(0.49)$$

$$= 0.060$$

Graphs of the preceding distributions illustrate that the binomial distribution is quite skewed when the proportion is 0.1 (as well as when the proportion is close to 1.0, such as 0.9 and 0.8). When the proportion is near 0.5, the distribution is nearly symmetric—perfectly so at 0.5.

8. **a.**

$$\text{Mean number of months} = \frac{(12 + 13 + 14 + 15 + 16)}{5}$$

$$= \frac{70}{5} = 14.0$$

and the standard deviation is

$$\sqrt{\frac{(12-14)^2 + (13-14)^2 + (14-14)^2 + (15-14)^2 + (16-14)^2}{5}} = 1.41$$

(Note that the standard deviation uses 5 in the denominator instead of 4 because we are assuming that these 5 observations make up the entire population.)

b.

$$\text{The mean of the mean number of months} = \frac{(12 + 12.5 + \cdots + 15.5 + 16)}{25}$$

$$= \frac{350}{25} = 14.0$$

and the standard deviation of the mean (or the standard error of the mean, *SE*) is

$$\sqrt{\frac{(12-14)^2 + (12.5-14)^2 + \cdots + (15.5-14)^2 + (16-14)^2}{25}} = 1.0$$

Note that the mean of the means found in part b is the same as the mean found in part a, and the *SE* is the same as

$$\frac{\sigma}{\sqrt{n}} = \frac{1.41}{\sqrt{2}}$$

$$= 1.0$$

9. **a.** This question refers to individuals and is equivalent to asking what proportion of the area under the curve is greater than $(103 - 100)/3 = +1.00$ and less than $(97 - 100)/3 = -1.00$, using the *z* distribution; the area is 0.317, or 31.7%, from Table A–2.

b. This question concerns means. The standard error with $n = 36$ is $3/6 = 0.5$. The critical ratio for a mean equal to 99 is $(99 - 100)/0.5 = -2.00$ and for 101 is $+2.00$. The area below -2.00 and above $+2.00$ is 0.046; therefore, 4.6% of the *means* are outside the limits of 99 and 101.

10. **a.** The standard deviation is

$$\sqrt{n}(SE) = \sqrt{131}(6.2)$$

$$= (11.45)(6.2) = 71.0$$

Then the probability that a patient is intoxicated more than 104 times per year is

$$P(X > 104) = P\left[z > \frac{(104 - 61.6)}{71}\right]$$

$$= P(z > 0.597)$$

From Table A–2, the $P(z > 0.60)$ is 0.274, so we know the probability is slightly more.

b. From Table A–2, the value of *z* that separates the upper 5% of the distribution from the lower 95% is 1.645. We need to find *X* so that

$$P[(X - \mu) / \sigma > 1.645] = 0.05$$

Solving for X gives $X = (1.645 \times 71.0) + 61.6 = 178.4$, or approximately 179 times a year.

11. Approximately 5% of medical students graduate with a debt of $200,000, and this is $96,000 above the mean of $104,000. The point in the normal distribution that separates the top 5% is 1.645. Therefore, $96,000 is 1.645 standard deviations; we divide by 1.645 to find that one standard deviation is $58,359.

CHAPTER 5

1. **a.**   Wider.
    b.   Increase the sample size to obtain a narrower confidence interval.
    c.   Narrower.

2. $H_0: \mu = 0.76$
    $H_1: \mu \neq 0.76$
    $\bar{x} = 0.68$
    $SE = 0.01$

    $t = \dfrac{0.68 - 0.76}{0.03} = -0.08$

    p-value < 0.001

    95% CI:

    $0.68 \pm 2.14 \times 0.01$

    $(0.66, 0.70)$

    Since the null value of 0.76 is not included in the 95% confidence interval, the null hypothesis is rejected at the 0.05 level. This is consistent with the p-value < 0.001 found in the hypothesis test.

3. The two-tailed z value for α of 0.05 is ± 1.96, and the lower one-tailed z value related to $\beta = 0.80$ is approximately -0.84. With a standard deviation of .03 and a 0.02 m difference, the sample size is approximately 18. This is much less than the sample needed to find a 0.01 m difference.

    $$n = \left[\frac{(z_\alpha - z_\beta)\sigma}{\mu_1 - \mu_0} \right]^2$$

    $$= \left[\frac{(1.96 - (-0.84)) \times 0.03}{0.68 - 0.67} \right]^2$$

    $$= \left[\frac{0.084}{0.01} \right]^2 = 70.56 \text{ or } 71$$

4. We found a needed sample size of 408 to detect a difference between 17% and 12%. For 80% power to find a difference between 17% and 10%, a sample of 200 is adequate. A smaller sample size is needed when the difference we want to detect is larger.

$$n = \left[\frac{z_\alpha \sqrt{\pi_0 \times (1 - \pi_0)} - z_\beta \sqrt{\pi_1 \times (1 - \pi_1)}}{\pi_0 - \pi_1} \right]^2$$

$$= \left[\frac{1.96\sqrt{0.17 \times 0.83} - (-0.84)\sqrt{0.10 \times 0.90}}{0.17 - 0.10} \right]^2$$

$$= \left[\frac{0.988}{0.07} \right]^2 = 199.20 \text{ or } 200$$

5. Our power calculations assumed $SD = 0.03$ m, and Rabago and coworkers (2015) had an SD of 0.04. This illustrates the role of the standard deviation in finding the sample size.

6. Solving for X:

    $$t = \frac{x}{1.7 / \sqrt{10}} > 2.179$$

    $$\frac{x}{1.7 / \sqrt{10}} > 2.179$$

    $$\frac{x}{0.538} > 2.179$$

    $$x > 1.17$$

7. See Table B–4.

    They agree by chance that $30/50 = 60\% \times 35/50 = 70\%$ or 42% were negative and $40\% \times 30\%$, or 12%, were positive, for a total of 54% of the mammograms. They actually agreed on $25 + 10$ or 35 of 50, or 70%.

    $$\kappa = \left(\frac{\text{Observed} - \text{Expected agreement}}{1 - \text{Expected agreement}} \right)$$

    $$= \frac{0.70 - 0.54}{1 - 0.54}$$

    $$= \frac{0.16}{0.46} = 0.348$$

Table B–4. Classification of a sample of 50 mammograms by two physicians.

Physician 1	Physician 2		
	Negative	**Positive**	
Negative	25	5	30
Positive	10	10	20
	35	15	50

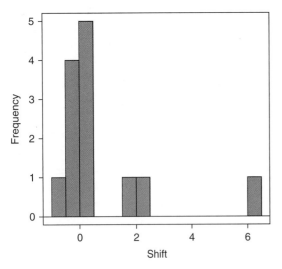

Figure B–4. Histogram of change in M-wave scores.

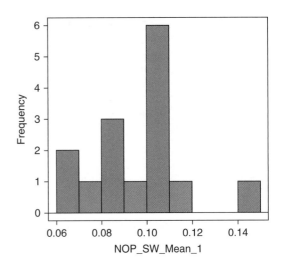

Figure B–5. Stride width for men with no perturbation.

8. a. A histogram of the change in M-wave scores in Figure B–4 shows a skewed distribution. The Wilcoxon test should be used.

b. Both the Wilcoxon and paired t-test result in the same conclusion—do not reject the null hypothesis that the difference is 0.

9. a. The distribution of stride width for men is skewed to the right (see Figure B–5). A nonparametric procedure is therefore recommended.

b. One-sample sign-test
data: sw$NOP_SW_Mean_1
s = 0, p value = 0.00006104
alternative hypothesis: true median is not equal to 0.15
95% confidence interval:
0.08189084   0.10500000
sample estimates:
median of x 0.104

Achieved and Interpolated Confidence Intervals:

	Conf.Level	L.E.pt	U.E.pt
Lower Achieved CI	0.8815	0.0860	0.105
Interpolated CI	0.9500	0.0819	0.105
Upper Achieved CI	0.9648	0.0810	0.105

One-sample t-test:
data: NOP_SW_Mean_1
t = −9.6922, df = 14, p value = 0.0000001374
alternative hypothesis: true mean is not equal to 0.15
95% confidence interval:
0.08592302   0.10914364
sample estimates:
mean of x

0.09753333
Both tests give the same conclusion—reject the null hypothesis with $p < 0.0001$. No solution for group exercises, so no solution for #10.

CHAPTER 6

1. The critical value of t is the same, 1.96 using interpolation, and the pooled standard deviation and standard error must be recalculated. The 95% confidence interval is

$$SD_p = \sqrt{\frac{(50-1)11.0^2 + (50-1)10.6^2}{50 + 50 - 2}} = 10.80$$

$$SE_{(\bar{x}_1 - \bar{x}_2)} = 10.80\sqrt{\frac{1}{50} + \frac{1}{50}} = 10.80 \times 0.2 = 2.16$$

$$1.9 \pm 1.96 \times 2.16$$

$$1.9 \pm 4.23$$

$$-2.33 \text{ to } 6.13$$

This CI is wider than the one in the Section "Decisions About Means in Two Independent" and now contains zero. We would, therefore, conclude that no difference exists in pulse oximetry if only 50 patients were in each group.

2. Pooled $SD = SD_p$

$$= \sqrt{\frac{(24-1)7.08^2 + (24-1)9.30^2}{24 + 24 - 2}}$$

$$= 8.26$$

3. If sample sizes are equal, $n_1 = n_2$, so we can use simply n in the formula for pooled SD. The result is that the pooled SD is the square root of the mean of SD_1^2 and SD_2^2.

$$\frac{(n_1 - 1)SD_1^2 + (n_2 - 1)SD_2^2}{n_1 + n_2 - 2}$$

$$= \frac{(n - 1)SD_1^2 + (n - 1)SD_2^2}{n + n - 2}$$

$$= \frac{(n - 1)(SD_1^2 + SD_2^2)}{2n - 2}$$

$$= \frac{(n - 1)(SD_1^2 + SD_2^2)}{2(n - 1)}$$

$$= \frac{SD_1^2 + SD_2^2}{2}$$

4. The null hypothesis is that the PAM scores were the same, and the alternative hypothesis is that they were not the same. The t test can be used for this research question; we use an α of 0.05 so results can be compared with the 95% confidence interval. The degrees of freedom are $422 + 732 - 2 = 1152$, so the critical value is 1.96. The pooled standard deviation calculated earlier in Chapter 6 is 10.75. So the t statistic is

$$t_{1152} = \frac{55.3 - 53.4}{10.75\sqrt{\dfrac{1}{422} + \dfrac{1}{732}}} = \frac{1.9}{0.66} = 2.87$$

$t = 2.87$ and is greater than the critical value of 1.96, so we reject the null hypothesis and conclude that, on the average, patients who had CRD had a higher PAM score than patients who did not have CRD.

5. Let N be the total number of observations, A the number of observations in a given row, and K the number of observations in a given column. For example, for a table with two rows and three columns, we have Table B–5, in which we want to find the expected value for the cell with the asterisk (*).

Table B–5. Contingency table with two rows and three columns.

	*		A
			B
J	K	L	N

The probability that an observation occurs in row A, $P(A)$, is A/N, and the probability that an observation occurs in column K, $P(K)$, is K/N. The null hypothesis being tested by chi-square is that the events represented by the rows and columns are independent. Using the multiplication rule for independent events, the probability that an observation occurs in row A *and* column K is $P(A)P(K) = A/N \times K/N = AK/N^2$. Multiplying this probability by the total number of observations N gives the number of observations that occur in both row A and column K; that is, $AK/N^2 \times N = AK\ N/N^2 = AK/N$ or the row total ÷ the column total ÷ the grand total.

6. The rule of thumb for α equal to 0.05 and power equal to 0.80 has $z_\alpha = 1.96$ and $z_\beta = -1.28$ for all computations; that is, only σ and $(\mu_0 - \mu_1)$ change. Therefore,

$$n = 2\left[\frac{(z_\alpha - z_\beta)\sigma}{\mu_1 - \mu_2}\right]^2$$

$$= 2\left\{\frac{[1.96 - (-1.28)]\sigma}{\mu_1 - \mu_2}\right\}^2$$

$$= 2\left[\frac{(3.24)\sigma}{\mu_1 - \mu_2}\right]^2$$

$$= 2 \times 10.5\left[\frac{\sigma}{\mu_1 - \mu_2}\right]^2$$

7. Output from G*Power (Figure B–6) indicates that 20 patients are needed for 80% power.

8. The 95% confidence interval, discussed earlier in Chapter 6, was $- 1.9 \pm (1.96)(0.66) = 1.9 \pm 1.29$, or 0.61 to 3.28. To have 90% and 99% confidence intervals, only the value for t with 919 degrees of freedom needs to be changed.

The 90% CI is $-1.9 \pm (1.645)(0.66) = 1.9 \pm 1.08$ or 0.81 to 2.99.

The 99% CI is $1.9 \pm (2.576)(0.66) = 1.9 \pm 1.70$ or 0.20 to 3.60.

Lower confidence gives a narrower interval, and higher confidence requires a wider interval.

9. Chances are good that more variation exists in the number of procedures done in the midsized centers. The t test requires that the variances (or standard deviations) not be different in the two groups. Because the sample sizes are quite different, 60 compared with 25, it is possible that violating the assumption of equal variances resulted in a nonsignificant t test.

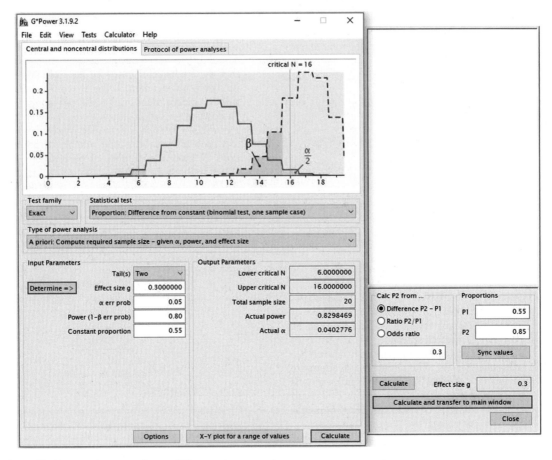

Figure B–6. Sample size to detect difference in proportions.

CHAPTER 7

1. The ANOVA results are given in Table B–6. The observed value for the *F* ratio is 11.09, with 2 and 107 degrees of freedom. The critical value from Table A–4 with 2 and 70 degrees of freedom (the closest value) is approximately 3.14 at $p = 0.05$; therefore, there is sufficient evidence to conclude that the mean ADMA levels are not the same for all three groups of patients.

2. Refer to Table B–6; the Tukey and Scheffé procedures indicate that groups HIV+ART+ group is different from both the HIV– and the HIV+ART– groups

3. Two comparisons are independent if they use nonoverlapping information.

   a. Independent because each comparison uses different data.

   b. Dependent because data on physicians are used in each comparison.

   c. Independent because each comparison uses different data.

   d. None of these three comparisons are independent from the other two because they all use data on medical students.

4. a. This is a one-way, or one-factor, ANOVA because only one nonerror term occurs, the among-groups term.

   b. Total variation is 2,000.

   c. There were four groups of patients because the degrees of freedom are 3. There were 40 patients because $n - 4 = 36$.

   d. The *F* ratio is $(800/3)/33.3 = 8.01$.

   e. The critical value with 3 and 30 degrees of freedom is 4.51; with 3 and 40 degrees of

Table B–6. ANOVA of ADMA by HIV Group

```
> ANOVA_HIV <- aov(ADMA ~ group, data=HIV)

> summary(ANOVA_HIV)
               Df Sum Sq Mean Sq F value   Pr(>F)
group           2 0.3962 0.19811   11.09 0.0000419 ***
Residuals     107 1.9110 0.01786
---
Signif. codes:  0 '***' 0.001 '**' 0.01 '*' 0.05 '.' 0.1 ' ' 1
1 observation deleted due to missingness

> with(HIV, numSummary(ADMA, groups=group, statistics=c("mean", "sd")))
              mean        sd data:n data:NA
HIV-     0.5964211 0.10614336     38       1
HIV+ART- 0.6244545 0.17334083     44       0
HIV+ART+ 0.4765000 0.08652018     28       0



        Simultaneous Tests for General Linear Hypotheses

Multiple Comparisons of Means: Tukey Contrasts


Fit: aov(formula = ADMA ~ group, data = HIV)

Linear Hypotheses:
                        Estimate Std. Error t value Pr(>|t|)
HIV+ART- - HIV- == 0     0.02803    0.02960   0.947  0.61114
HIV+ART+ - HIV- == 0    -0.11992    0.03328  -3.603  0.00138 **
HIV+ART+ - HIV+ART- == 0 -0.14795   0.03231  -4.580 < 0.0001 ***
---
Signif. codes:  0 '***' 0.001 '**' 0.01 '*' 0.05 '.' 0.1 ' ' 1
(Adjusted p values reported -- single-step method)
```

freedom is 4.31; interpolating for 3 and 36 degrees of freedom gives 4.39.

f. Reject the null hypothesis of no difference and conclude that mean blood pressure differs in groups that consume different amounts of alcohol. A post hoc comparison is necessary to determine specifically which of the four groups differ.

5. a. No, the p value is 0.545.
   b. Yes, the p value is $8.49 \times 10{-}6$, or 0.00000849.
   c. Yes, the interaction is also significant, with $p = 0.00000580$.
   d. A significant interaction means that the effect of one of the factors, such as type of psoriasis, depends on the level of the other factor, age at onset. Therefore, it is not possible to draw any conclusions about the factors independently; we cannot say simply that

%TBSA differs by familial versus sporadic type; we must note that the differences depend on age at onset.

CHAPTER 8

1. a. $$X^2 = \frac{(894 - 753.4)^2}{753.4} + \frac{(2873 - 3013.6)^2}{3013.6}$$
$$+ \frac{(902 - 1042.3)^2}{1042.3} + \frac{(4311 - 4170.4)^2}{4170.4}$$
$$= 26.24 + 6.56 + 18.88 + 4.74 = 54.499$$

With 1 degree of freedom, this value is much larger than the 3.841 associated with $p = 0.05$. We conclude that the evidence is sufficient to conclude that a significant relationship exists between exposure to benzodiazepine and the development of Alzheimer's disease.

b. $RR = \dfrac{894/3{,}767}{902/5{,}213} = \dfrac{0.237}{0.173} = 1.37$

95% CI:

$$exp\left[\ln(1.37) \pm 1.96\sqrt{\dfrac{1 - \left(894/3{,}767\right)}{894} + \dfrac{1 - \left(902/5{,}213\right)}{902}}\right]$$

$$exp\left[\ln(1.37) \pm 1.96 \times 0.042\right]$$

$$exp\left[0.315 \pm 0.082\right]$$

$$(1.26,\ 1.49)$$

Because the confidence interval does not contain 1, therefore, the evidence is sufficient to conclude that a significant risk of Alzheimer's disease exists in subjects taking benzodiazepine.

2. $r = b \times \dfrac{S_x}{S_y} = 0.97 \times \dfrac{3.80}{6.54} = 0.56$

3. a. Case–control.

   b. The odds ratio is $(20 \times 1{,}157)/(41 \times 121) = 4.66$; 95% confidence limits are the antilogarithms of

$$exp\left[\ln(4.66) \pm 1.96\sqrt{\dfrac{1}{20} + \dfrac{1}{41} + \dfrac{1}{1157} + \dfrac{1}{121}}\right]$$

$$= exp(0.97, 2.11)$$

$$= 2.65 \text{ to } 8.21$$

   c. The age-adjusted odds ratio is an estimate of the value of the odds ratio if the cases and controls had identical age distributions. Because the age adjustment increases the odds ratio from 4.66 to 8.1, the cases represented a younger group of women than the controls, and the age adjustment compensates for this difference. Thus, controlling for age, we have 95% confidence that the interval from 3.7 to 18 contains the true increase in risk of deep vein thrombosis (pulmonary embolism) with the use of oral contraceptives.

4. a and b.
   The solutions calculated using R for parts a and b are below.

```
            Pearson's product-moment correlation

data:  IPQ_Total_score and SF12_total_score
t = -10.276, df = 177, p-value < 2.2e-16
alternative hypothesis: true correlation is not equal to 0
95 percent confidence interval:
 -0.6955788 -0.5103537
sample estimates:
      cor
-0.6112695
```

5. a. BMI has the strongest relationship with age.

   b. BMI, because it has the highest correlation.

6. The regression line goes through the point $(\bar{X}, \bar{Y})$; therefore, the point at which X intersects the regression line, when projected onto the Y axis, is $\bar{Y}' = \bar{Y}$.

7. a. The questions addressed by the study were: Is the pathogenesis of steroid-responsive nephritis syndrome (SRNS) immune-complex-mediated? Does the clinical activity of the disease relate to the presence of circulatory immune complexes?

   b. Preexisting groups were used, patients with SRNS and patients with systemic lupus erythematosus (SLE), so the study was not randomized. No treatment was administered, so it was not a clinical trial. The observations on the variables of interest, IgG-containing complexes and C1q binding, were obtained at the same time, and the study question focused on "What is happening?" This study is therefore best described as cross-sectional.

   c. Patients with and without evidence of active disease were studied. Patients with SLE were also studied because immune complexes are known to have a pathogenetic role in this disease.

   d. According to Figure 8–21 the correlation between C1q-binding and IgG complexes for SLE patients is significant, $r = 0.91$, but this result in and of itself does not establish a cause-and-effect relationship. The correlation is not significant for patients with SRNS, but the sample size is relatively small, indicating low power to detect a significant relationship.

   e. Authors state that the lines are 95% confidence limits for the patients with lupus. However, the lines are parallel, instead of curved, as they should be. They probably relate to individuals, because (1) of the way they are described in the legend, and (2) limits for the mean would probably be closer to the regression line.

   f. It's not possible to tell for sure; however, it looks as if they might. First, the correlation for SRNS

Table B–7. Kaplan–Meier tables for patients who had kidney transplantation.

	Treatment = azathioprine				Treatment = cyclosporine		
Rank	Sample Size	Time	Survivorship S (t)	Rank	Sample Size	Time	Survivorship S (t)
1	31	1.0	0.967742	1	21	1.0	0.952381
2	30	1.0	0.935484	2	20	6.0	0.904762
3	29	1.0	0.903226	3	19	8.0	0.857143
4	28	1.0+		4	18	12.0+	
5	27	1.0+		5	17	12.0+	
6	26	2.0	0.868486	6	16	12.0+	
7	25	2.0+		7	15	13.0+	
8	24	3.0	0.832299	8	14	14.0+	
9	23	3.0	0.796112	9	13	15.0+	
10	22	3.0	0.759926	10	12	15.0+	
11	21	4.0+		11	11	16.0+	
12	20	5.0	0.721929	12	10	17.0+	
13	19	5.0+		13	9	17.0+	
14	18	5.0+		14	8	18.0+	
15	17	8.0+		15	7	19.0+	
16	16	8.0+		16	6	19.0+	
17	15	8.0+		17	5	20.0+	
18	14	10.0+		18	4	21.0+	
19	13	10.0+		19	3	22.0+	
20	12	12.0+		20	2	22.0+	
21	11	12.0+		21	1	22.0+	
22	10	13.0+					
23	9	14.0+					
24	8	15.0+					
25	7	17.0	0.618797				
26	6	18.0+					
27	5	18.0+					
28	4	19.0+					
29	3	20.0+					
30	2	23.0+					
31	1	23.0+					

Data from Dr. Alan Birtch.

patients is not significantly different from 0 and the correlation for SLE patients is 0.91; if correlations are different, so are the regression lines. The sample size of SRNS patients is very small, however, and may keep us from detecting a statistically significant difference.

g. No. The study population must be carefully defined to reduce the likelihood that patients with other disease processes are not included.

CHAPTER 9

1. a. See Table B–7 for the arrangements of the observations according to the length of time patients were in the study and survival probabilities.

b. The survival curve, produced with R, is given in Figure B–7.

c. Information for the logrank statistic is as shown in Table B–8.

2. a. The survival curves are given in Figure B–8. It appears that survival rates for the subjects with high serum MMP-14 (dashed lines in the figure) have shorter survival. This is consistent throughout the time period.

b. The logrank statistic is 10.2 (using the survdiff function in R). Because this is a chi-square statistic with 1 degree of freedom, we know that this value indicates statistical significance ($p = 0.001$). We therefore conclude that these observations do provide sufficient

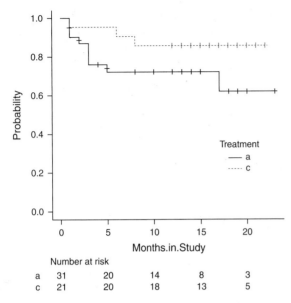

Figure B–7. Survival curve for patients with kidney transplants.

Table B–8. Information on the logrank statistic.

Treatment Value	Failed Count	Censored Count	Total Count
Azathioprine	9	22	31
Cyclosporine	3	18	21
Chi-square = 2.38	df = 1	p = 0.12	

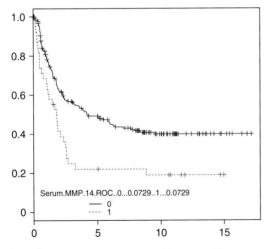

Figure B–8. Survival curve for patients with high vs low MMP-14.

evidence for a difference in survival in the two serum MMP-14 groups.

    c.   This study was observational and not randomized. Therefore, the difference found may be due to other covariates that may impact survival and/or the MMP-14 level.

3. The patients with combination treatment have a median survival of approximately 15 months. Those treated with regorafenib alone have a median survival of 10 months.

4. **a.** The Kaplan–Meier curves are given in Figure B–9.

    b.   The curves are widely separated, showing a large difference for those classified as intestinal tumors versus diffuse. The classification variable appears to be a valid indicator of risk and should be included as a covariate in the analysis.

5. The Mantel–Haenszel is an excellent procedure to compare two distributions. Note that it is possible

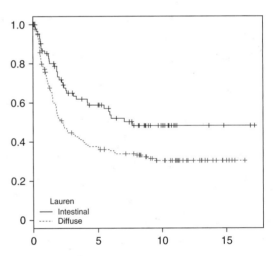

Figure B–9. Kaplan–Meier survival curves by Lauren classification.

to estimate the Mantel–Haenszel statistic from the study's Figure B–2.

6. **a.** Survival was best for patients whose disease was restricted to a single vessel.

    b.   The highest mortality rate was observed among patients with left main vessel or triple-vessel disease.

    c.   The median survival for group with single-vessel disease was approximately 18 years; for the other two groups it was approximately 12 years.

CHAPTER 10

1. For smokers, the adjusted mean is the mean in smokers, 3.33, minus the product of the regression coefficient, 0.0113, and the difference between the occlusion score in smokers and the occlusion score in the entire sample (estimated from Figure 10–3); that is,

$$-[0.0113 \times (198.33 - 151.67)] = 2.80$$

Similarly, the adjusted mean in nonsmokers is

$$1.00 - [0.0113 \times (105.00 - 151.67)] = 1.53$$

These are the same values we found (within round-off error) in Section "Controlling for Confounding."

2. Predicted value for a patient with an ASA = 1, poor functional status, severe hypertension undergoing an open surgical procedure of 1.5 hours:

$$-3.246 + 0.887$$
$$\times [ASA > 3]$$
$$+0.754 \times [\text{poor functional status}]$$
$$+0.632 \times [\text{No sHTN}]$$
$$+1.084 \times [\text{open approach}]$$
$$+0.838 \times [\text{longer than 2 hours}]$$

and we evaluate it as follows:

$$-3.246 +$$
$$0.887 \times [0]$$
$$+0.754 \times [1]$$
$$+0.632 \times [0]$$
$$+1.084 \times [1]$$
$$+0.838 \times [0]$$
$$= -1.408$$

and

$$p_x = \frac{1}{1 + \exp[-(b_0 + b_1 X_1 + b_2 X_2 + b_3 X_3)]}$$
$$= \frac{1}{1 + \exp[-(-1.408)]}$$
$$= \frac{1}{1 + 4.088} = 0.196$$

Therefore, there is a 19.6% chance of a LOS longer than 7 days.

Table B–9. Calculation of Kappa Statistic.

Observed		Predicted CORRECT LOS > 7		Total
		0	1	
CORRECT LOS >7	0	409	22	431
	1	90	26	116
Total		499	48	547

Expected		Predicted CORRECT LOS > 7		Total
		0	1	
CORRECT LOS >7	0	393.179159	37.820841	431
	1	105.820841	10.179159	116
Total		499	48	547

Expected	0.73740095
Observed	0.7952468
Kappa	0.22028203

3. See Table B–9

4. If the investigators want to distinguish among three groups of runners, using the numerical anthropometric measures, discriminant analysis should be used. Multiple regression can be used, however, if the actual running time of each runner was used instead of dividing the runners into three groups; in this situation, the outcome measure is numerical.

5. Given the patient is a woman and in the FFS payplan, the regression equation is

$$0.613 - [0.26 \times 1(\text{if a male})]$$
$$-[0.014 \times 1(\text{if in FFS payplan})]$$
$$-[0.0002 \times 80(\text{personal functioning})]$$
$$-[0.00006 \times 80(\text{mental health})]$$
$$-[0.002 \times 75(\text{health perceptions})]$$
$$-[0.0001 \times 70(\text{age})]$$
$$-[0.021 \times 10(\text{income scale value})]$$
$$+[0.002 \times 1(\text{if 3-year term})]$$
$$-[0.003 \times 1(\text{if took physical})]$$
$$+[0.105 \times 14(\text{number of bed days at time 00})]$$
$$0.613 - 0.014 - 0.016 - 0.0048 - 0.150 - 0.007$$
$$-0.210 + 0.002 - 0.003 + 1.470$$
$$= 1.680$$

which gives 1.68 predicted bed-days during a 30-day period.

6. **a.** The regression coefficient is 0.267, indicating a positive relationship.

   b. The negative regression coefficient indicates that older ages are associated with lower depression scores, indicating less depression. It is significant because the p value is 0.538. One possible interpretation is that people tend to be more able to deal with their physical conditions and circumstances that occur with increasing age, but this is purely speculative.

   c. The block on physical health increases R^2 by 0.174 or approximately 17%.

7. **a.** Your regression results should resemble those we produced in Table 10–13.

   b. Father's height was the variable included in model 1. Stepwise regression begins with the independent variable that has the highest correlation with the outcome, so father's height had the highest correlation with the child's final height.

   c. Mother's height, height for chronologic age, and dose are in the final model. Based on the standardized coefficients, the variable making the largest contribution is height for chronologic age.

   d. After the other variables entered the equation in model 4, the father's height was no longer significant. This can occur when the other variables are predicting the same portion of the outcome that father's height was predicting, once the values of all other variables are held constant.

   e. $-1.138 + (-0.575 \times -2.20)$

   $+ (1.325 \times -3.07) + (0.121 \times 20)$

   $= -1.138 + 1.265 - 4.068 + 2.42$

   $= -1.52$

   This child's final height is therefore predicted to be –1.52, compared with the child's actual height of –2.18.

CHAPTER 11

1. **a.** A nonrepresentative group; those that do not like the airline probably are not on the plane; the flight is not over.

   b. Response bias; only those that felt strongly in one direction or the other tend to respond.

   c. Typically, patient satisfaction questionnaires are very general in nature and provide little detail on real issues; the response rate is very low, often less than 10%. It may be better to concentrate resources on questionnaires on specific topics sent to random samples of patients with adequate follow-up to produce a reliable response rate.

   d. Students may fear that their response will in some way be identified and may hesitate to express their true feelings.

2. Depending on the question you want to answer, you could form confidence intervals for the means or examine correlations among responses to the different variables.

3. It might be easier for parents to estimate the number of hours their child watches TV in an average week rather than a month. Alternatively, the pediatrician could list a set of choices, such as 0–5, 6–10, 10–15, and so on.

4. Both sides of the issue should be represented in a question to keep from leading the respondent. It would be better to ask: "Do you agree or disagree that the new clinic hours are an improvement over the old ones?" Even better would be: "What is your opinion of the new clinic hours compared with the old clinic hours?" and provide five responses such as: much better, somewhat better, no difference, somewhat worse, much worse.

5. Either d or e, depending on the amount of resources you have to gather the membership list.

CHAPTER 12

1. **a.** With a baseline of 2% and 95% sensitivity, $0.95 \times 20 = 19$ true-positives; with 50% sensitivity, the false-positive rate is 50% and $0.50 \times 980 = 490$ false-positives occur. The probability of lupus with a positive test is $TP/(TP + FP) = 19/509 = 3.7\%$.

   b. With a baseline of 20%, 190 true-positives occur. Similarly, with 50% specificity, 400 false-positives occur. The chances of lupus with this index of suspicion is, therefore, $190/590 = 32.2\%$.

2. Using Bayes' theorem with $D =$ lupus and $T =$ test, we have

$$P(D^- \mid T^-) = \frac{P(T^- \mid D^-)P(D^-)}{P(T^- \mid D^-)P(D^-) + P(T^- \mid D^+)P(D^+)}$$

$$= \frac{0.50 \times 0.98}{(0.50 \times 0.98) + (0.05 \times 0.02)}$$

$$= \frac{0.49}{0.49 + 0.001} = 0.998$$

Using the likelihood ratio method requires us to redefine the pretest odds as the odds of *no* disease, that is, $0.98/(1 - 0.98) = 49$. The likelihood ratio for a negative test is the specificity divided by the false-negative rate (i.e., the likelihood of a negative test for persons without the disease versus persons with the disease); therefore, the likelihood ratio is $0.50/0.05 = 10$. Multiplying, we get $49 \times 10 = 490$, the posttest odds. Reconverting to the posttest probability, or the predictive value of a negative test, gives $490/(1 + 490) = 0.998$, the same result as with Bayes' theorem.

3. a. Increasing the threshold for a positive ESR from ≥ 20 mm/hr to ≥ 0 mm/hr will decrease the sensitivity.

  b. There will be more false-positives because the specificity will increase.

4. a. Positive results occurred 138 times in 150 known diabetics $= 138/150 = 92\%$ sensitivity.

  b. $150 - 24 = 126$ negative results in 150 persons without diabetes gives $126/150 = 84\%$ specificity.

  c. The false-positive rate is $24/150$, or $100\% -$ specificity $= 16\%$.

  d. 80% sensitivity in 150 persons with diabetes gives 120 true-positives. 4% false-positives in 150 persons without diabetes is 6 persons. The chances of diabetes with a positive fasting blood sugar is thus $120/126 = 95.2\%$.

  e. 80% sensitivity in 90 (out of 100) patients with diabetes $= 72$ true-positives; 4% false-positive rate in 10 patients without dia-

betes $= 0.4$ false-positive. Therefore, $72/72.4 = 0.9945$, or 99.45%, of patients like this man who have a positive fasting blood sugar actually have diabetes.

5. a. There are $80 \times 0.19 = 15.2$ true-positives, and $80 - 15.2 = 64.8$ false-negatives; $20 \times 0.82 = 16.4$ true-negatives and $20 - 16.4 = 3.6$ false-positives. Therefore, the probability of an MI with a positive ECG is $15.2/(15.2 + 3.6) = 80.9\%$.

  b. The probability of an MI even if the test is negative is $64.8/(64.8 + 16.4) = 79.8\%$.

  c. These calculations illustrate the uselessness of this criterion (ST elevation ≥ 5 mm in discordant leads) in diagnosing MI.

  d. The likelihood ratio is TP/FP or $19/18 = 1.06$.

  e. The pretest odds are $80/20$, or 4 to 1. The posttest odds are $4 \times 1.06 = 4.24$. As you can see, the test does very little to change the index of suspicion.

6. See Figure B–10 for the expected utilities for the decision tree.

7. a. 0.20, seen on the top branch.

  b. No, this is not obvious. Although the author provides the proportion of patients who have a positive examination, 0.26 (and negative examination, 0.74), these numbers include false-positives (and false-negatives) as well as true-positives (and true-negatives). The author also gives the predictive value of a positive test, 0.78 (and of a negative test,

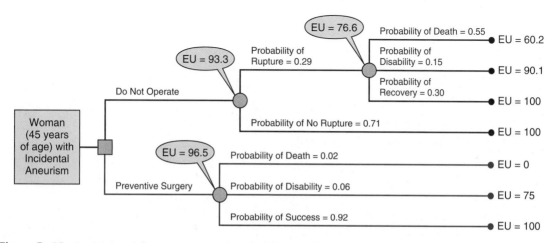

Figure B–10. Decision tree for aneurysms with probabilities and utilities included.
(EU = expected utility.) (Reproduced with permission from van Crevel H, Habbema JD, Braakman R: Decision analysis of the management of incidental intracranial saccular aneurysms, *Neurology*. 1986 Oct;36(10):1335-1339.)

0.997); and by using quite a bit of algebra, we can work backward to obtain the estimates of 0.989 for sensitivity and 0.928 for specificity. Readers of the article should not be expected to do these manipulations, however; authors should give precise values used in any analysis.

c. For no test or therapy: $(0.20)(48) + (0.80)(100) = 89.6$; for colectomy: $(0.03)(0) + (0.97) [(0.20)(78) + (0.80)(100)] = 92.7$. Therefore, colonoscopy is the arm with the highest utility, at 94.6.

CHAPTER 13

1. C
2. A
3. D
4. D
5. D
6. B
7. E
8. A
9. C
10. E
11. A
12. E
13. C
14. C
15. A
16. E
17. B
18. C
19. A
20. C
21. D
22. D
23. C
24. A
25. D
26. B
27. C
28. A
29. E
30. D
31. A
32. D
33. B
34. E
35. D
36. D
37. C
38. G
39. A
40. C
41. A
42. B
43. B
44. A
45. B
46. C
47. C
48. B
49. D
50. E
51. A
52. E
53. B
54. E
55. A
56. B
57. H
58. B
59. I
60. E
61. G

Appendix C: Flowcharts for Relating Research Questions to Statistical Methods

Flowchart to Use	Research Questions
C–1	Is there a difference in means or medians for ordinal or numerical measures?
C–2	Is there a difference in means or medians for ordinal or numerical measures, three or more groups?
C–3	Is there a difference in proportions for nominal measures?
C–4	Is there an association?
C–5	Is there a difference in measures of association?
C–6	Are there two or more independent variables?

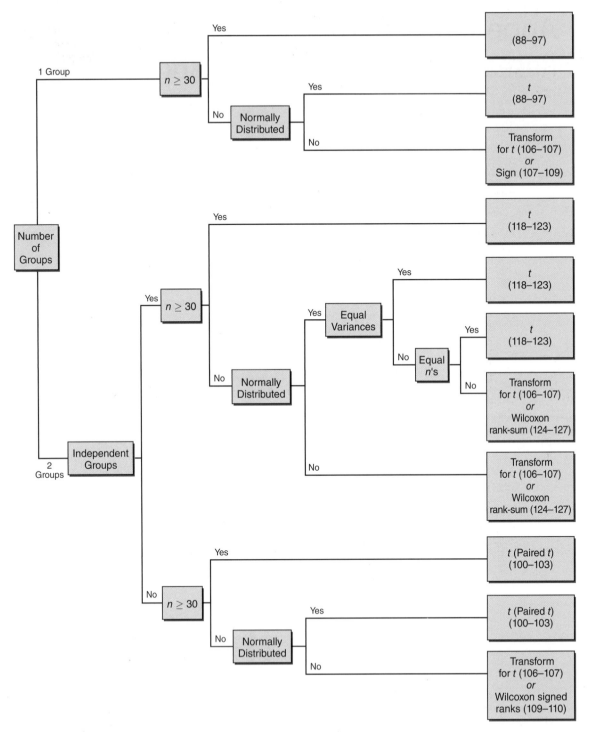

Figure C-1. Is there a difference in means or medians for ordinal or numerical measures?

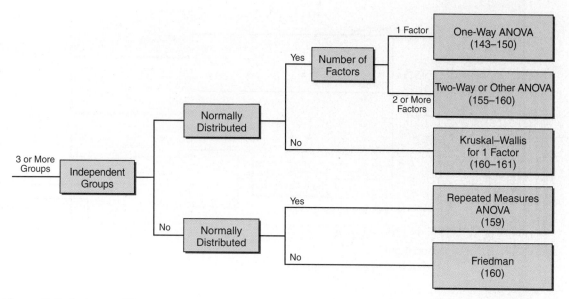

Figure C–2. Is there a difference in means or medians for ordinal or numerical measures, three or more groups?

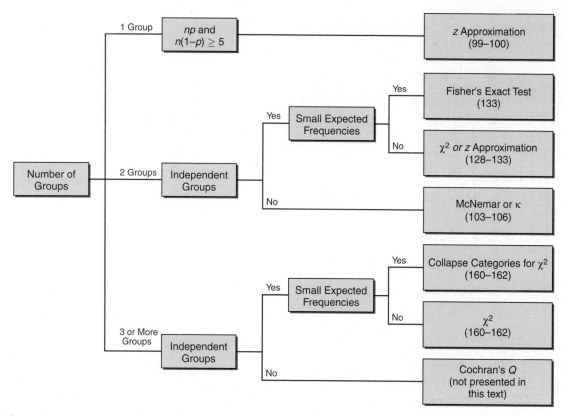

Figure C–3. Is there a difference in proportions for nominal measures?

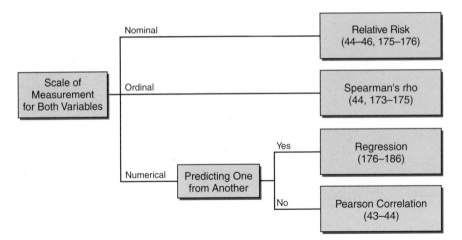

Figure C–4. Is there an association?

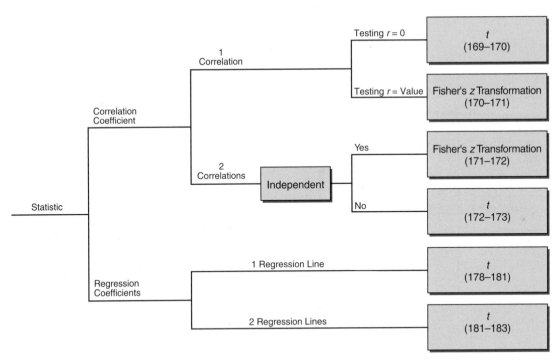

Figure C–5. Is there a difference in measures of association?

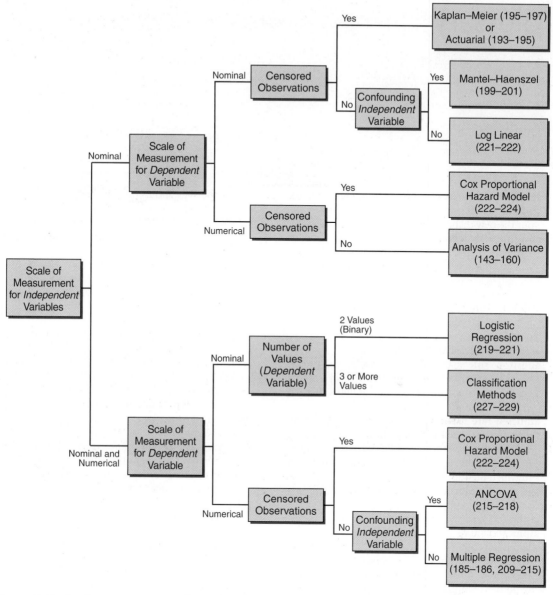

Figure C–6. Are there two or more independent variables?

Glossary

absolute risk increase (ARI) The increase in risk with a new therapy compared with the risk without the new therapy.

absolute risk reduction (ARR) The reduction in risk with a new therapy compared with the risk without the new therapy; it is the absolute value of the difference between the experimental event rate and the control event rate ($|EER - CER|$).

absolute value The positive value of a number, regardless of whether the number is positive or negative. The absolute value of a is symbolized $|a|$.

actuarial analysis See *life table analysis.*

addition rule The rule which states the probability that two or more mutually exclusive events all occur is the sum of the probabilities of each individual event.

adjusted rate A rate adjusted so that it is independent of the distribution of a possible confounding variable. For example, age-adjusted rates are independent of the age distribution in the population to which they apply.

age-specific mortality rate The mortality rate in a specific age group.

alpha (α) error See *type I error.*

alpha (α) value The level of alpha (α) selected in a hypothesis test.

alternative hypothesis The opposite of the null hypothesis. It is the conclusion when the null hypothesis is rejected.

analysis of covariance (ANCOVA) A special type of analysis of variance or regression used to control for the effect of a possible confounding factor.

analysis of residuals In regression, an analysis of the differences between Y and Y' to evaluate assumptions and provide guidance on how well the equation fits the data.

analysis of variance (ANOVA) A statistical procedure that determines whether any differences exist among two or more groups of subjects on one or more factors. The F test is used in ANOVA.

backward elimination A method to select variables in multiple regression that enters all variables into the regression equation and then eliminates the variable that adds the least to the prediction, followed by the other variables one at a time that decrease the multiple R by the least amount until all statistically significant variables are removed from the equation.

bar chart or bar graph A chart or graph used with nominal characteristics to display the numbers or percentages of observations with the characteristic of interest.

Bayes' theorem A formula for calculating the conditional probability of one event, $P(A|B)$, from the conditional probability of the other event, $P(B|A)$.

bell-shaped distribution A term used to describe the shape of the normal (Gaussian) distribution.

beta (β) error See *type II error.*

bias The error related to the ways the targeted and sampled populations differ; also called measurement error, it threatens the validity of a study.

binary observation A nominal measure that has only two outcomes (examples are gender: male or female; survival: yes or no).

binomial distribution The probability distribution that describes the number of successes X observed in n independent trials, each with the same probability of occurrence.

biometrics The study of measurement and statistical analysis in medicine and biology.

biostatistics The application of research study design and statistical analysis to applications in medicine and biology.

bivariate plot A two-dimensional plot or scatterplot of the values of two characteristics measured on the same set of subjects.

blind study An experimental study in which subjects do not know the treatment they are receiving; investigators may also be blind to the treatment subjects are receiving; see also *double-blind trial.*

block design In analysis of variance, a design in which subjects within each block (or stratum) are assigned to a different treatment.

Bonferroni *t* A method for comparing means in analysis of variance; also called the Dunn multiple-comparison procedure.

bootstrap A method for estimating standard errors or confidence intervals in which a small sample of observations is randomly selected from the original sample, estimates are calculated, and the sample is returned to the original sample. This process continues many times to produce a distribution upon which to base the estimates.

box plot A graph that displays both the frequencies and the distribution of observations. It is useful for comparing two distributions.

box-and-whisker plot The same as box plot.

canonical correlation analysis An advanced statistical method for examining the relationships between two sets of interval or numerical measurements made on the same set of subjects.

case–control An observational study that begins with patient cases who have the outcome or disease being investigated and control subjects who do not have the outcome or disease. It then looks backward to identify possible precursors or risk factors.

case–series study A simple descriptive account of interesting or intriguing characteristics observed in a group of subjects.

categorical observation A variable whose values are categories (an example is type of anemia). See also *nominal scale.*

cause-specific mortality rate The mortality rate from a specific disease.

cell A category of counts or value in a contingency table.

censored observation An observation whose value is unknown, generally because the subject has not been in the study long enough for the outcome of interest, such as death, to occur.

central limit theorem A theorem that states that the distribution of means is approximately normal if the sample size is large enough ($n \geq 30$), regardless of the underlying distribution of the original measurements.

chance agreement A measure of the proportion of times two or more raters agree in their measurement or assessment of a phenomenon.

chi-square (χ^2) distribution The distribution used to analyze counts in frequency tables.

chi-square (χ^2) test The statistical test used to test the null hypothesis that proportions are equal or, equivalently, that factors or characteristics are independent or not associated.

classes or class limits The subdivisions of a numerical characteristic (or the widths of the classes) when it is displayed in a frequency table or graph (an example is ages by decades).

classification and regression tree (CART) analysis A multivariate method used to detect significant relationships among variables which are then used to develop predictive models for classifying future subjects.

clinical epidemiology The application of the science of epidemiology to clinical medicine and decision-making.

clinical trial An experimental study of a drug or procedure in which the subjects are humans.

closed question A question on an interview or questionnaire in which a specific set of response options are provided.

cluster analysis An advanced statistical method that determines a classification or taxonomy from multiple measures of a set of objects or subjects.

cluster random sample A two-stage sampling process in which the population is divided into clusters, a random sample of clusters is chosen, and then random samples of subjects within the clusters are selected.

coefficient of determination (r^2) The square of the correlation coefficient. It is interpreted as the amount of variance in one variable that is accounted for by knowing the second variable.

coefficient of variation (CV) The standard deviation divided by the mean (generally multiplied by 100). It is used to obtain a measure of relative variation.

cohort A group of subjects who remain together in the same study over time.

cohort study An observational study that begins with a set of subjects who have a risk factor (or have been exposed to an agent) and a second set of subjects who do not have the risk factor or exposure. Both sets are followed prospectively through time to learn how many in each set develop the outcome or consequences of interest.

combination A formula in probability that it gives the number of ways a specific number of items, say *X,* can be selected from the total number of items, say *n,* in the entire population or sample.

complementary event An event opposite to the event being investigated.

computer package A set of statistical computer programs for analyzing data.

concurrent controls Control subjects assigned to a placebo or control condition during the same period that an experimental treatment or procedure is being evaluated.

conditional probability The probability of an event, such as *A,* given that another event, such as *B,* has occurred, denoted $P(A|B)$.

confidence bands Lines on each side of a regression line or curve that have a given probability of containing the line or curve in the population.

confidence coefficient The term in the formula for a confidence interval that determines probability level associated with the interval, such as 90%, 95%, and 99%.

confidence interval (CI) The interval computed from sample data that has a given probability that the unknown parameter, such as the mean or proportion, is contained within the interval. Common confidence intervals are 90%, 95%, and 99%.

confidence limits The limits of a confidence interval. These limits are computed from sample data and have a given probability that the unknown parameter is located between them.

confounded A term used to describe a study or observation that has one or more nuisance variables present that may lead to incorrect interpretations.

confounding variable A variable more likely to be present in one group of subjects than another that is related to the outcome of interest and thus potentially confuses, or "confounds," the results.

conservative A term used to describe a statistical test if it reduces the chances of a type I error.

construct validity A demonstration that the measurement of a characteristic is related to similar measures of the same characteristic and not related to measures of other characteristics.

content validity A measure of the degree to which the items on a test or measurement scale are representative of the characteristic being measured.

contingency table A table used to display counts or frequencies for two or more nominal or quantitative variables.

continuity correction An adaptation to a test statistic when a continuous probability distribution is used to estimate a discrete probability distribution; e.g., using the chi-square distribution for analyzing contingency tables.

continuous scale A scale used to measure a numerical characteristic with values that occur on a continuum (an example is age).

control event rate (CER) The number of subjects in the control group who develop the outcome being studied.

control subjects In a clinical trial, subjects assigned to the placebo or control condition; in a case–control study, subjects without the disease or outcome.

controlled for A term used to describe a confounding variable that is taken into consideration in the design or the analysis of the study.

controlled trial A trial in which subjects are assigned to a control condition as well as to an experimental condition.

corrected chi-square test A chi-square test for a 2×2 table that uses Yates' correction, making it more conservative.

correlation coefficient (r) A measure of the linear relationship between two numerical measurements made on the same set of subjects. It ranges from -1 to $+1$, with 0 indicating no relationship. Also called the Pearson product moment.

cost–benefit analysis A quantified methods to evaluate the trade-offs between the costs (or disadvantages) and the benefits (or *advantages*) of a procedure or management strategy.

cost-effectiveness analysis A quantitative method to evaluate the cost of a procedure or management strategy that takes into account the outcome as well in order to select the lowest-cost option.

covariate A potentially confounding variable controlled for in analysis of covariance.

Cox proportional hazard model or **Cox model** A regression method used when the outcome is censored. The regression coefficients are interpreted as adjusted relative risk or odds ratios.

criterion validity An indication of how well a test or scale predicts another related characteristic, ideally a "gold standard" if one exists.

criterion variable The outcome (or dependent variable) that is predicted in a regression problem.

critical ratio The term for the z score used in statistical tests.

critical region The region (or set of values) in which a test statistic must occur for the null hypothesis to be rejected.

critical value The value that a test statistic must exceed (in an absolute value sense) for the null hypothesis to be rejected.

crossover study A clinical trial in which each group of subjects receives two or more treatments, but in different sequences.

cross-product ratio See *relative risk*.

cross-sectional study An observational study that examines a characteristic (or set of characteristics) in a set of subjects at one point in time; a "snapshot" of a characteristic or condition of interest; also called survey or poll.

cross-validation A procedure for applying the results of an analysis from one sample of subjects to a new sample of subjects to evaluate how well they generalize. It is frequently used in regression.

crude rate A rate for the entire population that is not specific or adjusted for any given subset of the population.

cumulative frequency or **percentage** In a frequency table, the frequency (or percentage) of observations having a given value plus all lower values.

curvilinear relationship (between X and Y) A relationship that indicates that X and Y vary together, but not in constant increments.

decision analysis A formal model for describing and analyzing a decision; also called medical decision-making.

decision tree A diagram of a set of possible actions, with their probabilities and the values of the outcomes listed. It is used to analyze a decision process.

degrees of freedom (*df*) A parameter in some commonly used probability distributions; e.g., the *t* distribution and the chi-square distribution.

dependent groups or samples Samples in which the values in one group can be predicted from the values in the other group.

dependent variable The variable whose values are the outcomes in a study; also called response or criterion variable.

dependent-groups *t* test See *paired* t *test.*

descriptive statistics Statistics, such as the mean, the standard deviation, the proportion, and the rate, used to describe attributes of a set of data.

dichotomous observation A nominal measure that has only two outcomes (examples are gender: male or female; survival: yes or no); also called *binary.*

direct method of rate standardization A method of adjusting rates when comparing two or more populations; it requires knowledge of the specific rates for each category in the populations to be adjusted and the frequencies in at least one population.

directional test See *one-tailed test.*

discrete scale A scale used to measure a numerical characteristic that has integer values (an example is number of pregnancies).

discriminant analysis A regression technique for predicting a nominal outcome that has more than two values; a method used to classify subjects or objects into groups; also called discriminant function analysis.

distribution The values of a characteristic or variable along with the frequency of their occurrence. Distributions may be based on empirical observations or may be theoretical probability distributions (e.g., normal, binomial, chi-square).

distribution-free Statistical methods that make no assumptions regarding the distribution of the observations; that is, nonparametric.

dot plot A graphic method for displaying the frequency distribution of numerical observations for one or more groups.

double-blind trial A clinical trial in which neither the subjects nor the investigator(s) know which treatment subjects have received.

dummy coding A procedure in which a code of 0 or 1 is assigned to a nominal predictor variable used in regression analysis.

Dunnett's procedure A multiple-comparison method for comparing multiple treatment groups with a single control group following a significant *F* test in analysis of variance.

effect or effect size The magnitude of a difference or relationship. It is used for determining sample sizes and for combining results across studies in meta-analysis.

error mean square (MS_E) The mean square in the denominator of *F* in ANOVA.

error term See *residual.*

estimation The process of using information from a sample to draw conclusions about the values of parameters in a population.

event A single outcome (or set of outcomes) from an experiment.

evidence-based medicine (EBM) The application of the evidence based on clinical research and clinical expertise to decide optimal patient management.

expected frequencies In contingency tables, the frequencies observed if the null hypothesis is true.

expected value Used in decision-making to denote the probability of a given outcome over the long run.

experiment (in probability) A planned process of data collection.

experimental event rate (EER) The number of subjects in the experimental or treatment group who develop the outcome being studied.

experimental study A comparative study involving an intervention or manipulation. It is called a trial when human subjects are involved.

explanatory variable See *independent variable.*

exponential probability distribution A probability distribution used in models of survival or decay.

***F* distribution** The probability distribution used to test the equality of two estimates of the variance. It is the distribution used with the *F* test in ANOVA.

***F* test** The statistical test for comparing two variances. It is used in ANOVA.

face validity An interview or survey that has questions on it that look related to the purpose.

factor A characteristic that is the focus of inquiry in a study; used in analysis of variance.

factor analysis An advanced statistical method for analyzing the relationships among a set of items or indicators to determine the factors or dimensions that underlie them.

factorial design In ANOVA, a design in which each subject (or object) receives one level of each factor.

false-negative (FN) A test result that is negative in a person who has the disease.

false-positive (FP) A test result that is positive in a person who does not have the disease.

first quartile The 25th percentile.

Fisher's exact test An exact test for 2×2 contingency tables. It is used when the sample size is too small to use the chi-square test.

Fisher's z transformation A transformation of the correlation coefficient so that it is normally distributed.

focus groups A process in which a small group of people are interviewed about a topic or issue; often used to help generate questions for a survey, but may be used independently in qualitative research.

forward selection A model-building method in multiple regression that first enters into the regression equation the variable with the highest correlation, followed by the other variables one at a time that increase the multiple R by the greatest amount, until all statistically significant variables are included in the equation.

frequency The number of times a given value of an observation occurs. It is also called counts.

frequency distribution In a set of numerical observations, the list of values that occur along with the frequency of their occurrence. It may be set up as a frequency table or as a graph.

frequency polygon A line graph connecting the midpoints of the tops of the columns of a histogram. It is useful in comparing two frequency distributions.

frequency table A table showing the number or percentage of observations occurring at different values (or ranges of values) of a characteristic or variable.

functional status A measure of a person's ability to perform their daily activities, often called activities of daily living.

game theory A process of assigning subjective probabilities to outcomes from a decision.

Gaussian distribution See *normal distribution.*

Gehan's test A statistical test of the equality of two survival curves.

Generalized estimating equations (GEE) A complex multivariate method used to analyze situations in which subjects are nested within groups when observations between subjects are not independent.

generalized Wilcoxon test See *Gehan's test.*

geometric mean (GM) The nth root of the product of n observations, symbolized GM or G. It is used with logarithms or skewed distributions.

gold standard In diagnostic testing, a procedure that always identifies the true condition—diseased or disease-free—of a patient.

Hawthorne effect A bias introduced into an observational study when the subjects know they are in a study, and it is this knowledge that affects their behavior.

hazard function The probability that a person dies in a certain time interval, given that the person has lived until the beginning of the interval. Its reciprocal is mean survival time.

hazard ratio Similar to the risk ratio, it is the ratio of risk of the outcome (such as death) occurring at any time in one group compared with another group.

hierarchical design A study design in which one or more of the treatments is nested within levels of another factor, such as patients within hospitals.

hierarchical regression A logical model-building method in multiple regression in which the investigators group variables according to their function and add them to the regression equation as a group or block.

histogram A graph of a frequency distribution of numerical observations.

historical cohort study A cohort study that uses existing records or historical data to determine the effect of a risk factor or exposure on a group of patients.

historical controls In clinical trials, previously collected observations on patients that are used as the control values against which the treatment is compared.

homogeneity The situation in which the standard deviation of the dependent (Y) variable is the same, regardless of the value of the independent (X) variable; an assumption in ANOVA and regression.

homoscedasticity See *homogeneity.*

Hosmer and Lemeshow's Goodness of Fit Test A multivariate test used to test the significance of the overall results from a logistic regression analysis.

hypothesis test An approach to statistical inference resulting in a decision to reject or not to reject the null hypothesis.

incidence A rate giving the proportion of people who develop a given disease or condition within a specified period of time.

independent events Events whose occurrence or outcome has no effect on the probability of the other.

independent groups or samples Samples for which the values in one group cannot be predicted from the values in the other group.

independent observations Observations determined at different times or by different individuals without knowledge of the value of the first observation.

independent variable The explanatory or predictor variable in a study. It is sometimes called a factor in ANOVA.

independent-groups _t_ test See _two-sample t test._

index of suspicion See _prior probability._

inference (statistical) The process of drawing conclusions about a population of observations from a sample of observations.

intention-to-treat (principle) The statistical analysis of all subjects according to the group to which they were originally assigned or belonged.

interaction A relationship between two independent variables such that they have a different effect on the dependent variable; that is, the effect of one level of a factor _A_ depends on the level of factor _B_.

intercept In a regression equation, the predicted value of _Y_ when _X_ is equal to zero.

internal consistency (reliability) The degree to which the items on an instrument or test are related to each other and provide a measure of a single characteristic.

interquartile range The difference between the 25th percentile and the 75th percentile.

interrater reliability The reliability between measurements made by two different persons (or raters).

intervention The maneuver used in an experimental study. It may be a drug or a procedure.

intrarater reliability The reliability between measurements made by the same person (or rater) at two different points in time.

jackknife A method of cross-validation in which one observation at a time is left out of the sample; regression is performed on the remaining observations, and the results are applied to the original observation.

joint probability The probability of two events occurring at the same time.

Kaplan–Meier product limit method A method for analyzing survival for censored observations. It uses exact survival times in the calculations.

kappa (κ) A statistic used to measure interrater or intrarater agreement for nominal measures.

key concepts Concepts and topics identified in each chapter as being the key take-home messages.

least squares regression The most common form of regression in which the values for the intercept and regression coefficient(s) are found by minimizing the squared difference between the actual and predicted values of the outcome variable.

length of time to event A term used in outcome and cost-effectiveness studies; it measures the length of time from a treatment or assessment until the outcome of interest occurs.

level of significance The probability of incorrectly rejecting the null hypothesis in a test of hypothesis. Also see _alpha value_ and _p value._

Levene's test A test of the equality of two variances. It is less sensitive to departures from normality than the _F_ test and is often recommended by statisticians.

life table analysis A method for analyzing survival times for censored observations that have been grouped into intervals.

likelihood The probability of an outcome or event happening, given the parameters of the distribution of the outcome, such as the mean and standard deviation.

likelihood ratio In diagnostic testing, the ratio of true-positives to false-positives.

linear combination A weighted average of a set of variables or measures. For example, the prediction equation in multiple regression is a linear combination of the predictor variables.

linear regression (of _Y_ on _X_) The process of determining a regression or prediction equation to predict _Y_ from _X._

linear relationship (between _X_ and _Y_) A relationship indicating that _X_ and _Y_ vary together according to constant increments.

logarithm (ln) The exponent indicating the power to which _e_ (2.718) is raised to obtain a given number; also called the natural logarithm.

logistic regression The regression technique used when the outcome is a binary, or dichotomous, variable.

log-linear analysis A statistical method for analyzing the relationships among three or more nominal variables. It may be used as a regression method to predict a nominal outcome from nominal independent variables.

logrank test A statistical method for comparing two survival curves when censored observations occur.

longitudinal study A study that takes place over an extended period of time.

Mann-Whitney–Wilcoxon test See _Wilcoxon rank sum test._

Mantel–Haenszel chi-square test A statistical test of two or more 2×2 tables. It is used to compare survival distributions or to control for confounding factors.

marginal frequencies The row and column frequencies in a contingency table; that is, the frequencies listed on the margins of the table.

marginal probability The row and column probabilities in a contingency table; that is, the probabilities listed on the margins of the table.

matched-groups _t_ test See _paired t test._

matching (or matched groups) The process of making two groups homogeneous on possible confounding factors. It is sometimes done prior to randomization in clinical trials.

McNemar's test The chi-square test for comparing proportions from two dependent or paired groups.

mean ($\overline{X}$) The most common measure of central tendency, denoted by μ in the population and by in the sample. In a sample, the mean is the sum of the X values divided by the number n in the sample ($\Sigma X/n$).

mean square among groups (MS_A) An estimate of the variation in analysis of variance. It is used in the numerator of the F statistic.

mean square within groups (MS_W) An estimate of the variation in analysis of variance. It is used in the denominator of the F statistic.

measurement error The amount by which a measurement is incorrect because of problems inherent in the measuring process; also called bias.

measures of central tendency Index or summary numbers that describe the middle of a distribution. See *mean, median,* and *mode.*

measures of dispersion Index or summary numbers that describe the spread of observations about the mean. See *range; standard deviation.*

median (M or Md) A measure of central tendency. It is the middle observation; that is, the one that divides the distribution of values into halves. It is also equal to the 50th percentile.

medical decision-making or analysis The application of probabilities to the decision process in medicine. It is the basis for cost–benefit analysis.

MEDLINE A system that permits search of the bibliographic database of all articles in journals included in *Index Medicus.* Articles that meet specific criteria or contain specific key words are extracted for the researcher's perusal

meta-analysis A method for combining the results from several independent studies of the same outcome so that an overall p value may be determined.

minimally important clinical difference (MCID) The smallest amount a metric can change and be meaningful to clinicians and/or patients.

minimum variance A desirable characteristic of a statistic that estimates a population parameter, meaning that its variance or standard deviation is less than that of another statistic; that is, the sample mean (X) has a smaller standard deviation than the median, although both are estimators of the population mean μ.

modal class The interval (generally from a frequency table or histogram) that contains the highest frequency of observations.

mode The value of a numerical variable that occurs the most frequently.

model or modeling A statistical statement of the relationship among variables, sometimes based upon a theoretical model.

morbidity rate The number of patients in a defined population who develop a morbid condition over a specified period of time.

mortality rate The number of deaths in a defined population over a specified period. It is the number of people who die during a given period of time divided by the number of people at risk during the period.

multiple comparisons Comparisons resulting from many statistical tests performed for the same observations.

multiple R In multiple regression, the correlation between actual and predicted values of Y (i.e., $r_{YY'}$).

multiple regression A multivariate method for determining a regression or prediction equation to predict an outcome from a set of independent variables.

multiple-comparison procedure A method for comparing several means.

multiplication rule The rule that states the probability that two or more independent events all occur is the product of the probabilities of each individual event.

multivariate A term that refers to a study or analysis involving multiple independent or dependent variables.

multivariate analysis of variance (MANOVA) An advanced statistical method that provides a global test when there are multiple dependent variables and the independent variables are nominal. It is analogous to analysis of variance with multiple outcome measures.

mutually exclusive events Two or more events for which the occurrence of one event precludes the occurrence of the others.

natural log (ln) A logarithm with the base e ($e \approx$ 2.718) compared with the other well-known logarithm to base 10 (log). e describes population growth patterns and is very important in logistic and Cox regression where the inverse (the antilog) of the regression coefficients are adjusted odds ratios.

Newman–Keuls procedure A multiple-comparison method for making pairwise comparisons between means following a significant F test in analysis of variance.

nominal scale The simplest scale of measurement. It is used for characteristics that have no numerical values (examples are race and gender). It is also called a categorical or qualitative scale.

nondirectional test See *two-tailed test.*

nonmutually exclusive events Two or more events for which the occurrence of one event does not preclude the occurrence of the others.

nonparametric method A statistical test that makes no assumptions regarding the distribution of the observations.

nonprobability sample A sample selected in such a way that the probability that a subject is selected is unknown.

nonrandomized trial A clinical trial in which subjects are assigned to treatments on other than a randomized basis. It is subject to several biases.

normal distribution A symmetric, bell-shaped probability distribution with mean μ and standard deviation σ. If observations follow a normal distribution, the interval $(\mu \pm 2\sigma)$ contains 95% of the observations. It is also called the Gaussian distribution.

null hypothesis The hypothesis being tested about a population. *Null* generally means "no difference" and thus refers to a situation in which no difference exists (e.g., between the means in a treatment group and a control group).

number needed to harm (NNH) The number of patients that need to be treated with a proposed therapy in order to cause one undesirable outcome.

number needed to treat (NNT) The number of patients that need to be treated with a proposed therapy in order to prevent or cure one individual; it is the reciprocal of the absolute risk reduction (1/ARR).

numerical scale The highest level of measurement. It is used for characteristics that can be given numerical values; the differences between numbers have meaning (examples are height, weight, blood pressure level). It is also called an interval or ratio scale.

objective probability An estimate of probability from observable events or phenomena.

observational study A study that does not involve an intervention or manipulation. It is called case–control, cross-sectional, or cohort, depending on the design of the study.

observed frequencies The frequencies that occur in a study. They are generally arranged in a contingency table.

odds ratio (OR) An estimate of the relative risk calculated in case–control studies. It is the odds that a patient was exposed to a given risk factor divided by the odds that a control was exposed to the risk factor.

odds The probability that an event will occur divided by the probability that the event will not occur; that is, odds $= P/(1 - P)$, where P is the probability.

one-tailed test A test in which the alternative hypothesis specifies a deviation from the null hypothesis in one direction only. The critical region is located in one end of the distribution of the test statistic. It is also called a directional test.

open-ended question A question on an interview or questionnaire that has a fill-in-the-blank answer.

ordinal scale Used for characteristics that have an underlying order to their values; the numbers used are arbitrary (an example is Apgar scores).

orphan p A p value given without reference to the statistical method used to determine it.

orthogonal Independent, nonredundant, or non-overlapping, such as orthogonal comparisons in ANOVA or orthogonal factors in factor analysis.

outcome (in an experiment) The result of an experiment or trial.

outcome assessment The process of including quality-of-life or physical-function variables in clinical outcomes. Studies that focus on outcomes often emphasize how patients view and value their health, the care they receive, and the results or outcomes of this care.

outcome variable The dependent or criterion variable in a study.

p value The probability of observing a result as extreme as or more extreme than the one actually observed from chance alone (i.e., if the null hypothesis is true).

paired design See *repeated-measures design*.

paired t test The statistical method for comparing the difference (or change) in a numerical variable observed for two paired (or matched) groups. It also applies to before-and-after measurements made on the same group of subjects.

parameter The population value of a characteristic of a distribution (e.g., the mean μ).

patient satisfaction Refers to outcome measures of patient's liking and approval of health care facilities and operations, providers, and other components of the entities that provide patient care.

percentage A proportion multiplied by 100.

percentage polygon A line graph connecting the midpoints of the tops of the columns of a histogram based on percentages instead of counts. It is useful in comparing two or more sets of observations when the frequencies in each group are not equal.

percentile A number that indicates the percentage of a distribution that is less than or equal to that number.

person-years Found by adding the length of time subjects are in a study. This concept is frequently used in epidemiology but is not recommended by statisticians because of difficulties in interpretation and analysis.

piecewise linear regression A method used to estimate sections of a regression line when a curvilinear relationship exists between the independent and dependent variables.

placebo A sham treatment or procedure. It is used to reduce bias in clinical studies.

point estimate A general term for any statistic (e.g., mean, standard deviation, proportion).

Poisson distribution A probability distribution used to model the number of times a rare event occurs.

poll A questionnaire administered to a sample of people, often about a single issue.

polynomial regression A special case of multiple regression in which each term in the equation is a power of the independent variable X. Polynomial regression provides a way to fit a regression model to curvilinear relationships and is an alternative to transforming the data to a linear scale.

pooled standard deviation The standard deviation used in the independent-groups t test when the standard deviations in the two groups are equal.

population The entire collection of observations or subjects that have something in common and to which conclusions are inferred.

post hoc comparison Method for comparing means following analysis of variance.

post hoc method See *post hoc comparison*.

posterior probability The conditional probability calculated by using Bayes' theorem. It is the predictive value of a positive test (true-positives divided by all positives) or a negative test (true-negatives divided by all negatives).

posteriori method See *post hoc comparison*.

posttest odds In diagnostic testing, the odds that a patient has a given disease or condition after a diagnostic procedure is performed and interpreted. They are similar to the predictive value of a diagnostic test.

power The ability of a test statistic to detect a specified alternative hypothesis or difference of a specified size when the alternative hypothesis is true (i.e., $1 - \beta$, where β is the probability of a type II error). More loosely, it is the ability of a study to detect an actual effect or difference.

preattentive attributes visual properties that are processed much faster by the brain when presented. They include color, form, movement, and special positioning.

predictive value of a negative test (PV–) The proportion of time that a patient with a negative diagnostic test result does not have the disease being investigated.

predictive value of a positive test (PV+) The proportion of time that a patient with a positive diagnostic test result has the disease being investigated.

pretest odds In diagnostic testing, the odds that a patient has a given disease or condition before a diagnostic procedure is performed and interpreted. They are similar to prior probabilities.

prevalence The proportion of people who have a given disease or condition at a specified point in time. It is not truly a rate, although it is often incorrectly called prevalence rate.

prior probability The unconditional probability used in the numerator of Bayes' theorem. It is the prevalence of a disease prior to performing a diagnostic procedure. Clinicians often refer to it as the index of suspicion.

probability distribution A frequency distribution of a random variable, which may be empirical or theoretical (e.g., normal, binomial).

probability sample See *random sample*.

probability The number of times an outcome occurs in the total number of trials. If A is the outcome, the probability of A is denoted $P(A)$.

product limit method See *Kaplan–Meier product limit method*.

progressively censored A situation in which patients enter a study at different points in time and remain in the study for varying lengths of time. See *censored observation*.

propensity score An advanced statistical method to control for an entire group of confounding variables.

proportion The number of observations with the characteristic of interest divided by the total number of observations. It is used to summarize counts.

proportional hazards model See *Cox proportional hazard model*.

prospective study A study designed before data are collected.

PUBMED See *MEDLINE*.

qualitative observations Characteristics measured on a nominal scale.

quality of life (QOL) A measure of a person's subjective assessment of the value of their health and functional abilities.

quantitative observations Characteristics measured on a numerical scale; the resulting numbers have inherent meaning.

quartile The 25th percentile or the 75th percentile, called the first and third quartiles, respectively.

random assignment The use of random methods to assign different treatments to patients or vice versa.

random error or **variation** The variation in a sample that can be expected to occur by chance.

random sample A sample of n subjects (or objects) selected from a population so that each has a known chance of being in the sample.

random variable A variable in a study in which subjects are randomly selected or randomly assigned to treatments.

randomization The process of assigning subjects to different treatments (or vice versa) by using random numbers.

randomized block design A study design used in ANOVA to help control for potential confounding.

randomized controlled trial (RCT) An experimental study in which subjects are randomly assigned to treatment groups.

range The difference between the largest and the smallest observation.

ranking scale A question format on an interview or survey in which respondents are asked to rate (from 1 to . . .) the options listed.

rank-order scale A scale for observations arranged according to their size, from lowest to highest or vice versa.

ranks A set of observations arranged according to their size, from lowest to highest or vice versa.

rate A proportion associated with a multiplier, called the base (e.g., 1,000, 10,000, 100,000), and computed over a specific period.

ratio A part divided by another part. It is the number of observations with the characteristic of interest divided by the number without the characteristic.

regression (of Y on X) The process of determining a prediction equation for predicting Y from X.

regression coefficient The b in the simple regression equation $Y = a + bX$. It is sometimes interpreted as the slope of the regression line. In multiple regression, the bs are weights applied to the predictor variables.

regression toward the mean The phenomenon in which a predicted outcome for any given person tends to be closer to the mean outcome than the person's actual observation.

relative risk (RR) The ratio of the incidence of a given disease in exposed or at-risk persons to the incidence of the disease in unexposed persons. It is calculated in cohort or prospective studies.

relative risk reduction (RRR) The reduction in risk with a new therapy relative to the risk without the new therapy; it is the absolute value of the difference between the experimental event rate and the control event rate divided by the control event rate (|EER − CER|/CER).

reliability A measure of the reproducibility of a measurement. It is measured by kappa for nominal measures and by correlation for numerical measures.

repeated-measures design A study design in which subjects are measured at more than one time. It is also called a split-plot design in ANOVA.

representative population (or sample) A population or sample that is similar in important ways to the population to which the findings of a study are generalized.

residual The difference between the predicted value and the actual value of the outcome (dependent) variable in regression.

response variable See *dependent variable*.

retrospective cohort study See *historical cohort study*.

retrospective study A study undertaken in a post hoc manner, that is, after the observations have been made.

risk factor A term used to designate a characteristic that is more prevalent among subjects who develop a given disease or outcome than among subjects who do not. It is generally considered to be causal.

risk ratio See *relative risk*.

robust A term used to describe a statistical method if the outcome is not affected to a large extent by a violation of the assumptions of the method.

ROC (receiver operating characteristic) curve In diagnostic testing, a plot of the true-positives on the Y-axis versus the false-positives on the X-axis; used to evaluate the properties of a diagnostic test.

r-squared (r^2) The square of the correlation coefficient. It is interpreted as the amount of variance in one variable that is accounted for by knowing the second variable.

sample A subset of the population.

sampled population The population from which the sample is actually selected.

sampling distribution (of a statistic) The frequency distribution of the statistic for many samples. It is used to make inferences about the statistic from a single sample.

sampling frame A list of all possible subjects or objects in the population from which a random sample is to be drawn; required for some types of sampling, such as systematic sampling.

scale of measurement The degree of precision with which a characteristic is measured. It is generally categorized into nominal (or categorical), ordinal, and numerical (or interval and ratio) scales.

scatterplot A two-dimensional graph displaying the relationship between two numerical characteristics or variables.

Scheffé's procedure A multiple-comparison method for comparing means following a significant F test in analysis of variance. It is the most conservative multiple-comparison method.

self-controlled study A study in which the subjects serve as their own controls, achieved by measuring the characteristic of interest before and after an intervention.

sensitivity analysis In decision analysis, a method for determining the way the decision changes as a function of probabilities and utilities used in the analysis.

sensitivity The proportion of time a diagnostic test is positive in patients who have the disease or condition. A sensitive test has a low false-negative rate.

sex-specific mortality rate A mortality rate specific to either males or females.

sign test The nonparametric test used for testing a hypothesis about the median in a single group.

simple random sample A random sample in which each of the n subjects (or objects) in the sample has an equal chance of being selected.

skewed distribution A distribution in which a few outlying observations occur in one direction only. If the outlying observations are small, the distribution is skewed to the left, or negatively skewed; if they are large, the distribution is skewed to the right, or positively skewed.

slope (of the regression line) The amount Y changes for each unit that X changes. It is designated by b in the sample.

Spearman's rank correlation (rho) A nonparametric correlation that measures the tendency for two measurements to vary together.

specific rate A rate that pertains to a specific group or segment of the observations (examples are age-specific mortality rate and cause-specific mortality rate).

specificity The proportion of time that a diagnostic test is negative in patients who do not have the disease or condition. A specific test has a low false-positive rate.

standard deviation (SD) The most common measure of dispersion or spread, denoted by σ in the population and SD or s in the sample. It can be used with the mean to describe the distribution of observations. It is the square root of the average of the squared deviations of the observations from their mean.

standard error (SE) The standard deviation of the sampling distribution of a statistic.

standard error of the estimate ($S_{y.x}$) A measure of the variation in a regression line. It is based on the differences between the predicted and actual values of the dependent variable Y.

standard error of the mean (SEM) The standard deviation of the mean in a large number of samples.

standard normal distribution The normal distribution with mean 0 and standard deviation 1, also called the z distribution.

standardized mortality ratio The number of observed deaths divided by the number of expected deaths.

standardized regression coefficient A regression coefficient that has the effect of the measurement scale removed so that the size of the coefficient can be interpreted.

statistic A summary number for a sample (e.g., the mean), often used as an estimate of a parameter in the population.

statistical significance Generally interpreted as a result that would occur by chance, for example, 1 time in 20, with a p value less than or equal to 0.05. It occurs when the null hypothesis is rejected.

statistical test The procedure used to test a null hypothesis (e.g., t test, chi-square test).

stem-and-leaf plot A graphic display for numerical data. It is similar to both a frequency table and a histogram.

stepwise regression In multiple regression, a sequential method of selecting the variables to be included in the prediction equation.

stratified random sample A sample consisting of random samples from each subpopulation (or stratum) in a population. It is used so that the investigator can be sure that each subpopulation is appropriately represented in the sample.

structured abstract A journal article abstract that contains short, precise descriptions of the context of the study, the objective, design, setting and participants, the methods or interventions, main outcomes, results, and conclusions.

subjective probability An estimate of probability that reflects a person's opinion or best guess from previous experience.

sums of squares (SS) Quantities calculated in analysis of variance and used to obtain the mean squares for the F test.

suppression of zero A term used to describe a misleading graph that does not have a break (a jagged line) in the Y-axis to indicate that part of the scale is missing.

survey An observational study that generally has a cross-sectional design; a commonly used design to collect opinions.

survival analysis The statistical method for analyzing survival data when there are censored observations.

symbols Often Greek letters that stand for the population parameters and the Latin letters that stand for the sample statistics.

symmetric distribution A distribution that has the same shape on both sides of the mean. The mean, median, and mode are all equal. It is the opposite of a skewed distribution.

systematic error A measurement error that is the same (or constant) over all observations. See also *bias*.

systematic random sample A random sample obtained by selecting each kth subject or object.

t **distribution** A symmetric distribution with mean zero and a standard deviation larger than that for the normal distribution for small sample sizes. As *n* increases, the *t* distribution approaches the normal distribution.

t **test** The statistical test for comparing a mean with a norm or for comparing two means with small sample sizes ($n \le 30$). It is also used for testing whether a correlation coefficient or a regression coefficient is zero.

target population The population to which the investigator wishes to generalize.

test statistic The specific statistic used to test the null hypothesis (e.g., the *t* statistic or chi-square statistic).

testing threshold In diagnostic testing, the point at which the optimal decision is to perform a diagnostic test.

test–retest reliability A measure of the degree to which an instrument or test provides a consistent measure of a characteristic on different occasions.

third quartile The 75th percentile.

threshold model A model for deciding when a diagnostic test should be ordered, as opposed to doing nothing or treating the patient without performing the test.

transformation A change in the scale for the values of a variable.

treatment threshold In diagnostic testing, the point at which the optimal decision is to treat the patient without first performing a diagnostic test.

trial An experiment involving humans, commonly called a clinical trial. It is also a replication (repetition) of an experiment.

true-negative (TN) A test result that is negative in a person who does not have the disease.

true-positive (TP) A test result that is positive in a person who has the disease.

Tukey's HSD (honestly significant difference) test A post hoc test for making multiple pairwise comparisons between means following a significant *F* test in analysis of variance. It is a method highly recommended by statisticians.

two-sample *t* test The statistical test used to test the null hypothesis that two independent (or unrelated) groups have the same mean.

two-tailed test A test in which the alternative hypothesis specifies a deviation from the null hypothesis in either direction. The critical region is located in both ends of the distribution of the test statistic. It is also called a directional test.

two-way analysis of variance ANOVA with two independent variables.

type I error The error that results if a true null hypothesis is rejected or if a difference is concluded when no difference exists.

type II error The error that results if a false null hypothesis is not rejected or if a difference is not detected when a difference exists.

unbiasedness (of a statistic) A term used to describe a statistic whose mean based on a large number of samples is equal to the population parameter.

uncontrolled study An experimental study that has no control subjects.

utility The value of different outcomes in a decision tree.

validity The property of a measurement that indicates how well it measures the characteristic.

variable A characteristic of interest in a study that has different values for different subjects or objects.

variance (σ^2 in the population, s^2 in the sample) The square of the standard deviation.

variation (within subject) The variability in measurements of the same object or subject. It may occur naturally or may represent an error.

vital statistics Mortality and morbidity rates used in epidemiology and public health.

weighted average A number formed by multiplying each number in a set of numbers by a value called a weight, adding the resulting products, and then dividing by the sum of the weight.

Wilcoxon rank sum test A nonparametric test for comparing two independent samples with ordinal data or with numerical observations that are not normally distributed.

Wilcoxon signed ranks test A nonparametric test for comparing two dependent samples with ordinal data or with numerical observations that are not normally distributed.

Yates' correction The process of subtracting 0.5 from the numerator at each term in the chi-square statistic for 2×2 tables prior to squaring the term.

z **approximation** (to the binomial) The *z* test used to test the equality of two independent proportions.

z **distribution** The normal distribution with mean 0 and standard deviation 1. It is also called the standard normal distribution.

z **ratio** The test statistic used in the *z* test. It is formed by subtracting the hypothesized mean from the observed mean and dividing by the standard error of the mean.

z **score** The deviation of *X* from the mean divided by the standard deviation.

z **test** The statistical test for comparing a mean with a norm or comparing two means for large samples ($n \ge 30$).

z **transformation** A transformation that changes a normally distributed variable with mean and standard deviation *SD* to the *z* distribution with mean 0 and standard deviation 1.

References

Abraham A, Alabdali M, Alsulaiman A, et al. The sensitivity and specificity of the neurological examination in polyneuropathy patients with clinical and electrophysiological correlations. *PLoS One*. 2017;12(3):e0171597. https://doi.org/10.1371/journal.pone.0171597.

Alderman EL, Bourassa MG, Cohen LS, et al. Ten-year follow-up of survival and myocardial infarction in the randomized Coronary Artery Surgery Study. *Circulation*. 1990;82:1629–1646.

Alonso-Coello P, Irfan A, Solà I, et al. The quality of clinical practice guidelines over the last two decades: a systematic review of guideline appraisal studies. *Qual Saf Health Care*. 2010;19:e58.

Altman DG, De Stavola BL, Love SB, Stepniewska KA. Review of survival analysis published in cancer journals. *Br J Cancer*. 1995;72:511–518.

Anasetti C, Doney KC, Storb R, et al. Marrow transplantation for severe aplastic anemia. *Ann Intern Med*. 1986;104:461–466.

Anastasi A, Urbina S. *Psychological Testing*. 7th ed. London, UK: Macmillan; 1997.

Anderson KB, Simasathien S, Watanaveeradej V, et al. Clinical and laboratory predictors of influenza infection among individuals with influenza-like illness presenting to an urban Thai hospital over a five-year period. *PLoS One*. 2018;13(3):e0193050. https://doi.org/10.1371/journal.pone.0193050.

Andrewes D, Kaye A, Aitken S, Parr C, Bates L, Murphy M. The ESDQ: a new method of assessing emotional and social dysfunction in patients following brain surgery. *J Clin Exp Neuropsychol*. 2003;25:173–189.

Bagwell K, Wu X, Baum ED, et al. Cost-effectiveness analysis of intracapsular tonsillectomy and total tonsillectomy for pediatric obstructive sleep apnea. *Appl Health Econ Health Policy*. 2018;16:527. https://doi.org/10.1007/s40258-018-0396-4.

Bajwa K, Szabo E, Kjellstrand CM. A prospective study of risk factors and decision making in discontinuation of dialysis. *Arch Intern Med*. 1996;156:2571–2577.

Bale P, Bradbury D, Colley E. Anthropometric and training variables related to 10 km running performance. *Br J Sports Med*. 1986;20:170–173.

Barker DJP. Rise and fall of western diseases. *Nature*. 1989;338:371–372.

Bartko JJ. Rationale for reporting standard deviations rather than standard errors of the mean. *Am J Psychiatry*. 1985;142:1060.

Bellou V, Belbasis L, Tzoulaki I, Evangelou E. Risk factors for type 2 diabetes mellitus: an exposure-wide umbrella review of meta-analyses. *PLoS One*. 2018;13(3):e0194127. https://doi.org/10.1371/journal.pone.0194127.

Berkson J. Limitations of the application of four-fold table analyses to hospital data. *Biometrics Bull*. 1946;2:47–53.

Berry G, Matthews JNS, Armitage P. *Statistical Methods in Medical Research*. 4th ed. Oxford, UK: Blackwell Scientific; 2001.

Billioti de Gage S, Yola M, Thierry D, et al. Benzodiazepine use and risk of Alzheimer's disease: case-control study. *BMJ*. 2014;349:g5205.

Bordage G, Dawson B. Experimental study design and grant writing in eight steps and 28 questions. *Med Educ*. 2003;37:376–385.

Bos-Touwen I, Schuurmans M, Monninkhof EM, et al. Patient and disease characteristics associated with activation for self-management in patients with diabetes, chronic obstructive pulmonary disease, chronic heart failure and chronic renal disease: a cross-sectional survey study. *PLoS One*. 2015;10(5):e0126400. https://doi.org/10.1371/journal.pone.0126400.

Bottegoni C, Dei Giudici L, Salvemini S, et al. Homologous platelet-rich plasma for the treatment of knee osteoarthritis in selected elderly patients: an open-label, uncontrolled, pilot study. *Ther Adv Musculoskelet Dis*. 2016. https://doi.org/10.1177/1759720X16631188.

Box GEP. Non-normality and tests on variance. *Biometrika*. 1953;40:318–335.

Box GEP. Some theorems on quadratic forms applied in the study of the analysis of variance. *Ann Math Stat*. 1954;25:290–302.

Brtnikova M, Crane LA, Allison MA, Hurley LP, Beaty BL, Kempe A. A method for achieving high response rates in national surveys of U.S. primary care physicians. *PLoS One*. 2018;13(8):e0202755. https://doi.org/10.1371/journal.pone.0202755.

Buchsbaum DG, Buchanan RG, Centor RM, Schnoll SH, Lawton MJ. Screening for alcohol abuse using CAGE scores and likelihood ratios. *Ann Intern Med*. 1991;115:774–777.

Burns N, Grove SK. *Understanding Nursing Research*. 6th ed. Philadelphia, PA: WB Saunders; 2014.

Bush B, Shaw S, Cleary P, Delbanco TL, Aronson MD. Screening for alcohol abuse using the CAGE questionnaire. *Am J Med*. 1987;82:231–235.

Byrt T. How good is that agreement? (Letter to editor). *Epidemiology*. 1996;7:561.

Cai J, Karam JA, Parvizi J, Smith EB, Sharkey PF. Aquacel surgical dressing reduces the rate of acute pji following total joint arthroplasty: a case–control study. The Rothman Institute at Thomas Jefferson University Hospital, Philadelphia, PA. *J Arthroplasty*. 2014;29:1098–1100.

Caiola E, Litaker D. Factors influencing the selection of general internal medicine fellowship programs. *J Gen Intern Med*. 2000;15:656–658.

CASS Principal Investigators and Associates: Coronary Artery Surgery Study (CASS). A randomized trial of coronary bypass surgery. *Circulation*. 1983;68:951–960.

Centers for Disease Control and Prevention. Seasonal Influenza Vaccine Safety: A Summary for Clinicians. 2017. Accessed April 28, 2019. https://www.cdc.gov/flu/professionals/vaccination/vaccine_safety.htm.

Chatfield C. *Problem Solving: A Statistician's Guide*. 2nd ed. London, UK: Chapman & Hall; 1995.

Chaudhry M, Chan C, Su-Myat S, et al. Ascertaining cancer survivors in Ontario using the Ontario Cancer Registry and administrative data. *J Clin Oncol*. 2018;36:7(suppl):34–34

Chochinov HM, Hassard T, McClement S, et al. The Patient Dignity Inventory: a novel way of measuring dignity-related distress in palliative care. *J Pain Symptom Manage*. 2008;36(6):559–571.

Ciemins EL, Coon PJ, Coombs NC, et al. Intent-to-treat analysis of a simultaneous multisite telehealth diabetes prevention program. *BMJ Open Diabetes Res Care*. 2018;6:e000515. doi:10.1136/bmjdrc-2018-000515.

Cohen J. *Statistical Power Analysis for the Behavioral Sciences*. 2nd ed. Cambridge, MA: Academic Press; 1988.

Cohen J. A power primer. *Psychol Bull*. 1992;112(1):155–159.

Colditz GA, Manson JE, Hankinson SE. The Nurses' Health Study: 20-year contribution to the understanding of health among women. *J Womens Health*. 1997;6:49–62.

Collett D. *Modelling Survival Data in Medical Research*. 2nd ed. London, UK: Chapman & Hill; 2003.

Colton T. *Statistics in Medicine*. London, UK: Little, Brown Book Group; 1974.

Conover WJ. *Practical Nonparametric Statistics*. 3rd ed. Hoboken, NJ: Wiley; 1999.

Conover WJ, Iman RL. Rank transformations as a bridge between parametric and nonparametric statistics. *Am Stat*. 1981;35:124–129.

Cornelis E, Gorus E, Beyer I, Bautmans I, De Vriendt P. Early diagnosis of mild cognitive impairment and mild dementia through basic and instrumental activities of daily living: Development of a new evaluation tool. *PLoS Med*. 2017;14(3):e1002250. https://doi.org/10.1371/journal.pmed.1002250.

Cox DR. Regression models and life tables. *J R Stat Soc Series B*. 1972;34:187–220.

Cramer JA, Spilker B. *Quality of Life and Pharmacoeconomics: An Introduction*. 2nd ed. Philadelphia, PA: Lippincott-Raven; 1998.

Cutler S, Ederer F. Maximum utilization of the lifetable method in analyzing survival. *J Chronic Dis*. 1958;8:699–712.

D'Angio CT, Maniscalco WM, Pichichero ME. Immunologic responses of extremely premature infants to tetanus, Haemophilus influenzae, and polio immunizations. *Pediatrics*. 1995;96:18–22.

Dabi Y, Nedellec S, Bonneau C, Trouchard B, Rouzier R, Benachi A. Clinical validation of a model predicting the risk of preterm delivery. *PLoS One*. 2017;12(2):e0171801. https://doi.org/10.1371/journal.pone.0171801.

Daniel WW, Cross CL. *Biostatistics: A Foundation for Analysis in the Health Sciences*. 11th ed. Hoboken, NJ: Wiley; 2018.

Davidoff F. In the teeth of the evidence: The curious case of evidence-based medicine. *Mt Sinai J Med*. 1999;66:75–83.

Davids BO, Hutchins SS, Jones CP, et al. Disparities in life expectancy across US counties linked to county social factors, 2009 Community Health Status Indicators (CHSI). *J Racial Ethn Health Disparities*. 2014;1:2. https://doi.org/10.1007/s40615-013-0001-3.

Dawson B. Review of Multivariable Statistics. *Teach Learn Med*. 2000;12:108.

Dawson-Saunders B, Azen S, Greenberg R, Reed A. The instruction of biostatistics in medical schools. *Am Stat*. 1987;41(4):263–266. doi:10.1080/00031305.1987.10475497.

de Boer RA, Nayor M, deFilippi CR, et al. Association of cardiovascular biomarkers with incident heart failure with preserved and reduced ejection fraction. *JAMA Cardiol*. 2018; doi:10.1001/jamacardio.2017.4987.

Dennison BA, Rockwell HL, Baker SL. Excess fruit juice consumption by preschool-aged children is associated with short stature and obesity. *Pediatrics*. 1997;99:15–22.

Detsky AS, Abrams HB, McLaughlin JR, et al. Predicting cardiac complication in patients undergoing non-cardiac surgery. *J Gen Intern Med*. 1986;1:211–219.

Deyo RA, Diehl AK. Cancer as a cause of low back pain: Frequency, clinical presentation, and diagnostic strategies? *J Gen Intern Med*. 1988;3:230–238.

Deyo RA, Rainville J, Kent DL. What can the history and physical examination tell us about low back pain? *JAMA*. 1992;268:760–765.

Deyo RA, Jarvik JG, Chou R. Low back pain in primary care. *BMJ*. 2014;349:g4266.

Dillman DA, Smyth JD, Christian LM. *Mail & Internet Surveys*. 4th ed. Hoboken, NJ: Wiley; 2014.

Dittrich N, Agostino D, Antonini Philippe R, Guglielmo LGA, Place N. Effect of hypnotic suggestion on knee extensor neuromuscular properties in resting and fatigued states. *PLoS One*. 2018;13(4):e0195437. https://doi.org/10.1371/journal.pone.0195437.

Dixon MR, Haukoos JS, Udani SM, et al. Carcinoembryonic antigen and albumin predict survival in patients with advanced colon and rectal cancer. *Arch Surg*. 2003;138:962–966.

Dunn OJ, Clark VA. *Applied Statistics: Analysis of Variance and Regression*. 2nd ed. Hoboken, NJ: Wiley; 1987.

Durand MJ, Murphy SA, Schaefer KK, et al. Impaired hyperemic response to exercise post stroke. *PLoS One*. 2015;10(12):e0144023. https://doi.org/10.1371/journal.pone.0144023.

Dyrbye LN, Burke SE, Hardeman RR, et al. Association of clinical specialty with symptoms of burnout and career choice regret among us resident physicians. *JAMA*. 2018;320(11):1114–1130. doi:10.1001/jama.2018.12615

Dysangco A, Liu Z, Stein JH, Dubé MP, Gupta SK. HIV infection, antiretroviral therapy, and measures of endothelial function, inflammation, metabolism, and oxidative stress. *PLoS One.* 2017;12(8):e0183511. https://doi.org/10.1371/journal.pone.0183511.

Eckel N, Li Y, Kuxhaus O, Stefan N, Hu FB, Schulze MB. Transition from metabolic healthy to unhealthy phenotypes and association with cardiovascular disease risk across BMI categories in 90 257 women (the Nurses' Health Study): 30 year follow-up from a prospective cohort study. *Lancet Diabetes Endocrinol.* 2018;6(9):714–724. doi:10.1016/S2213-8587(18)30137-2. Epub 2018 May 31.

Eddy DM. *Clinical Decision Making: From Theory to Practice: A Collection of Essays.* Sudbury, MA: Jones & Bartlett; 1996.

Einarsson K, Nilsell K, Leijd B, Angelin B. Influence of age on secretion of cholesterol and synthesis of bile acids by the liver. *N Engl J Med.* 1985;313:277–282.

Elveback LR, Guillier CL, Keating FR. Health normality, and the ghost of Gauss. *JAMA.* 1970;211:69–75.

Enright PL, McBurnie MA, Bittner V, et al; Cardiovascular Health Study: The 6-min walk test: A quick measure of functional status in elderly adults. *Chest.* 2003;123:387–398.

Fagan TJ. Nomogram for Bayes' theorem. *N Engl J Med.* 1975;293:257.

Feinstein AR. *Clinical Epidemiology: The Architecture of Research.* Philadelphia, PA: WB Saunders; 1985.

Feinstein AR, Sosin DM, Wells CK. The Will Rogers phenomenon. *N Engl J Med.* 1985;312:1604–1608.

Few S. Effective_Chart_Design.pdf. 2018. http://www.perceptualedge.com/images/Effective_Chart_Design.pdf. Accessed January 5, 2019.

Few S. Visual Perception of Variation in Data Displays. *Visual Business Intelligence Newsletter.* 2016. http://www.perceptualedge.com/articles/visual_business_intelligence/the_visual_perception_of_variation.pdf. Accessed January 5, 2019.

Few S. *Now You See It: Simple Visualization Techniques for Quantitative Analysis.* San Francisco, CA: Analytics Press; 2009.

Fink A, Kosecoff J. *How to Conduct Surveys: A Step-by-Step Guide.* Thousand Oaks, CA: SAGE; 1998.

Finnerup N, Attal N, Haroutounian S, et al. Pharmacotherapy for neuropathic pain in adults: a systematic review and meta-analysis. *Lancet Neurol.* 2015;14(2):162–173. https://doi.org/10.1016/S1474-4422(14)70251-0.

Fisher LD, van Belle G. *Biostatistics: A Methodology for Health Sciences.* Hoboken, NJ: Wiley; 1996.

Fleiss JL. *Statistical Methods for Rates and Proportions.* 2nd ed. Hoboken, NJ: Wiley; 1981.

Fleiss JL. *Design and Analysis of Clinical Experiments.* Hoboken, NJ: Wiley; 1999.

Fox J., and Bouchet-Valat M. (2019). Rcmdr: R Commander. R package version 2.5-3.

Fox J, Carvalho M. The RcmdrPlugin.survival package: Extending the R Commander interface to survival analysis. *J Stat Softw.* 2012;49(7).

Gage TP. Managing the cancer risk in chronic ulcerative colitis. *J Clin Gastroenterol.* 1986;8:50–57.

Garb JL. *Understanding Medical Research.* London, UK: Little, Brown Book Group; 1996.

Gardner CD, Trepanowski JF, Del Gobbo LC, et al. Effect of low-fat vs low-carbohydrate diet on 12-month weight loss in overweight adults and the association with genotype pattern or insulin secretion. The DIETFITS randomized clinical trial. *JAMA.* 2018;319(7):667–679. doi:10.1001/jama.2018.0245

Gardner MJ, Altman DG. Confidence intervals rather than P values: estimation rather than hypothesis testing. *BMJ.* 1986;292:746–750.

Gardner MJ, Altman DG. *Statistics with Confidence.* London, UK: BMJ Books; 1989.

Gehan EA. A generalized Wilcoxon test for comparing arbitrarily singly-censored samples. *Biometrika.* 1965;52:15–21.

Gelber DA, Pfeifer M, Dawson B, Shumer M. Cardiovascular autonomic nervous system tests: determination of normative values and effect of confounding variables. *J Auton Nerv Syst.* 1997;62:40–44.

Gillings D, Koch G. The application of the principle of intention-to-treat to the analysis of clinical trials. *Drug Information J.* 1991;25:411–424.

Glass GV. Integrating findings: the meta-analysis of research. In Shulman LS, ed. *Review of Research in Education.* Australia: Peacock; 1977: 351–379.

Glass GV, Stanley JC. *Statistical Methods in Education and Psychology.* Upper Saddle River, NJ: Prentice Hall; 1970.

Glazer ES, Neill KG, Frakes JM, et al. Systematic review and case series report of acinar cell carcinoma of the pancreas. *Cancer Control.* 2016;446–454. https://doi.org/10.1177/107327481602300417.

Gold MR, Gold SR, Weinstein MC, eds. *Cost-Effectiveness in Health and Medicine.* Oxford, UK: Oxford University Press; 1996.

Goldman L. Cardiac risk in noncardiac surgery: an update. *Anesth Analg.* 1995;80:810–820.

Goldman L, Caldera DL, Nussbaum SR, et al. Multifactorial index of cardiac risk in non-cardiac surgical procedures. *N Engl J Med.* 1977;297:845–850.

Goldsmith JM, Kalish SB, Green D, Chmiel JS, Wallemark CB, Phair JP. Sequential clinical and immunologic abnormalities in hemophiliacs. *Arch Intern Med.* 1985;145:431–434.

Gonzalo MA, Grant C, Moreno I, et al. Glucose tolerance, insulin secretion, insulin sensitivity and glucose effectiveness in normal and overweight hyperthyroid women. *Clin Endocrinol (Oxf).* 1996;45:689–697.

Good DC, Henkle JQ, Gelber D, Welsh J, Verhulst S. Sleep-disordered breathing and poor functional outcome after stroke. *Stroke.* 1996;27:252–259.

Gordon T, Kannel WB. The Framingham, Massachusetts, Study twenty years later. In: Kessler IJ, Levin ML, eds. *The Community as an Epidemiologic Laboratory.* Baltimore, MA: Johns Hopkins Press; 1970.

Gordon T, Moore FE, Shurtleff D, Dawber TR. Some methodologic problems in the long term study of cardiovascular disease: observations on the Framingham Study. *J Chronic Dis.* 1959;10:186–206.

Goto T, Tsugawa Y, Faridi MK, Camargo CA, Hasegawa K. Reduced risk of acute exacerbation of copd after bariatric surgery: a self-controlled case series study. *Chest.* 2018;153(3):611–617. https://doi.org/10.1016/j.chest.2017.07.003.

Gotto AM. The Multiple Risk Factor Intervention Trial (MRFIT): a return to a landmark trial. *JAMA.* 1997;277:595–597.

Greenberg RS. Prospective studies. In Kotz S, Johnson NL, eds. *Encyclopedia of Statistical Sciences.* Vol 7. Hoboken, NJ: Wiley; 1986: 315–319.

Greenberg RS. Retrospective studies. In Kotz S, Johnson NL, eds. *Encyclopedia of Statistical Sciences.* Vol 8. Hoboken, NJ: Wiley; 1988: 120–124

Greenberg RS, Daniels SR, Flanders WD, Eley JW, Boring JR. *Medical Epidemiology: Population Health and Effective Health Care.* 5th ed. New York, NY: McGraw-Hill; 2015.

Greenhalgh T. How to read a paper: Papers that report diagnostic or screening tests. *BMJ.* 1997a;315:540–543.

Greenhalgh T. *How to Read a Paper: The Basics of Evidence Based Medicine.* London, UK: BMJ Publishing Group; 1997b.

Greenland S. Null misinterpretation in statistical testing and its impact on health risk assessment. *Prev Med.* 2011;53: 225–228.

Greenland S, Senn SJ, Rothman KJ, et al. Statistical tests, P values, confidence intervals, and power: a guide to misinterpretations. *Eur J Epidemiol.* 2016;31:337. https://doi.org/10.1007/s10654-016-0149-3.

Grucza RA, Przybeck TR, Spitznagel EL, Cloninger CR. Personality and depressive symptoms: a multi-dimensional analysis. *J Affect Disord.* 2003;74:123–130.

Guo Y, Bian J, Li Q, et al. A 3-minute test of cardiorespiratory fitness for use in primary care clinics. *PLOS ONE.* 2018;13(7):e0201598. https://doi.org/10.1371/journal.pone.0201598.

Gurusamy KS, Riviere D, van Laarhoven CJH, et al. Cost-effectiveness of laparoscopic versus open distal pancreatectomy for pancreatic cancer. *PLoS One.* 2017;12(12):e0189631. https://doi.org/10.1371/journal.pone.0189631.

Gurwitz JH, Field TS, Harrold LR, et al. Incidence and preventability of adverse drug events among older persons in the ambulatory setting. *JAMA.* 2003;289:1107–1116.

Guyatt GH, DiCenso A, Farewell V, Willan A, Griffith L. Randomized trials versus observational studies in adolescent pregnancy prevention. *J Clin Epidemiol.* 2000;53:167–174.

Hartz AJ, Anderson AJ, Brooks HL, Manley JC, Parent GT, Barboriak JJ. The association of smoking with cardiomyopathy. *N Engl J Med.* 1984;311:1201–1206.

Hays WL. *Statistics for the Social Sciences.* 5th ed. New York, NY: Holt, Rinehart and Winston; 1997.

He Y, Meng Z, Jia Q, et al. Sleep Quality of Patients with Differentiated Thyroid Cancer. *PLoS One.* 2015;10(6):e0130634. https://doi.org/10.1371/journal.pone.0130634.

Hébert R, Brayne C, Spiegelhalter D. Incidence of functional decline and improvement in a community-dwelling very elderly population. *Am J Epidemiol.* 1997;145:935–944.

Helmrich SP, Rosenberg L, Kaufman DW, Strom B, Shapiro S. Venous thromboembolism in relation to oral contraceptive use. *Obstet Gynecol.* 1987;69:91–95.

Henderson AS, Korten AE, Jacomb PA, et al. The course of depression in the elderly: a longitudinal community-based study in Australia. *Psychol Med.* 1997;27:119–129.

Hindmarsh PC, Brook CGD. Final height of short normal children treated with growth hormone. *Lancet.* 1996;348:13–16.

Hodgson LG, Cutler SJ. Anticipatory dementia and well-being. *Am J Alzheimer's Dis.* 1997;12:62–66.

Hoffman RM, Lo M, Clark JA, et al. Treatment decision regret among long-term survivors of localized prostate cancer: results from the prostate cancer outcomes study. *J Clin Oncol.* 2017;35(20):2306–2314. doi:10.1200/JCO.2016.70.6317.

Hollander M, Wolfe DA. *Nonparametric Statistical Methods.* 2nd ed. Hoboken, NJ: Wiley; 1998.

Hosmer DW, Lemeshow S. *Applied Survival Analysis.* Hoboken, NJ: Wiley; 1999.

Hosmer DW, Lemeshow S. *Applied Logistic Regression.* 2nd ed. Hoboken, NJ: Wiley; 2000.

Hotelling H. The selection of variates for use in prediction with some comments on the problem of nuisance parameters. *Ann Math Stat.* 1940;11:271–283.

Howcroft J, Lemaire ED, Kofman J, McIlroy WE. Elderly fall risk prediction using static posturography. *PLoS One.* 2017;12(2): e0172398. https://doi.org/10.1371/journal.pone.0172398.

Huang ES, Stafford RS. National patterns in the treatment of urinary tract infections in women by ambulatory care physicians. *Arch Intern Med.* 2002;162:41–47.

Hulley SB, Cummings SR, Browner WS, et al. ed. *Designing Clinical Research.* 4th ed. Philadelphia, PA: Lippincott Williams & Wilkins; 2013.

Ilango K, Vijayakumar T, Dubey G, Agrawal A. An Enlarged Vision on Various Types of Study Design in Human Subjects. *Global j pharmacol.* 2012;6(3):216–221.

Ingelfinger JA, Ware JH, Thibodeau LA. *Biostatistics in Clinical Medicine.* 3rd ed. Chicago, IL: McGraw-Hill; 1994.

International Committee of Medical Journal Editors. Uniform requirements for manuscripts submitted to biomedical journals. *Annals Intern Med.* 1997;126:36–47.

International Committee of Medical Journal Editors. *Recommendations for the Conduct, Reporting, Editing, and Publication of Scholarly Work in Medical Journals.* 2018. Available at: http://www.icmje.org/icmje-recommendations.pdf.

International Conference on Harmonization (ICH) E9 Expert Working Group. Statistical principles for clinical trials: ICH harmonized tripartite guideline. *Stat Med.* 1999;18:1905–1942.

Ioannidis JPA, Cappelleri JC, Lau J. Issues in comparisons between meta-analyses and large trials. *JAMA.* 1998;279:1089–1093.

Ioannidis JPA. Hijacked evidence-based medicine: stay the course and throw the pirates overboard. *J Clin Epidemiol.* 2017;84:11–13. https://doi.org/10.1016/j.jclinepi.2017.02.001.

Iribarren C, Reed DM, Burchfiel CM, Dwyer JH. Serum total cholesterol and mortality: confounding factors and risk modification in Japanese-American Men. *JAMA.* 1995;273(24):1926–1932. doi:10.1001/jama.1995.03520480046038.

Jackson AS, Stanforth PR, Gagnon J, et al. The effect of sex, age, and race on estimating percentage body fat from body mass index: the Heritage Family Study. *Int J Obes Relat Metab Disord.* 2002;26:789–796.

Jacobs CA, Christensen CP, Karthikeyan T. Patient and intraoperative factors influencing satisfaction two to five years after primary total knee arthroplasty. *J Arthroplasty.* 2014;29(8):1576–1579. https://doi.org/10.1016/j.arth.2014.03.022.

Johnston LD, Miech RA, O'Malley PM, Bachman JG, Schulenberg JE, Patrick ME. *Monitoring the Future National Survey Results on Drug Use: 1975–2017: Overview, Key Findings on Adolescent Drug Use.* Ann Arbor: Institute for Social Research, The University of Michigan; 2018.

Joines JD, McNutt RA, Carey TS, Deyo RA, Rouhani R. Finding cancer in primary care outpatients with low back pain. *J Gen Intern Med.* 2001;16:14–23.

Kaku DA, Lowenstein DH. Emergency of recreational drug abuse as a major risk factor for stroke in young adults. *Ann Intern Med.* 1990;113:821–827.

Kalbfleisch JD, Prentice RL. *The Statistical Analysis of Failure Time Data.* 2nd ed. Hoboken, NJ: Wiley; 2002.

Kasurinen A, Tervahartiala T, Laitinen A, et al. High serum MMP-14 predicts worse survival in gastric cancer. *PLoS One.* 2018;13(12):e0208800. https://doi.org/10.1371/journal.pone.0208800.

Katz MH. *Multivariable Analysis. A Practical Guide for Clinicians.* Cambridge, UK: Cambridge University Press; 1999.

Katzan IL, Cebul RD, Husak SH, Dawson NV, Baker DW. The effect of pneumonia on mortality among patients hospitalized for acute stroke. *Neurology.* 2003;60:620–625.

Kirk RE. *Experimental Design: Procedures for the Behavioral Sciences.* 3rd ed. Belmont, CA: Brooks/Cole; 1995.

Kleinbaum DG. *Survival Analysis: A Self-Learning Text.* Berlin, Germany: Springer; 1996.

Kleinbaum DG, Klein M. *Logistic Regression: A Self-Learning Text.* 3rd ed. Berlin. Germany: Springer; 2010.

Kluess HA, Neidert LE, Wainright KS, Zheng C, Babu JR. Plasma dipeptidyl peptidase IV activity and measures of body composition in apparently healthy people. *Dryad Digital Repository.* 2016. https://doi.org/10.5061/dryad.2680t.

Korn EL, Graubard BI. *Analysis of Health Surveys.* Hoboken, NJ: Wiley; 1999.

Kornak J, et al. Nonlinear N-Score estimation for establishing cognitive norms from the National Alzheimer's Coordinating Center dataset. *Alzheimers Dement.* 2018;14(7):390–391.

Kreder HJ, Grosso P, Williams JI, et al. Provider volume and other predictors of outcome after total knee arthroplasty: a population study in Ontario. *Can J Surg.* 2003;46:15–22.

Lamas GA, Pfeffer MA, Hamm P, Wertheimer J, Rouleau JL, Braunwald E. Do the results of randomized clinical trials of cardiovascular drugs influence medical practice? *N Engl J Med.* 1992;327:241–247.

Lawrie GM, Morris GC, Earle N. Long-term results of coronary bypass surgery. *Ann Surg.* 1991;213:377–385.

Lee ET, Wang JW. *Statistical Methods for Survival Data Analysis.* 3rd ed. Hoboken, NJ: Wiley; 2003.

LeLorier K, Gregoire G, Benhaddad A, Lapierre J, Derderian F. Discrepancies between meta-analysis and subsequent large randomized, controlled trials. *N Engl J Med.* 1997;337:536–542.

Leone MA, Raymkulova O, Lucenti A, et al. A reliability study of colour-Doppler sonography for the diagnosis of chronic cerebrospinal venous insufficiency shows low inter-rater agreement. *BMJ Open.* 2013;3(11):e003508. https://doi.org/10.1136/bmjopen-2013-003508.

Levinsky RJ, Malleson PN, Barratt TM, Soothill JF. Circulating immune complexes in steroid-responsive nephrotic syndrome. *N Engl J Med.* 1978;298:126–129.

Levy PS, Lemeshow S. *Sampling of Populations.* Hoboken, NJ: Wiley; 1999.

Li Y-C, Wang H-H, Ho C-H. Validity and reliability of the Mandarin version of Patient Dignity Inventory (PDI-MV) in cancer patients. *PLoS One.* 2018;13(9):e0203111. https://doi.org/10.1371/journal.pone.0203111.

Lin C-Y, Lin T-H, Chen C-C, Chen M-C, Chen C-P. Combination chemotherapy with Regorafenib in metastatic colorectal cancer treatment: a single center, retrospective study. *PLoS One.* 2018;13(1):e0190497. https://doi.org/10.1371/journal.pone.0190497.

Lissner L, Odell PM, D'Agostino RB, et al. Variability of body weight and health outcomes in the Framingham population. *N Engl J Med.* 1991;324:1839–1844.

Litwin M, Fink A. *Survey Kit. 9 volumes.* Thousand Oaks, CA: SAGE; 1995.

Locket T. *Evidence-Based and Cost-Effective Medicine for the Uninitiated.* Oxford, UK: Radcliff Medical Press; 1997.

Maisel AS, Krishnaswamy P, Nowak RM, et al. Rapid measurement of B-type natriuretic peptide in the emergency diagnosis of heart failure. *N Engl J Med.* 2002;347:161–167.

Marks RG, Dawson-Saunders EK, Bailar JC, Dan BB, Verran JA. Interactions between statisticians and biomedical journal editors. *Stat Med.* 1988;7:1003–1011.

Martínez ME, Unkart JT, Tao L, et al. Prognostic significance of marital status in breast cancer survival: a population-based study. *PLoS One.* 2017;12(5):e0175515. https://doi.org/10.1371/journal.pone.0175515.

Marwick TH, Shaw LJ, Lauer MS, et al. The noninvasive prediction of cardiac mortality in men and women with known or suspected coronary artery disease. *Am J Med.* 1999;106:172–178.

Mazanec DJ. Low back pain syndromes. In: Black ER, Bordley DR, Tape TG, Panzer RJ, eds. *Diagnostic Strategies for Common Medical Problems.* 2nd ed. Philadelphia, PA: American College of Physicians; 1999: 401–418.

McLean RR, Kiel DP, Berry SD, et al. Lower lean mass measured by dual-energy x-ray absorptiometry (DXA) is not associated with increased risk of hip fracture in women: the Framingham Osteoporosis Study. *Calcif Tissue Int.* 2018. doi:10.1007/s00223-017-0384-y.

McMaster University Health Sciences Centre, Department of Clinical Epidemiology and Biostatistics: clinical disagreement, I: how it occurs and why. *Can Med Assoc J.* 1980a;123:499–504.

McMaster University Health Sciences Centre, Department of Clinical Epidemiology and Biostatistics: clinical Disagreement, II: how to avoid it and learn from it. *Can Med Assoc J.* 1980b;123:613–617.

Meier P. The biggest public health experiment ever. In: Tanur JM, Pieters RS, Mosteller, eds. *Statistics: A Guide to the Unknown.* 3rd ed. Belmont, CA: Brooks/Cole; 1989.

Moore M, Link-Gelles R, Schaffner W, et al. Effectiveness of 13-valent pneumococcal conjugate vaccine for prevention of invasive pneumococcal disease in children in the USA: a matched case-control study. *Lancet Respir Med.* 2016;4(5):399–406. https://doi.org/10.1016/S2213-2600(16)00052-7.

Moore JG, Bjorkman DJ, Mitchell MD, Avots-Avotins A. Age does not influence acute aspirin-induced gastric mucosal damage. *Gastroenterology.* 1991;100:1626–1629.

Multiple Risk Factor Intervention Trial Research Group. Multiple risk factor intervention trial. *JAMA.* 1982;248:1465–1477.

Murphy JL, Wootton SA, Bond SA, Jackson AA. Energy content of stools in normal healthy controls and patients with cystic fibrosis. *Arch Dis Child.* 1991;66:495–500.

Neidert LE, Wainright KS, Zheng C, Babu JR, Kluess HA. Plasma dipeptidyl peptidase IV activity and measures of body composition in apparently healthy people. *Heliyon.* 2016;2(4):e00097. https://doi.org/10.1016/j.heliyon.2016. e00097.

Newcombe RG. Two-sided confidence intervals for the single proportion: comparison of seven methods. *Stat in Med.* 1998;17:857–872.

Nguyen CP, Adang EMM. Cost-effectiveness of breast cancer screening using mammography in Vietnamese women. *PLoS One.* 2018;13(3):e0194996. https://doi.org/10.1371/journal. pone.0194996.

Norman GR, Streiner DL. *PDQ Statistics.* 2nd ed. Hamilton, Ontario: Decker; 1996.

Ömeroglu H, Agus H, Biçimoglu A, Tümer Y. Analysis of a radiographic assessment method of acetabular cover in developmental dysplasia of the hip. *Arch Orthop Trauma Surg.* 2002;122:334–337.

Poblador-Plou B, Calderón-Larrañaga A, Marta-Moreno J, et al. Comorbidity of dementia: a cross-sectional study of primary care older patients. *BMC Psychiatry.* 2014;14(1):84.

Pauker SG, Kassirer JP. The threshold approach to clinical decision making. *N Engl J Med.* 1980;302:1109–1117.

Pauker SG, Kassirer JP. Decision analysis. *N Engl J Med.* 1987;316:250–258.

Pearson ES, Hartley HO, eds. *Biometrika Tables for Statisticians.* Vol 1. 3rd ed. Cambridge, UK: Cambridge University Press; 1966.

Pedhazur EJ. *Multiple Regression in Behavioral Research.* 3rd ed. New York, NY: Holt, Rinehart and Winston; 1997.

Penzel R, Hoegel J, Schmitz W, et al. Clusters of chromosomal imbalances in thymic epithelial tumours are associated with the WHO classification and the staging system according to Masaoka. *Int J Cancer.* 2003;105:494–498.

Pereira AJ, Corrêa TD, de Almeida FP, et al. Inaccuracy of venous point-of-care glucose measurements in critically ill patients: a cross-sectional study. *PLoS One.* 2015:10(6):e0129568. https://doi.org/10.1371/journal.pone.0129568.

Peto R, Peto J. Asymptotically efficient rank invariant test procedures (with discussion). *J R Stat Soc Series A.* 1972;135:185–206.

Poikolainen K, Reunala T, Karvonen J, Lauharanta J, Karkkainen P. Alcohol intake: a risk factor for psoriasis in young and middle aged men? *BMJ.* 1990;300:780–783.

Priede A, Andreu Y, Martínez P, Conchado A, Ruiz-Torres M, González-Blanch C. The factor structure of the Medical Outcomes Study–Social Support Survey: a comparison of different models in a sample of recently diagnosed cancer patients. *J Psychosom Res.* 2018;108:32–38. https://doi. org/10.1016/j.jpsychores.2018.02.008.

Prigerson HG, Bao Y, Shah MA, et al. Chemotherapy use, performance status, and quality of life at the end of life. *JAMA Oncol.* 2015;1(6):778–784. doi:10.1001/ jamaoncol.2015.2378.

Quinn T, Moskowitz J, Khan MW, et al. What families need and physicians deliver: contrasting communication preferences between surrogate decision-makers and physicians during outcome prognostication in critically ill TBI patients. *Neurocrit Care.* 2017;27:154. https://doi.org/10.1007/s12028-017-0427-2.

R Core Team. *R: A Language and Environment for Statistical Computing.* Vienna, Austria: R Foundation for Statistical Computing; 2019. http://www.R-project.org/.

Rabago CA, Dingwell JB, Wilken JM. Reliability and minimum detectable change of temporal-spatial, kinematic, and dynamic stability measures during perturbed gait. *PLoS One.* 2015;10(11):e0142083. https://doi.org/10.1371/journal. pone.0142083.

Raiffa H. *Decision Analysis.* New York, NY: McGraw-Hill; 1997.

Raurell-Torredà M, Olivet-Pujol J, Romero-Collado A, et al. Case-based learning and simulation: useful tools to enhance nurses' education? Nonrandomized controlled trial. *J Nurs Scholarsh.* 2014. https://doi.org/10.1111/jnu.12113.

Rea LM, Parker RA. *Designing and Conducting Survey Research: A Comprehensive Guide.* 2nd ed. San Francisco, CA: Jossey-Bass; 1997.

Robbins R, Seixas A, Jean-Louis G, et al. National patterns of physician management of sleep apnea and treatment among patients with hypertension. *PLoS One.* 2018;13(5):e0196981. https://doi.org/10.1371/journal.pone.0196981.

Roethlisberger FJ, Dickson WJ, Wright HA. *Management and the Worker.* Cambridge, MA: Harvard Univ Press; 1946.

Rogers WJ, Coggin CJ, Gersh BJ, et al. Ten-year follow-up of quality of life in patients randomized to receive medical therapy or coronary artery bypass graft surgery. The Coronary Artery Surgery Study. *Circulation.* 1990;82:1647–1658.

Rogers LQ, Bailey JE, Gutin B, et al. Teaching resident physicians to provide exercise counseling: a needs assessment. *Acad Med.* 2002;77:841–844.

Rubin DB. Estimating causal effects from large data sets using propensity scores. *Ann Intern Med.* 1997;127:757–763.

Rubin P, ed. *Clinical Oncology: A Multidisciplinary Approach.* 6th ed. Atlanta, GA: American Cancer Society; 1983.

Sackett DL. Bias in analytic research. *J Chronic Dis.* 1979;32:51–63.

Sackett DL, Haynes RB, Tugwell P. *Clinical Epidemiology: A Basic Science for Clinical Medicine.* 2nd ed. London, UK: Little, Brown Book Group; 1991.

Sacks HS, Berrier J, Reitman D, Ancona-Berk VA, Chalmers TC. Meta-analysis of randomized controlled trials. *N Engl J Med.* 1987;316:450–455.

Sgarbossa EB, Pinski SL, Barbagelata A, et al. Electrocardiographic diagnosis of evolving acute myocardial infarction in the presence of left bundle-branch block. *N Engl J Med.* 1996;334:481–487.

Schlesselman JJ. *Case-Control Studies: Design, Conduct, Analysis.* Oxford, UK: Oxford University Press; 1982.

Sekiya N, Nagasaki H. Reproducibility of the walking patterns of normal young adults: test-retest reliability of the walk ratio (step-length/step-rate). *Gait & Posture.* 1998;7(3): 225–227. https://doi.org/10.1016/S0966-6362(98)00009-5.

Serrano CW, Wright JW, Newton ER. Surgical glove perforation in obstetrics. *Obstet Gynecol.* 1991;77:525–528.

Shah AC, Ma K, Faraoni D, Oh DCS, Rooke GA, Van Norman GA. Self-reported functional status predicts post-operative outcomes in non-cardiac surgery patients with pulmonary hypertension. *PLoS One.* 2018;13(8):e0201914. https://doi. org/10.1371/journal.pone.0201914.

Shipley WU, Seiferheld W, Lukka HR, et al. Radiation with or without Antiandrogen Therapy in Recurrent Prostate Cancer. *N Engl J Med.* 2017;376(5):417–428. https://www.nejm.org/ doi/full/10.1056/NEJMoa1607529.

Shlipak MG, Lyons WL, Go AS, Chou TM, Evans GT, Browner WS. Should the electrocardiogram be used to guide therapy for patients with left bundle-branch block and suspected myocardial infarction? *JAMA*. 1999;281:714–719.

Snedecor GW, Cochran WG. *Statistical Methods*. 8th ed. Ames, IA: Iowa State University Press; 1989.

Springer. *Common Reasons for Rejection*. 2018. Available at: https://www.springer.com/gp/authors-editors/author andreviewertutorials/submitting-to-a-journal-and-peer-review/ what-is-open-access/10285582. Accessed April 28, 2019.

St Sauver JL, Boyd CM, Grossardt BR, et al. Risk of developing multimorbidity across all ages in an historical cohort study: differences by sex and ethnicity *BMJ Open* 2015;5:e006413. doi:10.1136/bmjopen-2014-006413.

Steering Committee of the Physicians' Health Study Research Group. Final report on the aspirin component of the ongoing Physicians' Health Study. *N Engl J Med*. 1989;321:129–135.

Stewart AL, Hays RD, Ware JE Jr. The MOS short-form general health survey. *Med Care*. 1988;26:724–735.

Stoline MR. The status of multiple comparisons: simultaneous estimation of all pairwise comparisons in one-way ANOVA designs. *Am Stat*. 1981;35:134–141.

Ström M, Uckelstam C, Andersson G, Hassmén P, Umefjord G, Carlbring P. Internet-delivered therapist-guided physical activity for mild to moderate depression: A randomized controlled trial. *PeerJ*. 2013;1:e178. https://doi.org/10.7717/peerj.178.

Stuart P, Malick F, Nair RP, et al. Analysis of phenotypic variation in psoriasis as a function of age at onset and family history. *Arch Dermatol Res*. 2002;294:207–213.

Tan EM, Cohen AS, Fries JF, et al. The 1982 revised criteria for the classification of systemic lupus erythematosus. *Arthritis Rheum*. 1982;25:1271–1277.

Tarlov AR, Ware JEJr, Greenfield S, Nelson EC, Perrin E, Zubkoff M. The Medical Outcomes Study: an application of methods for monitoring the results of medical care. *JAMA*. 1989;262:925–930.

Thiese MS, Arnold ZC, Walker SD. The misuse and abuse of statistics in biomedical research. *Biochemia Medica*. 2015;25(1):5–11. https://doi.org/10.11613/BM.2015.001.

Thompson IM, Goodman PJ, Tangen CM, et al. The influence of finasteride on the development of prostate cancer. *N Engl J Med*. 2003;349:213–222.

Tukey J. *Exploratory Data Analysis*. Boston, MA: Addision-Wesley; 1977.

van Crevel H, Habbema JDF, Braakman R. Decision analysis of the management of incidental intracranial saccular aneurysms. *Neurology*. 1986;36:1335–1339.

van Eersel MEA, Joosten H, Gansevoort RT, et al. Treatable vascular risk and cognitive performance in persons aged 35 years or older: longitudinal study of six years. *J Prev Alzheimers Dis*. 2019;6:42. https://doi.org/10.14283/jpad.2018.47.

van Lindert EJ, Bilsen MV, Flier MVD, Kolwijck E, Delye H, Oever JT. Topical vancomycin reduces the cerebrospinal fluid shunt infection rate: a retrospective cohort study. *PLoS ONe*. 2018;13(1):e0190249. https://doi.org/10.1371/journal.pone.0190249.

Walker H. *Studies in the History of Statistical Method*. Philadelphia, PA: Lippincott, Williams & Wilkins; 1931.

Ware C. *Information Visualization: Perception for Design*. Waltham, MA: Morgan Kaufman; 2013.

Ware JE, Brook RH, Rogers WH, et al. *Health Outcomes for Adults in Prepaid and Fee-for-service Systems of Care*. Santa Monica, CA: The RAND Corporation; 1987.

Wasserstein RL, Lazar NA. The ASA's Statement on p-Values: context, Process, and Purpose. *American Statistician*. 2016;70(2):129–133. doi:10.1080/00031305.2016.1154108.

Weiner DK, Rudy TE. Attitudinal barriers to effective treatment of persistent pain in nursing home residents. *J Am Geriatr Soc*. 2002;50:2035–2040.

Weingarten SR, Stone E, Green A, et al. A study of patient satisfaction and adherence to preventive care practice guidelines. *Am J Med*. 1995;99:590–596.

Weinstein JN. Clinical crossroads: a 45-year-old man with low back pain and a numb left foot. *JAMA*. 1998;280:730–736.

Weinstein MC, Fineberg HV. *Clinical Decision Analysis*. Philadelphia, PA: WB Saunders; 1998.

Xu JQ, Murphy SL, Kochanek KD, Bastian B, Arias E. *Deaths: Final data for 2016. National Vital Statistics Reports; vol 67 no 5*. Hyattsville, MD: National Center for Health Statistics; 2018. https://www.cdc.gov/flu/professionals/vaccination/vaccine_safety.htm.

Zamboni P, Morovic S, Menegatti E, et al. Screening for chronic cerebrospinal venous insufficiency (CCSVI) using ultrasound—recommendations for a protocol *Int Angiol*. 2011;30:571–97.

General Statistics and Miscellaneous Readings

Bailar JC, Mosteller F, eds. *Medical Uses of Statistics*. 2nd ed. Waltham, MA: Massachusetts Medical Society; 1992.

Briscoe MH. *Preparing Scientific Illustrations: A Guide to Better Posters, Presentations, and Publications*. 2nd ed. Berlin, Germany: Springer-Verlag; 1996.

Cummings SM, Savitz LA, Konrad TR. Reported response rates to mailed physician questionnaires. *Health Ser Res*. 2001;35:1347–1355.

Kleinbaum DG, Kupper LL, Muller KE, Nizam A, Kleinbaum DG, Nizati A. *Applied Regression Analysis and Other Multivariable Methods*. 3rd ed. California, CA: Duxbury Press; 1997.

Spirer HF, Spirer L, Jaffe AJ. Misused Statistics. New York, NY: Marcel Dekker; 1998.

Wainer H. How to display data badly. *Am Stat*. 1984;38:137–147.

Wainer H. Understanding graphs and tables. *Educ Researcher*. 1992;21:14–23.

Software

General Statistical Software

Decision Analysis by TreeAge, Version 4. TreeAge. Williamstown, MA, 2003.

JMP, Version 14.3. SAS Institute Inc. Cary, NC, 2019.

R, Version 3.6.0. R Core Team. http://www.R-project.org/, 2019.

SAS, Version 9.4. SAS Institute Inc. Cary, NC 2019.

SPSS, Version 26.0. IBM SPSS Statistics, 2019.

SYSTAT, Version 13.2. Systat Software Inc. San Jose CA 2019.

Power Analysis Programs

nQuery Advisor, Version 5. Statistical Solutions. Saugus, MA, 2003.

PASS (Power Analysis and Sample Size), Version 2019. NCSS, LLC. Kaysville, UT, 2019.

INDEX

Page numbers followed by *t* refer to tables; page numbers followed by *f* refer to figures.